Organometallic Compounds of Nickel, Palladium, Platinum, Copper, Silver and Gold

Organometallic Compounds of Nickel, Palladium, Platinum, Copper, Silver and Gold

Edited by

R. J. Cross
University of Glasgow

and

D. M. P. Mingos
University of Oxford

LONDON NEW YORK
CHAPMAN AND HALL

First published 1985 by Chapman and Hall Ltd
11 New Fetter Lane, London EC4P 4EE
733 Third Avenue, New York NY 10017

Phototypeset in the United States of America by
Mack Printing Company, Easton, Pennsylvania 18042
Printed in Great Britain by J.W. Arrowsmith Ltd, Bristol

ISBN 0 412 26840 X

Library of Congress Cataloging in Publication Data

Main entry under title:

Organometallic compounds of nickel,
palladium, copper, silver, and gold.
(Chapman and Hall chemistry
sourcebooks)
Includes index.
1. Organometallic compounds —
Handbooks, manuals, etc.
I. Cross, R.J., 1941- . II. Mingos,
D.M.P., 1944- . III. Series.
QD411.'72 1985 547'.05 84-29346

ISBN 0-412-26840-X

British Library Cataloguing in Publication Data

Organometallic compounds of nickel,
palladium, platinum, copper, silver and
gold. — (Chapman and Hall chemistry
sourcebooks)
1. Organometallic compounds
I. Cross, R.J. II. Mingos, D.M.P.
547'.05 QD411

ISBN 0-412-26840-X

Contents

Preface

This is one of the first volumes to be published in the series of *Chapman and Hall Chemistry Sourcebooks* which provides carefully tailored information to workers in specialized areas of chemistry. The information contained in this book is derived from the *Dictionary of Organometallic Compounds*, published in November 1984.

The organic compounds of the six metals in this volume are of great interest both to inorganic and organic chemists. Organonickel and organopalladium compounds are frequently used as selective reagents in synthesis and as catalysts for organic reactions. Organoplatinum compounds, however, are generally slower to react and lend themselves to mechanistic studies. A vast range of such compounds has been prepared. Whilst organometallics of the gold triad are fewer, they display a range of interesting structures, and organocopper compounds are widely used synthetic reagents. It is therefore anticipated that this particular compendium will reach a wide readership.

The databank on the properties of organometallic compounds, which is represented in its current form by the *Dictionary of Organometallic Compounds* and its subset publications such as this volume, will be kept continuously up-to-date. Supplements to the main *Dictionary* will appear annually and revised editions of this *Sourcebook* will be published from time to time as demands permits.

R.J. Cross
D.M.P. Mingos

Introduction

1. Using the Sourcebook

The *Sourcebook* is divided into element sections: within each section the arrangement of entries is in order of molecular formula according to the Hill convention (i.e. C, then H, then other elements in alphabetical sequence of element symbol; where no carbon is present, the elements including H are ordered strictly alphabetically).

Every entry is numbered to assist ready location and the entry number consists of a metal element symbol followed by a five-digit number.

Indexes

There are three printed indexes: a name index which lists every compound name or synonym in alphabetical order; a molecular formula index which lists all molecular formulae, including those of derivatives, in Hill convention order; and a CAS registry number index listing all CAS numbers included in the *Sourcebook* in serial order. All indexes refer to the entry number. In the name index an entry number which follows immediately upon an index term means that the term itself is used as the entry name but an entry number which is preceded by the word 'see' means that the term is a synonym to an entry name. In all three indexes an entry number which is preceded by the word 'in' refers the reader to a specified stereoisomer or derivative which is to be found embedded within the particular entry.

In addition to the three printed indexes, each element section is preceded by a graphical structure index allowing the rapid visual location of compounds of interest. The structure index reproduces all structure diagrams present in that element section in reduced size and printed in entry number order.

The following paragraphs summarize important considerations in compiling the information in this *Sourcebook*. For more detailed information, see the Introduction to the *Dictionary of Organometallic Compounds* from which this *Sourcebook* derives.

2. Compound Selection

In compiling this *Sourcebook* the aim has been to include from the primary literature up to mid 1983:

(1) Compounds representative of all important structural types (typically, the parent member of each series, where known, together with a selection of its homologues).

(2) Any compound with an established use, such as in catalysis, as a synthetic reagent or starting material.

(3) Other compounds of particular chemical, structural, biological or historical interest, especially those thought to exhibit unusual bonding characteristics.

Some compounds which are not considered sufficiently important to justify separate entries of their own have been included as derivatives in the entries of other compounds. These may include for example:

(1) Organic derivatives in the classical sense.

(2) Donor-acceptor complexes.

(3) The various salts of an anion or cation. In nearly every case, the entry for an ionic substance refers to the naked anion or cation, and the molecular formula, molecular weight and CAS registry number given for the main entry are those of the ion, in agreement with current CAS practice. Salts of the ion with various counterions are then treated as derivatives and the molecular formulae of all of these are given.

(4) Oligomeric compounds. Where a compound is known in several states of molecular aggregation these are all included in the one entry, which usually refers to the monomer. Compounds which are known only in dimeric form are entered as such, but the hypothetical monomers are included as derivatives to ensure that the names and molecular formulae of the monomeric forms occur in the indexes.

All names and molecular formulae recorded for derivatives occur in the Name and Molecular Formula Indexes respectively.

3. Chemical Names and Synonyms

The naming of organometallic compounds is frequently problematic and so in selecting the range of alternative names to present for each compound or derivative, editorial policy has been to report names which are found in the literature, including *Chemical Abstracts*, and not to attempt to impose a system of nomenclature. The editorial generation of new names has therefore been kept to a minimum required by consistency. Most names given in the *Sourcebook* are those given in the original paper(s) and in *Chemical Abstracts*.

Names corresponding to those used by CAS during

the 8th, 9th, and 10th collective index periods (1967-71, 1972-6 and 1977-81 respectively) are labelled with the suffixes 8CI, 9CI and 10CI respectively.

4. Toxicity and Hazard Information

Toxicity and hazard information is highlighted by the sign ▷ which also appears in the indexes.

All organometallic compounds should be treated as if they have dangerous properties.

The information contained in the *Sourcebook* has been compiled from sources believed to be reliable. No warranty, guarantee or representation is made by the Publisher as to the correctness or sufficiency of any information herein, and the Publisher assumes no responsibility in connection therewith.

The specific information in this publication on the hazardous and toxic properties of certain compounds is intended to alert the reader to possible dangers associated with the use of those compounds. The absence of such information should not, however, be taken as an indication of safety in use or misuse.

5. Bibliographic References

The selection of references is made with the aim of facilitating entry into the literature for the user who wishes to locate more detailed information about a particular compound. Reference contents are frequently indicated using mnemonic suffixes. In general recent references are preferred to older ones, and the number of references quoted does not necessarily indicate the relative importance of a compound.

Journal abbreviations generally follow the practice of *Chemical Abstracts Service Source Index* (CASSI). In patent references, no distinction is made between patent applications and granted patents.

6. Sources of Further Information

The following books and review series provide more information about various aspects of organometallic chemistry. Lists of reviews specific to organic compounds of particular metals may be found in the introductory sections of the metals concerned.

General

Comprehensive Organometallic Chemistry, Wilkinson, G. *et al.* Eds, Pergamon, Oxford, 1982. This book represents the most complete and up to date review of the whole subject. In addition to sections for each element there are chapters on the use of organometallics in organic synthesis and catalysis.

Comprehensive Inorganic Chemistry, Trotman-Dickenson, A.F. *et al.* Eds, Pergamon, Oxford, 1973. Contains information about organometallics as well as discussions of oxidation states, coordination chemistry and analysis of the metals.

Gmelins Handbuch der Anorganischen Chemie, 8th Edn, Springer-Verlag, Berlin. Some volumes of Gmelin covering organometallic compounds have been updated relatively recently and can therefore be consulted for comprehensive data on some types of organometallics. Some Gmelin element sections, however, are many years out of date.

Houben-Weyls Methoden der Organischen Chemie, 4th Edn, Band XIII, *Metallorganische Verbindungen*, Thieme-Verlag, Stuttgart.

The Chemistry of the Carbon-Metal Bond, Hartley, F.R. and Patai, S. Eds, Wiley, New York, 1982-. Contains sections on the synthesis, analysis and thermochemistry of various classes of organometallic compounds.

Transition-Metal Complexes of Phosphorus, Arsenic and Antimony Ligands, McAuliffe, C.A. Ed., Macmillan, London, 1973.

Methods of Elemento-Organic Chemistry, Kocheshkov, K.A. Ed., North Holland, Amsterdam, 1967.

MTP International Review of Science: Inorganic Chemistry, Series 2, Emeléus, H.J. Ed., Butterworths, London; University Park Press, Baltimore, 1974-5.

Advances in Organometallic Chemistry, Academic Press, 1964-.

Annual Surveys of Organometallic Chemistry, Elsevier, 1964-7.

Organometallic Chemistry Reviews, Elsevier, 1966-7.

Organometallic Chemistry Reviews, Section A: Subject Reviews 1968-72.

Organometallic Chemistry Reviews, Section B: Annual Surveys 1968-74.

Journal of Organometallic Chemistry: This incorporates reviews and surveys after the discontinuation of the two series of *Organometallic Chemistry Reviews*.

Organometallic Chemistry, 1972-, (Specialist Periodical Reports), RSC.

Coordination Chemistry Reviews, Elsevier, 1966-.

Progress in Inorganic Chemistry, Interscience, 1959-.

Advances in Inorganic Chemistry and Radiochemistry, Academic Press, 1959-.

Analysis

Scott's Standard Methods of Chemical Analysis, Furman, N.H. Ed., 6th Edn, Van Nostrand, New York, 1962.

Crompton, T.R., *Chemical Analysis of Organometallic Compounds*, Academic Press, London, 1973.

Spectroscopy

Nuclear Magnetic Resonance Spectroscopy of Nuclei Other than the Proton, Axenrod, T. and Webb, G.A. Eds, Wiley, London, 1974.

NMR and the Periodic Table, Harris, R.K. and Mann, B.E. Eds, Academic Press, London, 1978.

^{13}C NMR Data for Organometallic Compounds, Mann, B.E. and Taylor, B.F. Eds, Academic Press, London, 1981.

Spectroscopic Properties of Inorganic and Organometallic Compounds, 1968-, (Specialist Periodical Reports), RSC.

Handling

Shriver, D.F., *The Manipulation of Air-Sensitive Compounds*, McGraw-Hill, 1969.

Organometallic Syntheses, Academic Press, New York, 1965, Vol. 1.

Ag Silver

D. M. P. Mingos

Argent (Fr.), Silber (Ger.), Plata (Sp.), Argento (Ital.), Серебро (Sierebro) (Russ.), 銀 (Japan.)

Atomic Number. 47

Atomic Weight. 107.868

Electronic Configuration. [Kr] $4d^{10}\ 5s^{1}$

Oxidation States. Ag(I) is the commonest oxidation state for organometallic and related compounds, but Ag(II) and Ag(III) compounds are also known.

Coordination Number. Ag(I) compounds are typically linear, trigonal or tetrahedral, whilst those of Ag(II) are planar and those of Ag(III) are planar or octahedral.

Colour. Most organosilver(I) compounds are colourless with the exception of the highly coloured cluster compounds. Organosilver(III) compounds are commonly yellow.

Availability. Readily available starting materials include silver powder, Ag_2CO_3, $AgSbF_6$, $AgNO_3$, AgOAc, $AgBF_4$, $AgClO_4$, all of which are moderately expensive.

Handling. Organosilver compounds do not require any special handling techniques.

Isotopic Abundance. ^{107}Ag, 51.82%; ^{109}Ag, 48.18%.

Spectroscopy. ^{107}Ag, $I = \frac{1}{2}$, and ^{109}Ag, $I = \frac{1}{2}$, are rather insensitive nuclei with large T_1's; however there have been some reports of the use of ^{109}Ag nmr for organometallic compounds.

Analysis. EDTA titrations with disodium ethylbis(5-tetrazolylazo)acetate as indicator.

References. In addition to references listed in the introduction to the *Sourcebook*, the following provide further reading:

Godensky, L. M. *et al.*, *Engelhardt Tech. Bull.*, 1969, **9,** 117 (*thermodynamic data*)

Hartley, F. R., *Chem. Rev.*, 1973, **73,** 163 (*olefin and acetylene complexes*)

Singleton, E., *J. Organomet. Chem.*, 1978, **158,** 413 (*organometallic chemistry*)

Bruce, M. I., *J. Organomet. Chem.*, 1972, **44,** 209 (*carbonyl compounds*)

Henrichs, P. M. *et al.*, *J. Am. Chem. Soc.*, 1979, **101,** 3222 (*nmr*)

$AgC(NO_2)_3$
Ag-00001

$[MeAg]_n$
Ag-00002

$F_3CCFClAg$
Ag-00003

$Ag(CN)_2^{\ominus}$
Ag-00004

$[AgC{\equiv}CAg]_n$
Ag-00005

$Ag_2(OAc)_2$
Ag-00006

Me_2SAgNO_3
Ag-00007

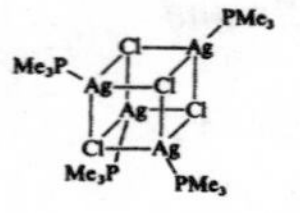

Ag-00008

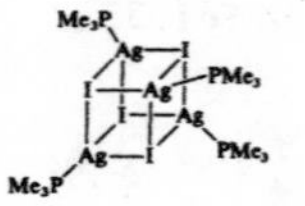

Ag-00009

$Ag(NCCH_3)_2^{\oplus}$
Ag-00010

$Ag(C_6F_5)$
Ag-00011

$[AgPh]_n$
Ag-00012

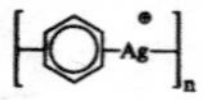

Ag-00013

$H_3C(CH_2)_3C{\equiv}CAg$
Ag-00014

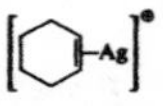

Ag-00015

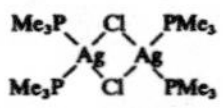

Ag-00016

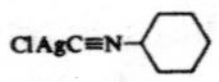

$ClAgC{\equiv}N$–cyclohexyl
Ag-00017

$[AgC{\equiv}CPh]_n$
Ag-00018

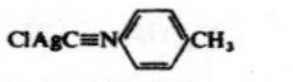

Ag-00019

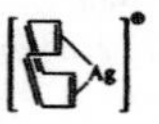

Ag-00020

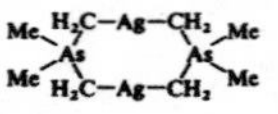

Ag-00021

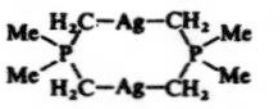

Ag-00022

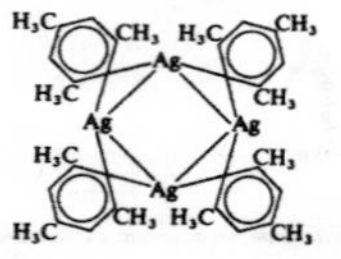

Ag-00023

$[Ag(C_6H_4CH_2NMe_2)]_n$
Ag-00024

$[Ag_2Br(C_6H_4CH_2NMe_2)]_n$
Ag-00025

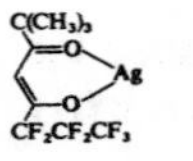

Ag-00026

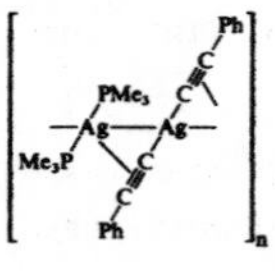

Ag-00027

$Me_3SiOAg(PMe_3)_3$
Ag-00028

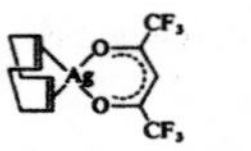

Ag-00029

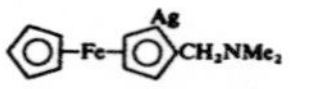

Ag-00030

$H_3C(CH_2)_3AgP(CH_2CH_2CH_2CH_3)_3$
Ag-00031

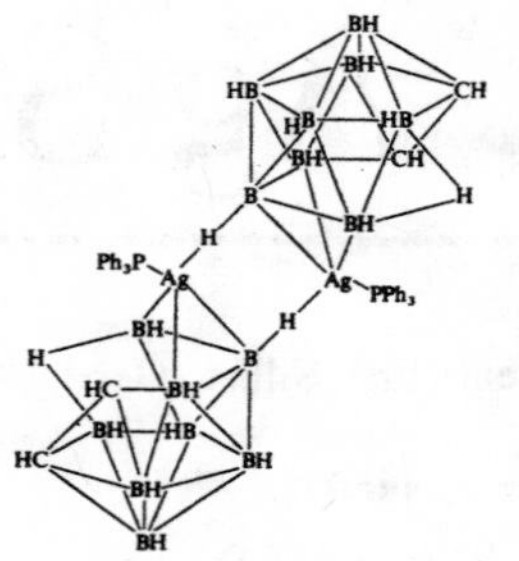

Ag-00032

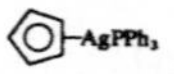

Ag-00033

$Ag^{\oplus}Ph_4B^{\ominus}$
Ag-00034

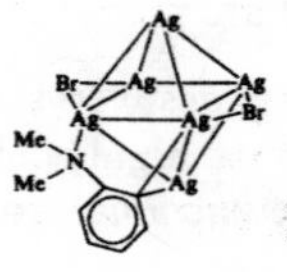

Only one of four amine groups shown
Ag-00035

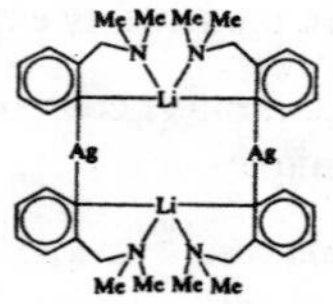

Ag-00036

$[Ph_3PCH_2{-}Ag{-}CH_2PPh_3]^{\oplus}$
Ag-00037

$(Ph_3P)_2Ag(C_2B_8H_{11})$
Ag-00038

$H_3B{-}H{-}Ag(PMePh_2)_3$
Ag-00039

$CAgN_3O_6$ Ag-00001

(Trinitromethyl)silver, 9CI

[41766-21-6]

$AgC(NO_2)_3$

M 257.896

Sol. MeCN. Light-sensitive.

Shevelev, S.A. *et al*, *Izv. Akad. Nauk SSSR*, *Ser. Khim.*, 1968, 382 (*synth*)
Erashko, V.I. *et al*, *Izv. Akad. Nauk SSSR*, *Ser. Khim.*, 1973, 344; 1977, 250 (*use*)

CH_3Ag Ag-00002

Methylsilver, 9CI

[75993-65-6]

$[MeAg]_n$

M 122.903

Polymeric. Yellow-brown. Dec. between −80° and −50°.

Semarano, G. *et al*, *Chem. Ber.*, 1941, **74**, 1089 (*synth*)
Beverwijk, C.D.M. *et al*, *Organomet. Chem. Rev.*, *Sect. A*, 1970, **5**, 215 (*rev*)

C_2AgClF_4 Ag-00003

(1-Chloro-1,2,2,2-tetrafluoroethyl)silver, 9CI

α-Chloroperfluoroethylsilver

[51102-98-8]

$F_3CCFClAg$

M 243.337

Miller, W.T. *et al*, *J. Am. Chem. Soc.*, 1968, **90**, 7367 (*synth*)
Dyatkin, B.L. *et al*, *J. Organomet. Chem.*, 1973, **57**, 423 (*synth*, *nmr*)

$C_2AgN_2^{\ominus}$ Ag-00004

Bis(cyano-*C*)argentate(1−), 9CI

Dicyanoargentate(1−)

[15391-88-5]

$Ag(CN)_2^{\ominus}$

M 159.903 (ion)

K salt: Potassium silver cyanide.
C_2AgKN_2 M 199.002
Used in silver plating and as bactericide. White, light-sensitive cryst. Sol. H_2O.

Bassett, H. *et al*, *J. Chem. Soc.*, 1924, 1660 (*synth*)
Staritzky, E., *Anal. Chem.*, 1956, **28**, 419 (*cryst struct*)
Chadwick, B.M. *et al*, *J. Mol. Struct.*, 1968, **2**, 281 (*raman*, *ir*)
Sharpe, A.G., *The Chemistry of Cyano Complexes of the Transition Metals*, Academic Press, 1976, 272 (*rev*)
Merck Index, 9th Ed., No. 7457.

C_2Ag_2 Ag-00005

Silver acetylide, 9CI

μ-1,2-Ethynediyldisilver, 10CI

[7659-31-6]

$[AgC{\equiv}CAg]_n$

M 239.758

Polymeric. Light-sensitive powder, v. explosive when dry. Sol. KCN with dec.

▷Explosive

Brauer, G., *Handb. Prep. Inorg. Chem.*, 1965, **2**, 1047 (*synth*)
Benham, R.A. *et al*, *Energy Res. Abstr.*, 1979, **4**, 8849; *CA*, **91**, 41556h (*use*)

$C_2H_3AgO_2$ Ag-00006

(Acetato)silver

Silver acetate

$Ag_2(OAc)_2$

M 166.913

Dimeric.

Dimer: [55906-24-6]. *Bis[μ-(acetato-O:O′)]disilver.*
$C_4H_6Ag_2O_4$ M 333.825
White to sl. greyish, light-sensitive solid. Spar. sol. H_2O.

Mathews, F.W. *et al*, *Anal. Chem.*, 1950, **22**, 514 (*synth*)
Kline, R.J. *et al*, *Inorg. Chem.*, 1966, **5**, 932 (*use*)
Adams, S.K. *et al*, *Inorg. Chim. Acta*, 1975, **12**, 163 (*ms*, *ir*)
Merck Index, 9th Ed., No. 8245.

$C_2H_6AgNO_3S$ Ag-00007

Dimethylsulfide(nitrato)silver

(Nitrato-O)[thiobis[methane]]silver, 9CI. *(Dimethylsulfide)silver nitrate*

[15171-27-4]

Me_2SAgNO_3

M 232.002

Useful starting material for synth. of alkoxy (*N*-alkylimino)methyl complexes. Cryst. (EtOH). Mp 120-3°.

Kubota, M. *et al*, *Inorg. Chem.*, 1966, **5**, 386 (*synth*, *ir*)
Minghetti, G. *et al*, *J. Organomet. Chem.*, 1973, **60**, C43 (*use*)
Minghetti, G. *et al*, *Inorg. Chem.*, 1975, **14**, 1974 (*synth*)

C_3H_9AgClP Ag-00008

Chloro(trimethylphosphine)silver

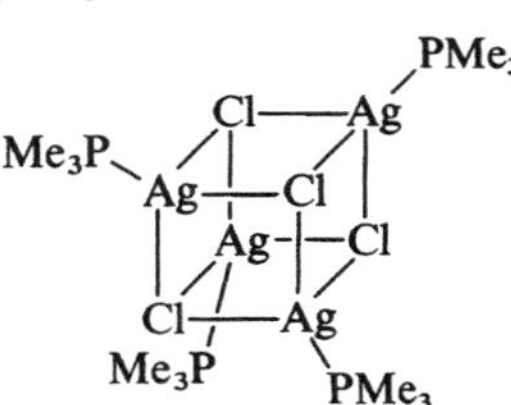

M 219.399

Tetrameric.

Tetramer: [40696-73-9]. *Tetra-μ₃-chlorotetrakis(trimethylphosphine)tetrasilver*, 9CI.
$C_{12}H_{36}Ag_4Cl_4P_4$ M 877.595
Cryst. (C_6H_6/pet. ether). Sol. C_6H_6. Mp 90-2°.

Schmidbaur, H. *et al*, *Chem. Ber.*, 1972, **105**, 3382 (*synth*)
Schmidbaur, H. *et al*, *Angew. Chem.*, *Int. Ed. Engl.*, 1973, **85**, 415 (*use*)

C_3H_9AgIP Ag-00009

Iodo(trimethylphosphine)silver

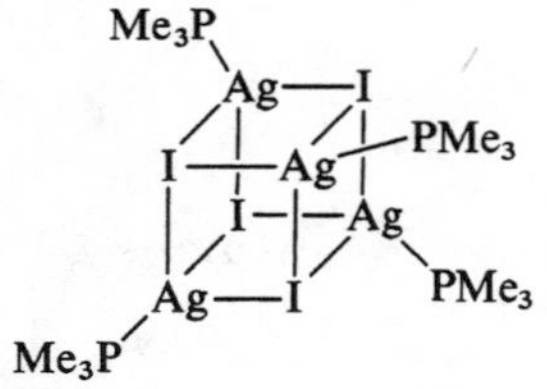

M 310.850

Tetrameric.

Tetramer: [12389-34-3]. *Tetra-μ_3-iodotetrakis(trimethylphosphine)tetrasilver.*

$C_{12}H_{36}Ag_4I_4P_4$ M 1243.401

Useful reagent for storing PMe_3. Mp 134-6°. Too unstable for recryst.

Mann, F.G. *et al*, *J. Chem. Soc.*, 1938, 702 (*synth*, *use*)
Inorg. Synth., 1967, **9**, 62; 1976, **16**, 153 (*synth*, *use*)
Pennington, B.T. *et al*, *J. Inorg. Nucl. Chem.*, 1978, **40**, 389 (*use*)

$C_4H_6AgN_2^{\oplus}$ Ag-00010

Bis(acetonitrile)silver(1+)

[55031-59-9]

$Ag(NCCH_3)_2^{\oplus}$

M 189.973 (ion)

Janz, G.J. *et al*, *J. Phys. Chem.*, 1967, **71**, 963 (*synth*, *ir*)
Roulet, R. *et al*, *Helv. Chim. Acta*, 1974, **57**, 2139 (*use*)

C_6AgF_5 Ag-00011

(Pentafluorophenyl)silver

[30123-12-7]

$Ag(C_6F_5)$

M 274.926

Sol. Et_2O, MeCN, DMF, Py. Mp 150°. Photosensitive in soln.

Sun, K.K. *et al*, *J. Am. Chem. Soc.*, 1970, **92**, 6985 (*synth*, *nmr*, *ir*)
Bennett, R.L. *et al*, *J. Chem. Soc., Dalton Trans.*, 1973, 2653 (*use*)

C_6H_5Ag Ag-00012

Phenylsilver, 9CI

[5274-48-6]

$[AgPh]_n$

M 184.974

Polymeric with bridging phenyl groups. Insol. aliphatic hydrocarbons, spar. sol. C_6H_6, $CHCl_3$, Py. Mp 74° dec. Not v. sensitive to O_2 and H_2O, sl. sensitive to light.

▷Explosive at r.t.

Beverwijk, C.D.M. *et al*, *J. Organomet. Chem.*, 1972, **43**, C11 (*synth*)
Hofstee, H.K. *et al*, *J. Organomet. Chem.*, 1978, **168**, 241 (*synth*, *nmr*, *ir*)
Bretherick, L., *Handbook of Reactive Chemical Hazards*, 2nd Ed., Butterworths, London and Boston, 1979, 569.
Sax, N.I., *Dangerous Properties of Industrial Materials*, 5th Ed., Van Nostrand-Reinhold, 1979, 907.
Hazards in the Chemical Laboratory, (Bretherick, L., Ed.), 3rd Ed., Royal Society of Chemistry, London, 1981, 439.

$C_6H_6Ag^{\oplus}$ Ag-00013

[(1,2-η)-Benzene]silver(1+), 10CI

[62969-28-2]

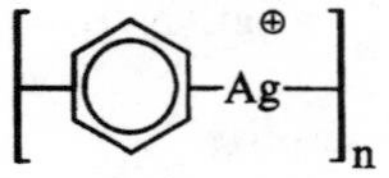

M 185.981 (ion)

Polymeric C_6H_6—Ag—C_6H_6—Ag chains with Ag ions lying above and below rings.

Perchlorate:

$C_6H_6AgClO_4$ M 285.432

Cryst. (C_6H_6). Sol. C_6H_6.

Rundle, R.E. *et al*, *J. Am. Chem. Soc.*, 1950, **72**, 5337 (*synth*, *cryst struct*)
Smith, H.G. *et al*, *J. Am. Chem. Soc.*, 1958, **80**, 5075 (*synth*, *cryst struct*)
Gmelin Handbuch der Anorg. Chem., 1975, **61**, **B5**, 90 (*rev*)
Gut, R. *et al*, *J. Organomet. Chem.*, 1977, **128**, 89 (*props*)

C_6H_9Ag Ag-00014

1-Hexynylsilver, 9CI

[60627-07-8]

$H_3C(CH_2)_3C{\equiv}CAg$

M 189.005

Reagent for synth. of acetylenic ketones. Prepd. *in situ* from $AgNO_3$. Sol. CCl_4, $CHCl_3$, C_6H_6.

Davis, R.B. *et al*, *J. Am. Chem. Soc.*, 1956, **78**, 1675 (*synth*, *use*)
Travkin, N.N. *et al*, *Zh. Obshch. Khim.*, 1976, **46**, 1088.

$C_6H_{10}Ag^{\oplus}$ Ag-00015

[(1,2-η)-Cyclohexene]silver(1+), 9CI

[45467-41-2]

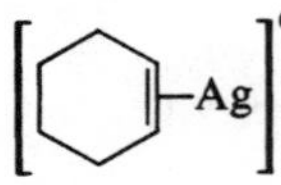

M 190.013 (ion)

Nitrate: [60447-73-6].

$C_6H_{10}AgNO_3$ M 252.018

Needle shaped cryst. (cyclohexene/MeOH). Mp 24-32°.

Perchlorate:

$C_6H_{10}AgClO_4$ M 289.464

Cryst. (cyclohexene/Me_2CO).

Comyns, A.E. *et al*, *J. Am. Chem. Soc.*, 1957, **79**, 4339 (*synth*)
Hosoya, H. *et al*, *Bull. Chem. Soc. Jpn.*, 1964, **37**, 249 (*ir*, *uv*)
Natarajan, G.S. *et al*, *Aust. J. Chem.*, 1974, **27**, 1209.
Inorg. Synth., 1976, **16**, 117 (*synth*, *use*)

$C_6H_{18}AgClP_2$ Ag-00016

Chlorobis(trimethylphosphine)silver

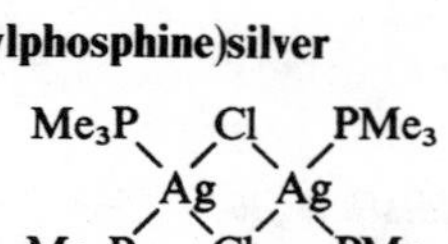

M 295.477

Dimeric.

Dimer: [40696-74-0]. *Di-μ-chlorotetrakis(trimethylphosphine)disilver*, 9CI.

$C_{12}H_{36}Ag_2Cl_2P_4$ M 590.953

Cryst. (C_6H_6/pet. ether). Sol. C_6H_6. Mp 75°.

Schmidbaur, H. *et al*, *Chem. Ber.*, 1972, **105**, 3382 (*synth*)

$C_7H_{11}AgClN$ Ag-00017

Chloro(isocyanocyclohexane)silver, 9CI

(Cyclohexyl isocyanide)chlorosilver

[55145-55-6]

ClAgC≡N–(cyclohexyl)

M 252.492

Solid. Insol. common org. solvs. Mp 93-5°.

Minghetti, G. *et al*, *Inorg. Chem.*, 1975, **14**, 1974 (*synth*)

C_8H_5Ag Ag-00018

(Phenylethynyl)silver, 9CI

[33440-88-9]

$[AgC{\equiv}CPh]_n$

M 208.996

Polymeric. Sol. Py, insol. most org. solvs.

Coates, G.E. *et al*, *Proc. Chem. Soc. London*, 1959, 396 (*use*)
Agawa, T. *et al*, *J. Am. Chem. Soc.*, 1961, **83**, 449 (*synth*, *use*)
Nast, R. *et al*, *Z. Anorg. Allg. Chem.*, 1963, **326**, 201 (*synth*)
Tsuda, T. *et al*, *J. Chem. Soc., Chem. Commun.*, 1974, 381 (*use*)
Aleksanyan, V.T. *et al*, *Spectrochim. Acta, Part A*, 1975, **31**, 517 (*ir*, *raman*)
Huang, S.J. *et al*, *J. Org. Chem.*, 1975, **40**, 124 (*synth*, *use*)
Travkin, N.N. *et al*, *Zh. Obshch. Khim.*, 1976, **46**, 1088.

C_8H_7AgClN Ag-00019

Chloro(1-isocyano-4-methylbenzene)silver

(p-Tolylisocyanide)chlorosilver

[41676-86-2]

ClAgC≡N–C_6H_4–CH_3

M 260.471

Insol. common org. solvs. Mp 153-6° dec.

Minghetti, G. *et al*, *J. Chem. Soc., Chem. Commun.*, 1973, 260 (*use*)
Minghetti, G. *et al*, *Inorg. Chem.*, 1975, **14**, 1974 (*synth*)

$C_8H_8Ag^{\oplus}$ Ag-00020

(1,3,5,7-Cyclooctatetraene)silver(1+), 9CI

[60447-72-5]

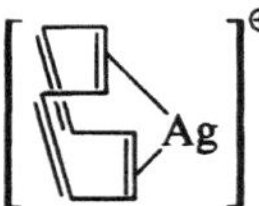

M 212.019 (ion)

Nitrate:

$C_8H_8AgNO_3$ M 274.024

Pale-yellow cryst. Mp 173-4° dec.

Cope, A.C. *et al*, *J. Am. Chem. Soc.*, 1950, **72**, 2515 (*synth*)
Mathews, F.S. *et al*, *J. Am. Chem. Soc.*, 1958, **80**, 4745 (*cryst struct*)
Mathews, F.S. *et al*, *J. Phys. Chem.*, 1959, **63**, 845 (*cryst struct*)

$C_8H_{20}Ag_2As_2$ Ag-00021

Bis[μ-(dimethylarsinidenio)bis[methylene]]disilver, 9CI

[56931-35-2]

M 481.825

Cryst. (toluene). Sol. toluene. Mp 180°. $Bp_{0.01}$ 150° subl.

Schmidbaur, H. *et al*, *Chem. Ber.*, 1975, **108**, 2656 (*synth*)

$C_8H_{20}Ag_2P_2$ Ag-00022

Bis[μ-[dimethyl(methylene)phosphoranyl]methyl]disilver, 9CI

[43064-38-6]

M 393.930

Cryst. (toluene/Et_2O or by subl.). Sol. C_6H_6, toluene. Mp 153-5°. $Bp_{0.001}$ 110-40° subl.

Schmidbaur, H. *et al*, *Chem. Ber.*, 1974, **107**, 3697 (*synth*)
Inorg. Synth., 1978, **18**, 142 (*synth*, *nmr*)

$C_9H_{11}Ag$ Ag-00023

(1,3,5-Trimethylbenzene)silver

Mesitylsilver

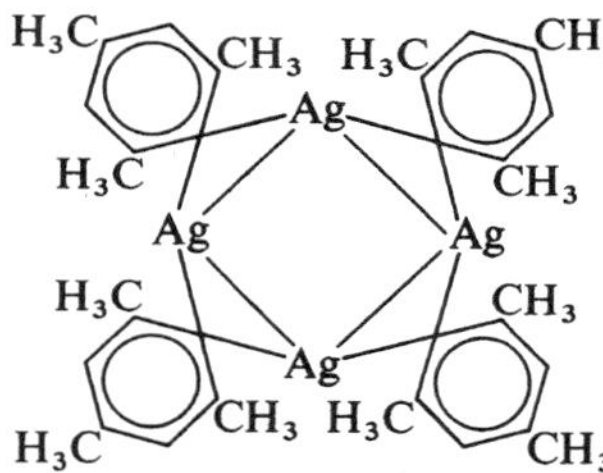

M 227.054

Tetrameric.

Tetramer: Tetrakis(1,3,5-trimethylbenzene)tetrasilver. Tetramesityltetrasilver.

$C_{36}H_{44}Ag_4$ M 908.216

Cryst. (toluene). V. sol. org. solvs. Dec. rapidly in air.

Gambarotta, S. *et al*, *J. Chem. Soc., Chem. Commun.*, 1983, 1087 (*synth*, *cryst struct*)

$C_9H_{12}AgN$ Ag-00024

[2-[(Dimethylamino)methyl]phenyl]silver, 9CI

[49771-93-9]

$[Ag(C_6H_4CH_2NMe_2)]_n$

M 242.069

Polymeric, possibly tetrameric in soln. Thermally stable cryst. (C_6H_6). Sol. C_6H_6. Mp 160-80° dec.

Leusink, A.J. *et al*, *J. Organomet. Chem.*, 1973, **56**, 379 (*synth*)

$C_9H_{12}Ag_2BrN$ **Ag-00025**

Bromo[2-[(dimethylamino)methyl]phenyl]disilver, 9CI

[50647-91-1]

$[Ag_2Br(C_6H_4CH_2NMe_2)]_n$

M 429.841

Polymeric. Rust brown solid. Dec. only slowly in air. Insol. C_6H_6. Mp 108° dec.

Leusink, A.J. *et al*, *J. Organomet. Chem.*, 1973, **56**, 379 (*synth*)

$C_{10}H_{10}AgF_7O_2$ **Ag-00026**

(6,6,7,7,8,8,8-Heptafluoro-2,2-dimethyl-3,5-octanedionato-*O,O'*)silver, 9CI

(1,1,1,2,2,3,3-Heptafluoro-7,7-dimethyl-4,6-octanedionato)silver(I). Ag(fod)

[76121-99-8]

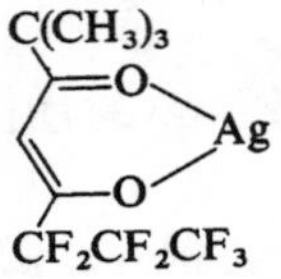

M 403.045

Used in conjunction with $Yb(fod)_3$ and $Pr(fod)_3$ as nmr shift reagent for aromatic protons. Light-sensitive, dec. on cryst. Insol. H_2O. Mp 134-5° dec.

Wenzel, T.J. *et al*, *J. Am. Chem. Soc.*, 1980, **102**, 5903 (*synth, use*)
Rackham, D.M. *et al*, *Spectrosc. Lett.*, 1981, **14**, 379, 639.
Wenzel, T.J. *et al*, *Anal. Chem.*, 1981, **53**, 343 (*synth, use*)

$C_{11}H_{14}AgP$ **Ag-00027**

(Phenylethynyl)(trimethylphosphine)silver

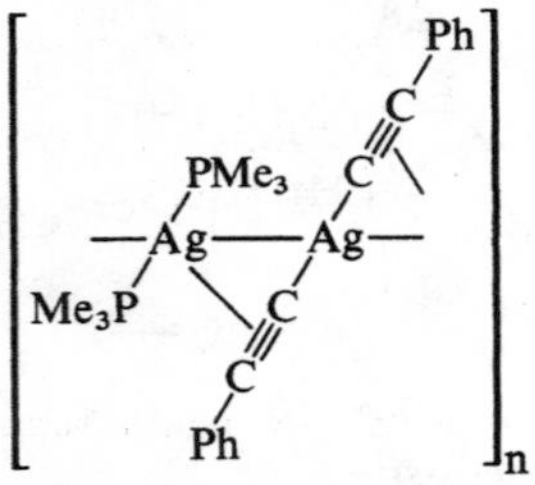

M 285.073

Polymeric with alternating $Ag(PMe_3)_2$ and $Ag(C{\equiv}CPh)$ units. Cryst. (Me_2CO). Sol. C_6H_6. Mp 130-40° dec.

Coates, G.E. *et al*, *J. Inorg. Nucl. Chem.*, 1961, **22**, 59 (*synth*)
Corfield, P.W.R. *et al*, *Acta Crystallogr.*, 1966, **20**, 502 (*cryst struct*)

$C_{12}H_{36}AgOP_3Si$ **Ag-00028**

Tris(trimethylphosphine)(trimethylsilanolato)silver, 9CI

[40696-91-1]

$Me_3SiOAg(PMe_3)_3$

M 425.291

Sol. C_6H_6. Mp 103-4°.

Schmidbaur, H. *et al*, *Chem. Ber.*, 1972, **105**, 3389.

$C_{13}H_{13}AgF_6O_2$ **Ag-00029**

[(1,2-η)-1,5-Cyclooctadiene](1,1,1,5,5,5-hexafluoro-2,4-pentanedionato-*O,O'*)silver, 9CI

(1,1,1,5,5,5-Hexafluoro-2,4-pentanedionato)(1,5-cyclooctadiene)silver. (1,5-Cycloctadiene)-(hexafluoroacetoacetonato)silver

[38892-25-0]

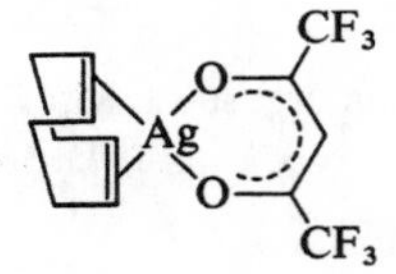

M 423.103

Relatively stable, nonionic, monomeric silver(I) olefin complex. Sol. halogenated solvs. Loses olefin when exposed to air.

Partenheimer, W. *et al*, *Inorg. Chem.*, 1972, **11**, 2840 (*synth*)
Inorg. Synth., 1976, **16**, 117 (*synth*)

$C_{13}H_{16}AgFeN$ **Ag-00030**

[2-[(Dimethylamino)methyl]ferrocenyl-*C,N*]silver, 10CI

1-[(Dimethylamino)methyl]-2-silverferrocene

[65286-18-2]

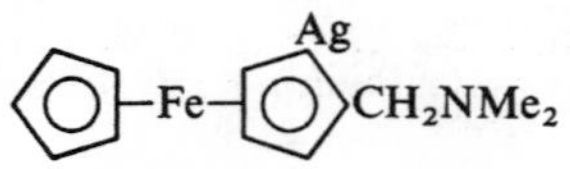

M 349.991

Precursor for biferrocenyl compounds. Isostructural with the Cu analogue.

Nesmeyanov, A.N. *et al*, *Izv. Akad. Nauk SSSR, Ser. Khim.*, 1977, 2354 (*synth, use*)
Nesmeyanov, A.N. *et al*, *J. Organomet. Chem.*, 1978, **153**, 115 (*synth, use, struct*)

$C_{16}H_{36}AgP$ **Ag-00031**

Butyl(tributylphosphine)silver, 9CI

[52543-55-2]

$H_3C(CH_2)_3AgP(CH_2CH_2CH_2CH_3)_3$

M 367.302

Dec. rapidly above −50°.

Whitesides, G.M. *et al*, *J. Am. Chem. Soc.*, 1974, **96**, 2806 (*synth*)
Bergbreiter, D.E. *et al*, *J. Org. Chem.*, 1981, **46**, 727.

$C_{20}H_{26}AgB_8P$ **Ag-00032**

Triphenylphosphine[(7,8,9-η)undecahydro-5,6-dicarbadecaborato(1−)]silver

[74354-46-4]

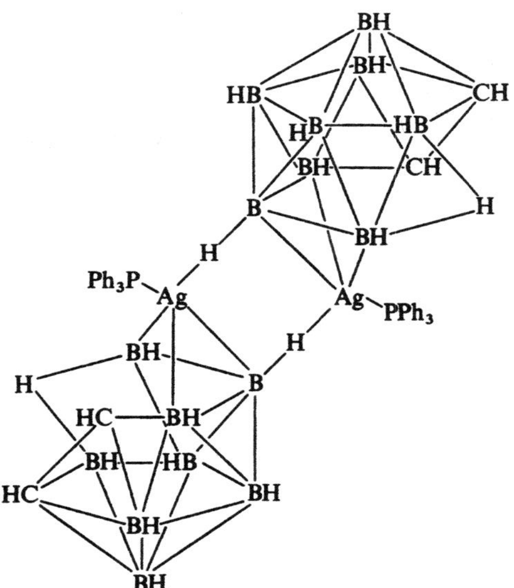

M 491.747

Dimeric in solid state with two *arachno*-AgC_2B_8 cages linked by a pair of Ag—H—B bridges.

Dimer: 11-Bis[triphenylphosphine-11-argenta-5,6-dicarbundecaborane(11)].

$C_{40}H_{52}Ag_2B_{16}P_2$ M 983.494

Cream cryst. ($CHCl_3$/hexane). Sol. $CHCl_3$.

Colquhoun, H.M. *et al*, *J. Chem. Soc., Chem. Commun.*, 1980, 192 (*synth, nmr, cryst struct*)

$C_{23}H_{20}AgP$ **Ag-00033**

(η^5-2,4-Cyclopentadien-1-yl)triphenylphosphinesilver, 9CI

[61374-56-9]

—AgPPh$_3$

M 435.253

Sol. DMF, insol. C_6H_6, Et_2O. Mp 75° dec. V. sensitive to moisture, dec. slowly at r.t.

Hofstee, H.K. *et al*, *J. Organomet. Chem.*, 1976, **120**, 313.

$C_{24}H_{20}AgB$ **Ag-00034**

Silver(1+) tetraphenylborate(1−), 10CI, 9CI, 8CI

Silver tetraphenylboride

[14637-35-5]

$Ag^{\oplus}Ph_4B^{\ominus}$

M 427.100

Used for gravimetric determination of $Ag^{\oplus}$ and in conductometric determinations of solubility and solubility prod. of Ag salts. Solid.

Mukherji, A.K. *et al*, *Anal. Chem.*, 1959, **31**, 608 (*props*)
Popovych, O., *Anal. Chem.*, 1966, **38**, 117 (*props*)
Costa, G. *et al*, *J. Organomet. Chem.*, 1967, **8**, 339 (*ir*)
Badoz-Lambling, J., *C.R. Hebd. Seances Acad. Sci.*, 1968, **266**, 95 (*props*)

$C_{32}H_{40}Ag_6Br_2N_4$ **Ag-00035**

Di-μ-bromotetrakis[μ_3-(2-dimethylamino)phenyl-*C,C,N*]hexasilver

[51231-89-1]

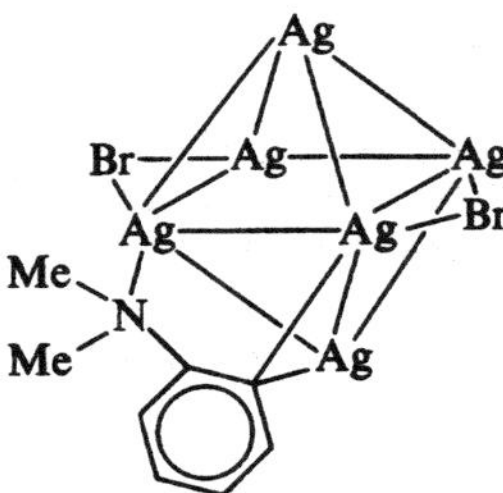

Only one of four amine groups shown

M 1287.711

Probably has octahedral cluster geometry analogous to that of Di-μ-bromotetrakis[μ_3-(2-dimethylaminophenyl-*C:C:N*)]hexacopper, Cu-00058. Cryst. (C_6H_6). Sol. C_6H_6. Mp 110-40° dec.

Leusink, A.J. *et al*, *J. Organomet. Chem.*, 1973, **56**, 379 (*synth*)

$C_{36}H_{48}Ag_2Li_2N_4$ **Ag-00036**

Tetrakis[μ-[2-[(dimethylamino)methyl]phenyl-*C,C,N*]bis(silver)dilithium, 9CI

[51005-77-7]

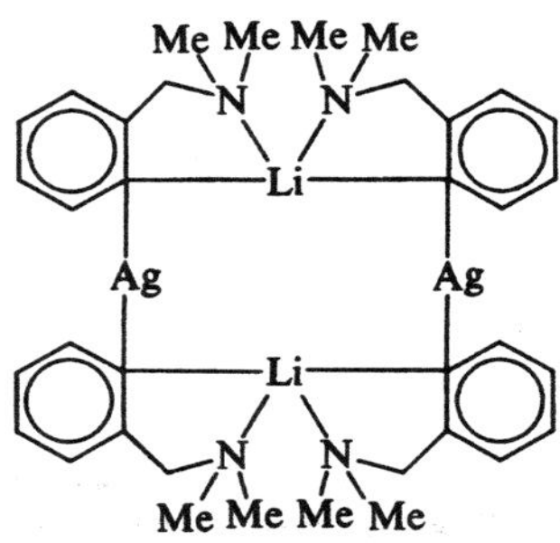

M 766.420

Cream solid, cryst. (C_6H_6/pentane). Sol. C_6H_6. Mp 180° dec. Water and O_2 sensitive.

Leusink, A.J. *et al*, *J. Organomet. Chem.*, 1973, **55**, 419 (*synth*)

$C_{38}H_{34}AgP_2^{\oplus}$ **Ag-00037**

Bis[(triphenylphosphonio)methyl]silver(1+), 9CI

[57111-08-7]

$[Ph_3PCH_2{-}Ag{-}CH_2PPh_3]^{\oplus}$

M 660.502 (ion)

Alkylidenetriphenylphosphorane complex.

Chloride:

$C_{38}H_{34}AgClP_2$ M 695.955

Cryst. (THF). Sol. CH_2Cl_2. Mp 192-4°. Shows high thermal stability.

Yamamoto, Y. *et al*, *J. Organomet. Chem.*, 1975, **96**, 133.

$C_{38}H_{41}AgB_8P_2$ **Ag-00038**

Bis(triphenylphosphine)[(7,8,9,-η)undecahydro-5,6-dicarbadecaborato(1−)]silver

[74354-45-3]

$$(Ph_3P)_2Ag(C_2B_8H_{11})$$

M 754.037

Struct. not known, probably monomeric. Cryst. ($CHCl_3$/hexane). Loses PPh_3 on recryst., giving Triphenylphosphine[(7,8,9-η)undecahydro-5,6-dicarbadecaborato(1−)]silver, Ag-00032 .

Colquhoun, H.M. *et al*, *J. Chem. Soc., Chem. Commun.*, 1980, 192 (*synth, nmr*)

$C_{39}H_{43}AgBP$ **Ag-00039**

Tris(methyldiphenylphosphine)[tetrahydroborato(1−)-*H*]silver

[72347-03-6]

$$H_3B{-}H{-}Ag(PMePh_2)_3$$

M 661.420

Cryst. (CH_2Cl_2/pentane). Sol. CH_2Cl_2, $CHCl_3$. Mp 90-3° dec.

Bommer, J.C. *et al*, *Inorg. Chem.*, 1980, **19**, 587 (*synth*)

Au Gold

D. M. P. Mingos

Or (Fr.), Gold (Ger.), Oro (Sp., Ital.), Золото (Zoloto) (Russ.), 金 (Japan.)

Atomic Number. 79

Atomic Weight. 196.9665

Electronic Configuration. [Xe] $5d^{10}\,6s^1$

Oxidation States. Au(I) and Au(III) are the common oxidation states in organometallic and related compounds; Au(II) compounds either tend to have Au—Au bonding or are mixed valence Au(I)—Au(III). Higher oxidation states found are usually with fluorine ligands.

Coordination Number. Au(I) compounds are generally linear, but sometimes trigonal and tetrahedral geometries are found in solid state. Au(II) and Au(III) complexes are square-planar.

Colour. Most Au(I) organometallics are colourless with the exception of the highly coloured cluster compounds. Au(III) compounds are typically yellow.

Availability. Starting materials available include gold metal, $HAuCl_4.nH_2O$, $NH_4AuCl_4.nH_2O$, $Au_2O_3.nH_2O$. The price of these is high and fluctuates with the price of gold metal on the world market.

Handling. Gold compounds do not require any special handling techniques.

Toxicity. Gold compounds are not generally regarded as being especially toxic. A range of gold compounds has been found to be biologically active, however, and so reasonable care should be taken.

Isotopic Abundance. ^{197}Au, 100%.

Spectroscopy. ^{197}Au has $I = \frac{3}{2}$ but its nuclear quadrupole and low sensitivity make it difficult to observe nmr spectra of this nucleus.

Mössbauer spectroscopy of ^{197}Au from 77.3 keV level of spin $\frac{1}{2}$ to ground state of spin $\frac{3}{2}$ is possible.

Analysis. Spectrophotometric methods generally depend on conversion to $[AuCl_4]^-$ or $[AuBr_4]^-$ in aqueous solution and measurement of the absorbance. If impurities interfere, solvent extraction into CH_2Cl_2—THF is undertaken. Rhodamine forms an intense red colour with $[AuCl_4]^-$. Atomic absorption spectrophotometry with a carbon rod atomiser is used for concentrations as low as 1 ppm.

References. In addition to references given in the introduction to the *Sourcebook*, the following provide further reading:

Puddephatt, R. J., *The Chemistry of Gold*, Elsevier, 1978 (*general review*)

Gedansky, L. M. *et al.*, *Engelhardt Tech. Bull.*, 1969, **10,** 5 (*thermochemistry and potential data*)

Schmidbaur, H., *Angew. Chem., Int. Ed. Engl.*, 1976, **15,** 728 (*organometallic compounds*)

Anderson, G. K., *Adv. Organomet. Chem.*, 1982, **20,** 40 (*organometallic compounds*)

Jones, P. G., *Gold Bull.*, 1981, **14,** 102, 159; 1983, **16,** 114 (*structural aspects*)

Parish, R. V., *Gold Bull.*, 1982, **15,** 51 (*Mössbauer*)

Hall, K. P. and Mingos, D. M. P., *Prog. Inorg. Chem.*, 1984, **32,** 237 (*metal-metal bonding and cluster compounds*)

Sadler, P. J., *Gold Bull.*, 1976, **9,** 110; *Struct. Bond.*, 1976, **29,** 171 (*biochemical aspects*)

Brown, D. H., *Chem. Soc. Rev.*, 1980, **9,** 217 (*biochemical aspects*)

Das, N. R. *et al.*, *Talanta*, 1976, **23,** 535 (*analysis*)

Fishkova, N. L., *Zh. Anal. Khim.*, 1974, **29,** 2121 (*atomic absorption*)

Schmidbaur, H. *et al.*, *Adv. Inorg. Chem. Radiochem.*, 1982, **25,** 239 (*oxidation states*)

$ClAuCO$
Au-00001

$AuCN$
Au-00002

$Au(CN)_2^{\ominus}$
Au-00003

$[AuC{\equiv}CAu]_n$
Au-00004

$ClAuCNMe$
Au-00005

$Cl_3AuNCCH_3$
Au-00006

$AuMe_2^{\ominus}$
Au-00007

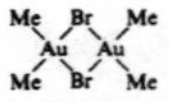

Au-00008

$BrAuSMe_2$
Au-00009

Br_3AuSMe_2
Au-00010

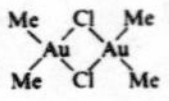

Au-00011

$ClAuSMe_2$
Au-00012

$ClAu(SeMe_2)$
Au-00013

Cl_3AuSMe_2
Au-00014

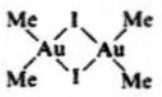

Au-00015

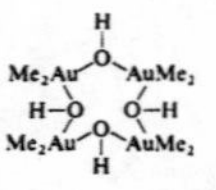

Au-00016

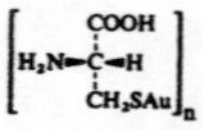

Au-00017

$ClAuC(OMe)NHMe$
Au-00018

$HOOCCH_2CH(SAu)COOH$
Au-00019

$ClAu(H_3CC{\equiv}CCH_3)$
Au-00020

$Au(NCCH_3)_2^{\oplus}$
Au-00021

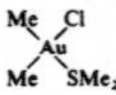

Au-00022

$MeAuP(OMe)_3$
Au-00023

$MeAuPMe_3$
Au-00024

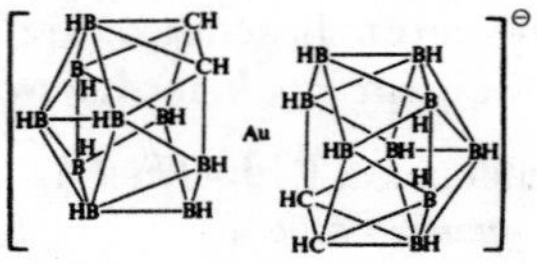

Au-00025

$Au(\eta\text{-}C_5H_5)$
Au-00027

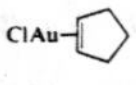

Au-00028

$MeAuCH_2PMe_3$
Au-00029

$PhAuCl_2$
Au-00030

$PhAuCl_3^{\ominus}$
Au-00031

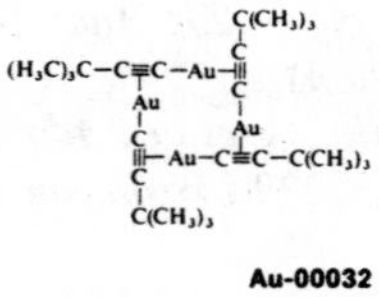

Au-00032

$Me_3PAuFe(CO)_3NO$
Au-00033

$(MeO)_3PAuFe(CO)_3NO$
Au-00034

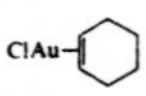

Au-00035

$[Au(CNEt)_2]^{\oplus}$
Au-00036

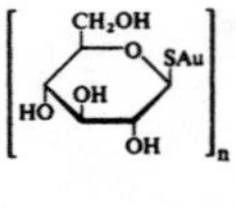

Au-00037

$BrAuPEt_3$
Au-00038

Br_3AuPEt_3
Au-00039

$ClAuP(OEt)_3$
Au-00040

$ClAuPEt_3$
Au-00041

Cl_3AuPEt_3
Au-00042

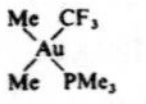

cis-form
Au-00043

$Me_2S(O)CH_2AuMe_3$
Au-00044

$Au[P(OMe)_3]_2^{\oplus}$
Au-00045

$Et_3PAuSCN$
Au-00046

$MeAuPEt_3$
Au-00047

$Me_3AuCH_2PMe_3$
Au-00048

$Me_3SiCH_2AuPMe_3$
Au-00049

$Me_3PAuCH_2PMe_3^{\oplus}$
Au-00050

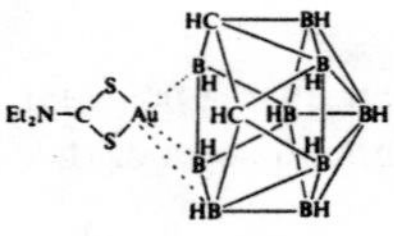

Au-00051

$[AuC{\equiv}CPh]_n$
Au-00052

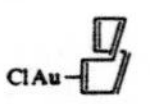

Au-00053

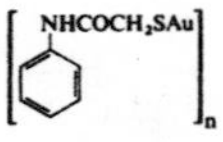

Au-00054

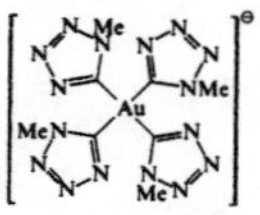

Au-00055

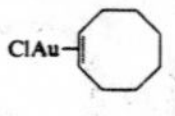

Au-00056

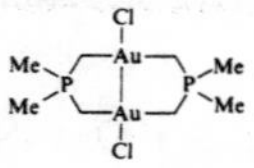

Au-00057

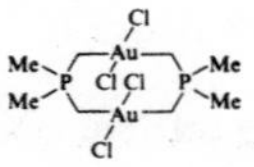

Au-00058

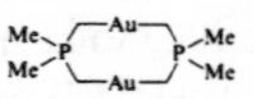

Au-00059

$[Me_3PCH_2AuCH_2PMe_3]^{\oplus}$
Au-00060

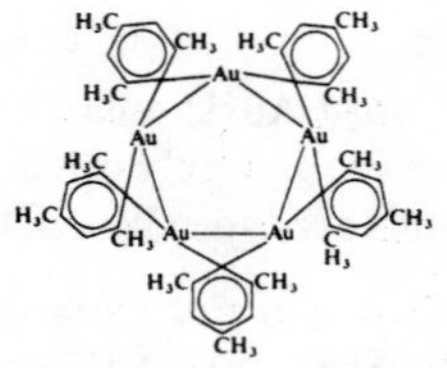

Au-00061

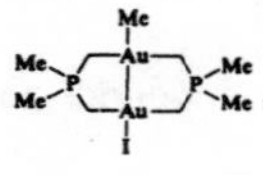

Au-00062

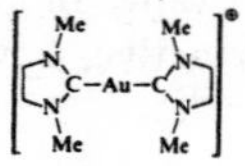

Au-00063

$[Et_3PAuSCH(COOH)CH_2COOH]_n$
Au-00064

$Au(C_6F_5)_2^{\ominus}$
Au-00065

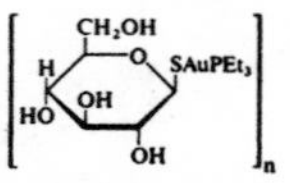

Au-00066

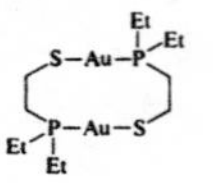

Au-00067

$ClAu(PhC{\equiv}CPh)$
Au-00068

Au-00069

Au-00070

Ph_3PAuCl

Au-00071

$MeAuPPh_3$

Au-00072

$Ph_3PAuCH{=}CH_2$

Au-00073

Au-00074

$Ph_3PAuFe(CO)_3NO$

Au-00075

Me_3AuPPh_3

Au-00076

$Ph_3PCH_2AuMe_3$

Au-00077

Au-00078

$Ph_3PAu[CH(COCH_3)_2]$

Au-00079

Au-00080

$PhAuPPh_3$

Au-00081

Au-00082

Au-00083

Au-00084

Au-00085

Au-00086

Au-00087

Au-00088

Au-00089

$[Au_2Li_2(C_6H_4CH_2NMe_2)_4]$

Au-00090

$Ph_3PAuFe(CO)_2(PPh_3)NO$

Au-00091

Au-00092

Au-00093

Au-00094

Au-00095

Au-00096

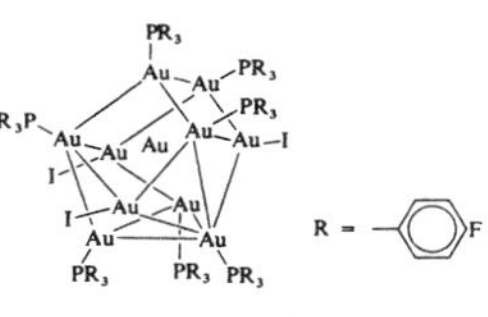

Au-00097

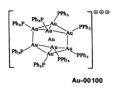

Au-00098

Au-00099

Au-00100

CAuClO **Au-00001**

Carbonylchlorogold, 9CI

[50960-82-2]

ClAuCO

M 260.430

Useful starting material for synthesising Au(I) compounds. Moisture-sensitive sublimable solid. Stable to 110°. Sol. $SOCl_2$, CCl_4, THF, CH_2Cl_2, C_6H_6. Mp 95° subl.

Manchot, W. *et al*, *Ber.*, 1925, **58**, 2175 (*synth*)
Kharasch, M.S. *et al*, *J. Am. Chem. Soc.*, 1930, **52**, 2919 (*synth*)
Belli Dell'Amico, D. *et al*, *Gazz. Chim. Ital.*, 1973, **103**, 1099.
Browning, J. *et al*, *J. Chem. Soc., Dalton Trans.*, 1977, 2061 (*nmr, ir*)
Jones, P.G. *et al*, *J. Chem. Soc., Dalton Trans.*, 1977, 1434 (*mossbauer*)

CAuN **Au-00002**

Gold cyanide, 9CI

Cyanogold

[506-65-0]

AuCN

M 222.984

Lemon-yellow cryst. powder. Stable in air. Unstable to light when moist. Spar. sol. H_2O, sol. alkali cyanide solns.

Brauer, G., *Handbook of Preparative Inorganic Chemistry*, Academic Press, 1965, **2**, 1064.
Chadwick, B.M. *et al*, *Adv. Inorg. Radiochem.*, 1968, **8**, 156 (*rev*)

$C_2AuN_2^{\ominus}$ **Au-00003**

Bis(cyano-*C*)aurate(1−), 9CI

Dicyanoaurate(1−)

[14950-87-9]

$Au(CN)_2^{\ominus}$

M 249.002 (ion)

K salt: Gold potassium cyanide.

C_2AuKN_2 M 288.100

Cryst. (H_2O), stable to air and light. Sol. H_2O, spar. sol. EtOH, insol. Et_2O, Me_2CO.

Chemnetius, F., *Chem. - Ztg.*, 1927, **51**, 823 (*synth*)
Rosenweig, A. *et al*, *Acta Crystallogr.*, 1959, **12**, 709 (*cryst struct*)
Jones, L.H., *Spectrochim. Acta*, 1963, **19**, 1675 (*ir*)
Brauer, G., *Handbook of Preparative Inorganic Chemistry*, Academic Press, 1965, **2**, 1065 (*synth*)
Faltens, M.O. *et al*, *J. Chem. Phys.*, 1970, **53**, 4249 (*mossbauer*)
Pesek, J.J. *et al*, *Inorg. Chem.*, 1979, **18**, 924 (*cmr*)

C_2Au_2 **Au-00004**

Gold acetylide, 9CI

[70950-00-4]

$[AuC{\equiv}CAu]_n$

M 417.955

Polymeric. Yellow powder. Insol. common org. solvs.

▷Explosive on heating or mechanical impact especially when dry

Mathews, A. *et al*, *J. Am. Chem. Soc.*, 1900, **22**, 108 (*synth, haz*)
Nast, R. *et al*, *Z. Anorg. Allg. Chem.*, 1964, **330**, 311.
Brauer, G., *Handbook of Preparative Inorg. Chem.*, Academic Press, 1965, **2**, 1063 (*synth*)
Nast, R., *Angew. Chem.*, 1965, **77**, 352 (*rev*)

C_2H_3AuClN **Au-00005**

Chloro(isocyanomethane)gold

Chloro(methyl isocyanide)gold

[37131-30-9]

ClAuCNMe

M 273.472

Useful starting material for synth. of carbene complexes. Cryst. (CH_2Cl_2 or Me_2CO). Sol. CH_2Cl_2, Me_2CO. Mp 211° (from CH_2Cl_2), 224° (from acetone).

Bonati, F. *et al*, *Gazz. Chim. Ital.*, 1973, **103**, 373 (*synth*)
Browning, J. *et al*, *J. Chem. Res. (S)*, 1978, 328; *J. Chem. Res. (M)*, 4201 (*nmr, ir*)

$C_2H_3AuCl_3N$ **Au-00006**

Acetonitriletrichlorogold, 9CI

Trichloro(acetonitrile)gold

[53747-67-4]

$Cl_3AuNCCH_3$

M 344.378

Orange-yellow cryst. (MeCN).

Kharasch, M.S. *et al*, *J. Am. Chem. Soc.*, 1934, **56**, 2057 (*synth, rev*)
Belli Dell'Amico, D. *et al*, *Gazz. Chim. Ital.*, 1973, **103**, 1099 (*synth, nmr*)

$C_2H_6Au^{\ominus}$ **Au-00007**

Dimethylaurate(1−), 9CI

[53863-37-9]

$AuMe_2^{\ominus}$

M 227.036 (ion)

Unstable above 0°, studied in soln. below this temp.

Li salt: [53863-37-9].

C_2H_6AuLi M 233.977

Obt. by addition of stoichiometric amount of LiMe to CH_3AuPPh_3. Unstable. Dec. >0°. Sol. Et_2O, dimethoxyethane. Has also been studied as deuterio-analogue.

Li salt, pentamethyldiethylenetriamine adduct: [57444-57-2]. [N-[*2-(dimethylimino)ethyl*]-N,N′,N′-*trimethyl-1,2-ethanediamine*-N,N′,N″]*lithium(1+) salt.*

$C_{11}H_{29}AuLiN_3$ M 407.278

Stable at r.t. V. sensitive to air and water. Mp 123° dec.

Li salt, Bis(Py) adduct: Stable at 0°, sensitive to air and water.

Tamaki, A. *et al*, *J. Chem. Soc., Dalton Trans.*, 1973, 2620 (*synth, nmr*)
Tamaki, A. *et al*, *J. Organomet. Chem.*, 1973, **51**, C39 (*synth, nmr*)
Rice, G.W. *et al*, *Inorg. Chem.*, 1975, **14**, 2402 (*nmr, ir, raman*)
Komiya, S. *et al*, *J. Am. Chem. Soc.*, 1977, **99**, 8440.

C_2H_6AuBr Au-00008

Bromodimethylgold, 9CI

Dimethylgold bromide

[42495-72-7]

```
Me   Br   Me
  \ /  \ /
  Au    Au
  / \  / \
Me   Br   Me
```

M 306.940

Dimeric.

Dimer: Di-μ-bromotetramethyldigold.

$C_4H_{12}Au_2Br_2$ M 613.880

Light-sensitive needles. Mp 68-9°.

Gibson, C.S. *et al*, *J. Chem. Soc.*, 1936, 324; 1939, 762 (*synth*)
Schmidbaur, H. *et al*, *Inorg. Chem.*, 1966, **5**, 2069 (*synth, ir, pmr*)
Scovell, W.M. *et al*, *Inorg. Chem.*, 1970, **9**, 2682 (*synth, ir, raman*)

C_2H_6AuBrS Au-00009

Bromo(dimethyl sulfide)gold

Bromo[thiobis[methane]]gold, 9CI

[37922-40-0]

$BrAuSMe_2$

M 339.000

Useful starting material for synth. of Au(I) compounds. Air stable cryst. (C_6H_6/Me_2CO). Mp 130-40° dec.

Allen, E.A. *et al*, *Spectrochim. Acta, Part A*, 1972, **28**, 2257 (*synth, ir*)
Goggin, P.L. *et al*, *J. Chem. Soc., Dalton Trans.*, 1972, 1904 (*synth, ir*)
Roulet, R. *et al*, *Chimia*, 1975, **29**, 346.

$C_2H_6AuBr_3S$ Au-00010

Tribromo(dimethyl sulfide)gold

Tribromo[thiobis[methane]]gold, 9CI

[39929-04-9]

Br_3AuSMe_2

M 498.808

Yellow, air stable.

Ray, P.C. *et al*, *Indian J. Chem.*, 1930, **7**, 67 (*synth*)
Allen, E.A. *et al*, *Spectrochim. Acta, Part A*, 1972, **28**, 2257 (*synth, ir*)

C_2H_6AuCl Au-00011

Chlorodimethylgold, 9CI

[42495-71-6]

```
Me   Cl   Me
  \ /  \ /
  Au    Au
  / \  / \
Me   Cl   Me
```

M 262.489

Dimeric.

Dimer: [30676-27-8]. *Di-μ-chlorotetramethyldigold.*

$C_4H_{12}Au_2Cl_2$ M 524.978

Cryst. (pet. ether). Mp 72-3°.

Scovell, W.M. *et al*, *Inorg. Chem.*, 1970, **9**, 2682 (*synth, ir, raman*)
Shiotani, A. *et al*, *Chem. Ber.*, 1971, **104**, 2838 (*synth, ir*)
Stocco, G.C. *et al*, *J. Am. Chem. Soc.*, 1971, **93**, 5057.

C_2H_6AuClS Au-00012

Chloro(dimethyl sulfide)gold

Chloro[thiobis[methane]]gold, 10CI, 9CI

[27892-37-3]

$ClAuSMe_2$

M 294.549

Useful starting material for synth. of Au(I) complexes. Air stable cryst. (C_6H_6/Me_2CO).

Ray, P.C. *et al*, *Indian J. Chem.*, 1930, **7**, 67 (*synth*)
Allen, E.A. *et al*, *Spectrochim. Acta, Part A*, 1972, **28**, 2257 (*synth, ir*)
Goggin, P.L. *et al*, *J. Chem. Soc., Dalton Trans.*, 1972, 1904 (*ir*)
Dash, K.C. *et al*, *Chem. Ber.*, 1973, **106**, 1221 (*synth, ir, nmr*)
Tamaki, A. *et al*, *J. Organomet. Chem.*, 1974, **64**, 411 (*synth*)
Roulet, R. *et al*, *Chimia*, 1975, **29**, 346 (*rev*)

$C_2H_6AuClSe$ Au-00013

Chloro[selenobis(methane)]gold, 9CI

Chloro(dimethylselenide)gold

[41867-97-4]

$ClAu(SeMe_2)$

M 341.449

Air stable. Cryst. (C_6H_6/Me_2CO). Mp 100° dec.

Dash, K.C. *et al*, *Chem. Ber.*, 1973, **106**, 1221 (*synth, nmr*)
Roulet, R. *et al*, *Chimia*, 1975, **29**, 346.

$C_2H_6AuCl_3S$ Au-00014

Trichloro(dimethylsulfide)gold

Trichloro[thiobis[methane]-S]gold, 9CI

[29826-91-3]

Cl_3AuSMe_2

M 365.455

Yellow, air-stable.

Ray, P.C. *et al*, *Indian J. Chem.*, 1930, **7**, 67 (*synth*)
Allen, E.A. *et al*, *Spectrochim. Acta, Part A*, 1972, **28**, 2257 (*synth, ir*)

C_2H_6AuI Au-00015

Iododimethylgold, 9CI

[42495-73-8]

```
Me   I    Me
  \ / \  /
  Au    Au
  / \ /  \
Me   I    Me
```

M 353.940

Dimeric.

Dimer: Di-μ-iodotetramethyldigold.

$C_4H_{12}Au_2I_2$ M 707.881

Mp 95-6° dec. forming red. liq.

▷Explosive melt

Miles, M.G. *et al*, *J. Am. Chem. Soc.*, 1966, **88**, 5738 (*synth*)
Scovell, W.M. *et al*, *Inorg. Chem.*, 1970, **9**, 2682.
Stocco, G. *et al*, *J. Am. Chem. Soc.*, 1971, **93**, 5057 (*nmr*)
Johnson, A. *et al*, *J. Organomet. Chem.*, 1975, **85**, 115 (*nmr*)

C_2H_7AuO Au-00016

Hydroxydimethylgold, 8CI

Dimethylgold(1+) hydroxide, 9CI

[14951-49-6]

Tetramer: Me_2Au and $AuMe_2$ units bridged by OH groups (H–O, O–H)

M 244.043

Tetrameric. Needles or plates (C_6H_6). Dec. above 120°.

▷Explodes on rapid heating

Miles, M.G. *et al*, *J. Am. Chem. Soc.*, 1966, **88**, 5738 (*synth*)
Glass, G.E. *et al*, *J. Am. Chem. Soc.*, 1968, **90**, 1131 (*ir, pmr, cryst struct*)
Harris, S.J. *et al*, *Inorg. Chem.*, 1969, **8**, 2259 (*synth*)

$C_3H_6AuNO_2S$ Au-00017

(Cysteinato-*O,S*)gold, 10CI

$[H_2N{-}C(COOH)(H){-}CH_2SAu]_n$

M 317.112

(*S*)-*form* [78990-41-7]

L-form

Has poss. role in metab. of Au(I) thiolates used in arthritis therapy. White to pale-yellow light-sensitive solid. V. sol. H_2O, sl. sol. aq. cysteine solns. Mp 180-230°.

Kowala, C. *et al*, *Aust. J. Chem.*, 1966, **19**, 547 (*synth*)
Danpure, C.J., *Biochem. Pharmacol.*, 1976, **25**, 2343 (*synth*)
Brown, D.H. *et al*, *J. Chem. Soc., Dalton Trans.*, 1978, 199.
Thompson, H.O. *et al*, *Bioinorg. Chem.*, 1978, **9**, 375 (*rev*)
Shaw, C.F. *et al*, *Inorg. Persp. Med. Biol.*, 1979, **2**, 287 (*rev*)
Inorg. Synth., 1982, **21**, 31 (*synth*)

$C_3H_7AuClNO$ Au-00018

Chloro[methoxy(methylamino)methylene]gold, 9CI

[51240-37-0]

ClAuC(OMe)NHMe

M 305.514

Example of general class of Au(I) carbene complexes. Cryst. (CH_2Cl_2/Et_2O), air stable. Mp 129-30° dec.

Minghetti, G. *et al*, *Inorg. Chem.*, 1974, **13**, 1600 (*synth*)
Parks, J.E. *et al*, *J. Organomet. Chem.*, 1974, **71**, 453 (*synth*)

$C_4H_5AuO_4S$ Au-00019

Mercaptobutanediato(1−)gold, 9CI

Gold thiomalate. [(1,2-Dicarboxyethyl)thio]gold. Aurothiomalic acid

$HOOCCH_2CH(SAu)COOH$

M 346.108

▷MD5435000.

Di-Na salt: [12244-57-4]. *Gold sodium thiomalate. Sodium aurothiomalate. Myochrysine. Myocrisin. Tauredon.*

$C_4H_3AuNa_2O_4S$ M 390.071

Antirheumatic drug. Yellowish-white powder. Sol. H_2O, insol. EtOH, Et_2O.

▷MD5435000.

Merck Index, 9th Ed., No. 4365.
Sadler, P.J., *Struct. Bonding (Berlin)*, 1976, **29**, 171 (*rev*)
Shaw, C.F. *et al*, *Inorg. Persp. Med. Biol.*, 1979, **2**, 287 (*rev*)
Brown, D.H. *et al*, *Chem. Soc. Rev.*, 1980, **9**, 217 (*rev*)
Brown, K. *et al*, *J. Am. Chem. Soc.*, 1981, **103**, 4943 (*mössbauer*)

C_4H_6AuCl Au-00020

[(2,3-η)-2-Butyne]chlorogold, 9CI

(η-Dimethylacetylene)chlorogold. Chloro(η-dimethylacetylene)gold

[37648-15-0]

$ClAu(H_3CC{\equiv}CCH_3)$

M 286.511

Cryst. (CH_2Cl_2/pentane). Thermally unstable above 0°. Sol. CH_2Cl_2, $CHCl_3$, nitrobenzene. Mp 0-5° dec.

Hüttel, R. *et al*, *Chem. Ber.*, 1972, **105**, 1664 (*synth*)

$C_4H_6AuN_2^{\oplus}$ Au-00021

Bis(acetonitrile)gold(1+), 9CI

[44606-68-0]

$Au(NCCH_3)_2^{\oplus}$

M 279.071 (ion)

Perchlorate: [51240-11-0].

$C_4H_6ClAuN_2O_4$ M 378.522

Cryst. (MeCN).

Bergerhoff, G., *Z. Anorg. Allg. Chem.*, 1964, **327**, 139 (*synth*)
Fenske, G.P. *et al*, *Inorg. Chem.*, 1974, **13**, 1783 (*use*)
Roulet, R. *et al*, *Chimia*, 1975, **29**, 346.
Johnson, P.R. *et al*, *J. Chem. Soc., Chem. Commun.*, 1978, 606.

$C_4H_{12}AuClS$ Au-00022

Chlorodimethyl(dimethyl sulfide)gold

Chlorodimethyl[thiobis[methane]]gold

[40587-17-5]

Au bonded to Me, Cl, Me, SMe_2

M 324.618

Heavy oil.

Schmidbaur, H., *Chem. Ber.*, 1972, **105**, 3662 (*synth, nmr*)

$C_4H_{12}AuO_3P$ Au-00023

Methyl(trimethyl phosphite-*P*)gold, 9CI

[38887-63-7]

$MeAuP(OMe)_3$

M 336.077

Colourless liq. Misc. most org. solvs. Bp 0-2°.

Schmidbaur, H. *et al*, *Chem. Ber.*, 1972, **105**, 2985 (*synth, ir, nmr*)

$C_4H_{12}AuP$ Au-00024

Methyl(trimethylphosphine)gold, 9CI

[32407-79-7]

$MeAuPMe_3$

M 288.079

Air- and moisture-stable solid, sl. photochemically unstable. Sol. common org. solvs. Mp 70-1°, 75.5°.

Coates, G.E. *et al*, *J. Chem. Soc.*, 1963, 421 (*synth*)
Schmidbaur, H. *et al*, *Chem. Ber.*, 1971, **104**, 2821 (*synth, nmr, raman*)
Shiotani, A. *et al*, *J. Am. Chem. Soc.*, 1971, **93**, 1555 (*nmr*)
Shaw, C.F. *et al*, *Inorg. Chem.*, 1973, **12**, 965 (*ir, raman*)
Behan, J. *et al*, *J. Chem. Soc., Chem. Commun.*, 1978, 444 (*pe*)

$C_4H_{22}AuB_{18}^{\ominus}$ Au-00025

Bis[undecahydro-1,2-dicarbaundecaborato(2−)]aurate(1−), 8CI
Bis(dicarbollide)aurate(1−)

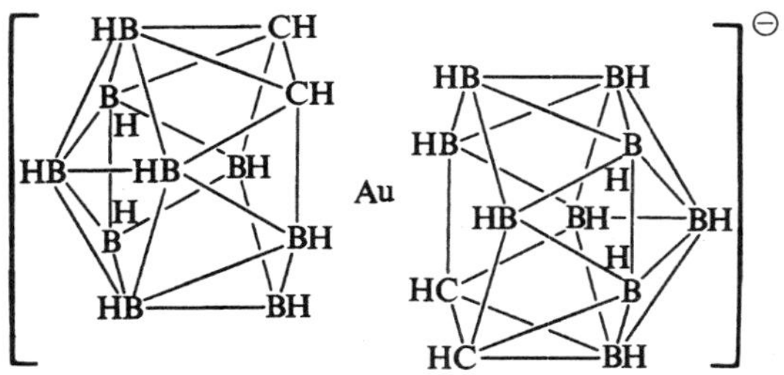

M 461.764 (ion)
"Slipped" sandwich struct. Large red cryst. (CH_2Cl_2/hexane).

Tetraethylammonium salt:
$C_{12}H_{42}AuB_{18}N$ M 592.017
Glittering red plates (CH_2Cl_2/hexane). Sol. Me_2CO, CH_2Cl_2, MeCN.

Methyltriphenylphosphonium salt:
$C_{23}H_{40}AuB_{18}P$ M 739.089
Large red cryst. (CH_2Cl_2/hexane).

Warren, L.F. *et al*, *J. Am. Chem. Soc.*, 1968, **90**, 4823 (*synth, nmr, pmr, ir*)
Wing, R.M., *J. Am. Chem. Soc.*, 1968, **90**, 4828 (*cryst struct*)

$C_4H_{22}AuB_{18}^{\ominus\ominus}$ Au-00026

Bis[undecahydro-1,2-dicarbaundecaborato(2−)]aurate(2−), 8CI
Bis(dicarbollide)aurate(2−)
M 461.764 (ion)
"Slipped" sandwich struct.

Bis(tetraethylammonium) salt:
$C_{20}H_{62}AuB_{18}N_2$ M 722.270
Blue, paramagnetic microcryst. Sol. THF, MeCN. μ_{eff} = 1.79 BM.

Warren, L.F. *et al*, *J. Am. Chem. Soc.*, 1968, **90**, 4823 (*synth*)

C_5H_5Au Au-00027

η-Cyclopentadienylgold

Au(η-C_5H_5)

M 262.061
Thermally unstable yellow powder, cryst. (pentane at −30°). Insol. EtOH, Et_2O.
▷Violent dec. at times

Hüttel, R. *et al*, *Angew. Chem.*, 1967, **79**, 859.

C_5H_8AuCl Au-00028

Chloro(cyclopentene)gold, 8CI

ClAu–(cyclopentene)

M 300.538
Thermally unstable above 55°. Sol. polar org. solvs., $CHCl_3$, THF. Mp 55-60° dec.

Hüttel, R. *et al*, *Chem. Ber.*, 1966, **99**, 462 (*synth*)

$C_5H_{14}AuP$ Au-00029

Methyl(trimethylphosphonium η-methylide)gold, 9CI
[55804-42-7]

$MeAuCH_2PMe_3$

M 302.106
Phosphonium methylide complex of gold(I). Air stable solid. Sol. polar org. solvs. Mp 119-21°. Dec. >150°.

Schmidbaur, H. *et al*, *Chem. Ber.*, 1975, **108**, 1321 (*synth, ir, nmr*)
Inorg. Synth., 1978, **18**, 141 (*synth*)

$C_6H_5AuCl_2$ Au-00030

Dichlorophenylgold, 9CI
[73060-08-9]

$PhAuCl_2$

M 344.978
Dimeric, chlorobridged.

Dimer: Bis[dichlorophenylgold]. Tetrachlorodiphenyldigold.
$C_{12}H_{10}Au_2Cl_4$ M 689.956
Yellow cryst. Sol. EtOH, sl. sol. C_6H_6, Et_2O. Mp 130° dec.

Kharasch, M.S. *et al*, *J. Am. Chem. Soc.*, 1931, **53**, 3053 (*synth*)
de Graaf, P.W.J. *et al*, *J. Organomet. Chem.*, 1976, **105**, 399 (*synth, ir, pmr*)

$C_6H_5AuCl_3^{\ominus}$ Au-00031

Trichlorophenylgold(1−)
Trichlorophenylaurate

$PhAuCl_3^{\ominus}$

M 380.431 (ion)

Tetrabutylammonium salt: [35798-01-7]. N,N,N-*Tributyl-1-butanaminium trichlorophenylaurate, 9CI.*
$C_{22}H_{41}AuCl_3N$ M 622.898
Yellow prisms. Mp 100° dec.

Tetraethylammonium salt: [51567-46-5]. N,N,N-*Triethylethanaminium trichlorophenylaurate, 9CI.*
$C_{14}H_{25}AuCl_3N$ M 510.684
Pale-cream prisms. Mp 154° dec.

Liddle, K.S. *et al*, *J. Chem. Soc., Chem. Commun.*, 1972, 26 (*synth, ir*)
Clark, R.J.H. *et al*, *Inorg. Chem.*, 1974, **13**, 2224 (*synth, ir, pmr*)

C_6H_9Au **Au-00032**

(3,3-Dimethyl-1-butyne)gold

tert-*Butylacetylidegold*

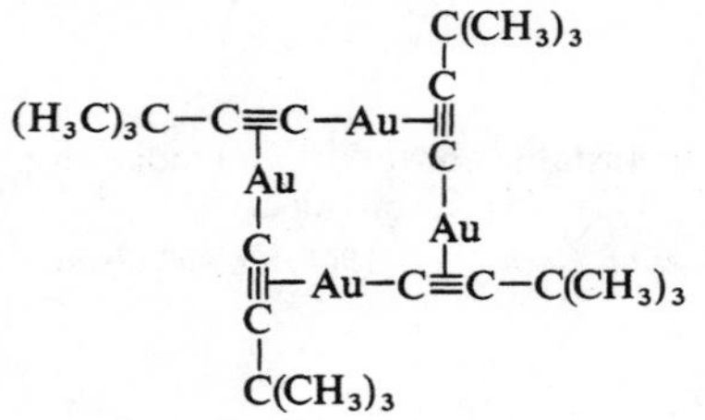

M 278.104

Tetrameric on basis of molecular mass determination in benzene.

Tetramer: Tetrakis(3,3-dimethyl-1-butyne)tetragold.

$C_{20}H_{36}Au_4$ M 1064.370

Yellow cryst. (hexane). Sol. hexane, propanol, C_6H_6, $CHCl_3$, insol. MeOH, EtOH. Mp 150° dec.

Coates, G.E. *et al*, *J. Chem. Soc.*, 1962, 3220 (*synth*)

$C_6H_9AuFeNO_4P$ **Au-00033**

Tricarbonylnitrosyl[(trimethylphosphine)aurio]iron, 8CI

[33989-32-1]

$Me_3PAuFe(CO)_3NO$

M 442.929

Mp 86-8° dec.

Casey, M. *et al*, *J. Chem. Soc.* (*A*), 1971, 2989 (*synth*, *ir*)

$C_6H_9AuFeNO_7P$ **Au-00034**

Tricarbonylnitrosyl[(trimethyl phosphite-*P*)aurio]iron

[34088-91-0]

$(MeO)_3PAuFe(CO)_3NO$

M 490.927

Mp 50-1° dec.

Casey, M. *et al*, *J. Chem. Soc.* (*A*), 1971, 2989 (*synth*, *ir*)

$C_6H_{10}AuCl$ **Au-00035**

Chloro(cyclohexene)gold

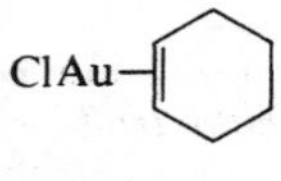

M 314.565

Thermally unstable above 55°. Sol. polar org. solvs., $CHCl_3$, THF. Mp 55-60° dec.

Hüttel, R. *et al*, *Chem. Ber.*, 1966, **99**, 462 (*synth*)

$C_6H_{10}AuN_2^{\oplus}$ **Au-00036**

Bis(isocyanoethane)gold(1+)

Bis(ethyl isocyanide)gold(1+)

[82582-20-5]

$[Au(CNEt)_2]^{\oplus}$

M 307.125 (ion)

Perchlorate:

$C_6H_{10}AuClN_2O_4$ M 406.576

Cryst. (Me_2CO/Et_2O). Sol. Me_2CO.

Chastain, S.K. *et al*, *Inorg. Chem.*, 1982, **21**, 3717 (*synth*, *mcd*)

$C_6H_{11}AuO_5S$ **Au-00037**

(1-Thioglucopyranosato)gold, 9CI

(1-Glucosylthio)gold. Aurothioglucose

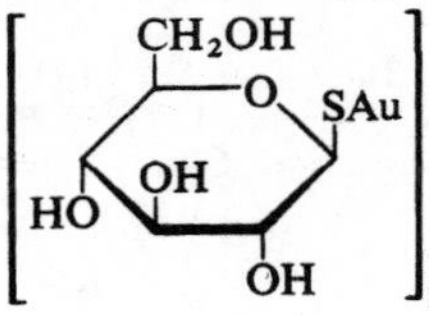

M 392.176

Polymeric.

***D*-form** [12192-57-3]

Aureotan. Solganol. Aurumine. Oronol

Antiarthritic drug. Yellow cryst. (EtOH aq.). Sol. H_2O, insol. org. solvs.

▷MD6475000.

Tetra-Ac: [69849-37-2]. (*1-Thioglucopyranosato-2,3,4,6-tetraacetato)gold*, 10CI.

$C_{14}H_{19}AuO_9S$ M 560.325

Antiarthritic drug. Polymeric.

Merck Index, 9th Ed., No. 902.
Sadler, P.J., *Struct. Bonding* (*Berlin*), 1976, **29**, 171 (*rev*)
Lorber, A. *et al*, *Gold. Bull.*, 1979, **12**, 149 (*rev*)
U.S.P., 4 133 952, (*1979*); *CA*, **90**, 152549g (*deriv*)
Brown, D.H. *et al*, *Chem. Soc. Rev.*, 1980, **9**, 217 (*rev*)
Brown, K. *et al*, *J. Am. Chem. Soc.*, 1981, **103**, 4943 (*mössbauer*)
Shaw, C.F. *et al*, *J. Inorg. Biochem.*, 1981, **14**, 267 (*rev*, *cmr*)

$C_6H_{15}AuBrP$ **Au-00038**

Bromo(triethylphosphine)gold, 9CI

[14243-60-8]

$BrAuPEt_3$

M 395.029

Cryst. (EtOH). Sol. $CHCl_3$, C_6H_6, EtOH. Mp 87°.

Mann, F.G. *et al*, *J. Chem. Soc.*, 1940, 1235 (*synth*)
Heaton, B.T. *et al*, *Inorg. Nucl. Chem. Lett.*, 1975, **11**, 363.
McAuliffe, C.A. *et al*, *J. Chem. Soc.*, *Dalton Trans.*, 1979, 1730 (*rev*)

$C_6H_{15}AuBr_3P$ **Au-00039**

Tribromo(triethylphosphine)gold, 9CI

[56213-25-3]

Br_3AuPEt_3

M 554.837

Deep-red needles (EtOH or C_6H_6). Sol. $CHCl_3$. Mp 129°.

Mann, F.G. *et al*, *J. Chem. Soc.*, 1940, 1235 (*synth*)
Heaton, B.T. *et al*, *Inorg. Nucl. Chem. Lett.*, 1975, **11**, 363 (*nmr*)
Brown, D.H. *et al*, *Inorg. Chim. Acta*, 1979, **32**, 117 (*uv*)
McNeillie, A. *et al*, *J. Chem. Soc.*, *Dalton Trans.*, 1980, 767 (*pe*)

$C_6H_{15}AuClO_3P$ **Au-00040**

Chloro(triethyl phosphite-*P*)gold, 9CI

Chloro(phosphorous acid triethyl ester)gold, 8CI

[33635-00-6]

$ClAuP(OEt)_3$

M 398.576

Antiarthritic drug.

Ger. Pat., 2 061 181, (*1971*); *CA*, **75**, 52818r (*use*)

Ger. Pat., 2 434 920, (*1975*); *CA*, **83**, 84857j
U.S.P., 3 903 274, (*1976*); *CA*, **84**, 17559w (*use*)
U.S.P., 3 947 565, (*1976*); *CA*, **85**, 5642a (*use*)
Lorber, A. *et al*, *Gold. Bull.*, 1979, **12**, 149 (*rev*)

$C_6H_{15}AuClP$ Au-00041

Chloro(triethylphosphine)gold, 9CI
[15529-90-5]

$ClAuPEt_3$

M 350.578
Shows antiarthritic activity. Cryst. (EtOH). Sol. C_6H_6, $CHCl_3$, EtOH. Mp 78°. $Bp_{0.03}$ 210°.
▷MD5431000.

Mann, F.G. *et al*, *J. Chem. Soc.*, 1937, 1828 (*synth*)
Walz, D.T. *et al*, *J. Pharmacol. Exp. Ther.*, 1972, **181**, 292 (*use*)
Schmidbaur, H. *et al*, *Z. Naturforsch., B*, 1976, **31**, 1607 (*nqr*)
Jones, P.G. *et al*, *J. Chem. Soc., Dalton Trans.*, 1977, 1434 (*mossbauer*)
Puddephatt, R.J. *et al*, *The Chemistry of Gold*, Elsevier, 1978, 248 (*rev*)
McAuliffe, C.A. *et al*, *J. Chem. Soc., Dalton Trans.*, 1979, 1730 (*synth*)
McNeillie, A. *et al*, *J. Chem. Soc., Dalton Trans.*, 1980, 767 (*pe*)

$C_6H_{15}AuCl_3P$ Au-00042

Trichloro(triethylphosphine)gold, 9CI
[56213-22-0]

Cl_3AuPEt_3

M 421.484
Pale-yellow needles (EtOH). Sol. Me_2CO, $CHCl_3$, spar. sol. EtOH, CCl_4. Mp 121°.

Mann, F.G. *et al*, *J. Chem. Soc.*, 1940, 1235 (*synth*)
Heaton, B.T. *et al*, *Inorg. Nucl. Chem. Lett.*, 1975, **11**, 363 (*nmr*)
Brown, D.H. *et al*, *Inorg. Chim. Acta*, 1979, **32**, 117 (*uv*)
McNeillie, A. *et al*, *J. Chem. Soc., Dalton Trans.*, 1980, 767 (*pe*)

$C_6H_{15}AuF_3P$ Au-00043

Dimethyl(trifluoromethyl)trimethylphosphinegold, 9CI
[50662-85-6]

Me, CF_3 / Au / Me, PMe_3 *cis-form*

M 372.120
cis- and *trans*-isomers observed in soln. by nmr. Cryst. (Et_2O). Mp 97-100°.

Johnson, A. *et al*, *J. Chem. Soc., Dalton Trans.*, 1976, 1360 (*synth, nmr*)

$C_6H_{17}AuOS$ Au-00044

(Dimethylsulfoxonium η-methylide)trimethylgold, 10CI
Trimethyl(dimethylsulfonium methylide)gold
[62931-77-5]

$Me_2S(O)CH_2AuMe_3$

M 334.226
Cryst. ($CHCl_3$). Sol. $CHCl_3$, CH_2Cl_2. Mp 83-5°.

Fackler, J.P. *et al*, *J. Am. Chem. Soc.*, 1977, **99**, 2363 (*synth*)
Stein, J. *et al*, *J. Am. Chem. Soc.*, 1981, **103**, 2192 (*synth, cryst struct, pe*)

$C_6H_{18}AuO_6P_2^{\oplus}$ Au-00045

Bis(trimethyl phosphite)gold(1+)
[82598-60-5]

$Au[P(OMe)_3]_2^{\oplus}$

M 445.119 (ion)
Perchlorate:
$C_6H_{18}AuClO_{10}P_2$ M 544.569
Cryst. ($CHCl_3/Et_2O$). Sol. $CHCl_3$.

Chastain, S.K. *et al*, *Inorg. Chem.*, 1982, **21**, 3717 (*synth, mcd*)

$C_7H_{15}AuNPS$ Au-00046

(Thiocyanato-*S*)(triethylphosphine)gold, 9CI
[14243-46-0]

$Et_3PAuSCN$

M 373.202
Shows antiarthritic activity. Cryst. (EtOH aq.). Sol. $CHCl_3$, EtOH, C_6H_6. Mp 50-1°.

Coates, G.E. *et al*, *Aust. J. Chem.*, 1966, **19**, 539 (*synth*)
Ger. Pat., 2 434 920, (*1975*); *CA*, **83**, 84857j (*synth, use*)

$C_7H_{18}AuP$ Au-00047

Methyl(triethylphosphine)gold, 8CI
[34275-23-5]

$MeAuPEt_3$

M 330.159
Air- and moisture-stable cryst. (pet. ether). Sol. most org. solvs. Mp 62°.

Calvin, G. *et al*, *Chem. Ind. (London)*, 1959, 1628 (*synth*)
Coates, G.E. *et al*, *J. Chem. Soc.*, 1962, 3220 (*synth, ir*)
Coates, G.E. *et al*, *J. Chem. Soc.*, 1963, 421.
Schmidbaur, H. *et al*, *Chem. Ber.*, 1971, **104**, 2821 (*synth, nmr, ir*)
Schmidbaur, H. *et al*, *Chem. Ber.*, 1975, **108**, 1321.

$C_7H_{20}AuP$ Au-00048

Trimethyl(trimethylphosphonium η-methylide)gold, 9CI
[55744-48-4]

$Me_3AuCH_2PMe_3$

M 332.175
Phosphonium methylide gold(III) complex. Air stable cryst. (Et_2O/pentane). Sol. most org. solvs. Mp 111-2°.

Schmidbaur, H. *et al*, *Inorg. Chim. Acta*, 1975, **13**, 79 (*synth*)

$C_7H_{20}AuPSi$ Au-00049

(Trimethylphosphine)[(trimethylsilyl)methyl]gold, 9CI
[55787-57-0]

$Me_3SiCH_2AuPMe_3$

M 360.261
Colourless waxy cryst. (THF/pentane). Thermally unstable. Sol. C_6H_6, THF. Mp 27-8°.

Schmidbaur, H. *et al*, *Chem. Ber.*, 1975, **108**, 1321 (*synth*)

$C_7H_{20}AuP_2^{\oplus}$ Au-00050

(Trimethylphosphine)(trimethylphosphonium η-methylide-)gold(1+), 9CI
[50323-06-3]

$Me_3PAuCH_2PMe_3^{\oplus}$

M 363.149 (ion)

Phosphonium methylide gold(I) complex.

Chloride:

$C_7H_{20}AuClP_2$ M 398.602

Air- and moisture-stable solid. Sol. $CHCl_3$, CH_2Cl_2, insol. C_6H_6, Et_2O. Mp 178-81°.

Schmidbaur, H. *et al*, *Angew. Chem., Int. Ed. Engl.*, 1973, **12**, 416 (*synth*)
Schmidbaur, H. *et al*, *Chem. Ber.*, 1975, **108**, 1321 (*synth, ir, nmr*)

$C_7H_{21}AuB_9NS_2$ Au-00051

(Diethylcarbamodithioato-*S,S'*)[(9,10,11-η)-undecahydro-7,8-dicarbaundecaborato(2−)]gold

[62572-50-3]

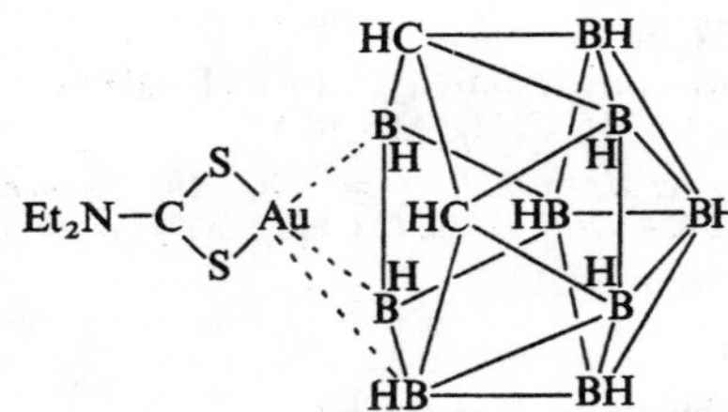

M 477.626

"Slipped" dicarbollide ligand in struct. Orange cryst. (CH_2Cl_2/pentane). Sol. CH_2Cl_2. Mp 115° dec.

Colquhoun, H.M. *et al*, *J. Chem. Soc., Dalton Trans.*, 1978, 303 (*synth, cryst struct, nmr*)

C_8H_5Au Au-00052

(Phenylethynyl)gold, 9CI

Phenylacetylidegold

[34679-27-1]

$[AuC{\equiv}CPh]_n$

M 298.094

Polymeric. Bright yellow; darkens above 150°, light sensitive but not explosive. Sol. donor solvs. (Py, DMF, DMSO). Mp 150° dec.

Coates, G.E. *et al*, *J. Chem. Soc.*, 1962, 3220 (*synth*)
Nast, R. *et al*, *Z. Anorg. Allg. Chem.*, 1964, **330**, 311 (*synth*)
Blues, E.T. *et al*, *J. Chem. Soc., Chem. Commun.*, 1974, 513 (*synth*)

C_8H_8AuCl Au-00053

Chloro[(1,2-η)-1,3,5,7-cyclooctatetraene]gold, 9CI

[55015-50-4]

ClAu—

M 336.571

Greenish-yellow cryst. (CH_2Cl_2/pentane). Thermally unstable above −20°. Sol. CH_2Cl_2, liq. SO_2.

Tauchner, P. *et al*, *Chem. Ber.*, 1974, **107**, 3761 (*synth, nmr*)

C_8H_8AuNOS Au-00054

[[(Phenylcarbamoyl)methyl]thio]gold

(2-Mercaptoacetanilide-S)gold, 9CI. Aurothioglycolic acid anilide. Lauron. Aurothioglycanide

[16925-51-2]

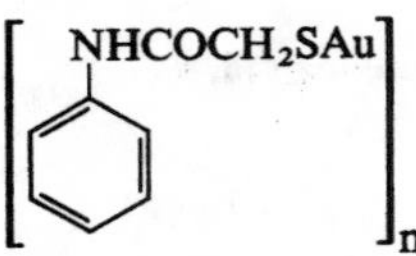

M 363.184

Polymeric. Antiarthritic drug. Greyish-yellow powder. Insol. H_2O, common org. solvs.

Merck Index, 9th Ed., 1976, No. 903.
Sadler, P.J., *Struct. Bonding*, 1976, **29**, 171 (*rev*)
Brown, D.H. *et al*, *Chem. Soc. Rev.*, 1980, **9**, 217 (*rev*)

$C_8H_{12}AuN_{16}^{\ominus}$ Au-00055

Tetrakis(1-methyl-1*H*-tetrazol-5-yl)aurate(1−), 8CI

Tetrakis(1-methyl-5-tetrazolato)aurate(1−)

[33461-24-4]

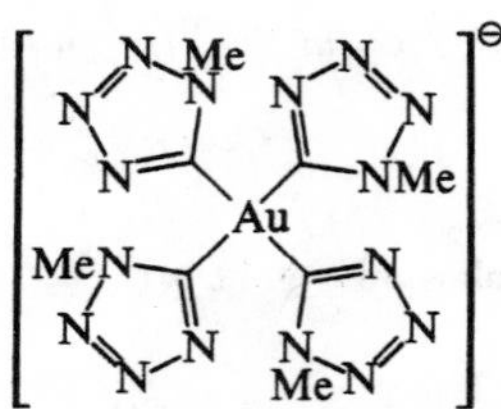

M 529.257 (ion)

Au(III) complex with four carbeniate ligands. Cryst. struct determination is on closely related isopropyl compd.

Tetraphenylarsonium salt:

$C_{32}H_{32}AsAuN_{16}$ M 912.600

Air-stable cryst. (CH_2Cl_2/Et_2O). Sol. CH_2Cl_2, $CHCl_3$, Me_2CO, spar. sol. THF, insol. Et_2O. Mp 167° dec.

Beck, W. *et al*, *Chem. Ber.*, 1972, **104**, 1816 (*synth*)
Fehlhammer, W.P. *et al*, *J. Am. Chem. Soc.*, 1972, **94**, 3370 (*cryst struct*)

$C_8H_{14}AuCl$ Au-00056

Chloro[(1,2-η)-cyclooctene]gold, 9CI

ClAu—

M 342.618

***cis*-form** [12145-57-2]

Thermally unstable above 81°. Sol. polar org. solvs. $CHCl_3$, THF. Mp 81-5° dec., 93-6° dec.

Hüttel, R. *et al*, *Chem. Ber.*, 1966, **99**, 462 (*synth*)

$C_8H_{20}Au_2Cl_2P_2$ **Au-00057**

Dichlorobis[μ-[(dimethylphosphinidenio)bis(methylene)]]digold, 9CI

[55744-44-0]

M 643.033

Example of Au(II) complex with Au-Au bond. Yellow, air stable. Spar. sol. polar org. solvs. Mp 197° dec.

Schmidbaur, H. *et al*, *Inorg. Chim. Acta*, 1975, **13**, 85 (*synth*)

$C_8H_{20}Au_2Cl_4P_2$ **Au-00058**

Tetrachlorobis[μ-[(dimethylphosphinidenio)bis[methylene]]]-digold, 9CI

[55744-46-2]

M 713.939

Dialkylphosphoniumbismethylide gold(III) complex. Yellow-orange air-stable compd. Mp 183° dec.

Schmidbaur, H. *et al*, *Inorg. Chim. Acta*, 1975, **13**, 85 (*synth*)

$C_8H_{20}Au_2P_2$ **Au-00059**

Bis[μ-[(dimethylphosphinidenio)bis(methylene)]]digold, 9CI

[50449-81-5]

M 572.127

Dialkylphosphoniumbismethylide complex. Air stable. Sol. CH_2Cl_2, $CHCl_3$. Mp 216-8°.

Schmidbaur, H. *et al*, *Angew. Chem., Int. Ed. Engl.*, 1973, **12**, 416 (*synth*)

Schmidbaur, H. *et al*, *Inorg. Chim. Acta*, 1975, **13**, 85 (*synth*)

$C_8H_{22}AuP_2^{\oplus}$ **Au-00060**

Bis(trimethylphosphonium η-methylide)gold(1+), 9CI

[50323-09-6]

$[Me_3PCH_2AuCH_2PMe_3]^{\oplus}$

M 377.176 (ion)

Tested for pharmacological activity in treatment of arthritis.

Chloride:

$C_8H_{22}AuClP_2$ M 412.629

Sol. CH_2Cl_2, $CHCl_3$, MeOH. Mp 170° dec. Air stable at r.t.

Schmidbaur, H. *et al*, *Chem. Ber.*, 1975, **108**, 1321 (*synth, nmr*)

Schmidbaur, H. *et al*, *Z. Naturforsch., B*, 1978, **33**, 1325 (*synth*)

$C_9H_{11}Au$ **Au-00061**

(1,3,5-Trimethylbenzene)gold

Mesitylgold

M 316.152

Pentameric.

Pentamer: Pentakis(1,3,5-trimethylbenzene)pentagold. Penta[μ-mesityl]pentagold.

$C_{45}H_{55}Au_5$ M 1580.762

Yellow cryst. (THF). Sol. THF, toluene.

Gambarotto, S. *et al*, *J. Chem. Soc., Chem. Commun.*, 1983, 1304 (*synth, cryst struct*)

$C_9H_{23}Au_2IP_2$ **Au-00062**

Bis[μ-(dimethylphosphinidenio)bis[methylene]iodomethyldigold, 9CI

[55927-69-0]

M 714.066

Product of oxidative addition of MeI to Bis[μ-[(dimethylphosphinidenio)bis(methylene)]]digold, Au-00059 . Red air-stable solid. Mp 143° dec.

Schmidbaur, H. *et al*, *Inorg. Chim. Acta*, 1975, **13**, 85 (*synth*)

$C_{10}H_{20}AuN_4^{\oplus}$ **Au-00063**

Bis(1,3-dimethyl-2-imidazolidinylidene)gold(1+), 9CI

[41630-44-8]

M 393.261 (ion)

Representative of general class of bis(carbene)gold(I) complexes.

Tetrafluoroborate:

$C_{10}H_{20}AuBF_4N_4$ M 480.065

Air-stable cryst. (CH_2Cl_2/Et_2O). Sol. polar org. solvs. Mp 218-25°.

Cetinkaya, B. *et al*, *J. Chem. Soc., Dalton Trans.*, 1974, 1827 (*synth, ir, nmr*)

$C_{10}H_{20}AuO_4PS$ **Au-00064**

[Mercaptobutanedioato(1−)]triethylphosphinegold, 9CI

$[Et_3PAuSCH(COOH)CH_2COOH]_n$

M 464.266
Polymeric. Antiarthritic drug.

U.S.P., 3 718 679, (*1973*); *CA*, **78**, 135672
U.S.P., 3 718 680, (*1973*); *CA*, **78**, 135673
Sadler, P.J., *Struct. Bonding*, 1976, **29**, 171 (*rev*)
Lorber, A. *et al*, *Gold Bulletin*, 1979, **12**, 149 (*rev*)
Brown, D.H. *et al*, *Chem. Soc. Rev.*, 1980, **9**, 217 (*rev*)

$C_{12}AuF_{10}^{\ominus}$ — Au-00065

Bis(pentafluorophenyl)aurate(1−), 9CI
[60748-81-4]

$Au(C_6F_5)_2^{\ominus}$

M 531.083 (ion)
Tetrabutylammonium salt:
$C_{28}H_{36}AuF_{10}N$ M 773.550
Sol. Me_2CO, CH_2Cl_2, sl. sol. Et_2O, C_6H_6. Mp 110°.

Uson, R. *et al*, *J. Organomet. Chem.*, 1977, **131**, 471 (*synth*)

$C_{12}H_{26}AuO_5PS$ — Au-00066

(1-Thioglucopyranosato-*S*)(triethylphosphine)gold, 9CI

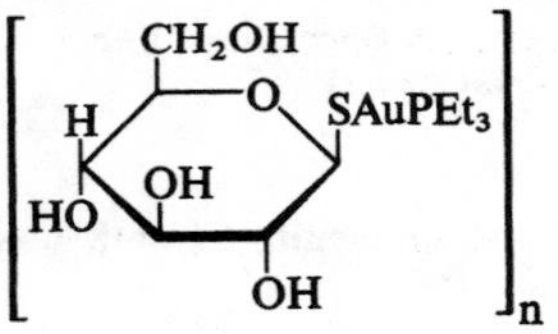

M 510.335
β-D-form [34031-29-3]
Antiarthritic drug. Polymeric.

Ger. Pat., 2 051 495, (*1971*); *CA*, **75**, 77223f
Sutton, B.M. *et al*, *J. Med. Chem.*, 1972, **15**, 1095 (*use*)
Sadler, P.J., *Struct. Bonding*, 1976, **29**, 171 (*rev*)
Lorber, A. *et al*, *Gold Bulletin*, 1979, **12**, 149 (*rev*)
U.S.P., 4 124 759, (*1979*); *CA*, **90**, 104297b (*use*)
Brown, D.H. *et al*, *Chem. Soc. Rev.*, 1980, **9**, 217 (*rev*)

$C_{12}H_{28}Au_2P_2S_2$ — Au-00067

Bis[*μ*-[2-(diethylphosphino)ethanethiolato-*P,S*]digold, 9CI
[51365-22-1]

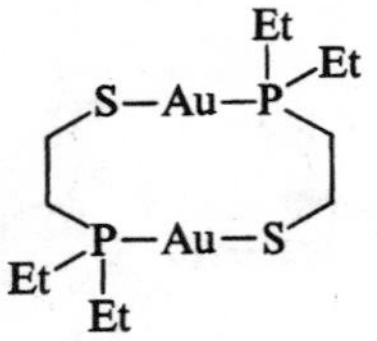

M 692.354
Shows antiarthritic props.

Weinstock, J. *et al*, *J. Med. Chem.*, 1974, **17**, 139.
Crane, W.S. *et al*, *Inorg. Chim. Acta*, 1978, **31**, L469 (*cryst struct*)

$C_{14}H_{10}AuCl$ — Au-00068

Chloro(diphenylacetylene)gold
Chloro[1,1′-(η^2-1,2-ethynediyl)bis[benzene]]gold, 9CI
[37048-17-2]

ClAu(PhC≡CPh)

M 410.653

Cryst. (CH_2Cl_2/pentane). Thermally unstable above 75°. Sol. CH_2Cl_2. Mp 75-8° dec.

Hüttel, R. *et al*, *Chem. Ber.*, 1972, **105**, 1664 (*synth*)

$C_{15}H_{16}AuClN_2$ — Au-00069

[Bis[(4-methylphenyl)amino]methylene]chlorogold, 9CI
[50870-66-1]

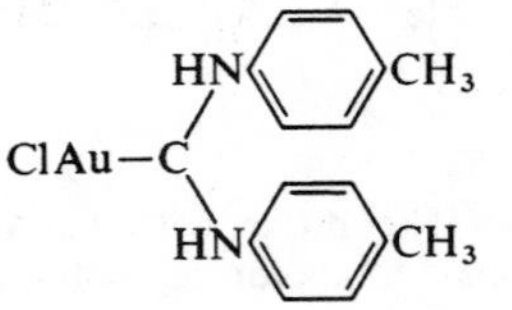

[Structure: ClAu–C(NH–C₆H₄–CH₃)₂]

M 456.724
Neutral carbene complex synth. from isonitrile complex and amine. Cryst. ($CHCl_3$/pet. ether). Air stable. Spar. sol. MeOH, Me_2CO. Mp 162° dec.

Bonati, F. *et al*, *J. Organomet. Chem.*, 1973, **59**, 403 (*synth*)

$C_{16}H_{20}AuIS$ — Au-00070

Iododimethyl(dibenzylsulfide)gold

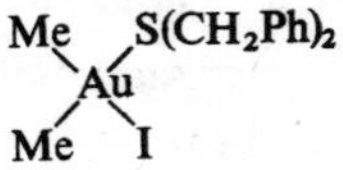

[Structure: Au with Me, Me, $S(CH_2Ph)_2$, I]

M 568.265
Mp 77-8° dec.

Bain, F.H. *et al*, *J. Chem. Soc.*, 1939, 762 (*synth*)

$C_{18}H_{15}AuClP$ — Au-00071

Chloro(triphenylphosphine)gold, 9CI
Triphenylphosphinegold chloride
[14243-64-2]

Ph_3PAuCl

M 494.710
Cryst. (EtOH). Sol. $CHCl_3$, Me_2CO. Mp 248-9°.

Jones, A.G. *et al*, *Spectrochim. Acta, Part A*, 1974, **30**, 563 (*synth, ir*)
Baenziger, N.C. *et al*, *Acta Crystallogr., Sect. B*, 1976, **32**, 962 (*cryst struct*)
Brown, D.H. *et al*, *J. Chem. Soc., Dalton Trans.*, 1977, 1874 (*uv*)
Jones, P.G. *et al*, *J. Chem. Soc., Dalton Trans.*, 1977, 1430, 1434 (*nqr, mössbauer*)
McAuliffe, C.A. *et al*, *J. Chem. Soc., Dalton Trans.*, 1979, 1730 (*synth, ir*)
McNeillie, A. *et al*, *J. Chem. Soc., Dalton Trans.*, 1980, 767 (*pe*)

$C_{19}H_{18}AuP$ — Au-00072

Methyl(triphenylphosphine)gold, 9CI
[23108-72-7]

$MeAuPPh_3$

M 474.291
Soft colourless cryst. (C_6H_6/pet. ether). Sol. Me_2CO, Et_2O, aromatics, halocarbons. Mp 175° dec.

Calvin, G. *et al*, *Chem. Ind. (London)*, 1959, 1628 (*synth, ir*)
Coates, G.E. *et al*, *J. Chem. Soc.*, 1962, 3220 (*synth*)
Tamaki, A. *et al*, *J. Am. Chem. Soc.*, 1974, **96**, 6140 (*synth*)
Johnson, A. *et al*, *J. Chem. Soc., Dalton Trans.*, 1975, 115 (*nmr*)

Gavens, P.D. *et al*, *Acta Crystallogr., Sect. B*, 1977, **33**, 137 (*cryst struct*)
Jones, P.G. *et al*, *J. Chem. Soc., Dalton Trans.*, 1977, 1434 (*mossbauer*)
Jordan, R.F. *et al*, *J. Am. Chem. Soc.*, 1979, **101**, 4853 (*cmr*)

$C_{20}H_{18}AuP$ Au-00073

(Triphenylphosphine)vinylgold
Ethenyl(triphenylphosphine)gold, 9CI
[37766-89-5]

$Ph_3PAuCH{=}CH_2$

M 486.302
Cryst. (C_6H_6/pet. ether). Stable at r.t. for several days. Sol. C_6H_6, CH_2Cl_2, THF, Et_2O. Mp 123-5°.

Nesmeyanov, A.N., *Izv. Akad. Nauk SSSR, Ser. Khim.*, 1972, 653.

$C_{20}H_{34}AuO_9PS$ Au-00074

[1-Thioglucopyranose-2,3,4,6-tetrakis(methylcarbamato)-*S*]triethylphosphinegold, 10CI
S-2,3,4,5-Tetraacetyl-1-thioglucopyranosato(triethylphosphine)gold. Auranofin

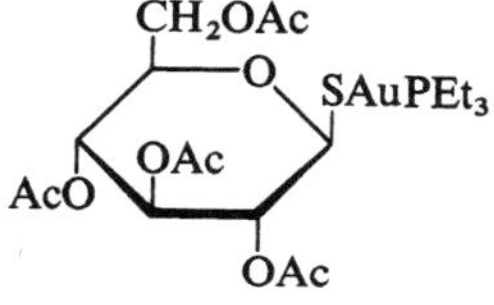

M 678.483
β-D-form [34031-32-8]
Antiarthritic drug.
▷MD6500000.

Sadler, P.J., *Struct. Bonding (Berlin)*, 1976, **29**, 171 (*rev*)
Walz, D.T. *et al*, *J. Pharmacol. Exp. Ther.*, 1976, **197**, 145.
U.S.P., 4 124 759, (*1979*); *CA*, **90**, 104297b (*synth*)
B.P., 1 586 996, (*1981*); *CA*, **95**, 169697e (*synth*)
Brown, D.H. *et al*, *Chem. Soc. Rev.*, 1980, **9**, 217 (*rev*)
Hill, D.T. *et al*, *Cryst. Struct. Commun.*, 1980, **9**, 676 (*cryst struct*)
Brown, K. *et al*, *J. Am. Chem. Soc.*, 1981, **103**, 4943 (*mössbauer*)

$C_{21}H_{15}AuFeNO_4P$ Au-00075

Tricarbonylnitrosyl[(triphenylphosphine)aurio]iron, 8CI
[33989-35-4]

$Ph_3PAuFe(CO)_3NO$

M 629.141
Yellow cryst. (pentane). Mp 98-9° dec.

Casey, M. *et al*, *J. Chem. Soc. (A)*, 1971, 2989 (*synth, ir*)

$C_{21}H_{24}AuP$ Au-00076

Trimethyl(triphenylphosphine)gold, 9CI
Trimethylgold triphenylphosphine
[33635-47-1]

Me_3AuPPh_3

M 504.361
Cryst. (hexane). Stable to air and moisture. Sol. CCl_4, C_6H_6, $CHCl_3$, dioxan. Mp 120° dec.

Gregory, B.J. *et al*, *J. Chem. Soc. (B)*, 1969, 276 (*synth*)
Schmidbaur, H. *et al*, *Chem. Ber.*, 1971, **104**, 2821 (*nmr*)
Stocco, G.C. *et al*, *J. Am. Chem. Soc.*, 1971, **93**, 5057 (*pmr*)
Tobias, R.S. *et al*, *Inorg. Chem.*, 1971, **10**, 1365 (*synth, ir, pmr*)

$C_{22}H_{26}AuP$ Au-00077

Trimethyl(triphenylmethylenephosphorane)gold
Trimethyl(triphenylphosphonium-η-methylide)gold
[77625-10-6]

$Ph_3PCH_2AuMe_3$

M 518.388
Cryst. ($CHCl_3$/pentane).

Stein, J. *et al*, *J. Am. Chem. Soc.*, 1981, **103**, 2192 (*cryst struct, pe*)

$C_{23}H_{20}AuP$ Au-00078

2,4-Cyclopentadien-1-yl(triphenylphosphine)gold, 9CI
[21135-20-6]

H AuPPh3

M 524.351
Fluxional molecule. Cryst. (THF/Me_2CO). Mp 100° dec.

Hüttel, R. *et al*, *Angew. Chem.*, 1967, **79**, 859 (*synth*)
Campbell, C.A. *et al*, *J. Chem. Soc. (A)*, 1971, 3282 (*nmr*)
Su, C.C., *J. Am. Chem. Soc.*, 1971, **93**, 5653.
Ortaggi, G., *J. Organomet. Chem.*, 1974, **80**, 275 (*nmr*)

$C_{23}H_{22}AuO_2P$ Au-00079

(1-Acetyl-2-oxopropyl)(triphenylphosphine)gold, 9CI
(Acetylacetonato)triphenylphosphine gold
[15454-04-3]

$Ph_3PAu[CH(COCH_3)_2]$

M 558.366
Cryst. (Me_2CO/Et_2O). Sol. most org. solvs. Mp 136-8°, 164-5°.

Gregory, B.J. *et al*, *J. Chem. Soc. (B)*, 1969, 276 (*synth, nmr*)
Gibson, D. *et al*, *J. Chem. Soc. (A)*, 1970, 367 (*synth*)

$C_{24}H_{20}AuFeO_3P$ Au-00080

Tricarbonyl($η^3$-2-propenyl)[(triphenylphosphine)gold]iron
Allyltricarbonyl[(triphenylphosphine)aurio]iron
[73891-25-5]

CO
—Fe CO
CO
AuPPh3

M 640.207
Small yellow cryst. (hexane). Mp 100-10° dec.

Simon, F.E. *et al*, *Inorg. Chem.*, 1980, **19**, 2338 (*synth, ir, pmr, struct*)

$C_{24}H_{20}AuP$ Au-00081

Phenyl(triphenylphosphine)gold, 9CI
[30142-19-9]

$PhAuPPh_3$

M 536.362
Cryst. (Et_2O). Mp 166° dec.

Glockling, F. *et al*, *J. Chem. Soc.*, 1962, 2658 (*synth*)
Coates, G.E. *et al*, *J. Chem. Soc.*, 1962, 3220 (*synth*)

$C_{25}H_{24}AuGeO_4PRu$ Au-00082

Tetracarbonyl(trimethylgermyl)[(triphenylphosphine)aurio]-ruthenium, 8CI

CO; OC; GeMe₃; Ru; OC; AuPPh₃; CO

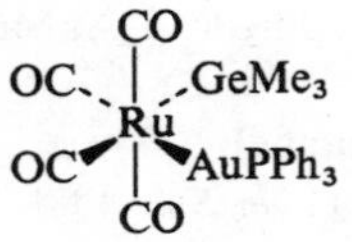

M 790.062

cis-form [34439-98-0]
Cream cryst. (CH_2Cl_2/hexane). Mp 95-105° dec.

Knox, S.A.R. *et al*, *J. Chem. Soc.* (*A*), 1971, 2874 (*synth*, *ir*, *pmr*)

$C_{25}H_{24}AuO_4PRuSi$ Au-00083

Tetracarbonyl(trimethylsilyl)[(triphenylphosphine)aurio]ruthenium, 8CI

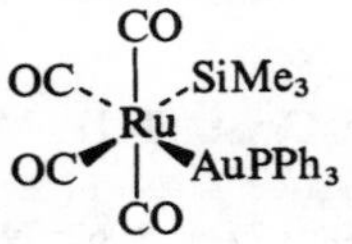

M 745.558

cis-form [26024-45-3]
Bronze cryst. Mp 106-7°.

Knox, S.A.R. *et al*, *J. Chem. Soc.* (*A*), 1969, 2559 (*synth*, *ir*)

$C_{27}H_{25}AuNOP$ Au-00084

[Methoxy[(4-methylphenyl)imino]methyl](triphenylphosphine)gold(I), 9CI
(*Triphenylphosphine*)(N-p-*tolyliminocarbomethoxy*)-*gold*(*I*)
[33637-36-4]

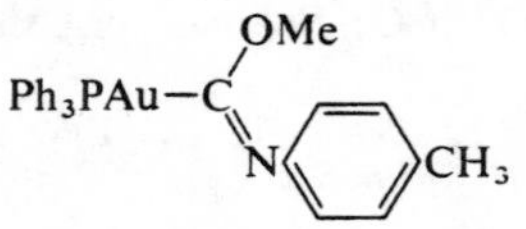

M 607.441
Example of alkoxy(imino)methylgold(I) complex. Cryst. (MeOH). Sol. polar org. solvs. Mp 169°.

Bonati, F. *et al*, *Gazz. Chim. Ital.*, 1972, **102**, 205 (*synth*)
Bonati, F. *et al*, *J. Organomet. Chem.*, 1973, **60**, C43.
Bonati, F. *et al*, *Synth. React. Inorg. Metal-Org. Chem.*, 1976, **6**, 383.

$C_{28}H_{24}AuFeP$ Au-00085

1-[(Triphenylphosphine)aurio]ferrocene, 9CI
(*Ferrocenyl*)(*triphenylphosphine*)*gold*
[35004-41-2]

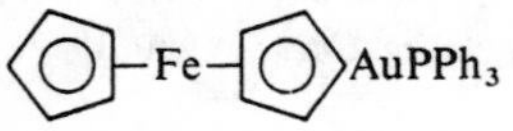

M 644.285
Orange air stable cryst. (THF/hexane). Sol. Et_2O, $CHCl_3$, THF, EtOH. Mp 150° dec.

Nesmeyanov, A.N. *et al*, *Izv. Akad. Nauk SSSR*, *Ser. Khim.*, 1969, 2030 (*synth*, *nmr*)
Nesmeyanov, A.N. *et al*, *J. Organomet. Chem.*, 1974, **65**, 131 (*nmr*)
Nesmeyanov, A.N. *et al*, *Izv. Akad. Nauk SSSR*, *Ser. Khim.*, 1976, 2844.
Jones, P.G. *et al*, *J. Chem. Soc.*, *Dalton Trans.*, 1977, 1434 (*mossbauer*)

$C_{28}H_{30}AuP_2^{\oplus}$ Au-00086

[1,2-Ethanediylbis[diphenylphosphine]-*P*,*P'*]dimethyl-gold(1+), 9CI
Dimethyl[*bis*(*diphenylphosphino*)*ethane*]*gold*(*1*+)

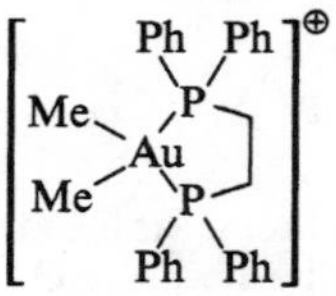

M 625.459 (ion)
Chloride: [34247-44-4].
$C_{28}H_{30}AuClP_2$ M 660.912
Air-stable solid. Sol. CH_2Cl_2, $CHCl_3$. Mp 163-72° dec.

Shiotani, A. *et al*, *Chem. Ber.*, 1971, **104**, 2838 (*nmr*)
Stocco, G.C. *et al*, *J. Am. Chem. Soc.*, 1971, **93**, 5057 (*synth*, *nmr*)
Shaw, C.F. *et al*, *J. Organomet. Chem.*, 1973, **51**, 365 (*raman*)

$C_{30}H_{32}AuI_2N_4^{\oplus}$ Au-00087

Bis[bis[(4-methylphenyl)amino]methylene]diiodogold(1+), 9CI
[58919-37-2]

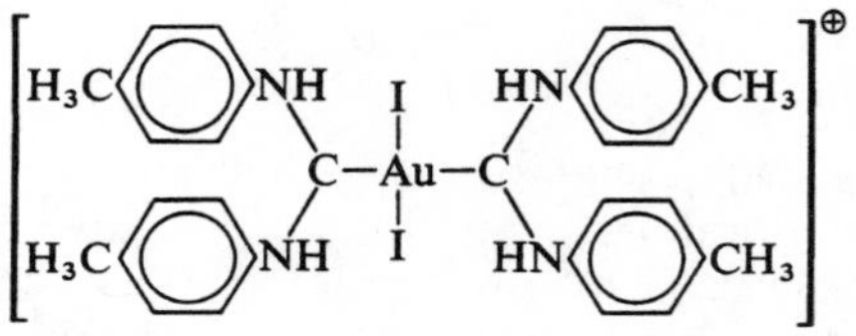

M 899.385 (ion)
Au(III) bis(carbene) complex.
Perchlorate:
$C_{30}H_{32}AuClI_2N_4O_4$ M 998.836
Orange cryst. (CH_2Cl_2/Et_2O). Mp 124°. Forms Et_2O solvate, Mp 133°.

Manojlovic-Muir, L., *J. Organomet. Chem.*, 1974, **73**, C45 (*cryst struct*)
Minghetti, G. *et al*, *Inorg. Chem.*, 1976, **15**, 1718 (*synth*, *nmr*)

$C_{36}H_{30}Au_2Zn_2$ Au-00088

Tetra-*μ*-phenylbis(phenylzinc)digold, 9CI
[54183-45-8]

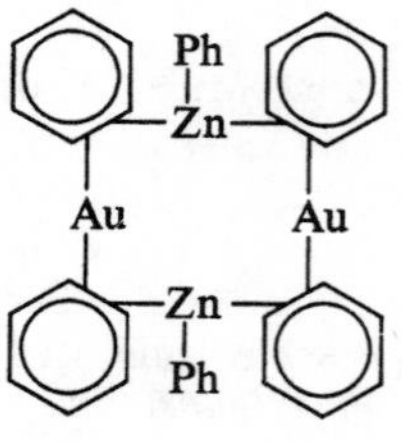

M 987.326
Orange-red air-sensitive cryst. (Et_2O). Sol. C_6H_6, CS_2, dec. in THF, DMF. Mp 114° dec.

De Graaf, P.W.J. *et al*, *J. Organomet. Chem.*, 1974, **78**, C19; 1977, **127**, 391 (*synth*, *nmr*)

$C_{36}H_{48}Au_2Cu_2N_4$ Au-00089

Tetrakis[2-[(dimethylamino)methyl]phenyl]bis(copper)digold, 9CI

[55466-93-8]

M 1057.827

Ochre solid. Sol. C_6H_6. Mp 137-9° dec.

van Koten, G. *et al*, *J. Organomet. Chem.*, 1974, **82**, C53; 1980, **186**, 427.

$C_{36}H_{48}Au_2Li_2N_4$ Au-00090

Tetrakis[μ-[2-[(dimethyamino)methyl]phenyl-*C*,*C*,*N*]]bis-(gold)dilithium

[54845-71-5]

$[Au_2Li_2(C_6H_4CH_2NMe_2)_4]$

M 944.617

White, thermally stable solid. Sol. C_6H_6, sl. sol. Et_2O. Mp 170-204° dec.

van Koten, G. *et al*, *J. Organomet. Chem.*, 1974, **82**, C53 (*synth*)
van Koten, G. *et al*, *J. Organomet. Chem.*, 1978, **148**, 317; 1980, **186**, 427 (*use*)

$C_{38}H_{30}AuFeNO_3P_2$ Au-00091

Dicarbonylnitrosyl(triphenylphosphine)[(triphenylphosphine)-aurio]iron, 8CI

[33989-39-8]

$Ph_3PAuFe(CO)_2(PPh_3)NO$

M 863.421

Red cryst. (C_6H_6/hexane). Dec. at 80°.

Casey, M. *et al*, *J. Chem. Soc. (A)*, 1971, 2989 (*synth, ir*)

$C_{40}H_{30}Au_2FeO_4P_2$ Au-00092

Tetracarbonylbis[(triphenylphosphine)aurio]iron, 8CI

Tetracarbonylbis[(triphenylphosphine)gold]iron, 10CI

M 1086.402

cis-form [16027-25-1]

Pale-yellow cryst. (Me_2CO aq.). Sol. nonpolar solvs., v. sl. sol. polar solvs. Mp ca. 150° dec.

Coffey, C.E. *et al*, *J. Chem. Soc.*, 1964, 1741 (*synth, ir*)
Forster, A. *et al*, *J. Chem. Soc., Chem. Commun.*, 1974, 1042 (*cmr*)
Jones, P.G. *et al*, *J. Chem. Soc., Dalton Trans.*, 1977, 1434 (*mössbauer*)

$C_{40}H_{30}Au_2O_4OsP_2$ Au-00093

Tetracarbonylbis[(triphenylphosphine)gold]osmium

M 1220.755

cis-form [41509-54-0]

Cream cryst. (CH_2Cl_2/hexane). Mp 155-65° dec.

George, R.D. *et al*, *J. Chem. Soc., Dalton Trans.*, 1973, 972 (*synth, ir*)

$C_{42}H_{35}Au_2P_2^{\oplus}$ Au-00094

μ-Phenylbis(triphenylphosphine)digold(1+), 9CI

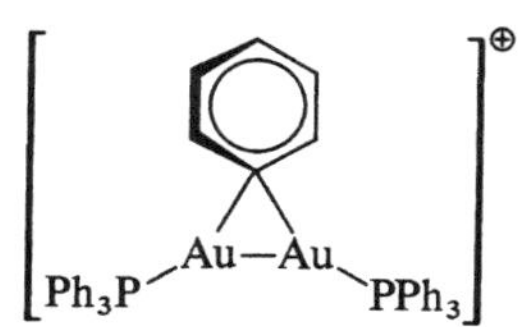

M 995.619 (ion)

Tetrafluoroborate: [50700-83-9].
$C_{42}H_{35}Au_2BF_4P_2$ M 1082.423
Beige cryst. (Me_2CO/Et_2O). Sol. CH_2Cl_2, Me_2CO. Mp 151-4° dec.

Grandberg, K.I. *et al*, *Dokl. Akad. Nauk SSSR, Ser. Sci. Khim.*, 1972, **206**, 1355 (*synth*)
Grandberg, K.I. *et al*, *Proc. Acad. Sci. USSR, Engl. Transl.*, 1972, **202/7**, 816 (*synth*)
Nesmeyanov, A.N. *et al*, *J. Organomet. Chem.*, 1974, **65**, 131 (*synth*)

$C_{46}H_{38}Au_2FeP_2$ Au-00095

1,1′-[Bis[triphenylphosphine]aurio]ferrocene, 9CI

[41559-20-0]

M 1102.534

Cryst. (THF/hexane). Sol. C_6H_6, Et_2O. Mp 104-5°. Dec. readily in soln. and solid state.

Perevelova, E.G. *et al*, *Izv. Akad. Nauk SSSR, Ser. Khim.*, 1972, 2594 (*synth*)

$C_{46}H_{39}Au_2FeP_2^{\oplus}$ Au-00096

[Bis(triphenylphosphine)digold](η⁵-2,4-cyclopentadien-1-yl)-[μ₃-[(1-η:1-η:1,2,3,4,5-η)-2,4-cyclopentadien-1-ylidene]]iron(1+), 9CI

[51900-72-2]

M 1103.542 (ion)

Tetrafluoroborate: [39453-01-5].
$C_{46}H_{39}Au_2BF_4FeP_2$ M 1190.345
Red cryst. Mod. sol. Me_2CO, $CHCl_3$, CH_2Cl_2, MeCN, insol. Et_2O, C_6H_6, THF. Mp 161-3° dec.

Sulfate:
$C_{92}H_{78}Au_4Fe_2O_4P_4S$ M 2303.141

Mp 160° dec.

Andrianov, V.G. *et al*, *J. Chem. Soc., Chem. Commun.*, 1973, 338 (*cryst struct*)
Nesmeyanov, A.N. *et al*, *Vestn. Mosk. Univ., Khim.*, 1973, **14**, 387; *CA*, **79**, 146613 (*synth, ir, uv, cryst struct, nmr*)
Nesmeyanov, A.N. *et al*, *J. Organomet. Chem.*, 1974, **65**, 131 (*synth*)
Lemenovskii, D.A. *et al*, *Izv. Akad. Nauk SSSR, Ser. Khim.*, 1975, 2105 (*pmr*)
Nesmeyanov, A.N. *et al*, *Izv. Akad. Nauk SSSR, Ser. Khim.*, 1978, 1122 (*nmr*)

$C_{50}H_{42}Au_2P_4$ Au-00097

Bis[μ-[methylenebis[diphenylphosphinato]](1−)-P:P′]digold, 10CI
[*Bis(diphenylphosphino)methanid*]*gold*
[77535-80-9]

M 1160.710
Air stable. Spar. sol. org. solvs. Mp 240° dec.

Schmidbaur, H. *et al*, *Chem. Ber.*, 1981, **114**, 433 (*synth, mossbauer*)
Briant, C.E. *et al*, *J. Organomet. Chem.*, 1982, **229**, C5 (*cryst struct*)

$C_{72}H_{60}Au_4I_2P_4$ Au-00098

Di-μ-iodotetrakis(triphenylphosphine)tetragold
[78519-63-8]

M 2090.836
Tetrahedral cluster. Pale-yellow cryst. ($CHCl_3/Me_2CO$). Sol. $CHCl_3$.

Demartin, F. *et al*, *J. Chem. Soc., Chem. Commun.*, 1981, 222 (*synth, cryst struct*)
Van Der Velden, J.W.A. *et al*, *Inorg. Chem.*, 1982, **21**, 4321 (*mossbauer, nmr*)

$C_{126}H_{84}Au_{11}F_{21}I_3P_7$ Au-00099

Triiodoheptakis[tris(4-fluorophenyl)phosphine]undecagold, 9CI
[37871-66-2]

M 4761.177
Example of high nuclearity gold cluster compound. Red cryst. (CH_2Cl_2/EtOH). Sol. CH_2Cl_2. Mp 215° dec.

McPartlin, M. *et al*, *J. Chem. Soc., Chem. Commun.*, 1969, 334 (*cryst struct*)
Cariati, F. *et al*, *Inorg. Chim. Acta*, 1971, **5**, 172 (*synth*)
Bellon, P.L. *et al*, *J. Chem. Soc., Dalton Trans.*, 1972, 1481 (*cryst struct*)
Mingos, D.M.P., *J. Chem. Soc., Dalton Trans.*, 1976, 1163.
Vollenbroek, F.A. *et al*, *Inorg. Chem.*, 1980, **19**, 2685 (*möss-bauer*)
Battistoni, G. *et al*, *J. Electron Spectrosc. Relat. Phenom.*, 1982, **28**, 23 (*pe*)

$C_{144}H_{120}Au_9P_8$⊕⊕⊕ Au-00100

Octakis(triphenylphosphine)nonagold(3+), 9CI
[60477-23-8]

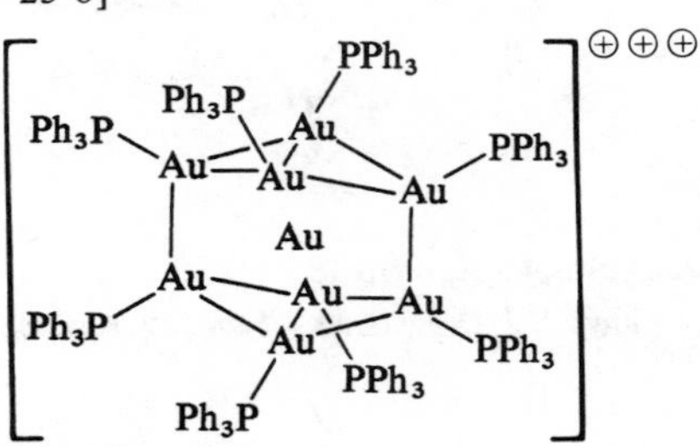

M 3871.021 (ion)
High nuclearity gold cluster.

Nitrate:
$C_{144}H_{120}Au_9N_3O_9P_8$ M 4057.035
Deep-green cryst. (CH_2Cl_2/hexane). Sol. CH_2Cl_2, EtOH. Mp 230° dec.

Bellon, P.L. *et al*, *J. Chem. Soc., Chem. Commun.*, 1971, 1423 (*cryst struct*)
Cariati, F. *et al*, *J. Chem. Soc., Dalton Trans.*, 1972, 2286 (*synth*)
Mingos, D.M.P., *J. Chem. Soc., Dalton Trans.*, 1976, 1163.
Battistoni, G. *et al*, *J. Electron Spectrosc. Relat. Phenom.*, 1982, **28**, 23 (*pe*)

Cu Copper

D. M. P. Mingos

Cuivre (Fr.), Kupfer (Ger.), Cobre (Sp.), Rame (Ital.), Медь (Mied') (Russ.), 銅 (Japan.)

Atomic Number. 29

Atomic Weight. 63.54(6) (variation in isotopic abundance limits precision).

Electronic Configuration. [Ar] $3d^{10}\,4s^{1}$

Oxidation States. +1, +2. In organometallic chemistry the former predominates. Higher oxidation states are found only with ligands such as O and F.

Coordination Number. Cu(I) compounds are linear, trigonal and tetrahedral. Cu(II) compounds are distorted tetrahedral, trigonal bipyramidal, square pyramidal and distorted octahedral.

Colour. Simple organocopper(I) compounds are colourless. Cluster compounds, however, are highly coloured.

Availability. Commonly available starting materials are copper powder, CuCl, $CuCl_2$, $CuBr(SMe_2)$, $CuSO_4{\cdot}5H_2O$.

Handling. Copper does not require any special handling techniques.

Toxicity. Most copper compounds are not considered to be toxic.

Isotopic Abundance. ^{63}Cu, 69%; ^{65}Cu, 31%.

Spectroscopy. The nuclear quadrupoles and low sensitivities of ^{63}Cu, $I = \frac{3}{2}$, and ^{65}Cu, $I = \frac{3}{2}$, have limited the applications in organometallic chemistry of direct nmr studies.

Analysis. EDTA titration with disodium ethylbis(5-tetrazolylazo)acetate as indicator, or iodometrically after addition of iodide.

References. In addition to the references listed in the introduction to the *Sourcebook* are the following:

Jardine, F. J., *Adv. Inorg. Chem. Radiochem.*, 1975, **17,** 117 (*general review*)

Bruce, M. I., *J. Organomet. Chem.*, 1972, **44,** 209 (*carbonyl compounds*)

Posner, G. H., *Organic Reactions*, 1972, 19 (*conjugate addition reactions*)

Kaufmann, T., *Angew. Chem., Int. Ed. Engl.*, 1974, **13,** 291 (*oxidative coupling using copper reagents*)

Saegusa, T. *et al.*, *Synthesis*, 1975, 291 (*synthesis of cyclic compounds via copper isonitriles*)

Normant, J. F., *Synthesis*, 1972, 63 (*organocuprates*)

$CuOSO_2CF_3$

Cu-00001

CuCN

Cu-00002

CuMe

Cu-00003

$Cu(CN)_2^{\ominus}$

Cu-00004

CuC≡CH

Cu-00005

$[CuOAc]_n$

Cu-00006

Me_2SCuBr

Cu-00007

$ICuSMe_2$

Cu-00008

$(Me_2Cu)Li$

Cu-00009

$CuC{\equiv}CCH_3$

Cu-00010

Cu-00011

Cu-00012

Cu-00013

n = 1

Cu-00014

As Cu-00014 with n = 2

Cu-00015

$H_2C{=}C(CH_3)C{\equiv}CCu$

Cu-00016

$CuC{\equiv}CCH_2CH_2CH_3$

Cu-00017

Cu-00018

$Cu(C_6F_5)$

Cu-00019

CuPh

Cu-00020

$(H_3C)_3CC{\equiv}CCu$

Cu-00021

$(H_3CCH{=}CH)_2CuLi$

Cu-00022

$Me_3SiC{\equiv}CCH_2Cu$

Cu-00023

$ICuP(OEt)_3$

Cu-00024

Cu-00025

only one of eight anisyl groups shown

Cu-00026

Cu-00027

CuC≡CPh

Cu-00028

Cu-00029

$(H_3CCN)_4Cu^{\oplus}$

Cu-00030

Cu-00031

$[Cu(CH_2SiMe_3)_2]^{\ominus}$

Cu-00032

Cu-00033

Cu-00034

Cu-00035

Cu-00036

Cu-00037

$(H_3C)_3CCuLiSPh$

Cu-00038

Cu-00039

Cu-00040

R = Et

Cu-00041

$(Ph_2Cu)Li$

Cu-00042

Cu-00043

$Me_3SiOCu(PMe_3)_3$

Cu-00044

Cu-00045

Cu-00046

R = Et

Cu-00047

$H_3C(CH_2)_3CuP(CH_2CH_2CH_2CH_3)_3$

Cu-00048

Cu-00049

6H atoms not shown

Cu-00050

$MeCuP(C_6H_{11})_3$

Cu-00051

$(Ph_3P)Cu(C_2B_8H_{11})$

Cu-00052

Cu-00053

Cu-00054

As Cu-00041 with R = Ph

Cu-00055

Struct. unknown

Cu-00056

As Cu-00047 with R = Ph

Cu-00057

Only one of four amine groups shown

Cu-00058

Cu-00059

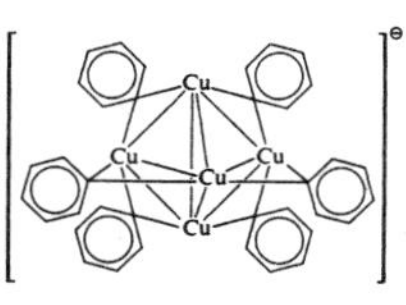

Cu-00060

$(Ph_3P)_2CuBH_4$

Cu-00062

Cu-00063

$H_3B{-}H{-}Cu(PMePh_2)_3$

Cu-00064

Cu-00065

only one of four μ_3-$C_6H_4NMe_2$ groups shown

Cu-00066

$MeCu(PPh_3)_3$

Cu-00067

$CCuF_3O_3S$ Cu-00001

Trifluoromethanesulfonic acid copper(1+) salt, 9CI

Copper(I) triflate. Copper(I) trifluoromethanesulfonate

[42152-44-3]

$CuOSO_2CF_3$

M 212.610

Catalyst for olefin dimerisation, cyclopropanation and carbene addn., for promotion of Grob-type fragmentations and in Ullmann reactions. Air- and moisture-sensitive.

Masamune, S. *et al*, *J. Am. Chem. Soc.*, 1977, **99**, 6756 (*use*)
Evers, J.Th.M. *et al*, *Tetrahedron Lett.*, 1978, 821, 2317, 2321 (*use*)
Salomon, R.G. *et al*, *J. Am. Chem. Soc.*, 1979, **101**, 3961 (*use*)
Org. Synth., 1980, **59**, 202 (*synth*, *use*)
Fieser, M. *et al*, *Reagents for Organic Synthesis*, Wiley, 1967-83, **8**, 125 (*use*)

CCuN Cu-00002

Copper cyanide, 9CI

Cuprous cyanide. Cupricin

[544-92-3]

CuCN

M 89.564

Insecticide, fungicide. White-cream powder, dark-green orthorhombic cryst. or dark-red monoclinic cryst. Sol. NH_3 aq., insol. H_2O, alcohols. Mp 474°.

▷Poisonous. GL7150000.

Barber, H.J., *J. Chem. Soc.*, 1943, 79 (*synth*)
Norberg, B. *et al*, *Acta Chem. Scand., Ser. A*, 1949, **3**, 174 (*synth*)
Vaughan, W.R. *et al*, *J. Am. Chem. Soc.*, 1954, **76**, 2504 (*use*)
Penneman, R.A. *et al*, *J. Chem. Phys.*, 1956, **24**, 293 (*ir*)
Chadwick, B.M. *et al*, *Adv. Inorg. Chem. Radiochem.*, 1966, **8**, 153 (*rev*, *synth*)
Merck Index, 9th Ed., 1976, No. 2666.
Sharpe, A.G., *The Chemistry of Cyano Complexes of the Transition Metals*, Interscience, New York, 1976, 266.

CH_3Cu Cu-00003

Methylcopper, 9CI

Copper methyl

[1184-53-8]

CuMe

M 78.581

Synthetic reagent. Unstable amorph. yellow solid. Air-sensitive.

▷Dry solid explodes violently

Gilman, H. *et al*, *J. Org. Chem.*, 1952, **17**, 1630 (*synth*)
Johnson, R. *et al*, *J. Chem. Soc.*, 1960, 3926 (*synth*)
Thiele, K.H. *et al*, *J. Organomet. Chem.*, 1968, **12**, 225 (*synth*)
Ikariya, T. *et al*, *J. Organomet. Chem.*, 1974, **72**, 145 (*synth*)
Fieser, M. *et al*, *Reagents for Organic Synthesis*, Wiley, 1967-83, **7**, 236.
Bretherick, L., *Handbook of Reactive Chemical Hazards*, 2nd Ed., Butterworths, London and Boston, 1979, 303.
Sax, N.I., *Dangerous Properties of Industrial Materials*, 5th Ed., Van Nostrand-Reinhold, 1979, 814.

$C_2CuN_2^{\ominus}$ Cu-00004

Bis(cyano-*C*)cuprate(1−), 9CI

Dicyanocuprate(1−)

[13682-73-0]

$Cu(CN)_2^{\ominus}$

M 115.581 (ion)

The anion forms helical chains with each copper atom 3-coordinate.

▷GS2168900.

K salt: Gold potassium cyanide.
C_2CuKN_2 M 154.680
Cryst. (KCN aq.). Spar. sol. H_2O.

Basset, H. *et al*, *J. Chem. Soc.*, 1924, 1660.
Staritzky, E. *et al*, *Anal. Chem.*, 1956, **28**, 419 (*synth*, *cryst struct*)
Merck Index, 9th Ed., No. 2672.
Sharpe, A.G., *The Chemistry of Cyano Complexes of the Transition Metals*, Interscience, New York, 1976, 266.

C_2HCu Cu-00005

Ethynylcopper, 9CI

Copper acetylide. Cuprous acetylide

[16753-36-9]

$CuC{\equiv}CH$

M 88.576

Catalyst for acetylene reactions. Unstable orange solid. Dec. at −45° → $C_2H_2 + Cu_2C_2$. Supported compd. is more stable.

▷Highly explosive when heated or shocked

Nast, R. *et al*, *Z. Anorg. Allg. Chem.*, 1957, **292**, 287; *CA*, **52**, 6996 (*synth*)
Bretherick, L., *Handbook of Reactive Chemical Hazards*, 2nd Ed., Butterworths, London and Boston, 1979, 340.

$C_2H_3CuO_2$ Cu-00006

(Acetato-*O,O′*)copper, 10CI

Cuprous acetate

[17203-87-1]

$[CuOAc]_n$

M 122.591

Polymeric planar chains in solid state. Transparent leafy cryst.

Angel, A. *et al*, *J. Chem. Soc.*, 1902, 1385 (*synth*)
Shimizu, H. *et al*, *J. Am. Chem. Soc.*, 1952, **74**, 4469 (*synth*)
Lin, D.C.K. *et al*, *Can. J. Chem.*, 1973, **51**, 2999 (*ms*)
Ogura, T. *et al*, *Inorg. Chem.*, 1973, **12**, 2611 (*ms*)
Drew, M.G.B. *et al*, *J. Chem. Soc., Chem. Commun.*, 1973, 124 (*synth*, *cryst struct*)
Merck Index, 9th Ed., No. 2663.

C_2H_6BrCuS Cu-00007

Bromo[thiobis(methane)]copper, 9CI

Cuprous bromide methyl sulfide

[54678-23-8]

Me_2SCuBr

M 205.579

Cryst. deriv. for prepn. of organocuprate reagents. Prisms (Me_2S/hexane). Mp ca. 135° dec. Dissociates in soln.

House, H.O. *et al*, *J. Org. Chem.*, 1975, **40**, 1460 (*use*)
Posner, G., *Org. React.*, 1975, **22**, 253 (*rev*)
San Filippo, J. *et al*, *Inorg. Chem.*, 1975, **14**, 1667 (*synth*)
Theis, A.B. *et al*, *Synth. Commun.*, 1981, **11**, 157 (*synth*, *use*)
Wuts, P.G.M., *Synth. Commun.*, 1981, **11**, 139 (*synth*, *use*)

C_2H_6CuIS Cu-00008

Iodo(dimethylsulfide)copper

Iodo[thiobis[methane]]copper, 9CI

[54678-24-9]

$ICuSMe_2$

M 252.580

Convenient precursor for the generation of lithium organocuprates. Cryst. (MeCN). Insol. most common org. solvs.

House, H.O., *J. Org. Chem.*, 1975, **40**, 1460 (*use*)
San Fillipo, J. *et al*, *Inorg. Chem.*, 1975, **14**, 1667 (*synth*)
Mansson, J.E., *Acta Chem. Scand.*, *Ser. B*, 1978, **32**, 543 (*synth, use*)

C_2H_6CuLi Cu-00009

Lithium dimethylcuprate(1–), 9CI

(Dimethylcopper)lithium, 9CI

[15681-48-8]

$(Me_2Cu)Li$

M 100.556

Methylating agent. Air- and moisture-sensitive. Prepd. and used *in situ*.

Gilman, H. *et al*, *J. Org. Chem.*, 1952, **17**, 1630 (*synth*)
House, H.L. *et al*, *J. Org. Chem.*, 1966, **31**, 3128 (*nmr*)
Corey, E.J. *et al*, *J. Am. Chem. Soc.*, 1967, **89**, 3911 (*synth, use*)
Whitesides, G.M. *et al*, *J. Am. Chem. Soc.*, 1969, **91**, 4871 (*synth, use*)
Normant, J.F., *Synthesis*, 1972, 63 (*rev*)
Posner, G.H., *Org. React.*, 1975, **22**, 253 (*rev*)
Pearson, R.G. *et al*, *J. Am. Chem. Soc.*, 1976, **98**, 4098 (*struct*)
Ashby, E.C. *et al*, *J. Am. Chem. Soc.*, 1977, **99**, 5312 (*pmr, struct*)
Ortiz, B. *et al*, *Chem. Ind. (London)*, 1979, 747 (*synth*)
Fieser, M. *et al*, *Reagents for Organic Synthesis*, Wiley, 1967-83, **7**, 120.

C_3H_3Cu Cu-00010

1-Propynylcopper, 9CI

Methylacetylide copper

[30645-13-7]

$CuC{\equiv}CCH_3$

M 102.603

Orange powder.

Schlubach, H.H. *et al*, *Justus Liebigs Ann. Chem.*, 1950, **568**, 141 (*synth*)
Nast, R. *et al*, *Chem. Ber.*, 1956, **89**, 415 (*synth*)
Coates, G.E. *et al*, *Proc. Chem. Soc., London*, 1959, 396 (*synth*)
Aleksanyan, V.T. *et al*, *Spectrochim. Acta, Part A*, 1975, **31**, 517 (*ir, raman*)

$C_4H_6Cl_2Cu_2$ Cu-00011

Dichloro-μ-1,4-butadienedicopper

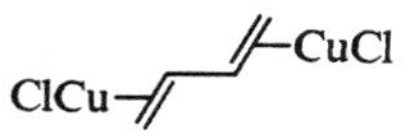

ClCu–CH=CH–CH=CH–CuCl

M 252.089

Pale-yellow solid, unstable in air.

Gilliland, E.R. *et al*, *J. Am. Chem. Soc.*, 1941, **63**, 2088 (*synth*)
Inorg. Synth., 1960, **6**, 216 (*synth*)

$C_4H_8CuN_2O_2S_2$ Cu-00012

Fluopsin *C*

Bis(N-hydroxy-N-methylmethanethioamidato-O,S)-copper, 9CI. *Bis(N-methylthioformohydroxamato)copper*, 8CI. *YC 73. Antibiotic YC 73*

[31323-25-8]

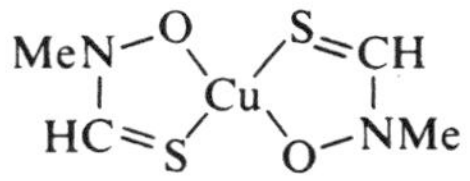

MeN–O–Cu(–S=CH–N(Me)–O–)–S=CH (bis-chelate)

M 243.785

Isol. from *Pseudomonas fluorescens*. Antibiotic. Dark-green cryst. (EtOH). Mp 199° dec. λ_{max} 231, 253, 267, 320 and 365 nm (MeOH).

▷GL6490000.

Shirahata, K. *et al*, *J. Antibiot.*, 1970, **23**, 546 (*isol, struct*)
Egawa, Y. *et al*, *J. Antibiot.*, 1971, **24**, 124 (*struct, synth*)
Shirahara, K. *et al*, *J. Antibiot.*, 1971, **24**, 140 (*synth, ir, nmr*)
Taylor, D., *Cryst. Struct. Commun.*, 1978, **7**, 237 (*cryst struct*)
Bell, S.J. *et al*, *Antimicrob. Agents Chemother.*, 1979, **15**, 384 (*rev*)

$C_4H_{11}CuSi$ Cu-00013

μ-[(Trimethylsilyl)methyl]copper

[50563-15-0]

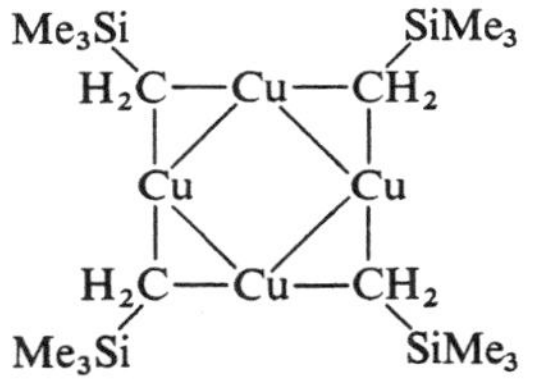

$[Me_3SiCH_2Cu]_4$ (cyclic tetramer: four Cu bridged by four CH_2SiMe_3 groups)

M 150.762

Tetrameric.

Tetramer: Tetrakis(μ-[(trimethylsilyl)methyl]tetracopper, 9CI.

$C_{16}H_{44}Cu_4Si_4$ M 603.050

Off-white needles (pentane at –70°). Sol. C_6H_6, pentane. Mp 78-9° dec.

Lappert, M.F. *et al*, *J. Chem. Soc., Chem. Commun.*, 1973, 24 (*synth*)
Jarvis, J.A.J. *et al*, *J. Chem. Soc., Dalton Trans.*, 1977, 999 (*synth, cryst struct*)
Middleton, A.R. *et al*, *J. Chem. Soc., Dalton Trans.*, 1981, 1898 (*props*)

$C_4H_{22}B_{18}Cu^{\ominus}$ Cu-00014

Bis[(7,8,9,10,11-η)-undecahydro-7,8-dicarbaundecaborato(2−)]cuprate(1−), 9CI
Bis(dicarbollide)cuprate(1−)
[51805-68-6]

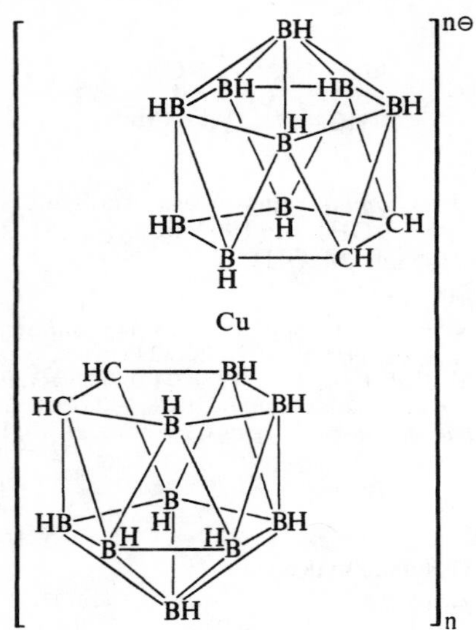

n = 1

M 328.344 (ion)
An example of a "slipped" sandwich complex.
Methyltriphenylphosphonium salt:
$C_{23}H_{40}B_{18}CuP$ M 605.669
Dark blood-red cryst. (CH_2Cl_2/hexane). Sol. CH_2Cl_2, Me_2CO.

Warren, L.F. *et al*, *J. Am. Chem. Soc.*, 1968, **90**, 4823 (*synth*)
Wing, R.M. *et al*, *J. Am. Chem. Soc.*, 1968, **90**, 4828 (*cryst struct*)
Mingos, D.M.P. *et al*, *J. Organomet. Chem.*, 1978, **146**, C37.

$C_4H_{22}B_{18}Cu^{\ominus\ominus}$ Cu-00015

Bis[(7,8,9,10,11-η)-undecahydro-7,8-dicarbaundecaborato(2−)]cuprate(2−), 9CI
Bis(dicarbollide)cuprate(2−)
As Bis[(7,8,9,10,11-η)-undecahydro-7,8-dicarbaundecaborato(2−)]cuprate(1−), Cu-00014 with

n = 2

M 328.344 (ion)
An example of a "slipped" sandwich complex.
Di-K salt: [42992-84-7].
$C_4H_{22}B_{18}CuK_2$ M 406.540
Blue cryst. (Me_2CO/hexane). Sol. CH_2Cl_2, Me_2CO.

Wing, R.M., *J. Am. Chem. Soc.*, 1967, **89**, 5599 (*cryst struct*)
Hawthorne, M.F. *et al*, *J. Am. Chem. Soc.*, 1968, **90**, 879 (*synth*)
Warren, L.F. *et al*, *J. Am. Chem. Soc.*, 1968, **90**, 4823 (*synth*)
Mingos, D.M.P. *et al*, *J. Organomet. Chem.*, 1978, **146**, C37.

C_5H_5Cu Cu-00016

3-Methyl-3-buten-1-ynylcopper, 9CI
Copper(I) isopropenylacetylide
[56964-06-8]

$H_2C{=}C(CH_3)C{\equiv}CCu$

M 128.641
Reagent used for coupling reactions. Bright-yellow ppt. Mp 187-91° dec.

Chini, P. *et al*, *Chim. Ind.* (*Milan*), 1964, **46**, 1049 (*synth*)
Schreiber, F.G. *et al*, *J. Chem. Soc., Perkin Trans. 1*, 1977, 90 (*synth, use*)
Schreiber, F.G. *et al*, *J. Chem. Res.* (*S*), 1978, 92 (*use*)
Schreiber, F.G. *et al*, *Org. Prep. Proced. Int.*, 1978, **10**, 177 (*use*)
Batu, G. *et al*, *J. Org. Chem.*, 1979, **44**, 3948 (*use*)
Ronald, R.C. *et al*, *J. Chem. Soc., Chem. Commun.*, 1979, 124 (*use*)
Fieser, M. *et al*, *Reagents for Organic Synthesis*, Wiley, 1967-83, **8**, 123 (*use*)

C_5H_7Cu Cu-00017

1-Pentynylcopper, 9CI
Copper pentyne
[19093-51-7]

$CuC{\equiv}CCH_2CH_2CH_3$

M 130.656
Used in prostaglandin synth. Canary-yellow solid.

Castro, C.E. *et al*, *J. Org. Chem.*, 1966, **31**, 4071 (*synth*)
Corey, E.J. *et al*, *J. Org. Chem.*, 1975, **40**, 2265 (*use*)
Caruthers, W., *Compr. Organomet. Chem.*, 1982, **7**, 661 (*rev*)

$C_5H_{13}CuN_3O^{\oplus}$ Cu-00018

[*N*-(2-Aminoethyl)-1,2-ethanediamine-*N*,*N′*,*N″*]carbonylcopper(1+)
Carbonyl(diethylenetriamine)copper
[65832-81-7]

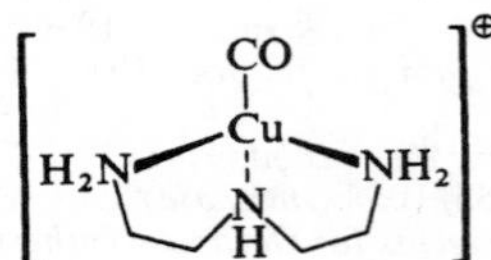

M 194.723 (ion)
Tetraphenylborate:
$C_{29}H_{33}BCuN_3O$ M 513.955
Cryst. (MeOH), mod. air-stable. Sl. sol. THF, Me_2CO.

Pasquali, M. *et al*, *Inorg. Chem.*, 1978, **17**, 1684 (*synth, cryst struct*)

C_6CuF_5 Cu-00019

(Pentafluorophenyl)copper, 9CI
[18206-43-4]

$Cu(C_6F_5)$

M 230.604
Probably tetrameric in solid state and soln.
Tetramer(?):
$C_{24}Cu_4F_{20}$ M 922.416
Nearly white cryst. (C_6H_6). Sol. C_6H_6, insol. alkanes. Mp 210-20° dec.

Cairncross, A. *et al*, *J. Am. Chem. Soc.*, 1968, **90**, 2186; 1971, **93**, 248 (*synth, ms, nmr*)
Gastinger, R.G. *et al*, *J. Org. Chem.*, 1978, **43**, 159 (*use*)

C_6H_5Cu Cu-00020

Phenylcopper, 9CI
Copper phenyl
[3220-49-3]

CuPh

M 140.652

Polymeric. Unstable amorph. solid. Mp 100° dec. Hydrol. by H_2O, dec. on heating in soln.

Gilman, H. *et al*, *Recl. Trav. Chim. Pays-Bas*, 1936, **55**, 821; *J. Org. Chem.*, 1952, **17**, 1630 (*synth*)
Costa, G. *et al*, *J. Organomet. Chem.*, 1966, **5**, 568 (*synth, ir*)
Hashimoto, S. *et al*, *J. Org. Chem.*, 1966, **31**, 891 (*synth*)
Camus, A. *et al*, *Inorg. Chim. Acta*, 1977, **23**, 131 (*rev*)
Hofstee, H.F. *et al*, *J. Organomet. Chem.*, 1978, **144**, 255 (*synth, nmr*)
Fieser, M. *et al*, *Reagents for Organic Synthesis*, Wiley, 1967-83, **7**, 282.

C_6H_9Cu Cu-00021

(3,3-Dimethyl-1-butynyl)copper, 9CI
Copper tert-*butylacetylide*
[40575-23-3]

$(H_3C)_3CC{\equiv}CCu$

M 144.683

Synthetic reagent. Orange-red. Sol. ethers, hydrocarbons.

House, H.O. *et al*, *J. Org. Chem.*, 1973, **38**, 3893 (*synth, use*)
Fieser, M. *et al*, *Reagents for Organic Synthesis*, Wiley, 1967-83, **5**, 148.

$C_6H_{10}CuLi$ Cu-00022

Di-1-propenylcopperlithium
Di-1-propenylcuprate(1−)lithium, 9CI

$(H_3CCH{=}CH)_2CuLi$

M 152.632

***(E,E)*-form** [33462-38-3]
Used in alkene synth.

Org. Synth., 1976, **55**, 103 (*synth, use*)
Fieser, M. *et al*, *Reagents for Organic Synthesis*, Wiley, 1967-83, **7**, 141.

$C_6H_{11}CuSi$ Cu-00023

[3-(Trimethylsilyl)-2-propynyl]copper, 9CI
(3-Cuprio-1-propynyl)trimethylsilane. Trimethylsilylpropargylcopper
[55630-32-5]

$Me_3SiC{\equiv}CCH_2Cu$

M 174.784

Ganem, B., *Tetrahedron Lett.*, 1974, 4467 (*synth, use*)
Commercon, A. *et al*, *J. Organomet. Chem.*, 1975, **93**, 415 (*synth*)
Fieser, M. *et al*, *Reagents for Organic Synthesis*, Wiley, 1967-83, **6**, 638 (*synth, use*)

$C_6H_{15}CuIO_3P$ Cu-00024

Iodo(triethyl phosphite-*P*)copper, 9CI
[51717-23-8]

$ICuP(OEt)_3$

M 356.607

Probably tetrameric in solid state.

Tetramer(?):
$C_{24}H_{60}Cu_4I_4O_{12}P_4$ M 1426.428
Reagent for Ullmann coupling of *o*-haloarylimines.
Cryst. (C_6H_6). Sol. C_6H_6. Mp 110-1°.

Nishizawa, Y., *Bull. Chem. Soc. Jpn.*, 1961, **34**, 1170 (*synth*)
Sato, T. *et al*, *Tetrahedron Lett.*, 1973, 4221 (*use*)
Ziegler, F.E. *et al*, *J. Am. Chem. Soc.*, 1976, **98**, 8282 (*use*)
Maryanoff, B.E. *et al*, *J. Org. Chem.*, 1979, **44**, 4410 (*use*)

$C_6H_{15}CuIP$ Cu-00025

Iodo(triethylphosphine)copper, 9CI
[56667-47-1]

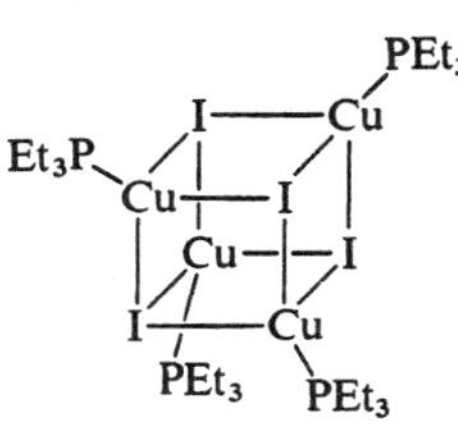

M 308.609

Tetrameric.

Tetramer: [51364-98-8]. *Tetra-μ_3-iodotetrakis(triethylphosphine)tetracopper.*
$C_{24}H_{60}Cu_4I_4P_4$ M 1234.435
Cryst. (C_6H_6). Mp 236-40° (softens at 230°).

Mann, F.G. *et al*, *J. Chem. Soc.*, 1936, 1503 (*synth*)
Churchill, M.R. *et al*, *Inorg. Chem.*, 1974, **13**, 1899 (*cryst struct*)
Bowmaker, G.A. *et al*, *Aust. J. Chem.*, 1978, **31**, 2137 (*ir, raman*)
Valigura, D. *et al*, *Bull. Soc. Chim. Belg.*, 1980, **89**, 831 (*nqr*)

C_7H_7CuO Cu-00026

2-Methoxyphenylcopper
o-*Anisylcopper*

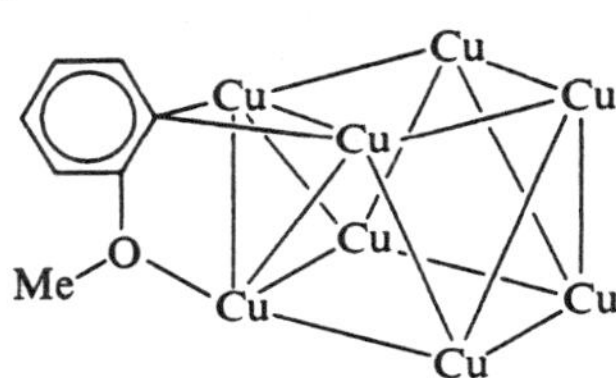

only one of eight anisyl groups shown

M 170.678

Octameric distorted square-antiprismatic cluster.

Octamer: [71344-04-2]. *Octakis[μ_3-(2-methoxyphenyl-C:C:O)]octacopper, 10CI. Octa-*o*-anisyloctacopper.*
$C_{56}H_{56}Cu_8O_8$ M 1365.422
Orange cryst. (toluene).

Camus, A. *et al*, *J. Organomet. Chem.*, 1968, **14**, 441; 1979, **174**, 121 (*synth, cryst struct*)
Costa, G. *et al*, *J. Organomet. Chem.*, 1978, **160**, 353.

C_7H_8CuN Cu-00027

(η^5-2,4-Cyclopentadien-1-yl)(isocyanomethane)copper
(Methyl isocyanide)(η^5-cyclopentadienyl)copper
[31921-94-5]

CpCuCNMe

M 169.693

Pale-yellow cryst. (pentane at −78°), unstable at r.t. Sol. pentane.

Cotton, F.A. *et al*, *J. Am. Chem. Soc.*, 1970, **92**, 5114 (*synth*)

C_8H_5Cu Cu-00028

(Phenylethynyl)copper, 9CI
Phenylacetylide copper
[13146-23-1]

CuC≡CPh

M 164.674
Used in Castro reaction for synthesising diarylacetylenes. Bright-yellow solid.

Castro, L.E. *et al*, *J. Org. Chem.*, 1966, **31**, 4071 (*synth*, *use*)
Tsuda, T. *et al*, *J. Am. Chem. Soc.*, 1972, **94**, 658 (*synth*)
Org. Synth., 1972, **52**, 128 (*synth*)
Aleksanyan, V.T. *et al*, *Spectrochim. Acta*, *Part A*, 1975, **31**, 517 (*ir*, *raman*)
Caruthers, W., *Compr. Organomet. Chem.*, 1982, **7**, 661 (*rev*)

$C_8H_{12}ClCu$ Cu-00029

Chloro[(1,2,5,6-η)-1,5-cyclooctadiene]copper, 10CI
[62389-79-1]

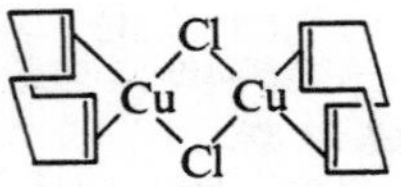

M 207.182
Dimeric.
Dimer: [32717-95-6]. *Di-μ-chlorobis[(1,2,5,6-η)-1,5-cyclooctadiene]dicopper*, 9CI.
$C_{16}H_{24}Cl_2Cu_2$ M 414.364
Yellow. Rapidly loses ligand in dry air at 20°.

van den Hende, J.H. *et al*, *J. Am. Chem. Soc.*, 1963, **85**, 1009 (*synth*, *cryst struct*)
Banthorpe, D.V. *et al*, *Chem. Ind. (London)*, 1973, 743 (*synth*)
Fitch, J.W. *et al*, *Synth. React. Inorg. Metal-Org. Chem.*, 1974, **4**, 1 (*use*)
Vinal, R.S., *Res. Discl.*, 1976, **152**, 43 (*use*)

$C_8H_{12}CuN_4^{\oplus}$ Cu-00030

Tetrakis(acetonitrile)copper(1+), 9CI

$(H_3CCN)_4Cu^{\oplus}$

M 227.756 (ion)
Hexafluorophosphate:
$C_8H_{12}CuF_6N_4P$ M 372.720
Used for synth. of Cu(I) complexes in nonaqueous media. Cryst. ($MeCN/Et_2O$ at −20°). Mod. sol. polar org. solvs. Air-sensitive as solid.

Maspero, F. *et al*, *J. Organomet. Chem.*, 1972, **38**, C43 (*use*)
Csoregh, I. *et al*, *Acta Crystallogr.*, *Sect. B*, 1975, **31**, 314 (*cryst struct*)
Eller, P.G. *et al*, *J. Am. Chem. Soc.*, 1977, **99**, 4346 (*use*)
Inorg. Synth., 1979, **19**, 90 (*synth*)

$C_8H_{20}As_2Cu_2$ Cu-00031

Bis[μ-[(dimethylarsinidenio)bis[methylene]]]dicopper, 9CI
[56870-45-2]

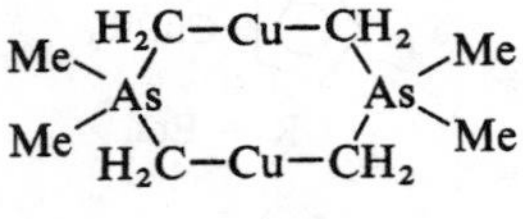

M 393.181
Cryst. (toluene). Sol. toluene. Mp 98°.

Schmidbaur, H. *et al*, *Chem. Ber.*, 1975, **108**, 2656 (*synth*)

$C_8H_{22}CuSi_2^{\ominus}$ Cu-00032

Bis[(trimethylsilylmethyl)]cuprate(1−), 9CI
[40988-97-4]

$[Cu(CH_2SiMe_3)_2]^{\ominus}$

M 237.979 (ion)
Li salt:
$C_8H_{22}CuLiSi_2$ M 244.920
Generally synth. *in situ* as THF soln. Solns. stable at r.t.

Lappert, M.F. *et al*, *J. Chem. Soc.*, *Chem. Commun.*, 1973, 24 (*synth*)
Kieft, R.L. *et al*, *J. Organomet. Chem.*, 1974, **77**, 289 (*synth*, *nmr*)
Jarvis, J.A.J. *et al*, *J. Chem. Soc.*, *Dalton Trans.*, 1977, 999 (*synth*)
Hannah, D.J. *et al*, *Aust. J. Chem.*, 1981, **34**, 181 (*use*)
Casey, C.P. *et al*, *J. Org. Chem.*, 1981, **46**, 2089 (*use*)

$C_8H_{24}Cu_2N_6O_2^{\oplus\oplus}$ Cu-00033

Dicarbonyl[μ-(1,2-ethanediamine-*N*,*N'*)]bis(1,2-ethanediamine-*N*,*N'*)dicopper(2+), 10CI
[69683-75-6]

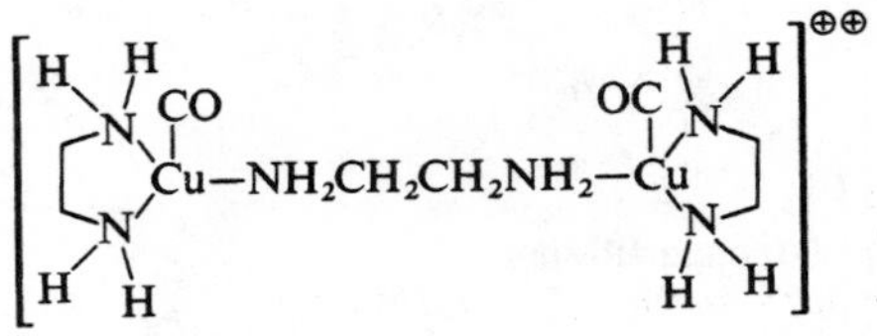

M 363.409 (ion)
Bis(tetraphenylborate):
$C_{56}H_{64}B_2Cu_2N_6O_2$ M 1001.873
Cryst. (MeOH). Mp 80° dec. Sensitive to moisture, rel. high thermal stability.

Pasquali, M. *et al*, *Inorg. Chem.*, 1980, **19**, 1191 (*synth*, *cryst struct*)

$C_9H_{10}CuLiS$ Cu-00034

Lithium phenylthio(cyclopropyl)cuprate
Lithium(benzenethiolato)cyclopropylcuprate

M 220.725
Synthetic reagent.

Piers, E. *et al*, *Tetrahedron Lett.*, 1976, 3233, 3237 (*synth*, *use*)
Fieser, M. *et al*, *Reagents for Organic Synthesis*, Wiley, 1967-83, **7**, 211.

$C_9H_{11}Cu$ Cu-00035

(1,3,5-Trimethylbenzene)copper

Mesitylcopper

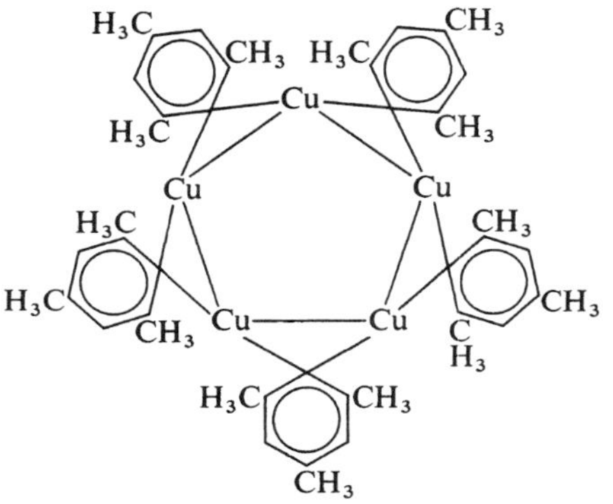

M 182.732

Pentameric.

Pentamer: Pentakis(1,3,5-trimethylbenzene)pentacopper. Penta(μ-mesityl)pentacopper.

$C_{45}H_{55}Cu_5$ M 913.660

Yellow cryst. (toluene). Sol. toluene.

Camus, A. *et al*, *J. Organomet. Chem.*, 1970, **21**, 249 (*use*)
Ikariya, T. *et al*, *J. Organomet. Chem.*, 1974, **72**, 145 (*use*)
Miyashita, N. *et al*, *Bull. Chem. Soc. Jpn.*, 1977, **50**, 1102 (*use*)
Tsuda, T. *et al*, *J. Org. Chem.*, 1981, **46**, 192 (*synth*)
Gambarotta, S. *et al*, *J. Chem. Soc., Chem. Commun.*, 1983, 1156 (*synth, cryst struct*)

$C_{10}H_8Cu_2Fe$ Cu-00036

1,1′-Ferrocenylenedicopper

1,1′-Dicuprioferrocene

[76082-12-7]

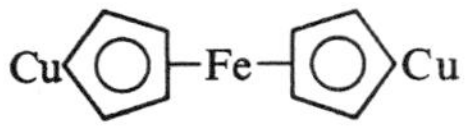

M 311.112

Thermally stable red-orange solid. Insol. common solvs. Dec. at 136°.

Sedova, N.N. *et al*, *J. Organomet. Chem.*, 1982, **224**, C53 (*synth*)

$C_{10}H_{10}BCuN_6O$ Cu-00037

Carbonyl[hydrotris(1*H*-pyrazolato-*N*^{1})borato(1–)-*N*^{2},*N*$^{2'}$-,*N*$^{2''}$]copper, 9CI

[52374-64-8]

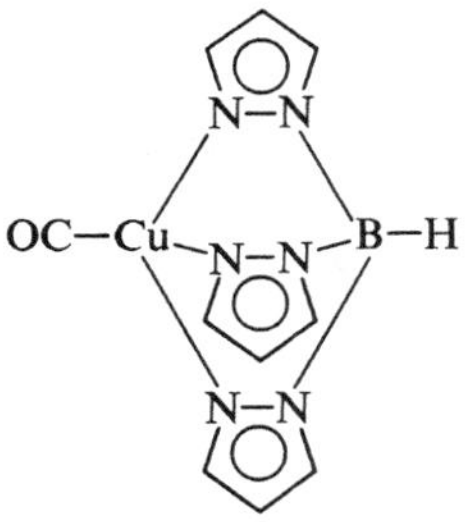

M 304.585

Cryst. (pet. ether). Sol. Me_2CO, THF. Mp 164-6°. Stable under CO atm. Rapid oxid. in soln.

Bruce, M.I. *et al*, *J. Chem. Soc., Dalton Trans.*, 1973, 2433 (*synth*)
Churchill, M.R. *et al*, *Inorg. Chem.*, 1975, **14**, 2051 (*cryst struct*)
Inorg. Synth., 1982, **21**, 108 (*synth*)

$C_{10}H_{14}CuLiS$ Cu-00038

Lithium phenylthio(*tert*-butyl)cuprate

Lithium(benzenethiolato)(1,1-dimethylethyl)cuprate, 9CI

[50281-66-8]

$(H_3C)_3CCuLiSPh$

M 236.768

Used in synth. of alkyl ketones from acid chlorides. Used in soln. Stable under N_2 at 0° at least 1 hr.

Posner, G.H. *et al*, *Synthesis*, 1974, 662 (*synth, use*)
Bennett, G.B. *et al*, *Org. Prep. Proced. Int.*, 1976, **8**, 13 (*use*)
Org. Synth., 1976, **55**, 122 (*synth, use*)
Fieser, M. *et al*, *Reagents for Organic Synthesis*, Wiley, 1967-83, **7**, 211.

$C_{10}H_{14}CuN$ Cu-00039

(η^5-2,4-Cyclopentadien-1-yl)(2-isocyano-2-methylpropane)-copper, 9CI

*(η-Cyclopentadienyl)(*tert*-butylisocyanide)copper*

[36222-40-9]

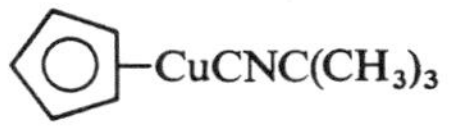

M 211.773

Catalyst for vinyl polymerisation. Cryst. (pentane). Sol. C_6H_6. Stable at r.t. for 1 month under N_2.

Saegusa, T. *et al*, *J. Am. Chem. Soc.*, 1971, **93**, 5656 (*synth, use*)
Tsuda, T. *et al*, *J. Am. Chem. Soc.*, 1974, **96**, 5930 (*synth*)
Takeo, H.S. *et al*, *Macromolecules*, 1975, **8**, 112 (*use*)

$C_{11}H_{15}CuO$ Cu-00040

Carbonyl(η^5-pentamethylcyclopentadienyl)copper

(η^5-Pentamethylcyclopentadienyl)(carbonyl)copper

[86045-48-9]

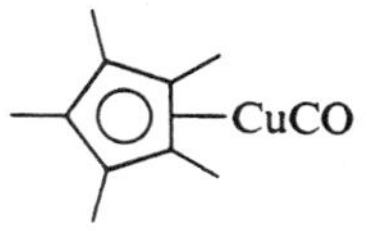

M 226.785

Cannot be isol. as pure solid because of limited stability. Stable at −78° under CO. Sol. Et_2O.

Macomber, D.W. *et al*, *J. Am. Chem. Soc.*, 1983, **105**, 5325 (*synth*)

$C_{11}H_{20}CuP$ Cu-00041

(η^5-2,4-Cyclopentadien-1-yl)(triethylphosphine)copper, 9CI

[12261-30-2]

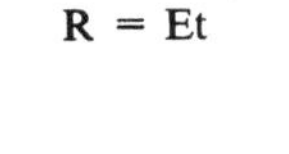

R = Et

M 246.799

η^5 in solid state and soln. Cryst. (pet. ether or by subl.). Sol. pet. ether, Et_2O, C_6H_6, liq. SO_2. Mp 122-4° dec. $Bp_{0.001}$ 55° subl. Solns. only moderately stable.

Wilkinson, G. *et al*, *J. Inorg. Nucl. Chem.*, 1956, **2**, 32 (*synth*)

Whitesides, G.M. *et al*, *J. Am. Chem. Soc.*, 1967, **89**, 2855 (*nmr*)
Cotton, F.A. *et al*, *J. Am. Chem. Soc.*, 1969, **91**, 7281; 1970, **92**, 5114 (*synth, ir*)
Delbaere, L.T.J. *et al*, *Acta Crystallogr., Sect. B*, 1970, **26**, 515 (*cryst struct*)
Tsuda, T. *et al*, *J. Am. Chem. Soc.*, 1972, **94**, 658 (*synth*)

$C_{12}H_{10}CuLi$ Cu-00042

Lithium diphenylcuprate(1−), 9CI
Diphenylcopperlithium
[23402-69-9]

$(Ph_2Cu)Li$

M 224.698
Phenylating agent. Prepd. and used *in situ*.

Whitesides, G.M. *et al*, *J. Am. Chem. Soc.*, 1969, **91**, 4871 (*synth, use*)
Normant, J.F. *et al*, *Synthesis*, 1972, 63 (*rev*)
Fuchs, P.L. *et al*, *J. Am. Chem. Soc.*, 1975, **97**, 7372 (*use*)

$C_{12}H_{27}CuIP$ Cu-00043

Iodo(tributylphosphine)copper

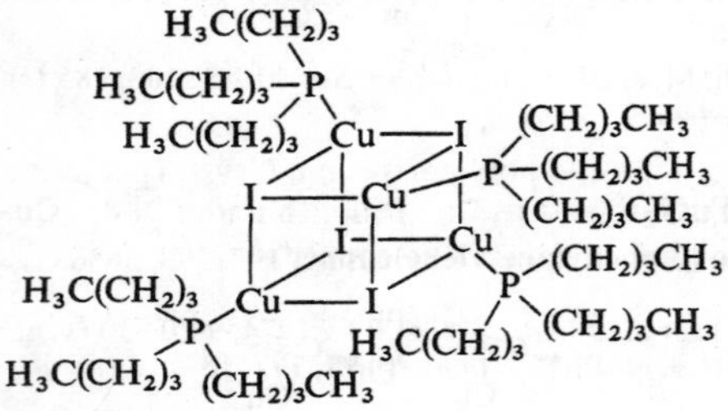

M 392.770
Tetrameric.
Tetramer: [59245-99-7]. *Tetraiodotetrakis(tributylphosphine)tetracopper*, *9CI.*
$C_{48}H_{108}Cu_4I_4P_4$ M 1571.078
Useful starting material for synth. of Li organocuprates. Cryst. ($EtOH/Me_2CO$). Sol. $CHCl_3$, C_6H_6, Et_2O. Mp 75°.
▷GL8942500.

Inorg. Synth., 1963, **7**, 10 (*synth*)
Cavazza, M. *et al*, *J. Chem. Soc., Chem. Commun.*, 1974, 501 (*use*)
Volkmann, R.A. *et al*, *J. Am. Chem. Soc.*, 1975, **97**, 4777 (*use*)

$C_{12}H_{36}CuOP_3Si$ Cu-00044

Tris(trimethylphosphine)(trimethylsilanolato)copper, 9CI
[40696-88-6]

$Me_3SiOCu(PMe_3)_3$

M 380.969
Sol. C_6H_6. Mp 72°.

Schmidbaur, H. *et al*, *Chem. Ber.*, 1972, **105**, 3389 (*synth*)

$C_{13}H_{16}CuFeN$ Cu-00045

[2-[(Dimethylamino)methyl]ferrocenyl-*C,N*]copper, 9CI
1-Copper-2-[(dimethylamino)methyl]ferrocene
[59612-86-1]

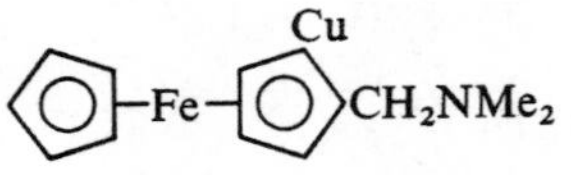

M 305.669
Intermed. for 2-arylferrocenes. Air-stable red-orange cryst. Insol. most org. solvs. Tetrameric struct. in solid state.

Nesmeyanov, A.N. *et al*, *Dokl. Akad. Nauk SSSR, Ser. Sci. Khim.*, 1976, **226**, 1092 (*synth, use, ir*)
Nesmeyanov, A.N. *et al*, *J. Organomet. Chem.*, 1977, **137**, 217 (*struct*)

$C_{13}H_{23}CuSi_2$ Cu-00046

[η-Bis(trimethylsilyl)acetylene](η^5-cyclopentadienyl)copper
[86024-12-6]

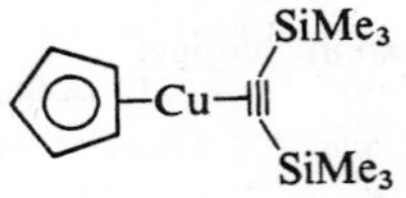

M 299.042
Pale-yellow cryst. (pentane at −78°). Sol. pentane, Et_2O, THF, C_6H_6. Air- and temp.-sensitive.

Macomber, D.W. *et al*, *J. Am. Chem. Soc.*, 1983, **105**, 5325 (*synth*)

$C_{16}H_{30}CuP$ Cu-00047

(η^5-Pentamethylcyclopentadienyl)(triethylphosphine)copper
[86024-10-4]

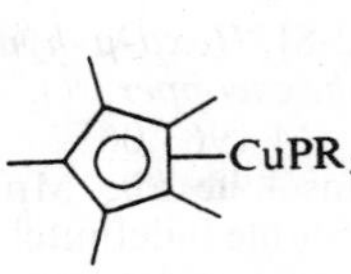

R = Et

M 316.933
Cryst. (pentane). Sol. pentane, Et_2O. Mp 152° dec. Air-sensitive in soln.

Macomber, D.W. *et al*, *J. Am. Chem. Soc.*, 1983, **105**, 5325 (*synth*)

$C_{16}H_{36}CuP$ Cu-00048

Butyl(tributylphosphine)copper, 9CI
[26679-41-4]

$H_3C(CH_2)_3CuP(CH_2CH_2CH_2CH_3)_3$

M 322.980
Dec. at 0° after 4h.

Whitesides, G.M. *et al*, *J. Am. Chem. Soc.*, 1970, **92**, 1426 (*synth*)
San Filippo, J. *et al*, *Inorg. Chem.*, 1978, **17**, 275 (*nmr*)
Bergbreiter, D.E. *et al*, *J. Org. Chem.*, 1981, **46**, 727.

$C_{18}H_{12}CuN_2O_2$ Cu-00049

Bis(8-quinolinolato-N^1,O^8)copper, 9CI
Oxine-copper, BSI
[10380-28-6]

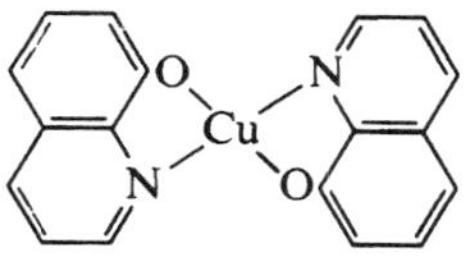

M 351.851
Protectant fungicide. Greenish-yellow cryst. powder. Insol. H_2O, common org. solvs. Dec. ca. 200°.
▷VC5250000.

Hollingshead, R.G.W., *Oxine and its Derivatives*, Butterworth, 1965, **1** (*synth, rev*)
Charalambous, J. *et al*, *Inorg. Chim. Acta*, 1977, **22**, 93 (*ms*)
Akaiwa, H. *et al*, *Bull. Chem. Soc. Jpn.*, 1979, **152**, 2453 (*ir*)
Pesticide Manual, 6th Ed., 396.

$C_{18}H_{16}CuP$ Cu-00050

Hydrido(triphenylphosphine)copper

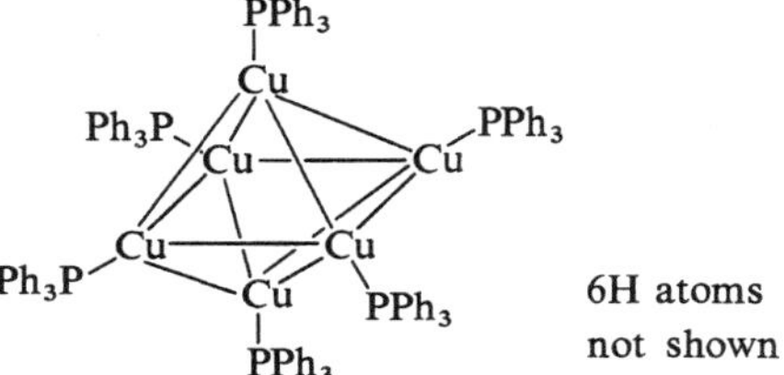

M 326.844
Octahedral hexameric cluster in solid state, oligomeric in soln.
Hexamer: [37702-12-8]. *Hexa-μ-hydridohexakis(triphenylphosphine)hexacopper*, 9CI.
$C_{108}H_{96}Cu_6P_6$ M 1961.065
Sol. C_6H_6, THF, insol. hexane. Mp 115° dec. Dec. in chlorinated solvs. Stable indefinitely under inert atmos.

Churchill, M.R. *et al*, *Inorg. Chem.*, 1972, **11**, 1818 (*synth, cryst struct*)
Inorg. Synth., 1979, **19**, 87 (*synth*)
Beguin, B. *et al*, *J. Organomet. Chem.*, 1981, **208**, C18 (*use*)

$C_{19}H_{36}CuP$ Cu-00051

Methyl(tricyclohexylphosphine)copper, 9CI
Methylcopper(tricyclohexylphosphine)
[53426-24-7]

$MeCuP(C_6H_{11})_3$

M 359.013
Air- and mositure-sensitive cryst. (Et_2O). Sol. Et_2O, THF, Me_2CO, toluene, C_6H_6, Py. Mp 105-10° dec.

Yamamoto, A. *et al*, *J. Organomet. Chem.*, 1974, **72**, 145 (*synth, pmr*)
Miyashita, A. *et al*, *Bull. Chem. Soc. Jpn.*, 1977, **50**, 1109 (*synth*)

$C_{20}H_{26}B_8CuP$ Cu-00052

(Triphenylphosphine)[(7,8,9-η)-undecahydro-5,6-dicarbadecaborato(1−)]copper, 10CI
[74354-44-2]

$(Ph_3P)Cu(C_2B_8H_{11})$

M 447.425
Struct. not known. Bright-yellow cryst. (Me_2CO). Sol. Me_2CO.

Colquhoun, H.M. *et al*, *J. Chem. Soc., Chem. Commun.*, 1980, 192 (*synth, nmr*)

$C_{20}H_{37}Cu_2N_4O_3^{\oplus}$ Cu-00053

(μ-Carbonyl)(μ-benzoato-*O,O'*)bis(*N,N,N',N'*-tetramethylethylenediamine)dicopper(1+)
[75812-17-8]

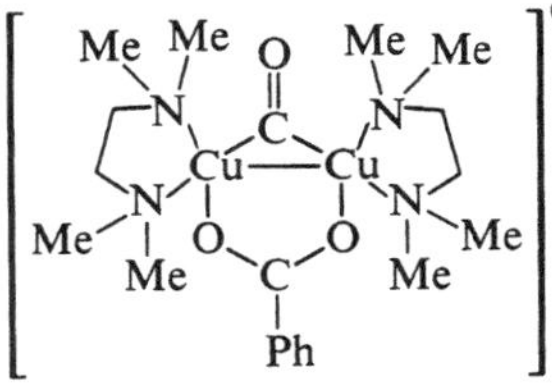

M 508.629 (ion)
Bridging carbonyl complex of Cu(I).
Tetraphenylborate:
$C_{44}H_{57}BCu_2N_4O_3$ M 827.861
Light-yellow cryst. (MeOH). Sol. THF, spar. sol. toluene.

Pasquali, M. *et al*, *J. Am. Chem. Soc.*, 1981, **103**, 185 (*synth, cryst struct*)

$C_{21}H_{15}CuO_2$ Cu-00054

(Benzoato)(diphenylacetylene)copper

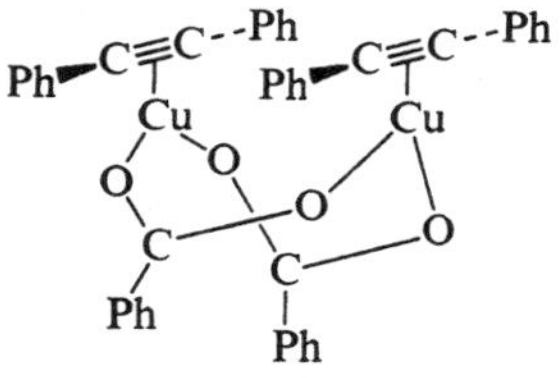

M 362.894
Dimeric.
Dimer: [82808-26-2]. *Bis[μ-(benzoato-O,O')]bis[1,1'-(η²-1,2-ethynediyl)bis[benzene]]dicopper*, 10CI. *Dibenzoatobis(diphenylacetylene)dicopper.*
$C_{42}H_{30}Cu_2O_4$ M 725.789
Cryst. (MeOH). Sol. MeOH.

Pasquali, M. *et al*, *Inorg. Chem.*, 1982, **21**, 4324 (*synth, cryst struct*)

$C_{23}H_{20}CuP$ Cu-00055

(η^5-2,4-Cyclopentadien-1-yl)triphenylphosphinecopper, 9CI
[31781-67-6]
As (η^5-2,4-Cyclopentadien-1-yl)(triethylphosphine)copper, Cu-00041 with

R = Ph

M 390.931
Cryst. (Et_2O at −78°). Mp 140° dec.

Colton, F.A. *et al*, *J. Am. Chem. Soc.*, 1969, **91**, 7281; 1970, **92**, 5114 (*synth*)
Colton, F.A. *et al*, *J. Am. Chem. Soc.*, 1970, **92**, 2353 (*cryst struct*)

$C_{26}H_{13}CuN_3O_6$ Cu-00056

Matchamycin, 8CI

Struct. unknown

M 526.951

Prod. by *Streptomyces E*-753. Copper-containing antibiotic active against gram-positive and -negative bacteria. Green cryst. (MeOH). Sol. $CHCl_3$, EtOH, insol. C_6H_6, Et_2O. Mp 150-6° dec. $[\alpha]_D^{25}$ +33° (c, 0.1 in DMSO).

Kimura, A. *et al*, *J. Antibiot.*, 1970, **23**, 461 (*isol*, *ir*, *uv*)

$C_{28}H_{30}CuP$ Cu-00057

(η^5-Pentamethylcyclopentadienyl)triphenylphosphinecopper

[86024-09-1]

As (η^5-Pentamethylcyclopentadienyl)(triethylphosphine)-copper, Cu-00047 with

R = Ph

M 461.065

Cryst. (Et_2O at −78°). Sol. Et_2O. Mp 145° dec. Air-sensitive in soln.

Macomber, D.W. *et al*, *J. Am. Chem. Soc.*, 1983, **105**, 5325 (*synth*)

$C_{32}H_{40}Br_2Cu_6N_4$ Cu-00058

Di-μ-bromotetrakis[μ_3-(2-dimethylaminophenyl-*C*:*C*:*N*)]hexacopper, 9CI

[58616-70-9]

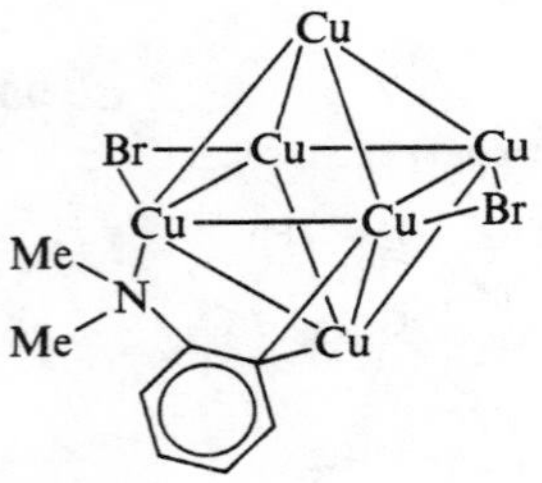

Only one of four amine groups shown

M 1021.779

Orange cryst. (C_6H_6). Sol. C_6H_6. Mp 198-202° dec.

Guss, J.M. *et al*, *J. Organomet. Chem.*, 1972, **40**, C79 (*cryst struct*)
van Koten, G. *et al*, *J. Organomet. Chem.*, 1975, **102**, 551 (*synth*)
van Koten, G. *et al*, *J. Org. Chem.*, 1977, **42**, 2047 (*use*)

$C_{36}H_{30}CuNO_3P_2$ Cu-00059

Nitratobis(triphenylphosphine)copper, 9CI

[23751-62-4]

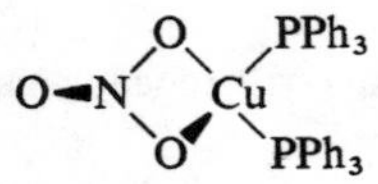

M 650.131

Cryst. (MeOH). Sol. $CHCl_3$, CH_2Cl_2, MeCN, DMF. Mp 248° dec.

Messmer, G.G., *Inorg. Chem.*, 1969, **8**, 2750 (*cryst struct*)
Jardine, F.H., *J. Inorg. Nucl. Chem.*, 1971, **33**, 2941 (*ir*)
Inorg. Synth., 1979, **19**, 93 (*synth*)

$C_{36}H_{30}Cu_5^{\ominus}$ Cu-00060

Hexa-μ-phenylpentacuprate(1−)

[81027-54-5]

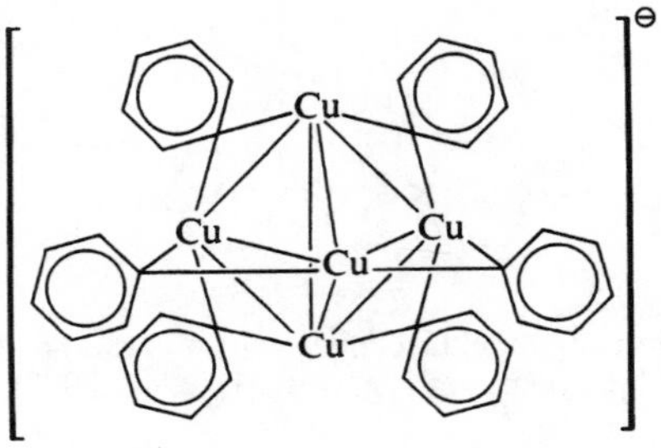

M 780.363 (ion)

Li salt, tetra-THF complex:
$C_{52}H_{62}Cu_5LiO_4$ M 1075.730
Pale-yellow cryst. (Et_2O). Sol. Et_2O.

Edwards, P.G. *et al*, *J. Am. Chem. Soc.*, 1982, **104**, 2072 (*synth*, *cryst struct*)

$C_{36}H_{34}BCuP_2$ Cu-00062

[Tetrahydroborato(1−)-*H*,*H'*]bis(triphenylphospine)copper, 9CI

Bis(triphenylphosphine)copper(I) borohydride

[16903-61-0]

$(Ph_3P)_2CuBH_4$

M 602.968

Reducing agent for converting RCOCl → RCHO. Cryst. ($CHCl_3$/EtOH). Sol. H_2O, org. solvs. Mp 164° dec., 177° dec. Forms C_6H_6 solvate, Mp 187°.

Davidson, J.M., *Chem. Ind.* (*London*), 1964, 2021 (*synth*)
Cariati, F. *et al*, *Gazz. Chim. Ital.*, 1965, **95**, 3 (*synth*)
Lippard, S.J. *et al*, *J. Am. Chem. Soc.*, 1967, **89**, 3929 (*cryst struct*)
Fleet, G.W.J. *et al*, *Tetrahedron Lett.*, 1978, 1437 (*use*)
Sorell, T.N. *et al*, *J. Org. Chem.*, 1980, **45**, 3449 (*synth*, *use*)
Fieser, M. *et al*, *Reagents for Organic Synthesis*, Wiley, 1967-83, **8**, 47.

Suggestions for new Entries are welcomed. Please write to the Editor, Dictionary of Organometallic Compounds, Chapman and Hall Ltd, 11 New Fetter Lane, London EC4P 4EE

$C_{36}H_{48}Au_2Cu_2N_4$ Cu-00063

Tetrakis[2-[(dimethylamino)methyl]phenyl]bis(copper)digold, 9CI

[55466-93-8]

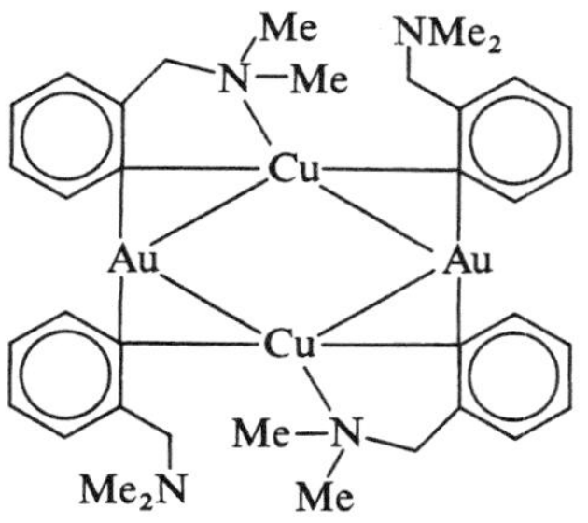

M 1057.827

Ochre solid. Sol. C_6H_6. Mp 137-9° dec.

van Koten, G. *et al*, *J. Organomet. Chem.*, 1974, **82**, C53; 1980, **186**, 427.

$C_{39}H_{43}BCuP$ Cu-00064

Tris(methyldiphenylphosphine)[tetrahydroborato(1−)-*H*]-copper

[63371-86-8]

$H_3B{-}H{-}Cu(PMePh_2)_3$

M 617.098

An example of monodentate $BH_4^{\ominus}$ ligand. Cryst. (CH_2Cl_2/pentane). Sol. CH_2Cl_2, $CHCl_3$. Mp 119-21° dec.

Bommer, J.C. *et al*, *Inorg. Chem.*, 1980, **19**, 587 (*synth*)
Takusagawa, F. *et al*, *J. Am. Chem. Soc.*, 1981, **103**, 5165 (*cryst struct, neutron struct*)

$C_{40}H_{56}Cu_4N_4$ Cu-00065

Tetrakis[μ-[2-[(dimethylamino)methyl]-5-methylphenyl-*C*:*C*,*N*]]tetracopper, 9CI

[37036-31-0]

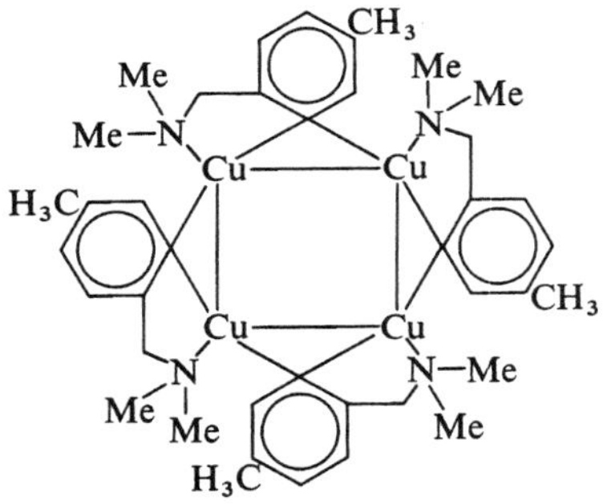

M 847.093

Distorted tetrameric cluster. Yellow cryst. (C_6H_6). Sol. C_6H_6, Et_2O. Mp 170-210° dec.

van Koten, G. *et al*, *J. Chem. Soc., Chem. Commun.*, 1970, 1107 (*synth*)
Guss, J.M. *et al*, *J. Chem. Soc., Chem. Commun.*, 1972, 446 (*cryst struct*)
van Koten, G. *et al*, *J. Organomet. Chem.*, 1975, **84**, 117, 129 (*synth*)
van Koten, G. *et al*, *J. Am. Chem. Soc.*, 1979, **101**, 6593 (*synth*)
van Koten, G. *et al*, *J. Organomet. Chem.*, 1979, **177**, 283 (*use*)

$C_{50}H_{54}Cu_6N_4$ Cu-00066

Tetrakis[μ_3-[2-(dimethylaminophenyl)-*C*:*C*:*N*]]bis[μ-[(4-methylphenyl)ethenyl]]hexacopper, 10CI

1,2,3;1,4,5;2,3,6;4,5,6-Tetrakis-μ_3-2-dimethylamino-phenyl-2,5;3,4-bis-μ_2-4-tolylethynyl-octahedro-*hexacopper*

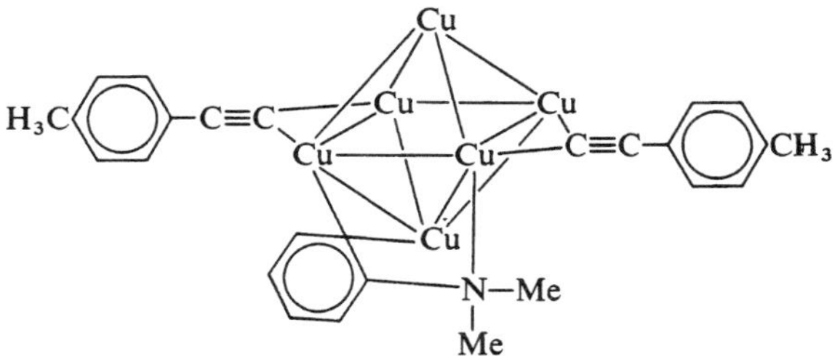

only one of four μ_3-$C_6H_4NMe_2$ groups shown

M 1092.279

Octahedral cluster of copper with bridging μ_2-ethynyl and μ_3-$C_6H_4NMe_2$. Yellow solid. Sol. C_6H_6. Mp 138° dec.

ten Hoedt, R.W.M. *et al*, *J. Organomet. Chem.*, 1977, **133**, 113 (*synth*)
van Koten, G. *et al*, *J. Org. Chem.*, 1977, **42**, 2705 (*use*)
ten Hoedt, R.W.M. *et al*, *J. Chem. Soc., Dalton Trans.*, 1978, 1800 (*cryst struct*)

$C_{55}H_{48}CuP_3$ Cu-00067

Methyltris(triphenylphosphine)copper, 9CI

Methylcoppertris(triphenylphosphine)

[38704-10-8]

$MeCu(PPh_3)_3$

M 865.451

Unstable yellow powder.

Toluene solvate: Light-sensitive yellow needles.

Et_2O solvate: Can be stored under N_2 in dark at r.t.

Costa, G. *et al*, *J. Inorg. Nucl. Chem.*, 1964, **26**, 961 (*synth*)
Yamamoto, A. *et al*, *Bull. Chem. Soc. Jpn.*, 1972, **45**, 1583 (*synth*)
Miyashita, A. *et al*, *Bull. Chem. Soc. Jpn.*, 1977, **50**, 1109 (*synth, props*)

$C_{56}H_{100}CuN_{18}O_{24}S_2$ Cu-00068

Zorbamycin

[11056-20-5]

M 1537.178

Isol. from *Streptomyces bikiniensis*. Shows antibiotic props. Blue amorph. solid. Probably related to Bleomycin family.

▷ZI2300000.

B,2HCl: $[\alpha]_D^{25}$ +247° (c, 0.6 in H_2O). λ_{max} 244, 290 sh, 298, 309 and 600 nm (MeOH).

Argoudelis, A.D. *et al*, *J. Antibiot.*, 1971, **24**, 543 (*isol*)
Issaq, H.J. *et al*, *J. Chromatogr.*, 1977, **133**, 291 (*tlc*)

$C_{58}H_{90}CuN_{18}O_{24}S_2$ **Cu-00069**
Zorbanomycin *B*

[12689-49-5]
M 1551.121
Isol. from *Streptomyces bikiniensis*. Antibiotic. Inhibits both gram-positive and -negative bacteria as well as various fungi. Disinfectant. Blue amorph. solid. Zorbanomycin *C* has similar props.

B,2HCl: [37299-61-9]. λ_{max} 243, 293, 308 sh, and 600 nm (MeOH).

Argoudelis, A.D. *et al*, *J. Antibiot.*, 1971, **24**, 543 (*isol*)

Ni Nickel

R. J. Cross

Nickel (Fr., Ger.), Niquel (Sp.), Nichel (Ital.), Никель (Nikiel) (Russ.), ニッケル (Japan.)

Atomic Number. 28

Atomic Weight. 58.70. Note that the limitation to accuracy is greater than the computed molecular weights of the entries suggest.

Electronic Configuration. [Ar] $3d^8\ 4s^2$

Oxidation States. The most common oxidation levels for organometallic compounds are +2 (d^8) and 0 (d^{10}). Both 16- and 18-electron compounds are common for each oxidation level.

Coordination Number. With conventional (η^1) ligands, four-coordinate square-planar geometry dominates oxidation level +2, whereas the zero-valent complexes are often tetrahedral.

Colour. Variable.

Availability. Common starting materials include $[Ni(OH_2)_6]Cl_2$, anhydrous $NiBr_2$ and nickel metal itself.

Handling. Although nickel compounds are the most prone to atmospheric or thermal degradation in the Ni, Pd, Pt triad, many of the compounds described are nevertheless air-stable and can be handled without precautions, at least as pure solids. Solutions are noticeably more prone to aerial oxidation or thermolysis, however, and it is wise both to protect them under an inert atmosphere, and to reduce time in solution to a minimum.

Toxicity. Nickel compounds, apart from the carbonyl complexes, are not especially toxic.

Isotopic Abundance. ^{58}Ni, 68.27%; ^{60}Ni, 26.10%; ^{61}Ni, 1.13%; ^{62}Ni, 3.59%; ^{64}Ni, 0.91%.

Spectroscopy. Nickel has no important magnetic isotopes (^{61}Ni at 1.13% natural abundance has $I = \frac{3}{2}$); most organometallic compounds are diamagnetic, making ^1H, ^{13}C, and ^{31}P nmr spectra valuable.

Analysis. Atomic absorption spectroscopy is now commonly used to analyse for nickel. Response is linear in the 0 – 5 ppm range, and sensitivity is 0.15 $\mu g\ cm^{-3}$.

Nickel can also be estimated gravimetrically as its bis(dimethylglyoximate). This is precipitated by adding dimethylglyoxime to ammoniacal solutions, after digesting the nickel compound in sulphuric acid.

The red precipitate of nickel bis(dimethylglyoximate) makes a sensitive spot test for nickel ions.

References. The low cost and high reactivity of nickel compounds contribute to their frequent use in organic synthetic and catalytic reactions. The reactions frequently exploit the easy transitions between 16- and 18-electron molecules.

In addition to reviews cited in the introduction to the *Sourcebook*, the reader is referred to the following:

Jolly, P. W. and Wilke, G., *The Organic Chemistry of Nickel*, Academic Press, New York, 1974, **1**; 1975, **2**.

$[Ni(CO)_3Cl]^{\ominus}$ (C_{3v})

Ni-00001

$[Ni(GeCl_3)(CO)_3]^{\ominus}$ (C_{3v})

Ni-00002

$Ni(CO)_3PCl_3$ (C_{3v})

Ni-00003

$Ni(CO)_3PF_3$ (C_{3v})

Ni-00004

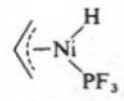

Ni-00005

$[Ni(CO)_3I]^{\ominus}$ (C_{3v})

Ni-00006

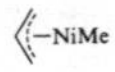

Ni-00007

$NiMe_4^{\ominus\ominus}$ (D_{4h})

Ni-00008

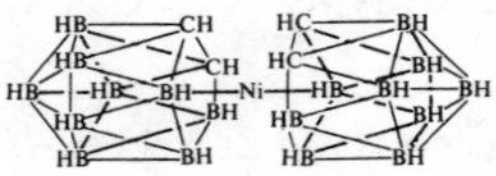

Ni-00009

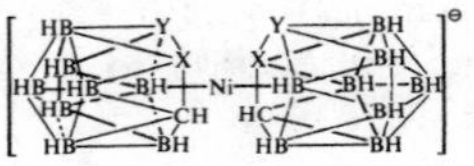

X = CH, Y = BH

Ni-00010

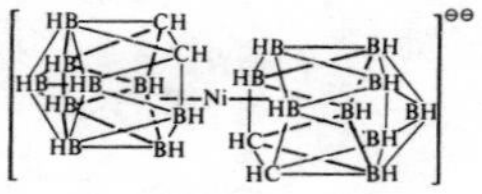

Ni-00011

As Ni-00010 with
X = B, Y = C

Ni-00012

$Ni(CN)_4^{\ominus\ominus}$ (D_{4h})

Ni-00013

$Ni(CO)_4$

Ni-00014

$Ni(CS)_4$ (T_d)

Ni-00015

$MeNCNi(CO)_3$ (C_{3v})

Ni-00016

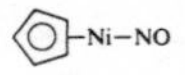

Ni-00017

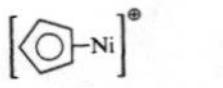

Ni-00018

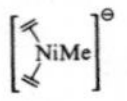

Ni-00019

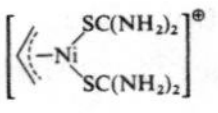

Ni-00020

$NiBr(C_6F_5)$

Ni-00021

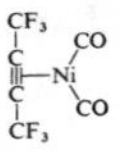

Ni-00022

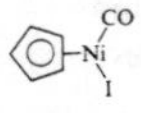

Ni-00023

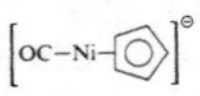

Ni-00024

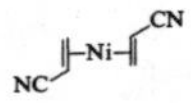

Ni-00025

$(MeNC)_2Ni(CO)_2$ (C_{2v})

Ni-00026

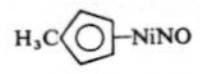

Ni-00027

$Ni(CO)_3P(OMe)_3$

Ni-00028

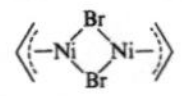

Ni-00029

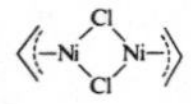

Ni-00030

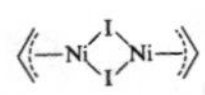

Ni-00031

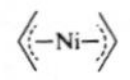

Ni-00032

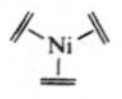

Ni-00033

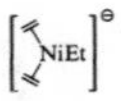

Ni-00034

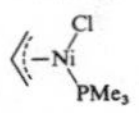

Ni-00035

$[(NC)_3Ni—Ni(CN)_3]^{\ominus\ominus\ominus\ominus}$

Ni-00036

$Ni_2(CO)_6^{\ominus\ominus}$

Ni-00037

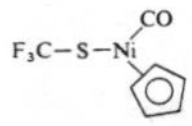

Ni-00038

$(MeNC)_3NiCO$ (C_{3v})

Ni-00039

$Ni(CO)_3(SEt_2)$

Ni-00040

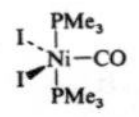

Ni-00041

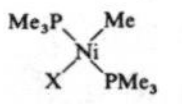

X = Cl

Ni-00042

As Ni-00042 with
X = I

Ni-00043

$[Ni(C{\equiv}CH)_4]^{\ominus\ominus}$ (D_{4h})

Ni-00044

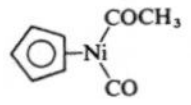

Ni-00045

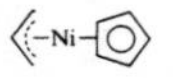

Ni-00046

$(MeNC)_4Ni$ (T_d)

Ni-00047

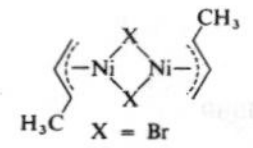

X = Br

Ni-00048

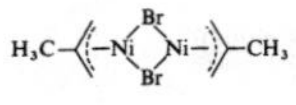

Ni-00049

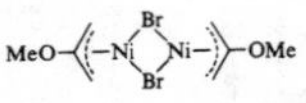

Ni-00050

As Ni-00048 with
X = Cl

Ni-00051

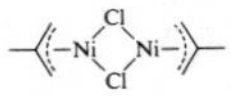

Ni-00052

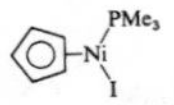

Ni-00053

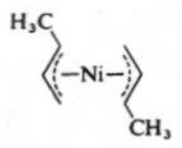

Ni-00054

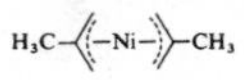

Ni-00055

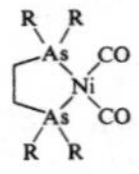

R = Me

Ni-00056

$[(H_2C{=}CH_2)_2Ni—H—Ni(H_2C{=}CH_2)_2]^{\ominus}$

Ni-00057

$Ni(CO)_2(PMe_3)_2$

Ni-00058

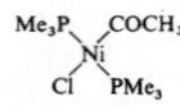

Ni-00059

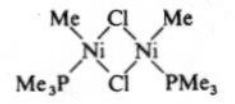

Ni-00060

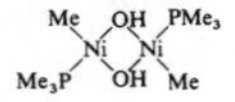

trans-form

Ni-00061

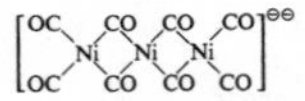

Ni-00062

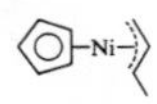

Ni-00063

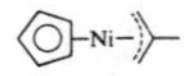

Ni-00064

Ni-00065

Ni-00066

L = R = Me

Ni-00067

Ni-00068

Ni-00069

Ni-00070

Ni-00071

Ni-00072

Ni-00073

Ni-00074

Ni-00075

As Ni-00066 with
L = $COCH_3$, R = Me

Ni-00076

$Ni(CO)(PMe_3)_3$ (C_{3v})

Ni-00077

Ni-00078

Ni-00079

Ni-00080

$Ni(C_6F_5)_2$

Ni-00081

Ni-00082

Ni-00083

Ni-00084

Ni-00085

Ni-00086

Ni-00087

Ni-00088

Ni-00089

Ni-00090

Ni-00091

Ni-00092

Ni-00093

Ni-00094

Ni-00095

trans-form

Ni-00096

R = Me

Ni-00097

$[(MeO)_3P]_4Ni$

Ni-00098

$(Me_3P)_4Ni$ (T_d)

Ni-00099

$[Ni_3Pt_3(CO)_{12}]^{\ominus\ominus}$

Ni-00100

Ni-00101

Ni-00102

Ni-00103

R = H

Ni-00104

Ni-00105

Ni-00106

Ni-00107

Ni-00108

Ni-00109

Ni-00110

Ni-00111

Ni-00112

Ni-00113

Ni-00114

Ni-00115

Ni-00116

Ni-00117

Ni-00118

As Ni-00104 with
R = CH_3

Ni-00119

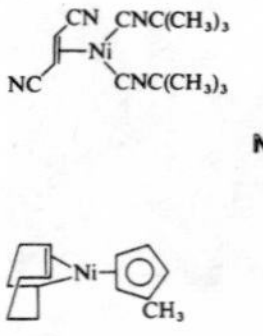

Ni-00120

Ni-00121

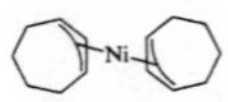

Ni-00122

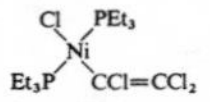

Ni-00123

$Ni(CO)_2(PEt_3)_2$ (T_d)

Ni-00124

$NiMe_2(PEt_3)_2$

Ni-00125

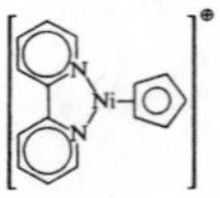

Ni-00126

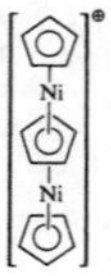

Ni-00127

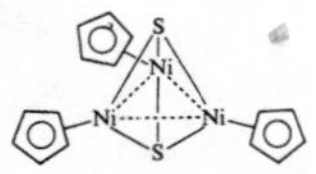

Ni-00128

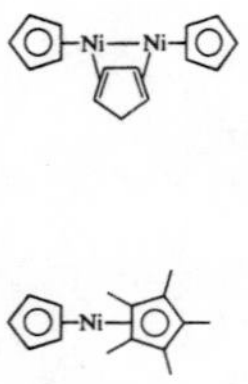

Ni-00129

Ni-00130

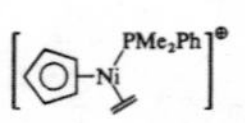

Ni-00131

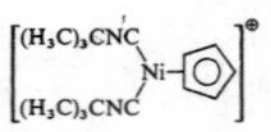

Ni-00132

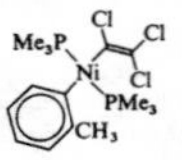

Ni-00133

$Ni(CO)_3P(CH_2CH_2CH_2CH_3)_3$ (T_d)

Ni-00134

$Ni(CO)_3P[C(CH_3)_3]_3$

Ni-00135

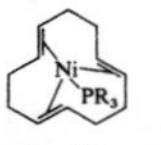

R = Me

Ni-00136

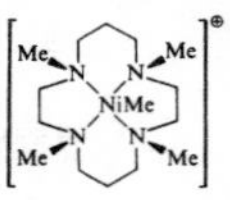

Ni-00137

$Ni[P(OMe)_3]_5^{\oplus\oplus}$ (D_{3h})

Ni-00138

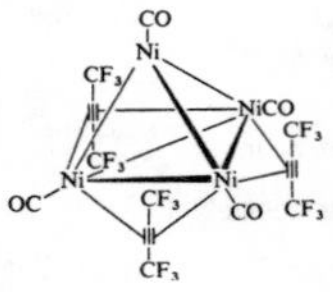

Ni-00139

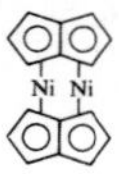

Ni-00140

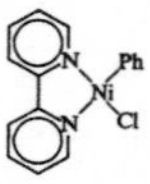

Ni-00141

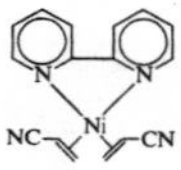

Ni-00142

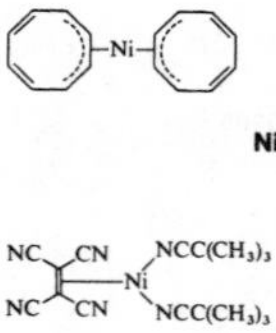

Ni-00143

Ni-00144

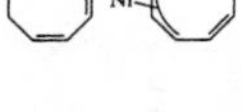

Ni-00145

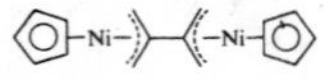

Ni-00146

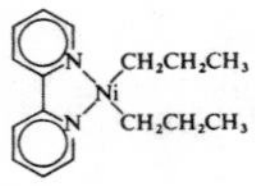

Ni-00147

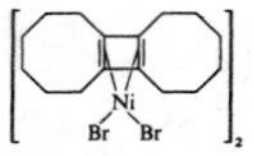

Ni-00148

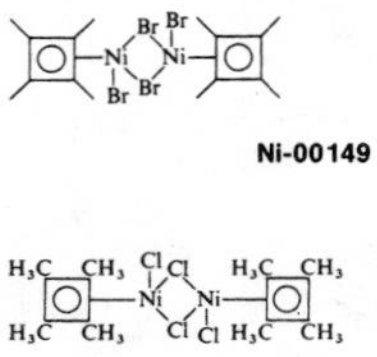

Ni-00149

Ni-00150

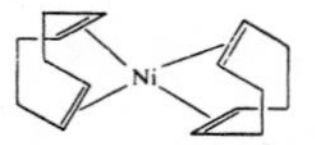

Ni-00151

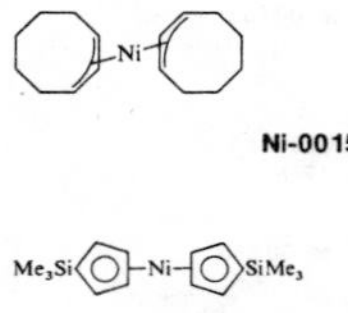

Ni-00152

Ni-00153

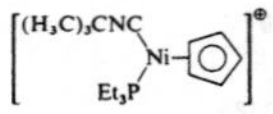

Ni-00154

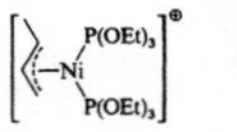

Ni-00155

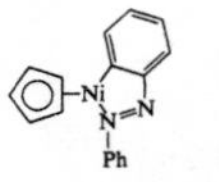

Ni-00156

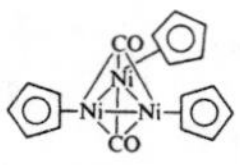

Ni-00157

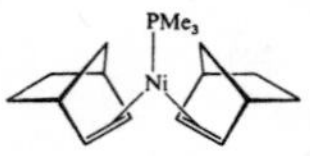

Ni-00158

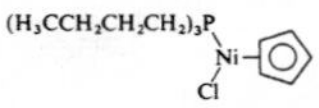

Ni-00159

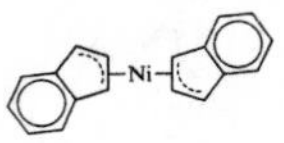

Ni-00160

$[NiPh_3]^{\ominus\ominus\ominus}$

Ni-00161

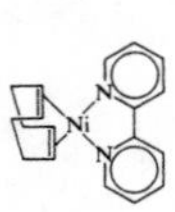

Ni-00162

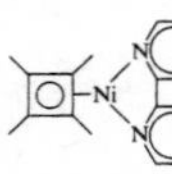

Ni-00163

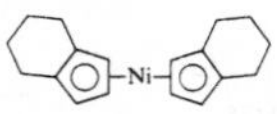

Ni-00164

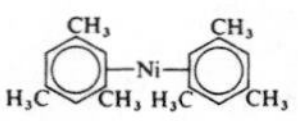

Ni-00165

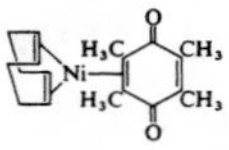

Ni-00166

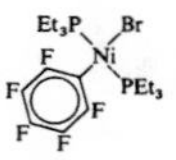

Ni-00167

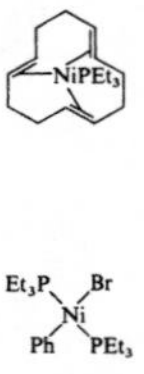

Ni-00168

Ni-00169

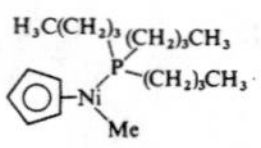

Ni-00170

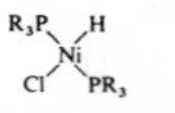

R = $(H_3C)_2CH-$

Ni-00171

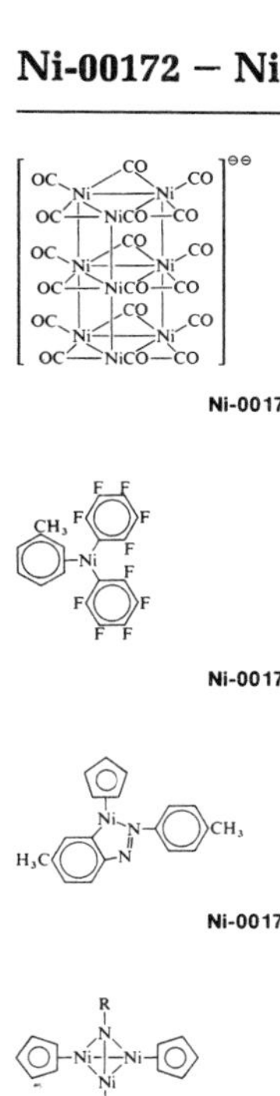

Ni-00172

Ni-00173

Ni-00174

Ni-00175

Ni-00176

Ni-00177

Ni-00178

Ni-00179

Ni-00180

Ni-00181

Ni-00182

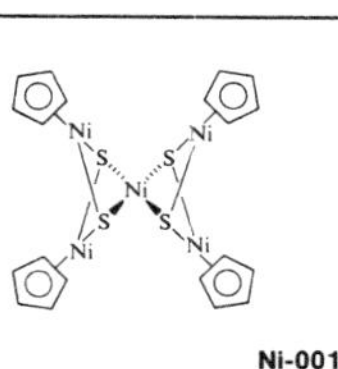

Ni-00183

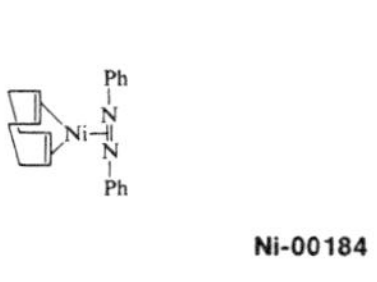

Ni-00184

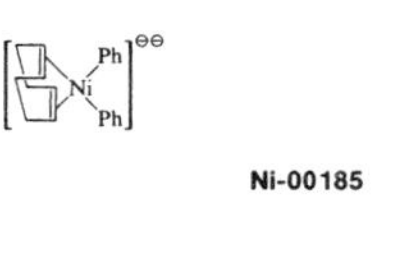

Ni-00185

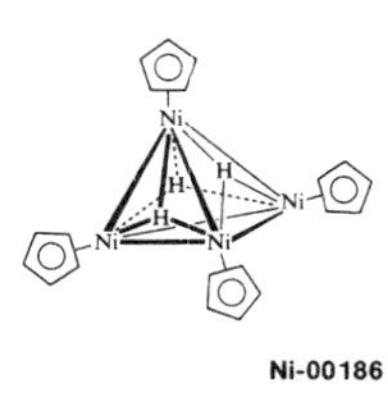

Ni-00186

Ni-00187

Ni-00188

Ni-00189

$[(H_3C)_3CNC]_4Ni$ (T_d)

Ni-00190

Ni-00191

Ni-00192

Ni-00193

Ni-00194

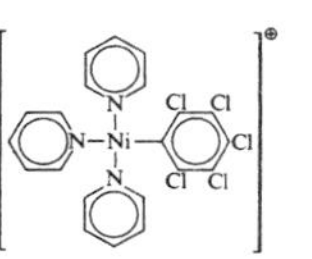

Ni-00195

$Ni(CO)_3(PPh_3)$ (C_{3v})

Ni-00196

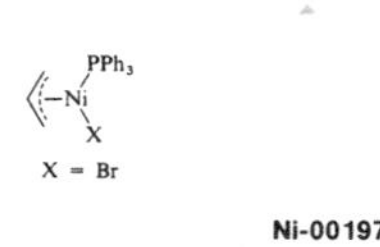

Ni-00197

As Ni-00197 with
X = Cl

Ni-00198

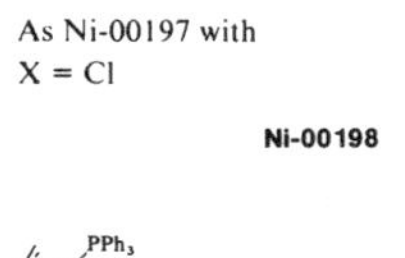

Ni-00199

Ni-00200

Ni-00201

Ni-00202

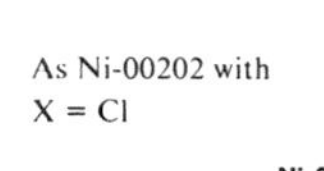

As Ni-00202 with
X = Cl

Ni-00203

Ni-00204

As Ni-00187 with
R = Ph

Ni-00205

Ni-00206

Ni-00207

Ni-00208

Ni-00209

Ni-00210

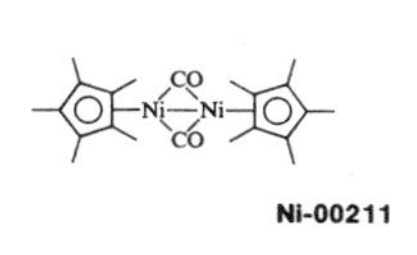

Ni-00211

Ni-00212

Ni-00213

Ni-00214

Ni-00215

Ni-00216

Ni-00217

Ni-00218

Ni-00219

Ni-00220

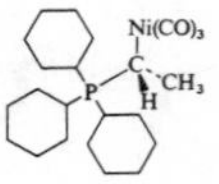

Ni-00221

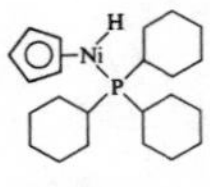

Ni-00222

$[Ni(C_6F_5)_4]^{\ominus\ominus}$ (D_{4h})

Ni-00223

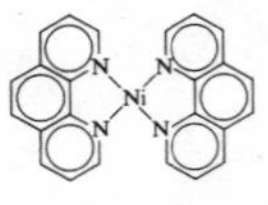

Ni-00224

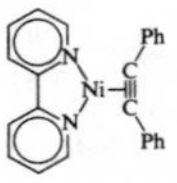

Ni-00225

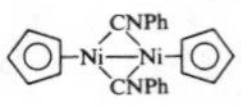

Ni-00226

$NiPh_4^{\ominus\ominus}$ (D_{4h})

Ni-00227

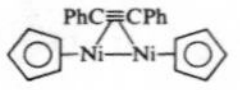

Ni-00228

$Ni(CH_2{=}CHCN)_2(PPh_3)$

Ni-00229

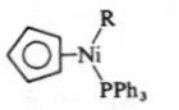

R = Me

Ni-00230

$(PhCH{=}CH_2)_3Ni$

Ni-00231

As Ni-00066 with
L = Me, R = Ph

Ni-00232

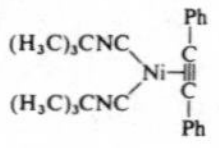

Ni-00233

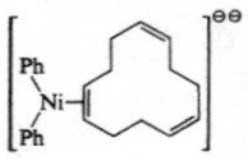

Ni-00234

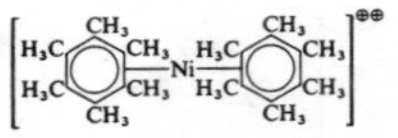

Ni-00235

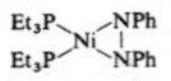

Ni-00236

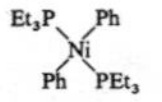

Ni-00237

As Ni-00066 with
L = Me, R = cyclohexyl

Ni-00238

$[(EtO)_3P]_4Ni$ (T_d)

Ni-00239

$(Et_3P)_4Ni$ (T_d)

Ni-00240

$[NiH[P(OEt)_3]_4]^{\oplus}$

Ni-00241

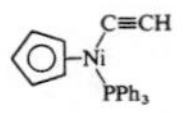

Ni-00242

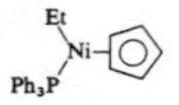

Ni-00243

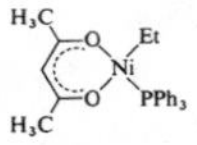

Ni-00244

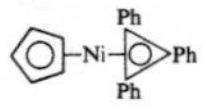

Ni-00245

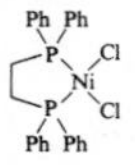

Ni-00246

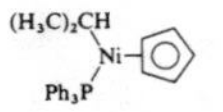

Ni-00247

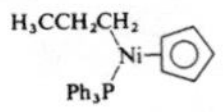

Ni-00248

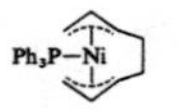

Ni-00249

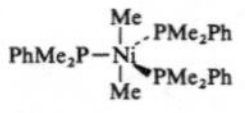

Ni-00250

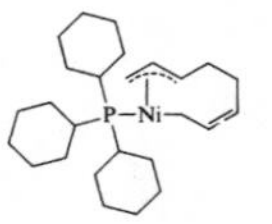

Ni-00251

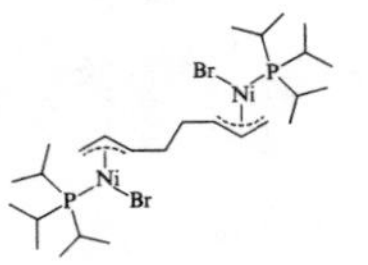

Ni-00252

As Ni-00230 with
R = $H_3C(CH_2)_3-$

Ni-00253

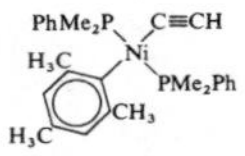

Ni-00254

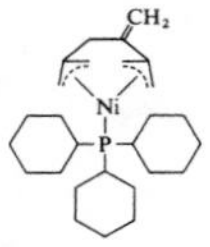

Ni-00255

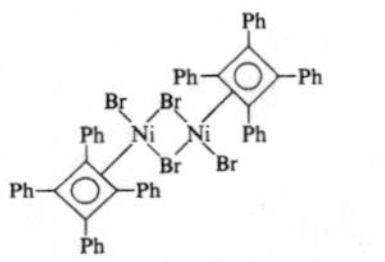

Ni-00256

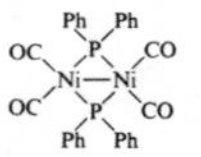

Ni-00257

As Ni-00056 with
R = Ph

Ni-00258

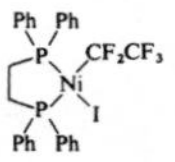

Ni-00259

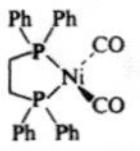

Ni-00260

$Ni(CO)_2(PMePh_2)_2$

Ni-00261

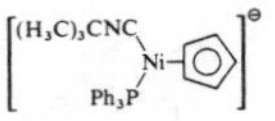

Ni-00262

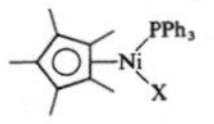

X = Br

Ni-00263

As Ni-00263 with
X = I

Ni-00264

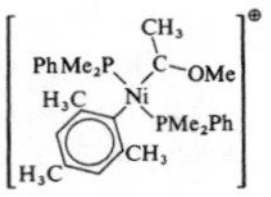

Ni-00265

$Ni(C{\equiv}CPh)_2(PEt_3)_2$

Ni-00266

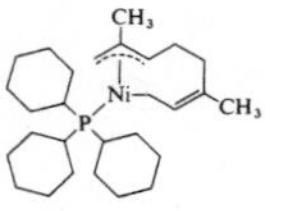

Ni-00267

$(C_6H_{11}NC)_4Ni$ (T_d)

Ni-00268

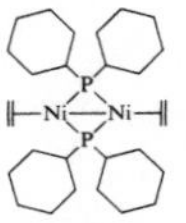

Ni-00269

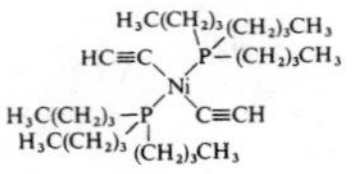

Ni-00270

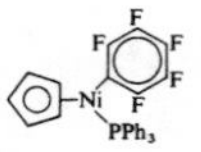

Ni-00271

As Ni-00230 with
R = Ph

Ni-00272

As Ni-00066 with
L = R = Ph

Ni-00273

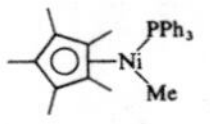

Ni-00274

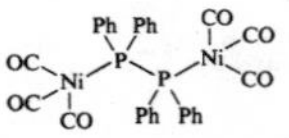

Ni-00275

As Ni-00066 with
L = COPh, R = Ph

Ni-00277

Struct. resembles Ni-00279 (neutral molecule)

Ni-00278

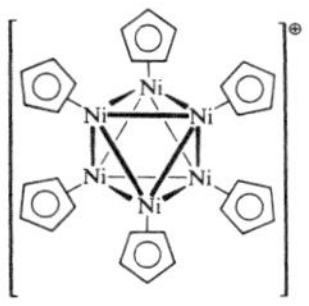

Ni-00279

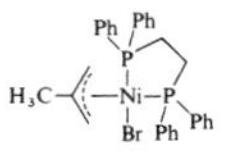

Ni-00280

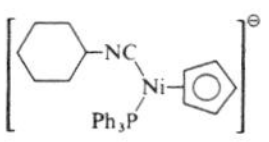

Ni-00281

As Ni-00136 with
R = Ph

Ni-00282

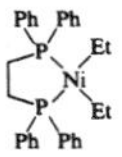

Ni-00283

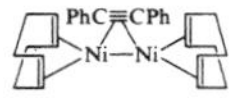

Ni-00284

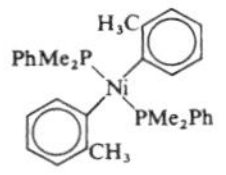

Ni-00285

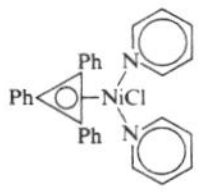

Ni-00286

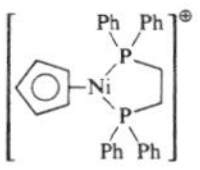

Ni-00287

$[Ni(C{\equiv}CPh)_4]^{\ominus\ominus}$ (D_{4h})

Ni-00288

$[Ni(C{\equiv}CPh)_4]^{\ominus\ominus\ominus\ominus}$ (T_d)

Ni-00289

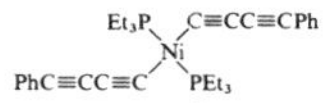

Ni-00290

$(Me_2PhP)_4Ni$ (T_d)

Ni-00291

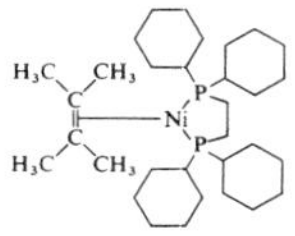

Ni-00292

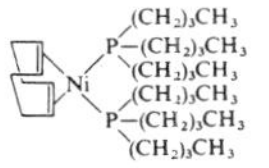

Ni-00293

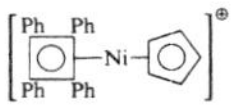

Ni-00294

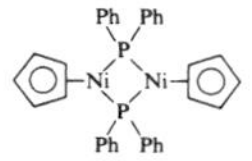

Ni-00295

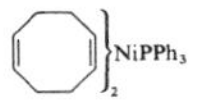

Ni-00296

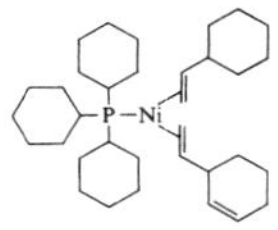

Ni-00297

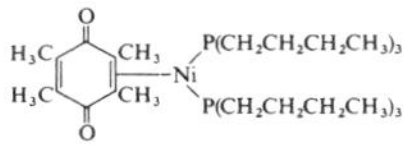

Ni-00298

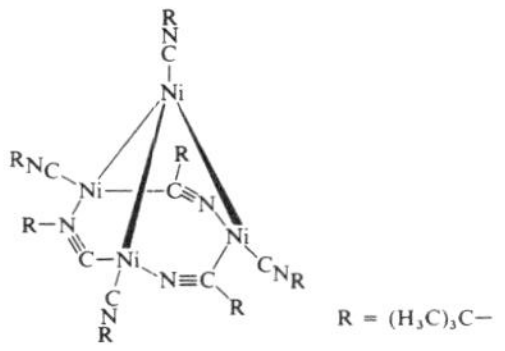

R = $(H_3C)_3C-$

Ni-00299

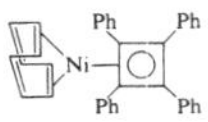

Ni-00300

$(Ph_3P)_2NiBr_2$ (T_d)

Ni-00301

$(Ph_3P)_2NiCl_2$

Ni-00302

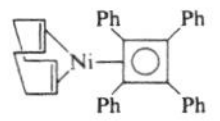

Ni-00303

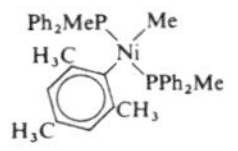

Ni-00304

As Ni-00171 with
R = cyclohexyl

Ni-00305

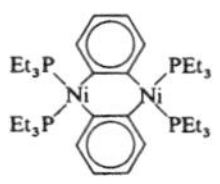

Ni-00306

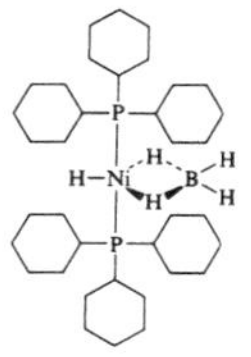

Ni-00307

$[[(H_3C)_2CHO]_3P_4Ni$ (T_d)

Ni-00308

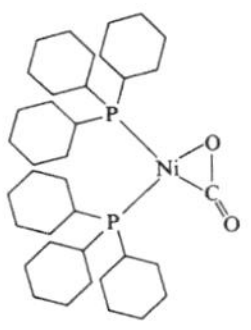

Ni-00309

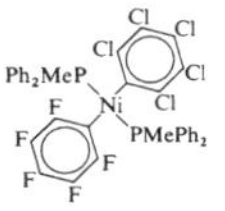

Ni-00310

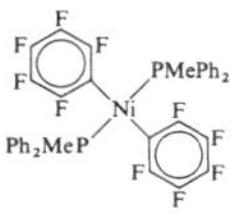

Ni-00311

$(Ph_3As)_2Ni(CO)_2$ (C_{2v})

Ni-00312

$Ni(PPh_3)_2(CO)_2$

Ni-00313

$(Ph_3Sb)_2Ni(CO)_2$ (C_{2v})

Ni-00314

$[(PhO)_3P]Ni(CO)_2PPh_3$

Ni-00315

$[(PhO)_3P]_2Ni(CO)_2$ (C_{2v})

Ni-00316

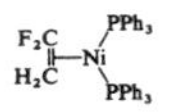

Ni-00317

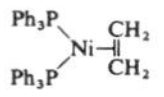

Ni-00318

$NiClEt(PPh_3)_2$

Ni-00319

$Ni(CO)_2[P(C_6H_{11})_3]_2$

Ni-00320

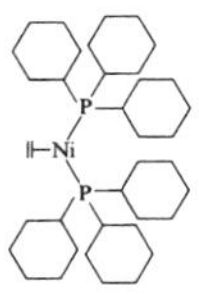

Ni-00321

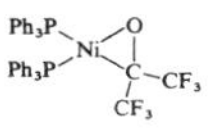

Ni-00322

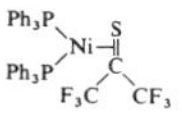

Ni-00323

$Ni(CH_2{=}CHCN)(PPh_3)_2$

Ni-00324

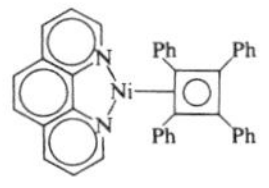

Ni-00325

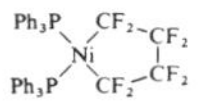

Ni-00326

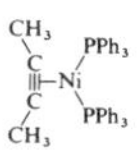

Ni-00327

$[Ph(EtO)_2P]_4Ni$ (T_d)

Ni-00328

$(Et_2PhP)_4Ni$

Ni-00329

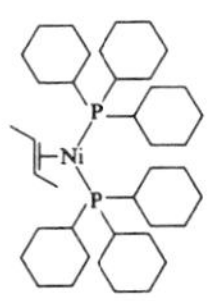

(*E*)-form

Ni-00330

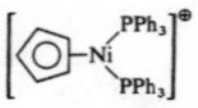

Ni-00331

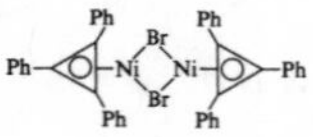

Ni-00332

$NiCl(C_6F_5)(PPh_3)_2$

Ni-00333

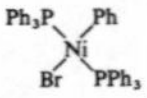

Ni-00334

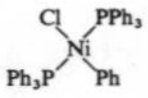

Ni-00335

$(PhCH{=}CHPh)_3Ni$

Ni-00336

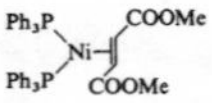

Ni-00337

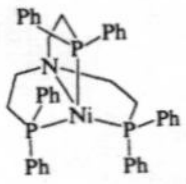

Ni-00338

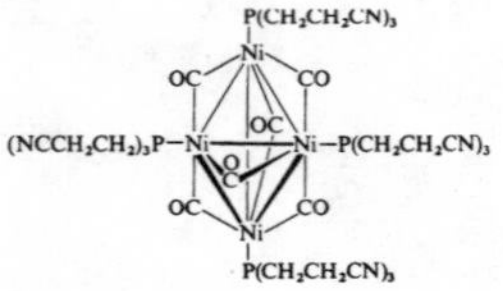

Ni-00339

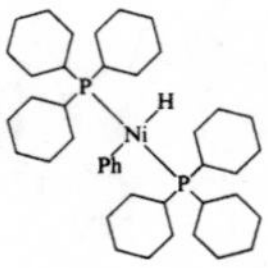

Ni-00340

$NiCl(COPh)(PPh_3)_2$

Ni-00341

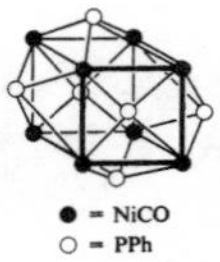

● = NiCO
○ = PPh

Ni-00342

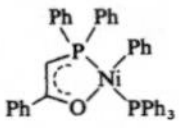

Ni-00343

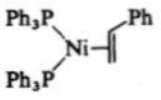

Ni-00344

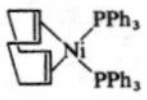

Ni-00345

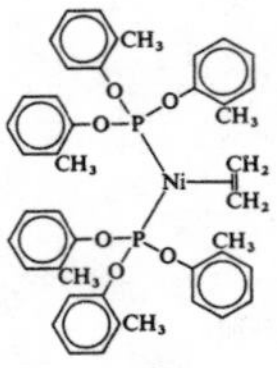

Ni-00346

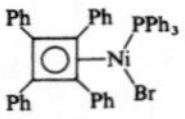

Ni-00347

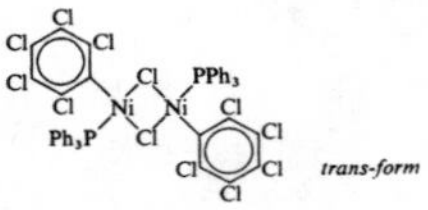

trans-form

Ni-00348

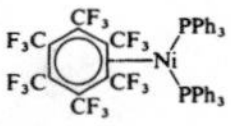

Ni-00349

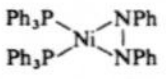

Ni-00350

$[NiPh_2(PPh_3)_2]^{\ominus\ominus}$

Ni-00351

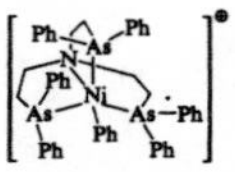

Ni-00352

$[(H_3CCH_2CH_2CH_2)_3P]_4Ni$

Ni-00353

As Ni-00299 with
R = cyclohexyl

Ni-00354

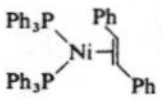

Ni-00355

As Ni-00097 with
R = Ph

Ni-00356

$[NiH(Ph_2PCH_2CH_2PPh_2)_2]^{\oplus}$

Ni-00357

$Ni[P(OMe)Ph_2]_4$ (T_d)

Ni-00358

$Ni(PMePh_2)_4$

Ni-00359

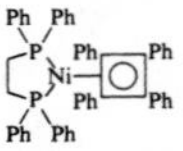

Ni-00360

$(Ph_3P)_3Ni$

Ni-00361

$[Ni(SiPh_3)_3]^{\ominus\ominus\ominus}$

Ni-00362

$NiBrH(PPh_3)_3$

Ni-00363

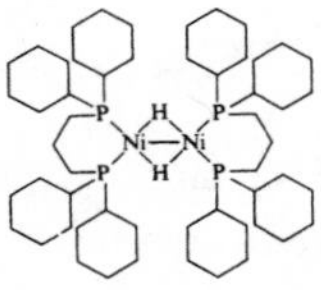

Ni-00364

$[Ni(CO)(PPh_3)_3]$ (C_{3v})

Ni-00365

$Ni(CO)[P(OPh)_3]_3$

Ni-00366

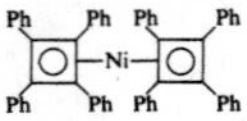

Ni-00367

$[NiH(CH_3CN)(PPh_3)_3]^{\oplus}$

Ni-00368

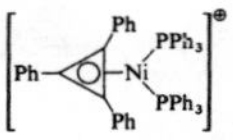

Ni-00369

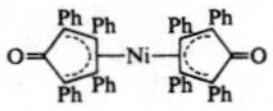

Ni-00370

$[Ni(C_6F_5)(PPh_3)_3]^{\oplus}$

Ni-00371

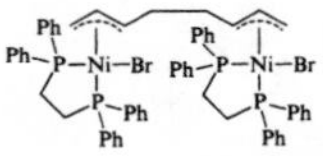

Ni-00372

$Ni[P(OC_6H_4CH_3)_3]_3$

Ni-00373

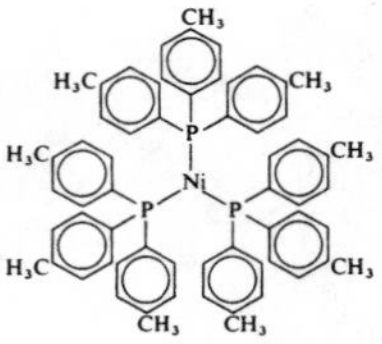

Ni-00374

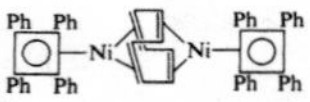

Ni-00375

$(Ph_3As)_4Ni$ (T_d)

Ni-00376

$Ni[P(OPh)_3]_4$

Ni-00377

$Ni(PPh_3)_4$ (T_d)

Ni-00378

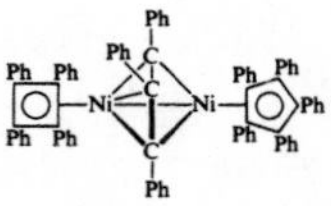

Ni-00379

$Ni(PCl_3)_4$ (T_d)

Ni-00380

$Ni(PF_3)_4$ (T_d)

Ni-00381

$C_3ClNiO_3^{\ominus}$ Ni-00001

Tricarbonylchloronickelate(1–), 8CI
Chlorotricarbonylnickelate(1–)

$[Ni(CO)_3Cl]^{\ominus}$ (C_{3v})

M 178.174 (ion)
Catalyst for carbonylation of benzyl chloride and carbonylation with acetylene insertion of acyl halides. Anion stable in air-free soln. even at 70-80°.
Tetrabutylammonium salt: [27116-03-6].
$C_{19}H_{36}ClNNiO_3$ M 420.641
Not stable in the pure state.
Benzyltrimethylammonium salt: [27116-04-7].
$C_{13}H_{16}ClNNiO_3$ M 328.417
Not stable in the pure state.

Cassar, L. *et al*, *Inorg. Nucl. Chem. Lett.*, 1970, **6**, 291 (*synth, ir*)

$C_3Cl_3GeNiO_3^{\ominus}$ Ni-00002

Tricarbonyl(trichlorogermyl)nickelate(1–), 9CI
Trichlorogermylnickelate(1–) tricarbonyl

$[Ni(GeCl_3)(CO)_3]^{\ominus}$ (C_{3v})

M 321.670 (ion)
Tetraethylammonium salt: [53426-17-8].
$C_{11}H_{20}Cl_3GeNNiO_3$ M 451.923
Orange cryst. (CH_2Cl_2/pentane). Mp 85°. Mod. unstable, even under N_2.

Kruck, T. *et al*, *Z. Naturforsch., B*, 1974, **29**, 198 (*synth*)

$C_3Cl_3NiO_3P$ Ni-00003

Tricarbonyl(phosphorous trichloride)nickel, 8CI
(Trichlorophosphine)nickel tricarbonyl. Tricarbonyl-(trichlorophosphine)nickel. (Phosphorous trichloride)-tricarbonylnickel
[18474-97-0]

$Ni(CO)_3PCl_3$ (C_{3v})

M 280.054
Compound obt. only in soln. Sol. toluene, $CHCl_3$.

Meriwether, L.S. *et al*, *J. Am. Chem. Soc.*, 1961, **83**, 3192 (*nmr*)
Tolman, C.A., *J. Am. Chem. Soc.*, 1970, **92**, 2956 (*nmr*)
Bodner, G.M., *Inorg. Chem.*, 1975, **14**, 1932 (*nmr*)

$C_3F_3NiO_3P$ Ni-00004

Tricarbonyl(phosphorous trifluoride)nickel, 9CI, 8CI
(Trifluorophosphine)nickel tricarbonyl. Tricarbonyl(trifluorophosphine)nickel. (Phosphorous trifluoride)-tricarbonylnickel
[14264-32-5]

$Ni(CO)_3PF_3$ (C_{3v})

M 230.690
Colourless, mobile liq. Sol. hexane. d 1.49. Mp –93°. V.p. 88mm at 0°.

Clark, R.J. *et al*, *Inorg. Chem.*, 1965, **4**, 651 (*synth, ir, nmr*)
Bouquet, G. *et al*, *J. Mol. Struct.*, 1968, **1**, 211 (*ir, raman*)
Mathieu, R. *et al*, *Inorg. Chem.*, 1970, **9**, 2030 (*nmr*)

$C_3H_6F_3NiP$ Ni-00005

η^3-(2-Propenyl)hydrido(trifluorophosphine)nickel
π-Allylhydro(phosphorous trifluoride)nickel, 8CI. *(η^3-Allyl)hydrido(trifluorophosphine)nickel*
[31902-26-8]

H, Ni, PF_3

M 188.739
Red-brown cryst.

Boennemann, H., *Angew. Chem., Int. Ed. Engl.*, 1970, **9**, 736 (*synth, pmr*)

$C_3INiO_3^{\ominus}$ Ni-00006

Tricarbonyliodonickelate(1–), 9CI, 8CI
Iodotricarbonylnickelate(1–)
[36830-71-4]

$[Ni(CO)_3I]^{\ominus}$ (C_{3v})

M 269.626 (ion)
Catalyst for carbonylation of benzyl chloride and carbonylation with acetylene insertion of acyl halides. Anion stable in air-free soln. even at 70-80°.
Na salt: [27122-29-8].
$C_3INaNiO_3$ M 292.615
Not stable in the pure state.
Tetrabutylammonium salt: [27122-27-6].
$C_{19}H_{36}INNiO_3$ M 512.093
Not stable in pure state.

Cassar, L. *et al*, *Inorg. Nucl. Chem. Lett.*, 1970, **6**, 291 (*synth, ir*)
Foa, M. *et al*, *Gazz. Chim. Ital.*, 1972, **102**, 85 (*synth, use*)

C_4H_8Ni Ni-00007

Methyl[(1,2,3-η)-2-propen-1-yl]nickel
Allylmethylnickel

–NiMe

M 114.797
Probably dimeric, though somewhat volatile even at –78°.
Dimer: Dimethylbis[(1,2,3-η)-2-propen-1-yl]dinickel. Bis(allyl)dimethyldinickel. Diallyldimethyldinickel.
$C_8H_{16}Ni_2$ M 229.594
Violet cryst. Sol. Et_2O. Dec. ~–35° even in an inert atm.

Bogdanovic, B. *et al*, *Angew. Chem., Int. Ed. Engl.*, 1966, **5**, 582 (*synth, pmr*)

$C_4H_{12}Ni^{\ominus\ominus}$ Ni-00008

Tetramethylnickelate(2–)

$NiMe_4^{\ominus\ominus}$ (D_{4h})

M 118.829 (ion)
Di-Li salt: [54688-83-4].
$C_4H_{12}Li_2Ni$ M 132.711
Small golden-yellow lustrous cryst. +2THF (THF). Mod. sol. Et_2O, sol. THF. Dec. at 129-30°. V. air- and moisture-sensitive.

Taube, R. *et al*, *Angew. Chem., Int. Ed. Engl.*, 1975, **14**, 261 (*synth*)

$C_4H_{22}B_{18}Ni$ Ni-00009

Bis[(7,8,9,10,11-η)-undecahydro-7,8-dicarbaundecaborato(2−)]nickel, 9CI

[36548-55-7]

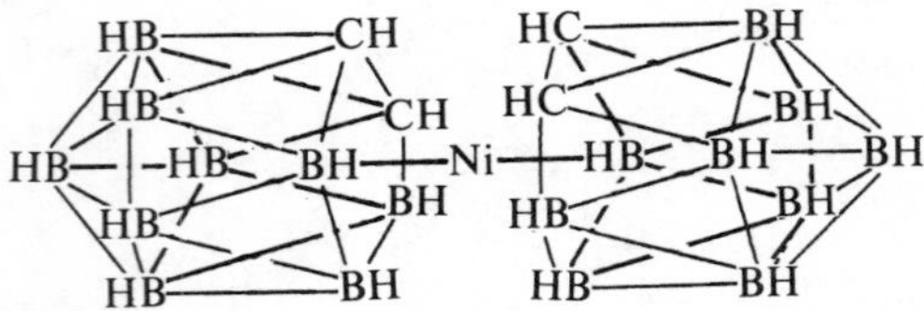

M 323.488

Air-stable orange cryst. Sol. most org. solvs. Subl. unchanged *in vacuo* at 150°, dec. ~265°.

Hawthorne, M.F. *et al, J. Am. Chem. Soc.*, 1968, **90**, 879 (*synth, ir, pmr*)
St Clair, D. *et al, J. Am. Chem. Soc.*, 1970, **92**, 1173 (*struct*)
Smith, D.E. *et al, J. Chem. Soc., Dalton Trans.*, 1971, 8 (*polarog*)

$C_4H_{22}B_{18}Ni^{\ominus}$ Ni-00010

Bis[(7,8,9,10,11-η)-undecahydro-7,8-dicarbaundecaborato(2−)]nickelate(1−), 9CI

[51159-91-2]

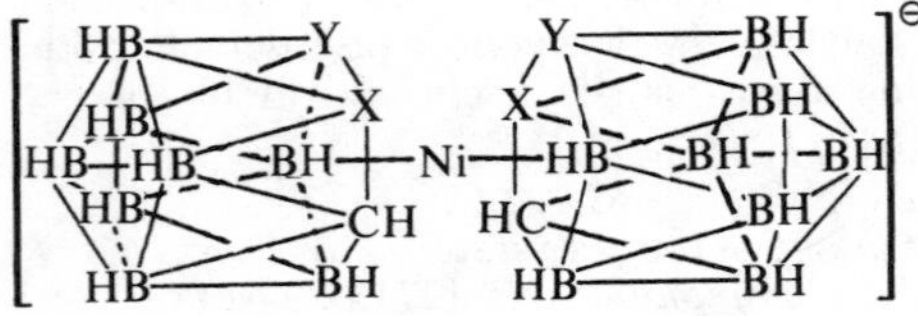

X = CH, Y = BH

M 323.488 (ion)

Rb salt:

$C_4H_{22}B_{18}NiRb$ M 408.956

Green-black lustrous cryst.

Tetramethylammonium salt: [51159-92-3].

$C_8H_{34}B_{18}NNi$ M 397.633

Yellow-brown solid. Mp >300°.

Hawthorne, M.F. *et al, J. Am. Chem. Soc.*, 1968, **90**, 879 (*synth, ir, pmr*)
Hansen, F.V. *et al, Acta Chem. Scand.*, 1973, **27**, 1210 (*struct*)

$C_4H_{22}B_{18}Ni^{\ominus\ominus}$ Ni-00011

Bis[(7,8,9,10,11-η)-undecahydro-7,8-dicarbaundecaborato(2−)]nickelate(2−), 9CI

[36733-09-2]

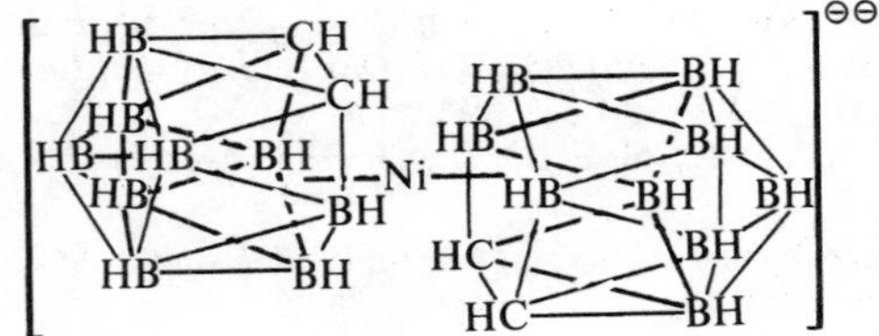

M 323.488 (ion)

Bis(tetramethylammonium) salt:

$C_{12}H_{46}B_{18}N_2Ni$ M 471.779

Pale-brown needles. Extremely air-sensitive.

Hawthorne, M.F. *et al, J. Am. Chem. Soc.*, 1968, **90**, 879 (*synth, ir, pmr*)
Wing, R.M., *J. Am. Chem. Soc.*, 1968, **90**, 4828 (*struct*)
Pavlik, I. *et al, CA*, 1976, **85**, 93221 (*pe*)

$C_4H_{22}B_{18}Ni^{\ominus}$ Ni-00012

Bis[(7,8,9,10,11-η)-undecahydro-7,9-dicarbaundecaborato(2−)]nickelate(1−), 9CI

As Bis[(7,8,9,10,11-η)-undecahydro-7,8-dicarbaundecaborato(2−)]nickelate(1−), Ni-00010 with

X = BH, Y = CH

M 323.488 (ion)

Tetramethylammonium salt:

$C_8H_{34}B_{18}NNi$ M 397.633

Olive-green cryst. (Me_2CO aq.). Mp >300°.

Rb salt: [42443-78-7].

$C_4H_{22}B_{18}NiRb$ M 408.956

No phys. details recorded.

Hawthorne, M.F. *et al, J. Am. Chem. Soc.*, 1968, **90**, 862, 879 (*synth, ir, pmr*)
Pont, L.O. *et al, Inorg. Chem.*, 1974, **13**, 483 (*pe*)

$C_4N_4Ni^{\ominus\ominus}$ Ni-00013

Tetrakis(cyano-*C*)nickelate(2−), 9CI

[15453-80-2]

$Ni(CN)_4^{\ominus\ominus}$ (D_{4h})

M 162.761 (ion)

Di-Na salt: [14038-85-8].

$C_4N_4Na_2Ni$ M 208.740

Catalyst for alkyne hydrogenation and hydrogenation-rearrangement of butene. Catalyst for vat dye printing.

Di-K salt: [14220-17-8].

$C_4K_2N_4Ni$ M 240.957

Used in indirect complexometric titration determination of silver, and titrimetric determination of phosphorus. Catalyst in polymerisation of vinyl compds. Red-orange cryst. + $1H_2O$ (H_2O). Monohydrate dehydrates at 100°.

▷QR8650000.

Bis(tetrabutylammonium) salt: [21518-38-7].

$C_{36}H_{72}N_6Ni$ M 647.695

Catalyst in ethylene polymerisation.

Inorg. Synth., 1946, **2**, 227 (*synth*)
Larsen, F.K. *et al, Acta Chem. Scand.*, 1967, **23**, 61 (*struct*)
Mason, W.R. *et al, J. Am. Chem. Soc.*, 1968, **90**, 5721 (*uv*)
Jones, D. *et al, Spectrochim. Acta, Part A*, 1968, **24**, 973.
Cowman, C.D. *et al, J. Am. Chem. Soc.*, 1973, **95**, 7873 (*uv*)
Matienzo, J. *et al, Inorg. Chem.*, 1973, **12**, 2762 (*pe*)

C_4NiO_4 Ni-00014

Nickel carbonyl, 9CI

Nickel tetracarbonyl. Tetracarbonylnickel

[13463-39-3]

$Ni(CO)_4$

M 170.732

Catalyst for carbonylations, organic halide couplings, polymerisations and oligomerisations of alkenes and alkynes. Intermed. in Mond process for purifn. of Ni. Liq. Mp −25°. Bp_{769} 43°.

▷Extremely toxic vapour. May ignite in air. Carcinogenic. Causes dermatitis. TLV 0.35. QR6300000.

Dewar, J. *et al, J. Chem. Soc.*, 1904, **85**, 203.
Manchot, W. *et al, Ber.*, 1929, **62**, 678 (*synth*)
Inorg. Synth., 1946, **2**, 234 (*synth*)
Bodner, G. *et al, Inorg. Chem.*, 1975, **14**, 1932 (*cmr*)
Fieser, M. *et al, Reagents for Organic Synthesis*, Wiley, 1967-83, **7**, 250.
Prasad, P.L. *et al, J. Chem. Phys.*, 1977, **67**, 4584 (*ir*)
Bretherick, L., *Handbook of Reactive Chemical Hazards*, 2nd Ed., Butterworths, London and Boston, 1979, 519.
Sax, N.I., *Dangerous Properties of Industrial Materials*, 5th Ed., Van Nostrand-Reinhold, 1979, 849.
Hazards in the Chemical Laboratory, (Bretherick, L., Ed.), 3rd Ed., Royal Society of Chemistry, London, 1981, 495.

C_4NiS_4 Ni-00015

Tetrakis(thiocarbonyl)nickel

Tetrakis(carbonothioyl)nickel, 9CI. *Nickel thiocarbonyl*

[51062-92-1]

$Ni(CS)_4$ (T_d)

M 234.974

Characterised spectroscopically.

Yarbrough, L.W., *J. Chem. Soc., Chem. Commun.*, 1973, 705 (*ms, ir*)

$C_5H_3NNiO_3$ Ni-00016

Tricarbonyl(isocyanomethane)nickel, 10CI

Tricarbonyl(methyl isocyanide)nickel, 8CI. *Methylisonitrilenickel tricarbonyl*

[16787-44-3]

$MeNCNi(CO)_3$ (C_{3v})

M 183.774

Solid. Sl. sol. hydrocarbons, mod. sol. Et_2O, $CHCl_3$.

Bignorgne, M., *J. Organomet. Chem.*, 1963, **1**, 101 (*synth, raman*)

Haas, H. *et al*, *J. Chem. Phys.*, 1967, **47**, 2996 (*ir*)

C_5H_5NNiO Ni-00017

(η^5-2,4-Cyclopentadien-1-yl)nitrosylnickel, 10CI

[12071-73-7]

Cp–Ni–NO

M 153.791

Red oil. Fp −41°. Bp_{15} 47-8°.

Gmelin's Handbuch der Anorg. Chem., 8th Ed., 1974, Suppl., **17**, 108.

$C_5H_5Ni^{\oplus}$ Ni-00018

(η^5-2,4-Cyclopentadien-1-yl)nickel(1+), 9CI

[52668-78-7]

$[CpNi]^{\oplus}$

M 123.785 (ion)

Tetrafluoroborate: [52668-79-8].

$C_5H_5BF_4Ni$ M 210.588

Dark-brown solid.

Court, T.L. *et al*, *J. Organomet. Chem.*, 1974, **65**, 245 (*synth, ir, pmr*)

$C_5H_{11}Ni^{\ominus}$ Ni-00019

Bis(ethylene)methylnickelate(1−)

Bis(η^2-ethene)methylnickelate(1−), 9CI. *Methylbis(ethylene)nickelate(1−)*

$[(C_2H_4)_2NiMe]^{\ominus}$

M 129.832 (ion)

Bis(tetramethylethylenediamine)lithium(1+) salt: [60349-34-0].

$C_{17}H_{43}LiN_4Ni$ M 369.185

Cryst. Stable under Ar at r.t.

Jonas, K. *et al*, *Angew. Chem., Int. Ed. Engl.*, 1976, **15**, 621 (*synth*)

$C_5H_{13}N_4NiS_2^{\oplus}$ Ni-00020

(η^3-2-Propenyl)bis(thiourea-*S*)nickel(1+), 9CI

(π-Allyl)bis(thiourea)nickel(1+), 8CI

$[(C_3H_5)Ni(SC(NH_2)_2)_2]^{\oplus}$

M 251.995 (ion)

Catalyses CO insertions.

Bromide: [32696-88-1].

$C_5H_{13}BrN_4NiS_2$ M 331.899

No props. recorded.

Guerreri, F., *J. Chem. Soc., Chem. Commun.*, 1968, 983 (*synth*)

Singer, A., *Inorg. Chem.*, 1970, **9**, 2245 (*struct*)

Eaton, D.R. *et al*, *Can. J. Chem.*, 1975, **53**, 633 (*pmr*)

C_6BrF_5Ni Ni-00021

Bromo(pentafluorophenyl)nickel, 9CI

(Pentafluorophenyl)bromonickel

[48133-12-6]

$NiBr(C_6F_5)$

M 305.652

Thermally stable only to −80°.

Klabunde, K.J., *Angew. Chem., Int. Ed. Engl.*, 1975, **14**, 287 (*synth*)

Habeeb, J.J. *et al*, *J. Organomet. Chem.*, 1977, **139**, C17 (*synth*)

$C_6F_6NiO_2$ Ni-00022

Dicarbonyl[(2,3-η)-1,1,1,4,4,4-hexafluoro-2-butyne]nickel, 9CI

Dicarbonyl[bis(trifluoromethyl)acetylene]nickel

[57903-03-4]

$(CF_3C{\equiv}CCF_3)Ni(CO)_2$

M 276.745

Colourless, volatile liq. Rapidly dec. at r.t. to give 99981-3.

Davidson, J.L. *et al*, *J. Am. Chem. Soc.*, 1975, **97**, 7490 (*synth*)

Davidson, J.L. *et al*, *J. Chem. Soc., Dalton Trans.*, 1979, 506 (*synth, ir, nmr*)

C_6H_5INiO Ni-00023

Carbonyl(η^5-2,4-cyclopentadien-1-yl)iodonickel, 9CI

(π-Cyclopentadienyl)carbonyliodonickel. Iodo(π-cyclopentadienyl)carbonylnickel

[55046-35-0]

CpNi(CO)I

M 278.699

Black-violet glistening cryst. Sol. all org. solvs. Extremely sensitive to air and moisture, and sensitive to light and heat. Dec. >20°.

Fischer, E.O. *et al*, *Chem. Ber.*, 1958, **91**, 1725 (*synth*)

$C_6H_5NiO^{\ominus}$ Ni-00024

Carbonyl(η^5-2,4-cyclopentadien-1-yl)nickelate(1−), 9CI

(π-Cyclopentadienyl)carbonylnickelate(1−)

[12127-99-0]

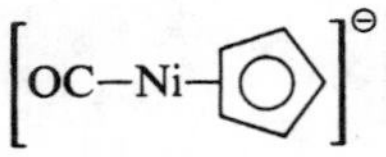

$[OC-Ni-C_5H_5]^{\ominus}$

M 151.795 (ion)

Orange soln. generated in THF from $Ni_2(C_5H_5)_2(CO)_2$ and K. Air-sensitive. Reacts readily with organic halides or unsaturated molecules to produce organonickel compds.

Brown, J.M. *et al*, *J. Chem. Soc.*, *Perkin Trans. 2*, 1974, 905 (*synth*)

$C_6H_6N_2Ni$ Ni-00025

Bis[(2,3-η)-2-propenenitrile]nickel, 10CI, 9CI

Bis(acrylonitrile)nickel, 8CI

[12266-58-9]

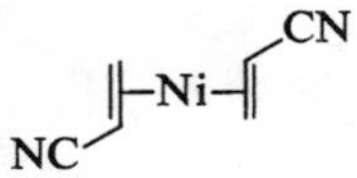

M 164.817

Catalyst for isomerisation and unusual [2 + 2] cycloadditions. Red cryst. Dec. above 100°. Adds phosphines etc.

▷Pyrophoric

Schrauzer, G.N., *J. Am. Chem. Soc.*, 1959, **81**, 5310 (*synth*, *ir*)
Fritz, H.P. *et al*, *Chem. Ber.*, 1961, **94**, 650 (*ir*)
Dubini, M. *et al*, *Chim. Ind. (Milan)*, 1967, **49**, 1283; *CA*, **68**, 74736 (*synth*)
Fieser, M. *et al*, *Reagents for Organic Synthesis*, Wiley, 1967-83, **6**, 45.

$C_6H_6N_2NiO_2$ Ni-00026

Dicarbonylbis(isocyanomethane)nickel, 10CI

Dicarbonylbis(methyl isocyanide)nickel, 8CI. *Bis(methylisonitrile)nickel dicarbonyl*

[16787-45-4]

$(MeNC)_2Ni(CO)_2$ (C_{2v})

M 196.816

White solid. V. sl. sol. org. solvs.

Bignorgne, M., *J. Organomet. Chem.*, 1963, **1**, 101 (*synth*, *raman*)
Haas, H. *et al*, *J. Chem. Phys.*, 1967, **47**, 2996 (*ir*)

C_6H_7NNiO Ni-00027

(η^5-1-Methyl-2,4-cyclopentadien-1-yl)nitrosylnickel, 9CI

Nitrosyl(methylcyclopentadienyl)nickel

[32714-42-4]

$H_3C-C_5H_4-NiNO$

M 167.817

Dark-red liq.

Bailey, R.T., *Spectrochim. Acta, Part A*, 1969, **25**, 1127 (*synth*, *ir*, *raman*)
Evans, S. *et al*, *J. Chem. Soc.*, *Faraday Trans. 2*, 1974, **70**, 417 (*synth*)

$C_6H_9NiO_6P$ Ni-00028

Tricarbonyl(trimethyl phosphite-*P*)nickel, 9CI

(Trimethyl phosphite)nickel tricarbonyl. Tricarbonyl(phosphorous acid)nickel trimethyl ester, 8CI

[17099-58-0]

$Ni(CO)_3P(OMe)_3$

M 266.797

Catalyst for dimerisation of pentyne, ethene and cycloalkadienes. Cryst. (pentane or MeOH).

Bignorgne, M., *Bull. Soc. Chim. Fr.*, 1960, 1986 (*synth*, *ir*)
Bouquet, G. *et al*, *J. Mol. Struct.*, 1968, **1**, 211 (*ir*, *raman*)
Mathieu, R. *et al*, *Inorg. Chem.*, 1970, **9**, 2030 (*nmr*)
Bodner, G.M., *Inorg. Chem.*, 1975, **14**, 1932 (*nmr*)

$C_6H_{10}Br_2Ni_2$ Ni-00029

Di-μ-bromobis(η^3-2-propenyl)dinickel, 9CI

Bis(π-allyl)di-μ-bromodinickel. Dibromodi-π-allyldinickel

[12012-90-7]

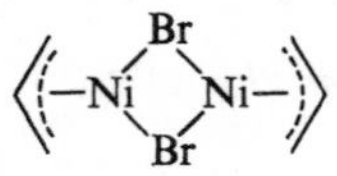

M 359.333

Catalyses polymerisation of olefins, and crosscoupling reaction of Grignard reagents and organic halides. Cryst.

Monomer: Bromo(2-propenyl)nickel. Allylbromonickel. Allylnickel bromide.
C_3H_5BrNi M 179.667
Unknown.

Fischer, E.O. *et al*, *Z. Naturforsch., B*, 1961, **16**, 77 (*synth*)
Nesmeyanov, A.N. *et al*, *Dokl. Akad. Nauk SSSR, Ser. Sci. Khim.*, 1974, **216**, 816 (*nmr*)
Chenskaya, T.B. *et al*, *J. Organomet. Chem.*, 1978, **148**, 85 (*ir*)

$C_6H_{10}Cl_2Ni_2$ Ni-00030

Di-μ-chlorobis(η^3-2-propenyl)dinickel, 10CI, 9CI

Di-π-allyldi-μ-chlorodinickel, 8CI. *Bis(allylchloronickel)*

[12145-00-5]

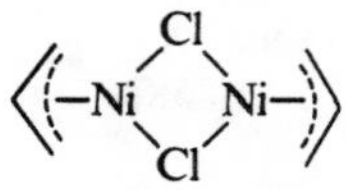

M 270.431

Bridged dimer. Catalyst for propene dimerisation and cocatalyst for isoprene trimerisation. Brown solid. Unstable.

Monomer: Chloro(2-propenylnickel). Allylchloronickel.
C_3H_5ClNi M 135.216
Unknown.

Heck, R.F. *et al*, *J. Am. Chem. Soc.*, 1963, **85**, 2013 (*synth*)
Wilke, G. *et al*, *Angew. Chem., Int. Ed. Engl.*, 1966, **5**, 151 (*synth*)
Piper, M.J. *et al*, *J. Chem. Soc., Chem. Commun.*, 1972, 50 (*synth*)
Chenskaya, T.B. *et al*, *Zh. Strukt. Khim.*, 1974, **15**, 31; *CA*, **80**, 107537 (*ir*)
Nesmeyanov, A.N. *et al*, *Dokl. Akad. Nauk. SSSR*, 1974, **216**, 816; *CA*, **81**, 70680 (*cmr*)

$C_6H_{10}I_2Ni_2$ Ni-00031

Di-μ-iodobis(η³-2-propenyl)dinickel, 9CI
Bis(allyl)diiododinickel. Diallyldiiododinickel

M 453.334
Bridged dimer. Diene polymerisation catalyst. Dark-red cryst. Subl. unchanged *in vacuo*.
Monomer: Iodo(η³-2-propenylnickel). Allyliodonickel.
C_3H_5INi M 226.667
Unknown.

Fischer, E.O. *et al*, *Chem. Ber.*, 1961, **94**, 2409 (*synth*)
Nesmeyanov, A.N. *et al*, *Dokl. Akad. Nauk SSSR, Ser. Sci. Khim.*, 1974, **216**, 816 (*nmr*)
Chenskaya, T.B. *et al*, *J. Organomet. Chem.*, 1978, **148**, 85 (*ir, raman*)

$C_6H_{10}Ni$ Ni-00032

Bis(η³-2-propenyl)nickel, 9CI
Bisallylnickel. Diallylnickel
[12077-85-9]

M 140.835
Exists and *syn* and *anti* stereoisomers in soln. Cocatalyst for polymerisation of alkenes, oligomerisation and cyclooligomerisation of butadienes. Yellow needles. Fp 1°. Subl. at 1mm.

Inorg. Synth., 1972, **13**, 79 (*synth*)
Gmelin's Handbuch der Anorg. Chem., 8th Ed., 1974, Suppl., **17**, 46.
Henc, B. *et al*, *J. Organomet. Chem.*, 1980, **191**, 425 (*pmr, cmr, raman*)

$C_6H_{12}Ni$ Ni-00033

Tris(η²-ethene)nickel, 10CI, 9CI
Tris(ethylene)nickel
[50696-82-7]

M 142.851
Catalyst for ethylene dimerisations. Needles (Et_2O). Mp >0° dec.

Fischer, K. *et al*, *Angew. Chem., Int. Ed. Engl.*, 1973, **12**, 565 (*synth, pmr, ir*)
Huber, H. *et al*, *J. Am. Chem. Soc.*, 1976, **98**, 6508 (*synth, ir, uv*)
Ozin, G.A. *et al*, *J. Am. Chem. Soc.*, 1978, **100**, 4750 (*ir, uv*)
Ozin, G.A. *et al*, *Inorg. Chem.*, 1978, **17**, 2836 (*uv*)
Gmelin Suppl., **16**, 417.

$C_6H_{13}Ni^{\ominus}$ Ni-00034

Ethylbis(ethylene)nickelate(1−)
Bis(η²-ethene)ethylnickelate(1−), 9CI

$[(C_2H_4)_2NiEt]^{\ominus}$

M 143.859 (ion)
Li salt:
$C_6H_{13}LiNi$ M 150.800
Cryst. + 4THF (THF).

Jonas, K. *et al*, *Angew. Chem., Int. Ed. Engl.*, 1976, **15**, 621; 1979, **18**, 488 (*synth*)

$C_6H_{14}ClNiP$ Ni-00035

Chloro(η³-2-propenyl)(trimethylphosphine)nickel
Allylchloro(trimethylphosphine)nickel

M 211.293
Catalyst for oligomerisation of alkenes. No phys. details recorded.

Bogdanovic, B., *Adv. Organomet. Chem.*, 1979, **17**, 105 (*use*)

$C_6N_6Ni_2^{\ominus\ominus\ominus\ominus}$ Ni-00036

Hexakiscyanodinickelate(4−), 9CI
Hexakis(cyano-C)di(Ni-Ni)nickelate(4−), 10CI. Hexacyanodinickelate(4−)
[12552-49-7]

$[(NC)_3Ni—Ni(CN)_3]^{\ominus\ominus\ominus\ominus}$

M 273.486 (ion)
Tetrapotassium salt: [40810-33-1].
$C_6K_4N_6Ni_2$ M 429.879
Red solid (EtOH). Dec. slowly in air to yellow solid.

Eastes, J.W. *et al*, *J. Am. Chem. Soc.*, 1942, **64**, 1187 (*synth*)
Inorg. Synth., 1957, **5**, 197 (*synth*)
de Haas, K.S. *et al*, *Inorg. Chim. Acta*, 1977, **24**, 269 (*ir*)

$C_6Ni_2O_6^{\ominus\ominus}$ Ni-00037

Hexacarbonyldinickelate(2−), 9CI
[80790-08-5]

$Ni_2(CO)_6^{\ominus\ominus}$

M 285.442 (ion)
Na salt:
$C_6Na_2Ni_2O_6$ M 331.422
Obt. only in NH_3 soln. on reduction of $Ni(CO)_4$ by Na. Readily condenses further by CO loss, or undergoes ammonolysis to $Ni_2(CO)_6H_2$.

Behrens, H. *et al*, *Chem. Ber.*, 1964, **94**, 1391 (*synth*)
Pacchoni, G. *et al*, *J. Organomet. Chem.*, 1982, **224**, 89.

$C_7H_5F_3NiOS$ Ni-00038

Carbonyl(η⁵-2,4-cyclopentadien-1-yl)(trifluoromethanethiolato)nickel, 9CI
(π-Cyclopentadienyl)carbonyl(trifluoromethylthiolato)-nickel
[50980-24-0]

$F_3C—S—Ni(CO)(C_5H_5)$

M 252.861
Compound not isol.

Davidson, J.L. *et al*, *J. Chem. Soc., Dalton Trans.*, 1973, 1957 (*synth*)

$C_7H_9N_3NiO$ Ni-00039

Carbonyltris(isocyanomethane)nickel, 10CI
Carbonyltris(methyl isocyanide)nickel, 8CI. Tris(methyl-isonitrile)nickel carbonyl
[15625-54-4]

$(MeNC)_3NiCO$ (C_{3v})

M 209.858
Yellow-white cryst.

Hieber, W. *et al*, *Z. Anorg. Allg. Chem.*, 1950, **262**, 344 (*synth*)
Bignorgne, M., *J. Organomet. Chem.*, 1963, **1**, 101 (*raman*)
Haas, H. *et al*, *J. Chem. Phys.*, 1967, **47**, 2996 (*ir*)

$C_7H_{10}NiO_3S$ Ni-00040

Tricarbonyl(diethylsulfide)nickel
Tricarbonyl(ethyl sulfide)nickel

$Ni(CO)_3(SEt_2)$

M 232.904
No phys. props. recorded.

Bouquet, G. *et al*, *Bull. Soc. Chim. Fr.*, 1962, 433 (*synth, ir*)

$C_7H_{18}I_2NiOP_2$ Ni-00041

Carbonyldiiodobis(trimethylphosphine)nickel, 9CI
Bis(trimethylphosphine)carbonylnickel diiodide
[35872-05-0]

I, I, PMe₃, PMe₃ on Ni–CO

M 492.665
Dark-brown cryst. Fairly stable in solid state and in soln. under CO. Sol. C_6H_6, CH_2Cl_2, insol. EtOH. Solns. slowly dec. under inert atm., can be handled briefly in air.

Pankowski, M. *et al*, *J. Organomet. Chem.*, 1976, **110**, 331 (*synth, ir*)
Saint-Joly, C. *et al*, *Inorg. Chem.*, 1980, **19**, 2403 (*synth, struct*)

$C_7H_{21}ClNiP_2$ Ni-00042

Chloro(methyl)bis(trimethylphosphine)nickel, 9CI
Bis(trimethylphosphine)methylnickel chloride
[38883-63-5]

Me_3P, Me, X, PMe_3 on Ni

X = Cl

M 261.333

trans-form

Air-sensitive cryst. (hexane). Water-stable, can be recovered from aq. solns. Dec. at 125-6°.

Klein, H.F. *et al*, *Chem. Ber.*, 1976, **105**, 2628; 1976, **109**, 2515 (*synth, pmr, ir*)

$C_7H_{21}INiP_2$ Ni-00043

Iodo(methyl)bis(trimethylphosphine)nickel, 9CI
[38883-68-0]

As Chloro(methyl)bis(trimethylphosphine)nickel, Ni-00042 with

X = I

M 352.785

trans-form

Brown air-sensitive leaflets (hexane). Mp 99-100°. Water-stable, can be recovered from aq. soln.

Klein, H.F. *et al*, *Chem. Ber.*, 1972, **105**, 2628 (*synth, ir, pmr*)

$C_8H_4Ni^{\ominus\ominus}$ Ni-00044

Tetraethynylnickelate(2−)
Tetrakis(acetylenyl)nickelate(2−).
Tetrakisethynylnickelate(2−)

$[Ni(C{\equiv}CH)_4]^{\ominus\ominus}$ (D_{4h})

M 158.810 (ion)

Di-Na salt:
$C_8H_4Na_2Ni$ M 204.789
Yellow cryst. + $2NH_3$. Insol. EtOH, MeOH, Me_2CO, Et_2O. Compound stable only below −10° under NH_3. Free salt cannot be obt.

Di-K salt:
$C_8H_4K_2Ni$ M 237.006
Yellow cryst. Fairly stable in dry air, dec. over several days on standing, even under N_2.

▷Detonates on impact or in a flame

Nast, R. *et al*, *Z. Anorg. Allg. Chem.*, 1955, **279**, 146 (*synth*)

$C_8H_8NiO_2$ Ni-00045

Acetylcarbonyl(η^5-2,4-cyclopentadien-1-yl)nickel, 10CI
Acetyl(π-cyclopentadienyl)carbonylnickel. (π-Cyclopentadienyl)acetylcarbonylnickel. Carbonyl(acetyl)cyclopentadienylnickel
[73643-66-0]

Cp–Ni(COCH₃)(CO)

M 194.840
Yellow oil. $Bp_{0.1\text{-}0.01}$ 50-60°.

Gompper, R. *et al*, *Justus Liebigs Ann. Chem.*, 1980, 229 (*synth, ir, pms, ms*)

$C_8H_{10}Ni$ Ni-00046

(η^5-2,4-Cyclopentadien-1-yl)(η^3-2-propenyl)nickel, 9CI
π-Allyl-π-cyclopentadienylnickel, 8CI.
Cyclopentadienylallylnickel
[12107-46-8]

allyl–Ni–Cp

M 164.857
Red-violet solid or liq. Mp 7-9°. Bp_{12} 73-5°. Subl. readily.

Fischer, E.O. *et al*, *Chem. Ber.*, 1961, **94**, 2409 (*synth, ir*)
McClellan, W.R. *et al*, *J. Am. Chem. Soc.*, 1961, **83**, 1601 (*synth, pmr*)
Nesmeyanov, A.N. *et al*, *Dokl. Akad. Nauk. SSSR*, 1974, **214**, 816; *CA*, **81**, 70680 (*cmr*)

$C_8H_{12}N_4Ni$ Ni-00047

Tetrakis(isocyanomethane)nickel, 9CI
Tetrakis(methyl isocyanide)nickel, 8CI
[16787-47-6]

$(MeNC)_4Ni$ (T_d)

M 222.900
V. sensitive to air.

Bigorgne, M., *J. Organomet. Chem.*, 1963, **1**, 101 (*synth*)

Bigorgne, M. *et al*, *CA*, 1967, **67**, 59211 (*ir, raman*)

$C_8H_{14}Br_2Ni_2$ Ni-00048

Di-μ-bromobis[(1,2,3-η)-2-butenyl]dinickel, 9CI
Di-μ-bromobis(1-methyl-π-allyl)dinickel, 8CI
[12145-58-3]

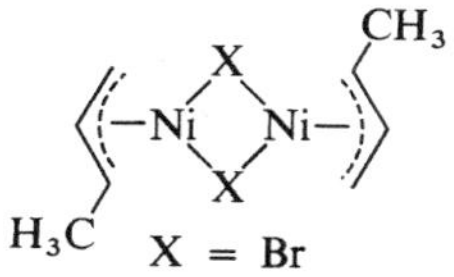

X = Br

M 387.387
Industrial catalyst for polymerisations.
Monomer: Bromo(1,2,3-η-2-butenyl)nickel. Bromo(1-methyl-π-allyl)nickel.
C_4H_7BrNi M 193.693
Unknown.

Fischer, E.O. *et al*, *Z. Naturforsch., B*, 1961, **16**, 77 (*synth*)
Churlyaeva, L.A. *et al*, *J. Organomet. Chem.*, 1972, **39**, C23 (*nmr*)

$C_8H_{14}Br_2Ni_2$ Ni-00049

Di-μ-bromobis[(1,2,3-η)-2-methyl-2-propenyl]dinickel, 9CI
Di-μ-bromobis(2-methylallyl)dinickel
[12300-62-8]

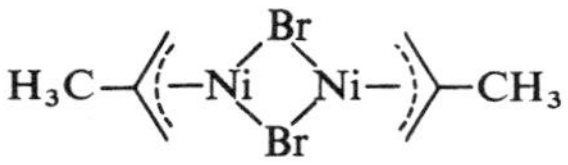

M 387.387
Olefin polymerisation catalyst. Dark-red cryst.
Monomer: Bromo(2-methyl-2-propenyl)nickel. Bromo(2-methylallyl)nickel.
C_4H_7BrNi M 193.693
Unknown.

Corey, E.J. *et al*, *J. Am. Chem. Soc.*, 1967, **89**, 2755 (*synth*)
Org. Synth., 1972, **52**, 115 (*synth, pmr*)

$C_8H_{14}Br_2Ni_2O_2$ Ni-00050

Di-μ-bromobis[(1,2,3-η)-2-methoxy-2-propenyl]dinickel, 9CI
Di-μ-bromobis(2-methoxyallyl)dinickel
[53401-78-8]

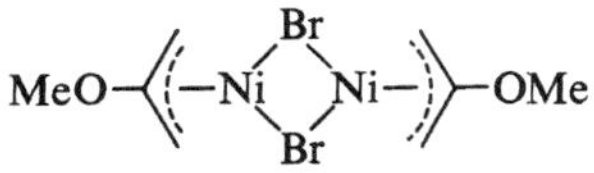

M 419.385
Brick-red cryst.; mod. air-sensitive as solid, but in soln. dec. immediately on exp. to air. Sol. C_6H_6, Et_2O, THF, DMF, $CHCl_3$. Insol. alkanes. Mp 96-8° (sealed tube under Ar).

Hegedus, L.S. *et al*, *J. Am. Chem. Soc.*, 1974, **96**, 3250 (*synth*)

$C_8H_{14}Cl_2Ni_2$ Ni-00051

Di-μ-chlorobis[(1,2,3-η)-2-butenyl]dinickel, 9CI
Di-μ-chlorobis(1-methyl-π-allyl)dinickel, 8CI
[12145-59-4]
As Di-μ-bromobis[(1,2,3-η)-2-butenyl]dinickel, Ni-00048 with

X = Cl

M 298.485
Catalyst for polymerisation of hydrocarbons.
Monomer:
C_4H_7ClNi M 149.242
Unknown.

Fischer, E.O. *et al*, *Z. Naturforsch., B*, 1961, **16**, 77 (*synth*)
Sharaev, O.K. *et al*, *Dokl. Akad. Nauk SSSR, Ser. Sci. Khim.*, 1965, **164**, 119 (*synth*)

$C_8H_{14}Cl_2Ni_2$ Ni-00052

Di-μ-chlorobis[(1,2,3,-η)-2-methyl-2-propenyl]dinickel, 9CI
Di-μ-chlorobis(2-methyl-π-allyl)dinickel, 8CI
[12145-60-7]

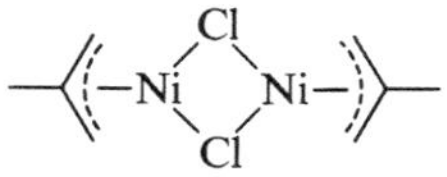

M 298.485
Bridged dimer. Catalyst for butadiene polymerisation. Red-brown solid.
Monomer: Chloro(2-methyl-2-propenyl)nickel. Chloro(2-methylallyl)nickel.
C_4H_7ClNi M 149.242
Unknown.

Netherlands Pat., 6 409 180, (*1965*); *CA*, **63**, 11617 (*synth, use*)
Wilke, G., *Angew. Chem., Int. Ed. Engl.*, 1966, **5**, 151 (*synth*)

$C_8H_{14}INiP$ Ni-00053

(η^5-2,4-Cyclopentadien-1-yl)iodo(trimethylphosphine)nickel, 9CI
Iodo(π-cyclopentadienyl)(trimethylphosphine)nickel
[55997-54-1]

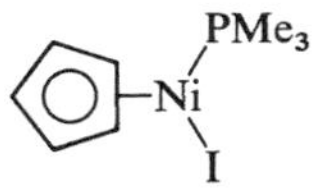

M 326.767
Solid. Mp 145° dec.

Mathey, F., *J. Organomet. Chem.*, 1975, **87**, 371 (*synth, pmr*)

$C_8H_{14}Ni$ Ni-00054

Bis[(1,2,3-η)-(1-methyl-2-propenyl)]nickel, 9CI
Bis(1-methyl-π-allyl)nickel, 8CI. Bis[(1,2,3-η)-2-buten-1-yl]nickel
[12145-63-0]

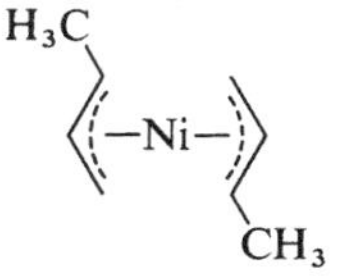

M 168.889
Orange-yellow solid. Mp −5°.

Wilke, G. *et al*, *Angew. Chem., Int. Ed. Engl.*, 1966, **5**, 151 (*synth*)
Nesmeyanov, A.N. *et al*, *Dokl. Akad. Nauk SSSR, Ser. Sci. Khim.*, 1974, **216**, 816 (*nmr*)
Batich, C.D., *J. Am. Chem. Soc.*, 1976, **98**, 7585 (*pe*)
Henc, B. *et al*, *J. Organomet. Chem.*, 1980, **191**, 425 (*pmr, raman*)

$C_8H_{14}Ni$ Ni-00055

Bis[(1,2,3-η)-2-methyl-2-propenyl]nickel, 9CI

Bis(2-methyl-π-allyl)nickel, 8CI

[12261-14-2]

H_3C–⟨–Ni–⟩–CH_3

M 168.889

Orange-yellow cryst. Mp 33° dec.

Dietrich, H., *Z. Kristallogr.*, 1965, **122**, 60 (*struct*)
Wilke, G. *Angew. Chem., Int. Ed. Engl.*, 1966, **5**, 151 (*synth*)
Boennemann, B. *et al*, *Angew. Chem., Int. Ed. Engl.*, 1967, **6**, 804 (*pmr*)
Boehm, M.C. *et al*, *Helv. Chim. Acta*, 1980, **63**, 990 (*pe*)
Henc, B. *et al*, *J. Organomet. Chem.*, 1980, **191**, 425 (*pmr*, *raman*)

$C_8H_{16}As_2NiO_2$ Ni-00056

Dicarbonyl[1,2-ethanediylbis[dimethylarsine]]nickel

Dicarbonyl[ethylenebis[dimethylarsine]]nickel

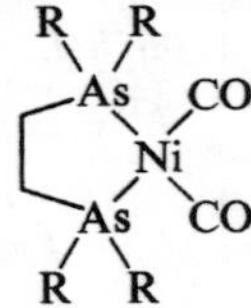

R = Me

M 352.746

Not isol.

Plankey, B.J. *et al*, *Inorg. Chem.*, 1979, **18**, 957.

$C_8H_{17}Ni_2^{\ominus}$ Ni-00057

Tetrakis(ethylene)(μ-hydrido)dinickelate(1−)

$[(H_2C{=}CH_2)_2Ni{-}H{-}Ni(H_2C{=}CH_2)_2]^{\ominus}$

M 230.602 (ion)

Formed from $Ni(C_2H_4)_3$ in tetramethylethylenediamine, the counterion is $[Li(TMEDA)_2]^{\oplus}$. No phys. details recorded.

Jonas, K. *et al*, *Angew. Chem., Int. Ed. Engl.*, 1980, **19**, 520 (*synth*)

$C_8H_{18}NiO_2P_2$ Ni-00058

Dicarbonylbis(trimethylphosphine)nickel, 9CI, 8CI

Bis(trimethylphosphine)dicarbonylnickel

[16787-34-1]

$Ni(CO)_2(PMe_3)_2$

M 266.867

Catalyst for hydrosilylation of isoprene and dimethylbutadiene. Cryst. (pentane or MeOH).

Bignorgne, M. *et al*, *Bull. Soc. Chim. Fr.*, 1960, 1986 (*synth*, *ir*)
Bouquet, G. *et al*, *J. Mol. Struct.*, 1968, **1**, 211 (*ir*, *raman*)
Mathieu, R. *et al*, *Inorg. Chem.*, 1970, **9**, 2030 (*nmr*)
Koenig, M.F. *et al*, *Spectrochim. Acta, Part A*, 1972, **28**, 1693 (*raman*)
Grobe, J. *et al*, *Z. Naturforsch., B*, 1981, **36**, 8 (*synth*)

$C_8H_{21}ClNiOP_2$ Ni-00059

Acetylchlorobis(trimethylphosphine)nickel, 9CI

Chloro(acetyl)bis(trimethylphosphine)nickel

[42481-73-2]

Me_3P, $COCH_3$, Ni, Cl, PMe_3

M 289.344

trans-form

Orange-yellow needles, stable to dry air. Mp 98-9°. Dec. >108°.

Klein, H.F. *et al*, *Chem. Ber.*, 1976, **109**, 2524 (*synth*, *ir*, *pmr*)
Huttner, G. *et al*, *Chem. Ber.*, 1976, **109**, 2533 (*struct*)

$C_8H_{24}Cl_2Ni_2P_2$ Ni-00060

Di-μ-chlorodimethylbis(trimethylphosphine)dinickel, 9CI

Bis(trimethylphosphine)dichlorodimethyldinickel

[42562-12-9]

Me, Cl, Me, Ni, Ni, Me_3P, Cl, PMe_3

M 370.511

Red-brown cryst. Dec. >93°. Mod. sol. toluene, Et_2O.

Klein, H.F. *et al*, *Chem. Ber.*, 1973, **106**, 1433 (*synth*, *ir*, *pmr*)

$C_8H_{26}Ni_2O_2P_2$ Ni-00061

Di-μ-hydroxydimethylbis(trimethylphosphine)dinickel, 9CI

[42531-32-8]

Me, OH, PMe_3, Ni, Ni, Me_3P, OH, Me *trans-form*

M 333.620

Bridged dimer. Brown cryst. Sol. toluene, mod. sol. Et_2O, pentane. Dec. >100° without melting. *Cis-* and *trans-*forms equilibrate in soln.

Monomer: Hydroxy(methyl)trimethylphosphinenickel.
$C_4H_{13}NiOP$ M 166.810
Unknown.

Klein, H.F. *et al*, *Chem. Ber.*, 1973, **106**, 1433 (*synth*, *ir*, *pmr*)

$C_8Ni_3O_8^{\ominus\ominus}$ Ni-00062

Tetra-μ-carbonyltetracarbonyltrinickelate(2−), 9CI

Octacarbonyltrinickelate(2−)

$[(OC)_2Ni(\mu\text{-}CO)_2Ni(\mu\text{-}CO)_2Ni(CO)_2]^{\ominus\ominus}$

M 400.153 (ion)

Bis(tetrabutylammonium) salt: [41948-83-8].
$C_{40}H_{72}N_2Ni_3O_8$ M 885.087
Insol. H_2O. Pure salt not isol.

Sternberg, H.W. *et al*, *J. Am. Chem. Soc.*, 1960, **82**, 3638 (*synth*)
Cassar, L., *J. Organomet. Chem.*, 1973, **51**, 381 (*synth*)

$C_9H_{12}Ni$ Ni-00063

[(1,2,3-η)-2-Butenyl](η⁵-2,4-cyclopentadien-1-yl)nickel, 9CI

π-Cyclopentadienyl(1-methylallyl)nickel, 8CI

[51733-18-7]

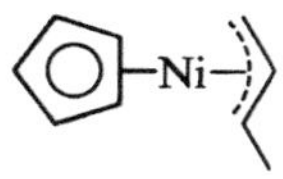

M 178.884

Known in *syn* and *anti* forms, but phys. details not available. Catalyst for polymerisation of butadiene. Red, air-sensitive liq.

McBride, D.W. *et al*, *J. Chem. Soc.*, 1964, 1752 (*synth*, *ir*, *pmr*)
Lehmkuhl, H. *et al*, *Justus Liebigs Ann. Chem.*, 1980, 744 (*synth*)
Benn, R. *et al*, *Org. Magn. Reson.*, 1980, **14**, 435 (*nmr*)

$C_9H_{12}Ni$ Ni-00064

(η⁵-2,4-Cyclopentadien-1-yl)[(1,2,3-η)-2-methyl-2-propenyl-]nickel, 10CI

(π-Cyclopentadienyl)(2-methylallyl)nickel

[74558-79-5]

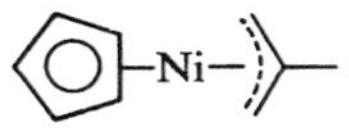

M 178.884

No phys. props. recorded.

Benn, R. *et al*, *Org. Magn. Reson.*, 1980, **14**, 435 (*nmr*)
Lehmkuhl, H. *et al*, *Justus Liebigs Ann. Chem.*, 1980, 744 (*synth*)

$C_9H_{14}NiOSn$ Ni-00065

Carbonyl(η⁵-2,4-cyclopentadien-1-yl)(trimethylstannyl)nickel, 9CI

Trimethylstannyl(π-cyclopentadienyl)nickel carbonyl.
Carbonyl(π-cyclopentadienyl)(trimethyltin)nickel.
π-Cyclopentadienylcarbonyl(trimethylstannyl)nickel

[31985-06-5]

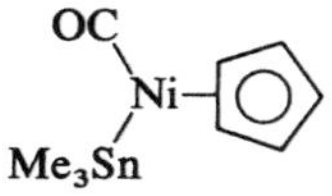

OC, Ni, Me_3Sn

M 315.589

Air-sensitive evil-smelling orange-red liq. $Bp_{0.01}$ 60°.

Abel, E.W. *et al*, *J. Organomet. Chem.*, 1970, **24**, 687 (*synth*, *ir*)
Abel, E.W. *et al*, *J. Organomet. Chem.*, 1973, **49**, 435 (*synth*, *nmr*)

$C_9H_{19}NiO_2P$ Ni-00066

Methyl(2,4-pentanedionato-*O,O'*)(trimethylphosphine)nickel, 9CI

Acetylacetonato(methyl)(trimethylphosphine)nickel

[42562-13-0]

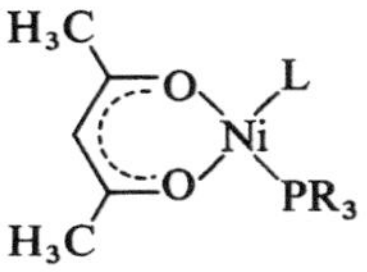

H_3C, O, L, Ni, PR_3, H_3C

L = R = Me

M 248.912

Light-brown cryst. (pentane). Stable in soln. for a considerable time. Air-sensitive both as solid and in soln. V. sol. Et_2O, toluene, mod. sol. pentane. Mp 72-4°. Dec. >150°.

Klein, H.F. *et al*, *Chem. Ber.*, 1973, **106**, 1433 (*synth*, *pmr*, *ir*)

$C_{10}H_{10}F_6Ni_2O_4$ Ni-00067

Bis(η³-2-propenyl)bis[μ-(trifluoroacetato-*O:O'*)]dinickel, 9CI

Bisallylbis(trifluoroacetato)dinickel

[32823-77-1]

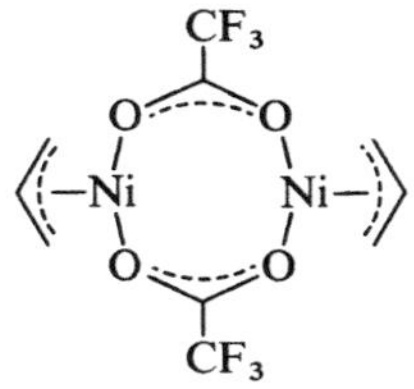

CF_3, O, O, Ni, Ni, O, O, CF_3

M 425.557

Catalyst for polymerisation of isoprene and styrene, and for stereospecific polymerisation of 1,3-butadiene. Orange-brown solid. Stable under Ar for several weeks at r.t. V. sol. Et_2O.

Monomer: (η³-Propenyl)(trifluoroacetato)nickel.
Allyl(trifluoroacetato)nickel.
$C_5H_5F_3NiO_2$ M 212.779
Unknown.

Dawans, F. *et al*, *J. Organomet. Chem.*, 1970, **21**, 259 (*synth*, *ir*, *pmr*)
Sourisseau, C. *et al*, *Can. J. Chem.*, 1974, **19**, 11 (*ir*)

$C_{10}H_{10}Ni$ Ni-00068

Nickelocene, 9CI

Di-π-cyclopentadienylnickel, 8CI. Bis(cyclopentadienyl)nickel

[1271-28-9]

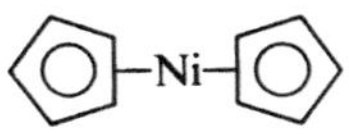

M 188.879

Catalyst for cross-coupling reacns. Dark-green needles (pet. ether). Mp 171-3°. Sublimes *in vacuo*. Paramagnetic.

▷QR6500000.

Fischer, E.O. *et al*, *Z. Naturforsch.*, 1953, **8**, 217 (*synth*)
Wilkinson, G. *et al*, *J. Am. Chem. Soc.*, 1954, **76**, 1970 (*synth*, *ir*)
Friedman, L. *et al*, *J. Am. Chem. Soc.*, 1955, **77**, 3689 (*ms*)
Knox, G.R. *et al*, *J. Chem. Soc.*, 1961, 4619 (*synth*)
Koehler, F.H., *J. Organomet. Chem.*, 1976, **110**, 235 (*cmr*, *pmr*)
Seiler, P. *et al*, *Acta Crystallogr., Sect. B*, 1980, **36**, 2255 (*struct*)

$C_{10}H_{11}Ni^{\oplus}$ Ni-00069

(η⁴-Cyclopentadiene)(η⁵-2,4-cyclopentadien-1-yl)nickel(1+), 9CI

Cyclopentadienyl(cyclopentadiene)nickel(1+)

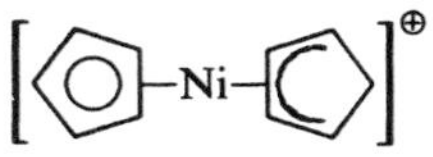

M 189.887 (ion)

No salts isol. Cation observed in HF solns. of nickelocene.

Turner, G.K. *et al*, *J. Organomet. Chem.*, 1975, **102**, C9 (*pmr*)

$C_{10}H_{12}Ni$ Ni-00070

(η^5-2,4-Cyclopentadien-1-yl)[(1,2,3-η)-2-cyclopenten-1-yl]nickel

[31811-17-3]

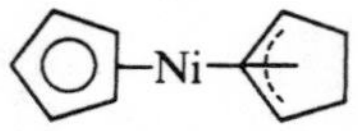

M 190.895

Dark-red prisms. Mp 43-4°.

Fischer, E.O. *et al*, *Chem. Ber.*, 1959, **92**, 1423 (*synth, ir*)
Dubeck, M. *et al*, *J. Am. Chem. Soc.*, 1961, **83**, 1257 (*synth, pmr*)
U.S.P., 3 088 960, (*1963*); *CA*, **59**, 10127 (*synth*)
McBride, D.W. *et al*, *J. Chem. Soc.*, 1964, 1752 (*synth*)

$C_{10}H_{12}NiO_2$ Ni-00071

(2,3,5,6-Tetramethyl-2,5-cyclohexadiene-1,4-dione)nickel

(*Tetramethyl*-p-*benzoquinone*)*nickel*. (*Duroquinone*)-*nickel*

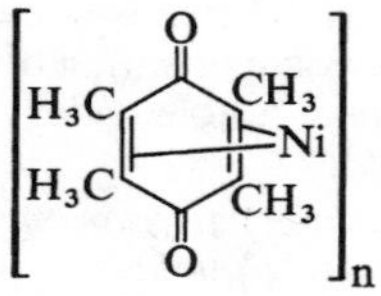

M 222.894

Polymeric. Violet solid. Insol. all comon solvs.

▷Pyrophoric

Schrauzer, G.N., *Z. Naturforsch., B*, 1962, **17**, 73 (*synth*)
Schrauzer, G.N., *Adv. Organomet. Chem.*, 1964, **2**, 2 (*synth*)

$C_{10}H_{14}NiO_4$ Ni-00072

Bis(2,4-pentanedionato-*O,O'*)nickel, 9CI

Bis(*acetylacetonato*)*nickel*

[3264-82-2]

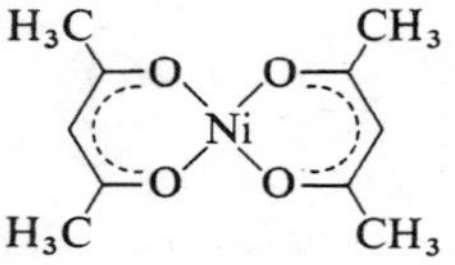

M 256.908

Many applications as a catalyst in polymerisation of organic compds. Blue-green solid.

▷SA2100000.

Fernelius, W.E. *et al*, *Inorg. Synth.*, 1957, **5**, 105 (*synth*)
Johnson, A. *et al*, *J. Am. Chem. Soc.*, 1972, **94**, 1419 (*synth*)
Schildcrout, S.M., *J. Phys. Chem.*, 1976, **80**, 2834 (*ms*)
Fragala, I. *et al*, *Inorg. Chim. Acta*, 1980, **40**, 15 (*pe*)

$C_{10}H_{14}Ni_2$ Ni-00073

Bis[μ-(π-1-vinylallyl)dinickel, 8CI

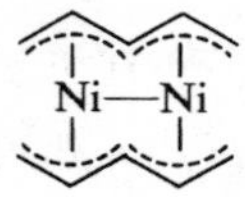

M 251.601

Golden-yellow cryst. (pentane). Extremely air-sensitive. Spar. sol. aprotic solvs.

Krueger, Ch., *Angew. Chem., Int. Ed. Engl.*, 1969, **8**, 678 (*struct*)
Rienaecker, R. *et al*, *Angew. Chem., Int. Ed. Engl.*, 1969, **8**, 677 (*synth, ir*)

$C_{10}H_{15}Cl_2N_2NiS_2Tl$ Ni-00074

Bis[(2-mercaptoethylamine)nickel]dichlorophenylthallium

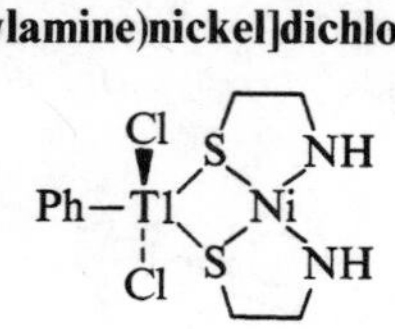

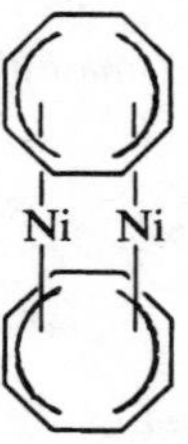

M 561.341

Trigonal bipyramidal struct. proposed. Pale-yellow solid. Mp 193-5° dec.

Pellerito, L. *et al*, *J. Organomet. Chem.*, 1974, **70**, C27 (*synth, ir*)

$C_{10}H_{16}Ni_2$ Ni-00075

Bis[μ-(η^3,η^3-1,3,5,7-cyclooctatetraene)]dinickel, 9CI

Dicyclooctatetraenedinickel

[61583-79-7]

M 253.616

Black cryst. Ni atoms disordered, but struct. compatible with allylic bonding to each ring.

Lehmkuhl, H. *et al*, *Justus Liebigs Ann. Chem.*, 1973, 692 (*synth*)
Brauer, D. *et al*, *J. Organomet. Chem.*, 1976, **122**, 265 (*struct*)

$C_{10}H_{19}NiO_3P$ Ni-00076

Acetyl(2,4-pentanedionato-*O,O'*)(trimethylphosphine)nickel, 9CI

Acetylacetonato(*acetyl*)(*trimethylphosphine*)*nickel*

[60767-31-9]

As Methyl(2,4-pentanedionato-*O,O'*)-(trimethylphosphine)nickel, Ni-00066 with

$$L = COCH_3, R = Me$$

M 276.922

Yellow cryst. (pentane). Sl. sol. polar solvs., mod. sol. covalent solvs. Mp 61-2°. Dec. >130°.

Klein, H.F. *et al*, *Chem. Ber.*, 1976, **109**, 2524 (*synth, ir, pmr*)

$C_{10}H_{27}NiOP_3$ Ni-00077

Carbonyltris(trimethylphosphine)nickel, 9CI, 8CI

Tris(*trimethylphosphine*)*carbonylnickel*

[15376-84-8]

$$Ni(CO)(PMe_3)_3\ (C_{3v})$$

M 314.934

White gummy solid, stable in dry air. Compound solidifies to a transparent glass after melting. Dec. begins at 120°/0.01 mm.

Bignorgne, M. *et al*, *Bull. Soc. Chim. Fr.*, 1960, 1986 (*synth, ir*)
Bouquet, G. *et al*, *J. Mol. Struct.*, 1968, **1**, 211 (*ir, raman*)
Mathieu, R. *et al*, *Inorg. Chem.*, 1970, **9**, 2030 (*nmr*)

$C_{11}H_{12}F_6Ni$ Ni-00078

[(1,2,5,6-η)-1,5-Cyclooctadiene][(1,2-η)-hexafluoropropene]nickel

(1,5-Cyclooctadiene)(hexafluoropropylene)nickel, 8CI

[31760-68-6]

M 316.896

Yellow cryst. (pet. ether), dec. >50°.

Cundy, C.S. *et al*, *J. Chem. Soc. (A)*, 1970, 1647 (*synth, pmr*)

$C_{11}H_{15}INiO$ Ni-00079

Carbonyl(iodo)(pentamethylcyclopentadienyl)nickel

(Pentamethylcyclopentadienyl)carbonyliodonickel

M 348.833

Compound not isol.

Mise, T. *et al*, *J. Organomet. Chem.*, 1979, **164**, 391 (*synth*)

$C_{11}H_{17}ClNi$ Ni-00080

[(2,3-η)-Bicyclo[2.2.1]hept-2-ene]chloro[(1,2,3-η)-2-methyl-2-propenyl]nickel, 9CI

(η-Norbornene)chloro(π-2-methylallyl)nickel

[36005-15-9]

M 243.398

Red cryst., air-sensitive. Insol. EtOH, sl. sol. C_6H_6, chlorinated solvs.

Gallazzi, M.C. *et al*, *J. Organomet. Chem.*, 1971, **33**, C45; 1975, **97**, 131 (*synth*)

$C_{12}F_{10}Ni$ Ni-00081

Bis(pentafluorophenyl)nickel

[68972-57-6]

$Ni(C_6F_5)_2$

M 392.806

Compound not isol. Yellow soln. in THF/dioxan, stable for several weeks under dry N_2. Red soln. in THF.

Arcas, A. *et al*, *Inorg. Chim. Acta*, 1978, **30**, 205 (*synth*)

$C_{12}H_8N_2NiO_2$ Ni-00082

(2,2′-Bipyridine)dicarbonylnickel, 10CI, 8CI

Dicarbonyl(2,2′-bipyridine)nickel

[14917-14-7]

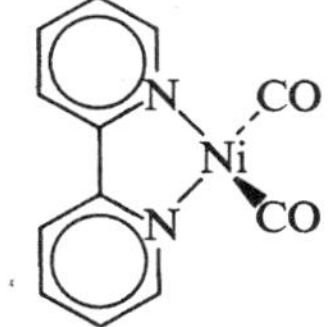

M 270.897

Catalyst for polymerisation of acetylenic compounds, and for reductive dimerisation of propionitrile halo derivs. Red solid. Insol. most solvs.

Nyholm, R.S. *et al*, *J. Chem. Soc.*, 1953, 2670 (*synth, ir*)
Kohara, T. *et al*, *Chem. Lett.*, 1979, 1513 (*synth, ir*)

$C_{12}H_{10}Br_2Ni_2O_2Sn$ Ni-00083

Dicarbonylbis(η^5-2,4-cyclopentadien-1-yl)[μ-(dibromostannylene)]dinickel, 9CI

Dicarbonyldi-π-cyclopentadienyl(μ-dibromostannylene)dinickel, 8CI. *Di(π-cyclopentadienyl)dicarbonyl)(μ-dibromotin)dinickel*

[36180-76-4]

M 582.088

Green cryst. ($CHCl_3$/hexane). Mp 107-8°. Slowly oxid. in the dry state and in soln.

Edmondson, R.C. *et al*, *J. Organomet. Chem.*, 1972, **35**, 119 (*synth, pmr, ir*)

$C_{12}H_{10}Ni_2O_2$ Ni-00084

Di-μ-carbonylbis(η^5-2,4-cyclopentadien-1-yl)dinickel, 9CI

Bis(cyclopentadienylcarbonylnickel). *Di-μ-carbonyldi-π-cyclopentadienyldinickel*, 8CI. *Bis(carbonylcyclopentadienylnickel)*

[12170-92-2]

M 303.590

Dark-red cryst. Mp 143°.

Fischer, E.O. *et al*, *Chem. Ber.*, 1958, **91**, 1725 (*synth*)
Fischer, E.O. *et al*, *Z. Naturforsch., B*, 1958, **13**, 456 (*synth, ir*)
Ger. Pat., 1 060 397, (*1959*); *CA*, **55**, 8431 (*synth*)
Manning, A.R. *et al*, *J. Chem. Soc. (A)*, 1971, 717 (*ir*)
Gansow, O.A. *et al*, *J. Am. Chem. Soc.*, 1976, **98**, 5817 (*cmr*)
Blake, M.R. *et al*, *Org. Mass Spectrom.*, 1978, **13**, 20 (*ms*)
Madach, T. *et al*, *Chem. Ber.*, 1980, **113**, 3235 (*struct*)

$C_{12}H_{12}Ni_2$ Ni-00085

Bis(η^5-2,4-cyclopentadien-1-yl)[μ-(η^2:η^2-ethyne)dinickel], 10CI, 9CI

[52445-55-3]

M 273.607

Green cryst. (pet. ether or by subl. *in vacuo*). Mp 143-4°.

Dubeck, M., *J. Am. Chem. Soc.*, 1960, **82**, 502 (*synth*)
Randall, E.W. *et al*, *J. Organomet. Chem.*, 1974, **64**, 271 (*synth, ir, pmr, cmr*)
Rossetti, R. *et al*, *Inorg. Chim. Acta*, 1975, **15**, 149 (*ms*)
Wang, Y. *et al*, *Inorg. Chem.*, 1976, **15**, 1122 (*struct*)

$C_{12}H_{13}BrN_2Ni$ Ni-00086

(2,2′-Bipyridine)bromo(ethyl)nickel, 10CI

Ethylbromo(2,2′-bipyridine)nickel

[79268-70-5]

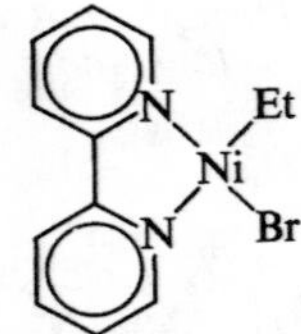

M 323.842

No phys. props. recorded. No analytically pure sample was obt.

Yamamoto, T. *et al*, *Bull. Chem. Soc. Jpn.*, 1981, **54**, 2010 (*synth*)

$C_{12}H_{13}Ni^{\oplus}$ Ni-00087

[(2,3,5,6-η)-Bicyclo[2.2.1]hepta-2,5-diene](η^5-2,4-cyclopentadien-1-yl)nickel(1+), 9CI

π-Cyclopentadienyl(norbornadiene)nickel(1+)

[48131-24-4]

M 215.925 (ion)

Tetrafluoroborate: [42088-00-6].
$C_{12}H_{13}BF_4Ni$ M 302.728
No phys. props. recorded.

Salzer, A. *et al*, *J. Organomet. Chem.*, 1973, **54**, 325 (*synth, pmr, ir*)
Court, T.L. *et al*, *J. Organomet. Chem.*, 1974, **65**, 224 (*nmr*)

$C_{12}H_{14}F_6Ni_2O_4$ Ni-00088

Bis[(1,2,3-η)-2-butenyl]bis[μ-trifluoroacetato-*O*:*O′*]dinickel, 9CI

Bis(1-methyl-π-allyl)bis(μ-trifluoroacetato)dinickel, 8CI. *Bis-μ-trifluoroacetatobis(1-methylallyl)dinickel. Bis[(1,2,3-η)-2-butenyl]bis(μ-trifluoroethanoato)dinickel*

[32964-71-9]

M 453.611

Catalyst for polymerisation of butadiene and cycloalkenes. Orange-brown solid.

Monomer: *(2-Butenyl)(trifluoroacetato)nickel. (1-Methylallyl)(trifluoroacetato)nickel.*
$C_6H_7F_3NiO_2$ M 226.805
Unknown.

Kormer, V.A. *et al*, *J. Polym. Sci., Part A-1*, 1972, **10**, 251 (*synth*)
Bourdauducq, P. *et al*, *J. Polym. Sci, Part A-1*, 1972, **10**, 2527 (*synth*)
Warin, R. *et al*, *J. Polym. Sci., Polym. Lett. Ed.*, 1973, **11**, 177 (*pmr*)

$C_{12}H_{14}N_2Ni$ Ni-00089

(2,2′-Bipyridine-*N*,*N′*)dimethylnickel, 9CI

Dimethyl(2,2′-bipyridine)nickel

[32370-42-6]

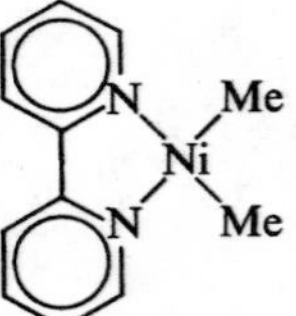

M 244.946

Catalyst for stereospecific polymerisation of acetaldehyde. Green cryst. (C_6H_6).

Wilke, G. *et al*, *Angew. Chem., Int. Ed. Engl.*, 1966, **5**, 581 (*synth*)
Yamamoto, T. *et al*, *J. Am. Chem. Soc.*, 1971, **93**, 3350 (*synth*)
Tolman, C.A. *et al*, *Inorg. Chem.*, 1973, **12**, 2770 (*pe*)

$C_{12}H_{14}Ni$ Ni-00090

Bis(η^5-1-methyl-2,4-cyclopentadien-1-yl)nickel

1,1′-Dimethylnickelocene, 9CI

[1293-95-4]

M 216.933

Can be used as catalyst in polymerisation of acetylenes. Green cryst. Mp 36-8°. Subl. *in vacuo*. Paramagnetic.

Anderson, S.E. *et al*, *Chem. Phys. Lett.*, 1972, **13**, 150 (*nmr*)
Evans, S. *et al*, *J. Chem. Soc., Faraday Trans. 2*, 1974, **70**, 356 (*pe*)
Koehler, F.H., *J. Organomet. Chem.*, 1976, **110**, 235 (*synth, pmr, nmr*)
Gordon, K.R. *et al*, *Inorg. Chem.*, 1978, **17**, 987 (*props*)

$C_{12}H_{18}Br_2Ni_2O_4$ Ni-00091

Di-μ-bromobis[(1,2,3-η)-2(ethoxycarbonyl)-2-propenyl]dinickel, 9CI

Di-μ-bromobis(2-carboxy-π-allyl)dinickel diethyl ester, 8CI. Di-μ-bromobis(2-carbethoxyallylnickel)

[12288-88-9]

M 503.460

Red cryst., extremely air-sensitive.

Monomer: Bromo(2-ethoxycarbonyl-2-propenyl)nickel.
$C_6H_9BrNiO_2$ M 251.730
Unknown.

Churchill, M.A. *et al*, *Inorg. Chem.*, 1967, **6**, 1386 (*synth, struct*)
Hegedus, L.S. *et al*, *J. Org. Chem.*, 1975, **40**, 593 (*synth*)

$C_{12}H_{18}Ni$ Ni-00092

Bis[(1,2,3-η)-2-cyclohexen-1-yl]nickel, 10CI

[75104-81-3]

M 220.964

Yellow cryst. (pentane). Mp −35° dec.

Henc, B. *et al*, *J. Organomet. Chem.*, 1980, **191**, 425 (*synth, pmr, cmr, ir, raman*)

$C_{12}H_{18}Ni$ Ni-00093

[(1,2,5,6,9,10-η)-1,5,9-Cyclododecatriene]nickel, 10CI, 9CI

[12126-69-1]

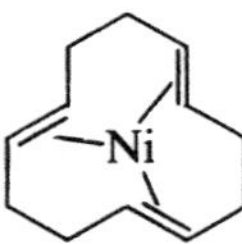

M 220.964

Metallic red cryst. Mp 102°. Two stereoisomers identified in soln.

Dietrich, H. *et al*, *Naturwissenschaften*, 1965, **52**, 301 (*struct*)
Bogdanovic, B. *et al*, *Justus Liebigs Ann. Chem.*, 1966, **699**, 1 (*synth*)
Nesmeyanov, A.N. *et al*, *Dokl. Akad. Nauk SSSR*, 1974, **216**, 816 (*cmr*)

$C_{12}H_{18}Ni$ Ni-00094

[(1,2,3,10,11,12-η)-2,6,10-Dodecatriene-1,12-diyl]nickel, 9CI

[36835-51-5]

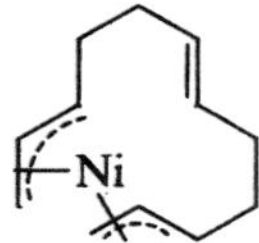

M 220.964

Formerly formulated as $\eta^{1\text{-}3,6\text{-}7,10\text{-}12}$. Has been formulated both with and without Ni-olefin bonding. Soln. pmr indicates central C atoms attached to Ni. Two stereoisomers present in soln. Red solid or dark-red volatile liq. Mp 15-6°. Subl. at 0.01 mm.

Bogdanovic, B. *et al*, *Justus Liebigs Ann. Chem.*, 1969, **727**, 143 (*synth, pmr*)
Heimbach, P. *et al*, *Adv. Organomet. Chem.*, 1970, **8**, 29.
Baker, R. *et al*, *J. Chem. Soc., Perkin Trans. 1*, 1978, 480.
Inorg. Synth., 1979, **19**, 80 (*synth*)
Henc, B. *et al*, *J. Organomet. Chem.*, 1980, **191**, 425 (*pmr, raman*)

$C_{12}H_{20}GeNiO$ Ni-00095

Carbonyl(η^5-2,4-cyclopentadien-1-yl)(triethylgermyl)nickel, 10CI

(Triethylgermyl)cyclopentadienylcarbonylnickel

[33196-00-8]

M 311.569

Liq. d^{20} 1.320. $Bp_{0.2}$ 79-80°. n_D^{20} 1.5932.

Gladyshev, E.N. *et al*, *Dokl. Akad. Nauk SSSR, Ser. Sci. Khim.*, 1968, **179**, 1333 (*synth*)

$C_{12}H_{30}Cl_2NiP_2$ Ni-00096

Dichlorobis(triethylphosphine)nickel, 9CI, 8CI

Bis(triethylphosphine)nickel dichloride. Bis(triethylphosphine)dichloronickel

[17523-24-9]

trans-form

M 365.913

Cocatalyst in olefin oligomerisations.

trans-form [15638-51-4]
Purple solid.

Jensen, K.A. *et al*, *Acta Chem. Scand.*, 1963, **17**, 1115 (*synth*)
Ekkehard, F. *et al*, *Z. Naturforsch., B*, 1967, **22**, 1095 (*nmr*)
Boorman, P.M. *et al*, *Inorg. Nucl. Chem. Lett.*, 1968, **4**, 101 (*ir*)
Fergusson, J.E. *et al*, *Inorg. Chim. Acta*, 1978, **31**, 145 (*ir, pmr*)

$C_{12}H_{32}NiP_4$ Ni-00097

Bis[1,2-bis(dimethylphosphino)ethane]nickel

Bis[1,2-ethanediylbis(dimethylphosphine)-P,P′]nickel, 9CI. Bis[ethylenebis(dimethylphosphine)]nickel, 8CI

[32104-66-8]

R = Me

M 358.970

White solid by subl., air-sensitive. Mp 120° (under N_2).

Chatt, J. *et al*, *J. Chem. Soc.*, 1962, 2537 (*synth*)
Tolman, C.A., *J. Am. Chem. Soc.*, 1970, **92**, 2956 (*pmr*)
Tolman, C.A., *Inorg. Chem.*, 1973, **12**, 2770 (*pe*)
Inorg. Synth., 1977, **17**, 117 (*synth*)

$C_{12}H_{36}NiO_{12}P_4$ Ni-00098

Tetrakis(trimethylphosphite-*P*)nickel, 9CI

Tetrakis(phosphorous acid)nickel dodecamethyl ester, 8CI

[14881-35-7]

$[(MeO)_3P]_4Ni$

M 554.994

Cryst. (pentane). V. sol. all org. solvs. Mp 130°.

Jensen, K.A. *et al*, *Acta Chem. Scand.*, 1965, **19**, 768 (*synth*)
Coskran, R.J. *et al*, *J. Am. Chem. Soc.*, 1967, **89**, 4535 (*nmr*)
Loutellier, A. *et al*, *J. Chim. Phys. Physicochim. Biol.*, 1970, **67**, 99 (*ir*, *raman*)
Tolman, C.A. *et al*, *Inorg. Chem.*, 1973, **12**, 2770 (*pe*)
Inorg. Synth., 1977, **17**, 117 (*synth*)
Crocker, C. *et al*, *J. Chem. Res. (S)*, 1979, 378 (*synth*, *nmr*)

$C_{12}H_{36}NiP_4$ Ni-00099

Tetrakis(trimethylphosphine)nickel, 9CI, 8CI

[28069-69-4]

$(Me_3P)_4Ni$ (T_d)

M 363.001

Light-yellow cryst. (pentane), dec. >160°. Stable indefinitely under N_2 at r.t. Sol. Et_2O, hydrocarbons, insol. H_2O. Mp 198°. Reacts rapidly with CCl_4, $CHCl_3$, more slowly with CH_2Cl_2.

Tolman, C.A., *J. Am. Chem. Soc.*, 1970, **92**, 2956 (*synth*)
Loutellier, A. *et al*, *J. Organomet. Chem.*, 1977, **133**, 201 (*ir*, *nmr*)
Inorg. Synth., 1977, **17**, 117 (*synth*)

$C_{12}Ni_3O_{12}Pt_3^{\ominus\ominus}$ Ni-00100

Dodecacarbonyltrinickelatetriplatinate(2−)

Tri-μ-carbonyltricarbonyl(tri-μ-carbonyltricarbonyltrinickelate)triplatinate(2−), 10CI

[72669-24-0]

$[Ni_3Pt_3(CO)_{12}]^{\ominus\ominus}$

M 1097.435 (ion)

Formed from mixt. of $[Pt_6(CO)_{12}]^{\ominus\ominus}$ and $[Ni_6(CO)_{12}]^{\ominus\ominus}$. Compd. not isol. in solid state. Sol. Me_2CO. Struct. is probably prismatic with Ni_3 and Pt_3 units retaining their identities.

Brown, C. *et al*, *J. Organomet. Chem.*, 1979, **181**, 233 (*nmr*)

$C_{12}Ni_5O_{12}^{\ominus\ominus}$ Ni-00101

Dodecacarbonylpentanickelate(2−)

[56938-71-7]

M 629.575 (ion)

Yellow soln.

Bis(triphenylphosphine)imminium salt: [57108-14-2]. Dark-yellow cryst. (toluene under CO).

Bis(tetramethylammonium) salt: [60464-16-6].
$C_{20}H_{24}N_2Ni_5O_{12}$ M 777.866
Brown cryst. (MeOH).

Bis(tetraethylammonium) salt: [60464-15-5].
$C_{28}H_{52}N_2Ni_5O_{12}$ M 902.175
Brown solid (MeOH).

Lower, L. *et al*, *J. Am. Chem. Soc.*, 1975, **97**, 5034 (*synth*, *struct*)
Longoni, G. *et al*, *Inorg. Chem.*, 1976, **15**, 3025 (*synth*, *ir*, *struct*)

$C_{12}Ni_6O_{12}^{\ominus\ominus}$ Ni-00102

Dodecacarbonylhexanickelate(2−)

[52261-68-4]

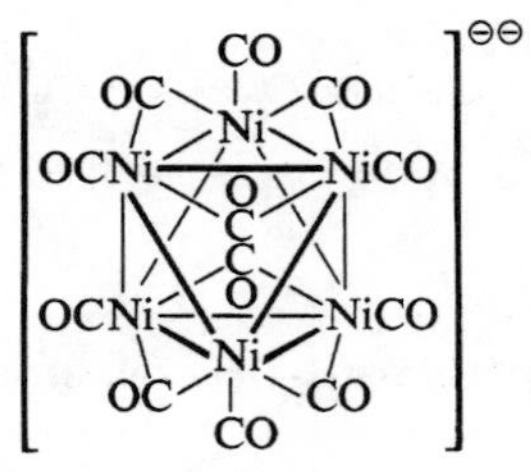

M 688.265 (ion)

Red soln.

Di-K salt: [60464-09-7].
$C_{12}K_2Ni_6O_{12}$ M 766.461
Red cryst. (THF).

Bis(tetraphenylphosphonium) salt: [60464-17-7].
$C_{60}H_{40}Ni_6O_{12}P_2$ M 1367.056
Dark-red cryst. (2-propanol).

Bis(tetramethylammonium) salt: [60464-19-9].
$C_{20}H_{24}N_2Ni_6O_{12}$ M 836.556
Red cryst. (Me_2CO/2-propanol).

Longoni, G. *et al*, *Inorg. Chem.*, 1976, **15**, 3025 (*synth*, *ir*, *struct*)

$C_{13}H_{14}Ni_2$ Ni-00103

Bis(η⁵-2,4-cyclopentadien-1-yl)[μ-[(1,2-η:1,2-η)-1-propyne]]dinickel, 9CI

[52445-53-1]

M 287.634

Deep-green cryst. Mod. stable as solid, dec. rapidly in soln. on exp. to air. V. sol. common org. solvents.

Randall, E.W. *et al*, *J. Organomet. Chem.*, 1974, **64**, 271 (*synth*, *ir*, *pmr*, *cmr*)
Rossetti, R. *et al*, *Inorg. Chim. Acta*, 1975, **15**, 149 (*ms*)

$C_{13}H_{17}Ni^{\oplus}$ Ni-00104

[(1,2,5,6-η)-1,5-Cyclooctadiene](η⁵-2,4-cyclopentadien-1-yl)nickel(1+), 9CI

(π-Cyclopentadienyl)(1,5-cyclooctadiene)nickel(1+)

[48138-38-1]

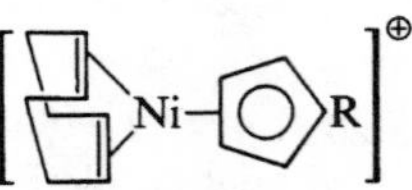

R = H

M 231.967 (ion)

Tetrafluoroborate: [42088-01-7].
$C_{13}H_{17}BF_4Ni$ M 318.771
No phys. props. recorded.

Salzer, A. *et al*, *J. Organomet. Chem.*, 1973, **54**, 325 (*synth, pmr, ir*)
Court, T.L. *et al*, *J. Organomet. Chem.*, 1974, **65**, 245 (*pmr*)

$C_{13}H_{20}NiO_2$ **Ni-00105**

(1,4,5-η)-4-Cycloocten-1-yl(2,4-pentanedionato-*O,O'*)nickel, 10CI
(Acetylacetonato)[(1,4,5-η)-4-cycloocten-1-yl]nickel
[12086-04-3]

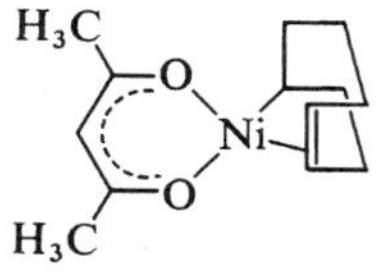

M 266.990
Brown-red cryst. Mp 73-5° dec. Subl. *in vacuo* at ca. 60°.

Bogdanovic, B. *et al*, *Justus Liebigs Ann. Chem.*, 1966, **699**, 1 (*synth*)
Mills, O.S. *et al*, *J. Chem. Soc., Chem. Commun.*, 1966, 738 (*struct*)

$C_{13}H_{30}Br_2NiOP_2$ **Ni-00106**

Dibromo(carbonyl)bis(triethylphosphine)nickel, 10CI
Carbonyldibromobis(triethylphosphine)nickel
[73687-97-5]

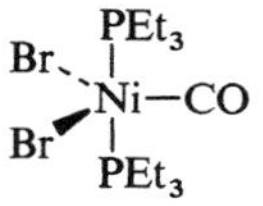

M 482.825
V. air-sensitive, unstable orange cryst. Sol. CH_2Cl_2. Dec. in soln.

Saint-Joly, C. *et al*, *Inorg. Chem.*, 1980, **19**, 2403 (*synth, nmr, ir, uv*)

$C_{13}H_{30}NiO_2P_2$ **Ni-00107**

[(*C,O*-η)-Carbon dioxide]bis(triethylphosphine)nickel, 10CI
Bis(triethylphosphine)(carbon dioxide)nickel
[63816-42-2]

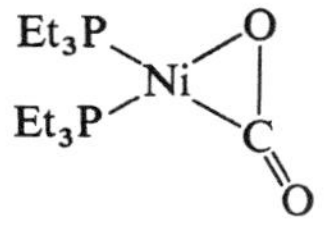

M 339.016
Yellow cryst. Mod. stable to air in solid state. Dec. >134°.

Aresta, M. *et al*, *J. Chem. Soc., Dalton Trans.*, 1977, 708 (*synth, ir, uv*)

$C_{13}H_{39}NiP_4^{\oplus}$ **Ni-00108**

Methyltetrakis(trimethylphosphine)nickel(1+), 9CI
Tetrakis(trimethylphosphine)methylnickel(1+)

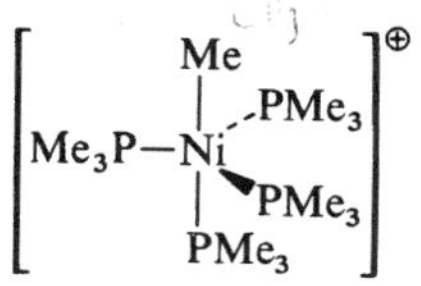

M 378.036 (ion)
Chloride: [52166-15-1].
$C_{13}H_{39}ClNiP_4$ M 413.489
Red-brown cryst. Dec. >58°.
Thiocyanate: [52166-19-5].
$C_{14}H_{39}NNiP_4S$ M 436.114
Dark-red cryst. Mp 94-8° dec.
Tetraphenylborate: [52166-20-8].
$C_{37}H_{59}BNiP_4$ M 697.268
Cryst. (Me_2CO/MeOH). Dec. >100°.

Klein, H.F. *et al*, *Chem. Ber.*, 1974, **107**, 537; 1976, **109**, 2515 (*synth, nmr, struct*)
Gleizes, A. *et al*, *Inorg. Chem.*, 1981, **20**, 2372 (*struct*)

$C_{14}H_8N_2NiO_2$ **Ni-00109**

Dicarbonyl(1,10-phenanthroline-N^1,N^{10})nickel, 9CI
Dicarbonyl(o-phenanthroline)nickel. (1,10-Phenanthroline)dicarbonylnickel
[36454-23-6]

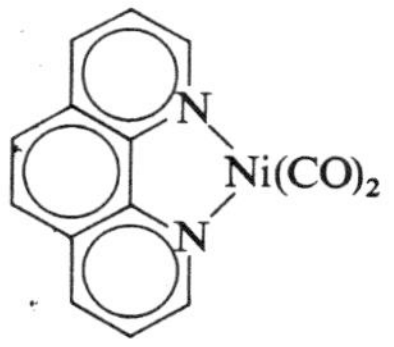

M 294.919
Catalyses oligomerisation of diacetyl.

Walther, D., *Z. Chem.*, 1977, **17**, 188 (*use*)
Walther, D. *et al*, *Z. Anorg. Allg. Chem.*, 1978, **440**, 22 (*use*)
Plankey, B.J. *et al*, *Inorg. Chem.*, 1979, **18**, 957 (*synth, ir*)

$C_{14}H_{10}F_6Ni_2$ **Ni-00110**

Bis(η^5-2,4-cyclopentadien-1-yl)[μ-[(2,3-η:2,3-η)-1,1,1,4,4,4-hexafluoro-2-butyne]]dinickel, 9CI
μ-Hexafluoro-2-butynebis(π-cyclopentadienylnickel)
[52445-59-7]

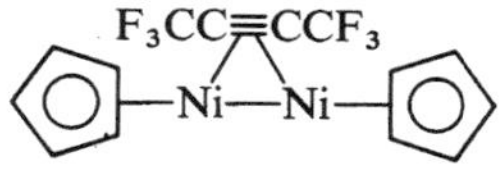

M 409.603
No phys. details recorded.

Randall, E.W. *et al*, *J. Organomet. Chem.*, 1974, **64**, 271 (*synth*)
Rossetti, R. *et al*, *Inorg. Chim. Acta*, 1975, **15**, 149 (*ms*)

$C_{14}H_{10}F_{12}Ni_2P_2$ **Ni-00111**

Bis[μ-[bis(trilfluoromethyl)phosphino]]di-π-cyclopentadienyldinickel, 8CI

Bis(η⁵-2,4-cyclopentadien-1-yl)bis[μ-[bis(trifluoromethyl)phosphine]]dinickel

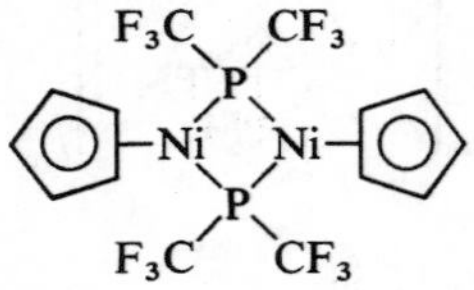

M 585.541

Bridged dimer. Black, air-stable cryst. (pet. ether). Spar. sol. org. solvs. Mp 297-9°.

Monomer: [*Bis(trifluoromethyl)phosphino*]-(*cyclopentadienyl*)*nickel.*
$C_7H_5F_6NiP$ M 292.771
Unknown.

Dobbie, R.C. *et al*, *J. Chem. Soc. (A)*, 1969, 1881 (*synth*, *ms*, *pmr*, *nmr*)

$C_{14}H_{14}Ni^{\ominus\ominus}$ **Ni-00112**

Ethylenediphenylnickelate(2−)

Ethenediphenylnickelate(2−). Bis(ethenediphenylnickelate)(4−)

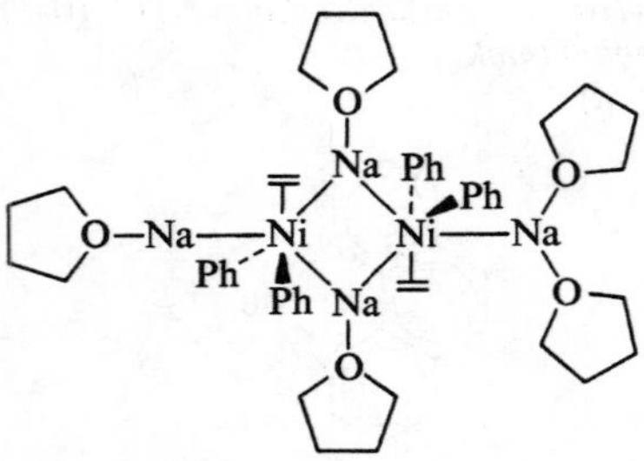

M 240.955 (ion)

Dimer, di-Na salt, pentakis-THF complex: [57774-33-1]. *Bis*[(η²-*ethene*)*diphenylnickel*]*pentakis*(*tetrahydrofuran*)*tetrasodium*, 9CI.
$C_{48}H_{68}Na_4Ni_2O_5$ M 934.401
Air-sensitive red cryst.

Jonas, K., *Angew. Chem., Int. Ed. Engl.*, 1976, **15**, 47 (*synth*)
Brauer, D.J. *et al*, *Angew. Chem., Int. Ed. Engl.*, 1976, **15**, 48 (*struct*)

$C_{14}H_{14}Ni_2O_2$ **Ni-00113**

Di-μ-carbonylbis[(1,2,3,4,5-η)-1-methyl-2,4-cyclopentadien-1-yl]dinickel, 10CI

Bis(π-methylcyclopentadienyl)di-μ-carbonyldinickel

[32028-28-7]

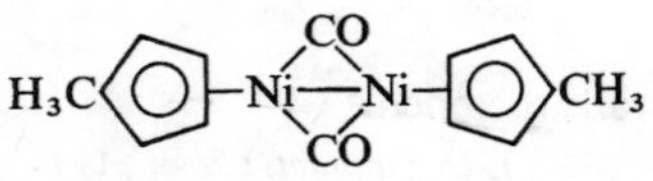

M 331.643

Catalyst in butadiene dimerization. Bright-orange cryst. Mp 85-8°.

U.S.P., 3 086 036, (*1963*); *CA*, **59**, 8792 (*synth*)
Gmelins Handbuch der Anorg. Chem., 1974, **B17**, 344 (*synth*)
Byers, L.R. *et al*, *Inorg. Chem.*, 1980, **19**, 680 (*struct*, *ir*, *nmr*, *ms*)

$C_{14}H_{16}N_2Ni$ **Ni-00114**

(2,2′-Bipyridine-*N*,*N*′)-1,4-butanediylnickel, 9CI

(*2,2′-Bipyridine*)*tetramethylenenickel. Tetramethylene-*(*bipyridyl*)*nickel. α,α′-Dipyridylnickelacyclopentane*

[62320-23-4]

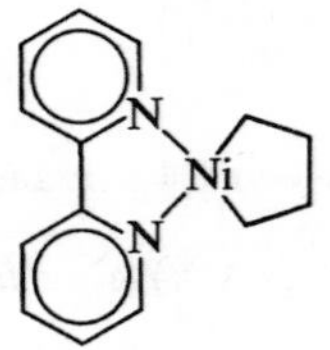

M 270.984

Used to prepare cycloalkanes from *αω*- and *gem*-dihalides. Air-sensitive dark-green cryst. Dec. at ~120°.

Takahashi, S. *et al*, *J. Chem. Soc., Chem. Commun.*, 1976, 839 (*use*)
Binger, P. *et al*, *Z. Naturforsch., B*, 1979, **34**, 1289 (*synth*, *ms*, *struct*)

$C_{14}H_{16}N_2Ni_2$ **Ni-00115**

Bis(η⁵-2,4-cyclopentadien-1-yl)bis[μ-(isocyanomethane)]dinickel, 9CI

Bis(η⁵-2,4-cyclopentadien-1-yl)bis(μ-methylisocyanide]dinickel. Bis(π-cyclopentadienyl)bis[μ-methylisonitrile]dinickel

[38979-69-0]

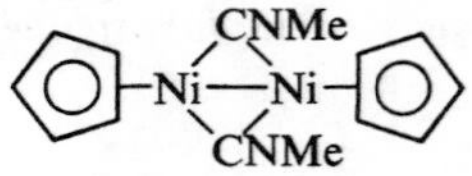

M 329.674

Cryst. No other physical data recorded.

Adams, R.D. *et al*, *J. Coord. Chem.*, 1972, **1**, 275 (*struct*)

$C_{14}H_{16}Ni_2$ **Ni-00116**

[μ-[(2,3-η:2,3-η)-2-Butyne]]bis(η⁵-2,4-cyclopentadien-1-yl-)dinickel, 9CI

(2-Butyne)dicyclopentadienyldinickel

[12147-37-4]

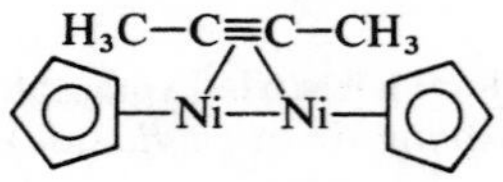

M 301.660

Black cryst.; oxid. by air. Mp 55°.

Tilney-Bassett, J.F., *J. Chem. Soc.*, 1961, 577 (*synth*)
Mills, O.S. *et al*, *Acta Crystallogr.*, 1965, **18**, 562 (*struct*)
Randall, E.W. *et al*, *J. Organomet. Chem.*, 1974, **64**, 271 (*spectra*)
Rossetti, R. *et al*, *Inorg. Chim. Acta*, 1975, **15**, 149 (*ms*)

$C_{14}H_{16}Ni_2$ **Ni-00117**

[μ-[(1,2,3,3a,6a-η:3a,4,5,6,6a-η)-pentalene]]bis(η³-2-propenyl)dinickel, 9CI

[36593-86-9]

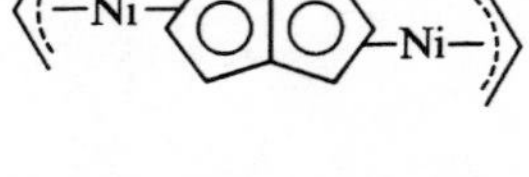

M 301.660

Deep-green cryst. (Et_2O), stable at r.t. Mp >145° dec. (sinters).

Miyake, A. *et al*, *Angew. Chem., Int. Ed. Engl.*, 1971, **10**, 801 (*synth, pmr, struct*)

$C_{14}H_{18}N_2Ni$ Ni-00118

(2,2′-Bipyridine-*N,N′*)diethylnickel, 9CI
Diethyl(bipyridyl)nickel
[15218-76-5]

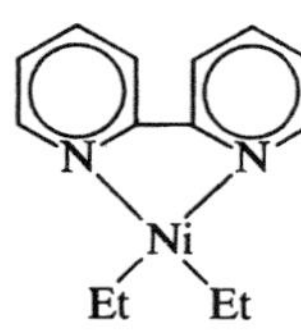

M 273.000
Catalyses oligomerisation of butadiene. Cryst. (C_6H_6, Me_2CO or Et_2O).

Yamamoto, A. *et al*, *J. Am. Chem. Soc.*, 1965, **87**, 4652 (*synth*)
Castellano, S. *et al*, *J. Phys. Chem.*, 1967, **71**, 2368 (*pmr*)
Saito, T., *J. Phys. Chem.*, 1967, **71**, 2370 (*pmr*)

$C_{14}H_{19}Ni^{\oplus}$ Ni-00119

[(1,2,5,6-η)-1,5-Cyclooctadiene](η⁵-1-methyl-2,4-cyclopentadien-1-yl)nickel(1+), 9CI
(Methylcyclopentadienyl)(1,5-cyclooctadiene)-nickel(1+)
As [(1,2,5,6-η)-1,5-Cyclooctadiene](η⁵-2,4-cyclopentadien-1-yl)nickel(1+), Ni-00104 with

R = CH_3

M 245.994 (ion)
Tetrafluoroborate: [42187-62-2].
$C_{14}H_{19}BF_4Ni$ M 332.798
No phys. props. recorded.

Salzer, A. *et al*, *J. Organomet. Chem.*, 1973, **54**, 325 (*synth, ir, pmr*)

$C_{14}H_{20}N_4Ni$ Ni-00120

[(1,2-η)-Ethene-1,2-biscarbonitrile]bis(2-isocyano-2-methylpropane)nickel, 10CI
(2,3-η)-2-Butenedinitrilebis(2-isocyano-2-methylpropane)nickel, 9CI. *Bis(*tert*-butylisocyanide)(fumaronitrile)nickel*, 8CI. *1,2-Dicyanoethylenebis(*tert*-butylisonitrile)nickel*
[32612-10-5]

CN $CNC(CH_3)_3$
Ni
NC $CNC(CH_3)_3$

M 303.029
Yellow cryst. (Et_2O), extremely air-sensitive.

Otsuka, S. *et al*, *J. Am. Chem. Soc.*, 1971, **93**, 6462 (*synth*)
Ittel, S.D., *Inorg. Chem.*, 1977, **16**, 2589 (*ir*)

$C_{14}H_{20}Ni$ Ni-00121

4-Cycloocten-1-yl(methyl-π-cyclopentadienyl)nickel, 8CI
(Methylcyclopentadienyl)(4-cycloocten-1-yl)nickel

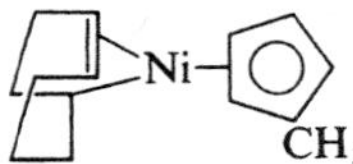

M 247.002

Viscous air-sensitive red liq. Sol. org. solvs.

Barnett, K.W., *J. Organomet. Chem.*, 1970, **21**, 477 (*synth, pmr, ms*)

$C_{14}H_{22}Ni$ Ni-00122

Bis[(1,2,3-η)-2-cyclohepten-1-yl]nickel, 10CI, 9CI
[38816-29-4]

M 249.018
Catalyses butadiene oligomerisation. Yellow cryst. (pentane). Mp 0-10° dec.

Henc, B. *et al*, *J. Organomet. Chem.*, 1980, **191**, 425 (*synth, pmr, cmr, ir, raman*)

$C_{14}H_{30}Cl_4NiP_2$ Ni-00123

Chloro(trichlorovinyl)bis(triethylphosphine)nickel, 8CI
Chloro(trichloroethenyl)bis(triethylphosphine)nickel, 9CI
[22853-51-6]

Cl PEt_3
Ni
Et_3P $CCl{=}CCl_2$

M 460.841
trans-form
Catalyst for hydrocarbon dimerisations. Yellow solid, fairly stable towards atm. O_2 and acids. Sol. Et_2O. Mp 92-92.8°. Dec. at 190-200°.

Miller, R.G. *et al*, *J. Am. Chem. Soc.*, 1968, **90**, 6248 (*synth, ir*)
Miller, R.G. *et al*, *J. Am. Chem. Soc.*, 1970, **92**, 1511 (*nmr*)
Fahey, D.R. *et al*, *Inorg. Chim. Acta*, 1979, **36**, 269 (*pe*)

$C_{14}H_{30}NiO_2P_2$ Ni-00124

Dicarbonylbis(triethylphosphine)nickel, 9CI, 8CI
Bis(triethylphosphine)nickel dicarbonyl
[16787-33-0]

$Ni(CO)_2(PEt_3)_2$ (T_d)

M 351.027
Catalyst for oligomerisation of alkenes and hydrogenation of butadiene. Sol. CH_2Cl_2.

Bignorgne, M. *et al*, *Bull. Soc. Chim. Fr.*, 1960, 1986 (*synth*)
Tolman, C.A. *et al*, *J. Am. Chem. Soc.*, 1970, **92**, 2953 (*ir*)
Bodner, G.M., *Inorg. Chem.*, 1975, **14**, 1932 (*nmr*)

$C_{14}H_{36}NiP_2$ Ni-00125

Dimethylbis(triethylphosphine)nickel, 9CI
Bis(triethylphosphine)dimethylnickel
[60542-85-0]

$NiMe_2(PEt_3)_2$

M 325.076
Catalyst for insertion reaction between CO, Grignard reagents and aryl halides to give ketones and tertiary alcohols. Unstable at r.t.

Yamamoto, A. *et al*, *Organotransition-Met. Chem., Proc. Jpn.-Am. Semin., 1st*, 1974 (*pub. 1975*), Plenum, New York, 265 (*synth*)

Yamamoto, T. *et al*, *Chem. Lett.*, 1976, 1217 (*use*)

$C_{15}H_{13}N_2Ni^{\oplus}$ **Ni-00126**

(2,2′-Bipyridine-*N,N′*)(η^5-2,4-cyclopentadien-1-yl)nickel(1+), 9CI

(π-Cyclopentadienyl)(2,2′-bipyridine)nickel(1+)

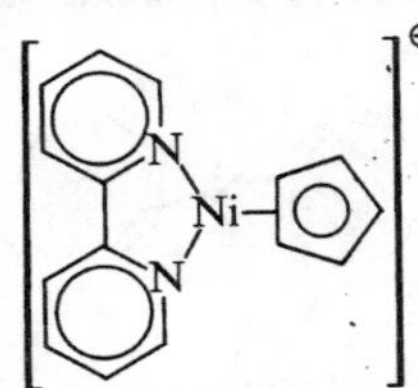

M 279.971 (ion)

Tetrafluoroborate: [38904-10-8].
$C_{15}H_{13}BF_4N_2Ni$ M 366.775
Light-red solid.

Salzer, A. *et al*, *Synth. React. Inorg. Metal-Org. Chem.*, 1972, **2**, 249 (*synth, ir, uv*)

$C_{15}H_{15}Ni_2^{\oplus}$ **Ni-00127**

[μ-(η^5:η^5-2,4-Cyclopentadien-1-yl)]bis(η^5-2,4-cyclopentadien-1-yl)dinickel(1+), 10CI

[53664-04-3]

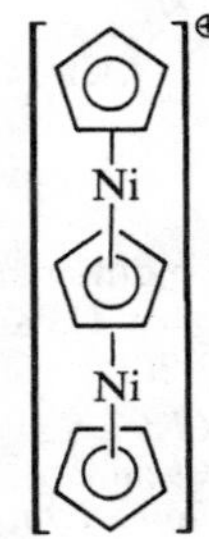

M 312.664 (ion)

Tetrafluoroborate: [37298-59-2].
$C_{15}H_{15}BF_4Ni_2$ M 399.467
Black-violet cryst. (propionic acid).

Hexafluorophosphate: [37298-60-5].
$C_{15}H_{15}F_6Ni_2P_2$ M 488.601
No phys. props. recorded.

Werner, H. *et al*, *Synth. Inorg. Met.-Org. Chem.*, 1972, **2**, 239 (*synth*)
Werner, H. *et al*, *J. Organomet. Chem.*, 1977, **141**, 339 (*synth*)
Dubler, E. *et al*, *Acta Crystallogr., Sect. B*, 1983, **39**, 607 (*struct*)

$C_{15}H_{15}Ni_3S_2$ **Ni-00128**

Tris(η^5-2,4-cyclopentadien-1-yl)di-μ_3-thioxotrinickel, 10CI

Tris(π-cyclopentadienyl)di(μ_3-sulfido)trinickel

[58396-47-7]

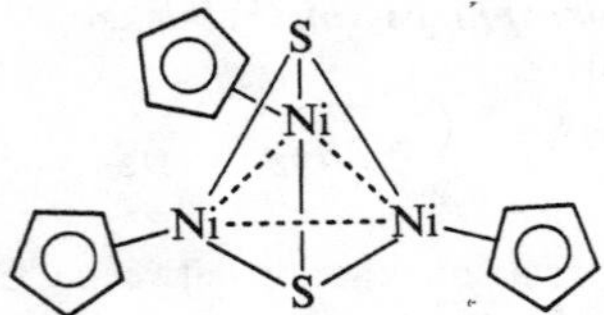

M 435.474
No phys. props. recorded.

Vahrenkamp, H. *et al*, *J. Am. Chem. Soc.*, 1968, **90**, 3272 (*struct*)

Oxton, I.A. *et al*, *Inorg. Chim. Acta*, 1981, **47**, 177 (*ir*)

$C_{15}H_{16}Ni_2$ **Ni-00129**

[μ-[(1,2-η:3,4-η)-1,3-Cyclopentadiene]]bis(η^5-2,4-cyclopentadien-1-yl)dinickel, 9CI

Bis(cyclopentadienyl)(μ-cyclopentadiene)dinickel

[38599-73-4]

M 313.671
Black cryst. Mp 140°.

Fischer, E.O. *et al*, *Chem. Ber.*, 1972, **105**, 3014 (*synth*)
Paquette, M.S. *et al*, *J. Am. Chem. Soc.*, 1980, **102**, 6621 (*synth*)

$C_{15}H_{20}Ni$ **Ni-00130**

η^5-Cyclopentadienyl(η^5-pentamethylcyclopentadienyl)nickel

1,2,3,4,5-Pentamethylnickelocene, 10CI

[75730-73-3]

M 259.013
Dark-green cryst. Subl. without observable dec.

Werner, H. *et al*, *J. Organomet. Chem.*, 1980, **198**, 97 (*synth, ms*)

$C_{15}H_{20}NiP^{\oplus}$ **Ni-00131**

[η^5-2,4-Cyclopentadien-1-yl](dimethylphenylphosphine)(η^2-ethene)nickel(1+), 10CI

(η^5-2,4-Cyclopentadien-1-yl)ethene(dimethylphenylphosphine)nickel(1+). Ethylene(cyclopentadienyl)(dimethylphenylphosphine)nickel(1+). Cyclopentadienyl(ethylene)(dimethylphenylphosphine)nickel(1+)

M 289.987 (ion)

Perchlorate: [64065-88-9].
$C_{15}H_{20}ClNiO_4P$ M 389.437
Red solid, stable at r.t. Gradually dec. in CH_2Cl_2 or Me_2CO soln.

Majuma, T. *et al*, *J. Organomet. Chem.*, 1977, **134**, C45 (*synth, ir, pmr*)

The first digit of the Entry number defines the Supplement in which the Entry is found. 0 indicates the Main Work

$C_{15}H_{23}N_2Ni^{\oplus}$ Ni-00132

(η^5-2,4-Cyclopentadien-1-yl)bis(2-isocyano-2-methylpropane)nickel(1+), 9CI

Bis(tert-*butylisocyanide*)-*π-cyclopentadienylnickel(1+)*, *8CI*. (*π-Cyclopentadienyl*)*bis*(tert-*butylisonitrilenickel(1+)*

M 290.050 (ion)

Bromide:
$C_{15}H_{23}BrN_2Ni$ M 369.954
Mp 118-9° dec.

Iodide:
$C_{15}H_{23}IN_2Ni$ M 416.955
Mp 124° dec.

Tetraphenylborate:
$C_{39}H_{43}BN_2Ni$ M 609.282
Mp 145-9° dec.

Yamamoto, Y. *et al*, *J. Organomet. Chem.*, 1969, **18**, 189 (*synth*)

$C_{15}H_{25}Cl_3NiP_2$ Ni-00133

(2-Methylphenyl)(trichlorovinyl)bis(trimethylphosphine)nickel

(*2-Methylphenyl*)(*trichloroethenyl*)*bis*(*trimethylphosphine*)*nickel*, *10CI*. o-*Tolyl*(*trichlorovinyl*)-*bis*(*trimethylphosphine*)*nickel*

M 432.359

***trans*-form** [77170-49-1]
Cryst. (EtOH). Mp 168-9° dec.

Wada, M. *et al*, *J. Chem. Soc., Dalton Trans.*, 1981, 240 (*synth*, *pmr*)

$C_{15}H_{27}NiO_3P$ Ni-00134

Tricarbonyl(tributylphosphine)nickel, 9CI, 8CI

Tributylphosphinenickel tricarbonyl

[15698-54-1]

$Ni(CO)_3P(CH_2CH_2CH_2CH_3)_3$ (T_d)

M 345.040

Used as catalyst in oligomerisation of butadiene. Compound obt. in soln. and not isol. Sol. $CHCl_3$.

Meriwether, L.S. *et al*, *J. Am. Chem. Soc.*, 1959, **81**, 4200.
Strohmeier, W. *et al*, *Chem. Ber.*, 1967, **100**, 2812 (*ir*)
Bodner, G.M., *Inorg. Chem.*, 1975, **14**, 1932 (*nmr*)

$C_{15}H_{27}NiO_3P$ Ni-00135

Tricarbonyl(tri-*tert*-butylphosphine)nickel, 8CI

Tricarbonyl[*tris*(*1,1-dimethylethyl*)*phosphine*]*nickel*, *9CI*

$Ni(CO)_3P[C(CH_3)_3]_3$

M 345.040

Cryst. (pentane). Sol. THF. Dec. at 105°.

Schumann, H. *et al*, *J. Organomet. Chem.*, 1969, **16**, P64 (*synth*)
Schumann, H. *et al*, *Chem. Ber.*, 1975, **108**, 1630 (*ir*, *raman*, *pmr*, *nmr*)
Pickardt, J. *et al*, *Z. Anorg. Allg. Chem.*, 1976, **426**, 66 (*struct*)

$C_{15}H_{27}NiP$ Ni-00136

[(1,2,5,6,9,10-η)-1,5,9-Cyclododecatriene](trimethylphosphine)nickel, 10CI

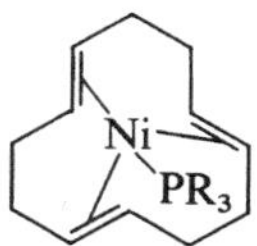

R = Me

M 297.042

(*E,E,E*)-*form* [62745-31-7]
No phys. props. reported.

Hoffmann, E.G. *et al*, *Z. Naturforsch., B*, 1976, **31**, 1712 (*nmr*)

$C_{15}H_{35}N_4Ni^{\oplus}$ Ni-00137

Methyl(1,4,8,11-tetramethyl-1,4,8,11-tetraazacyclotetradecane-N^1,N^4,N^8,N^{11})nickel(1+), 9CI

[*Tetra*(N-*methyl*)-*1,4,8,11-tetraazacyclotetradecane*]-*methylnickel(1+)*

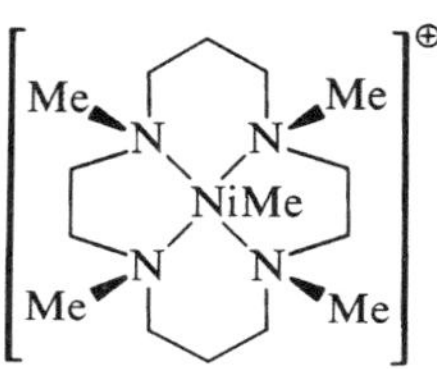

M 330.158 (ion)

Trifluoromethanesulphonate: [59419-75-9].
$C_{16}H_{35}F_3N_4NiO_3S$ M 479.223
Cryst. (THF/Et_2O). Stable for several days at r.t. under N_2, slowly dec. on exp. to air.

D'Aniello, M.J. *et al*, *J. Am. Chem. Soc.*, 1976, **98**, 1610 (*synth*)

$C_{15}H_{45}NiO_{15}P_5^{\oplus\oplus}$ Ni-00138

Pentakis(trimethylphosphite)nickel(2+), 9CI

[53701-87-4]

$Ni[P(OMe)_3]_5^{\oplus\oplus}$ (D_{3h})

M 679.070 (ion)

Orange soln., slightly air-sensitive.

Bis(*tetrafluoroborate*)*:* [53701-91-0].
$C_{15}H_{45}B_2F_8NiO_{15}P_5$ M 852.678
White cryst.

Diperchlorate: [55009-50-2].
$C_{15}H_{45}Cl_2NiO_{23}P_5$ M 877.972
Orange cryst. (MeOH/Et_2O).

Hexafluorosilicate: [54171-39-0].
$C_{15}H_{45}F_6NiO_{15}P_5Si$ M 821.146
Orange oil.

Coskran, K.J. *et al*, *Adv. Chem. Ser.*, 1966, **62**, 590 (*synth*, *uv*)
Coskran, K.J. *et al*, *J. Am. Chem. Soc.*, 1967, **89**, 4535 (*nmr*)
Ludmann, M.F. *et al*, *Bull. Soc. Chim. Fr.*, 1974, 2771 (*uv*)
Meakin, P. *et al*, *J. Am. Chem. Soc.*, 1974, **96**, 5751 (*synth*, *stereochem*)
Jesson, J.P. *et al*, *J. Am. Chem. Soc.*, 1974, **96**, 5760 (*pmr*)
Lukosius, E.J. *et al*, *Inorg. Chem.*, 1975, **14**, 1922, 1926 (*ir*, *uv*, *pmr*)

$C_{16}F_{18}Ni_4O_4$ **Ni-00139**

Tetracarbonyltris[μ_3-[(1-η:1,2-η:1,2-η)-1,1,1,4,4,4-hexafluoro-2-butyne]]tetranickel, 9CI

[58034-09-6]

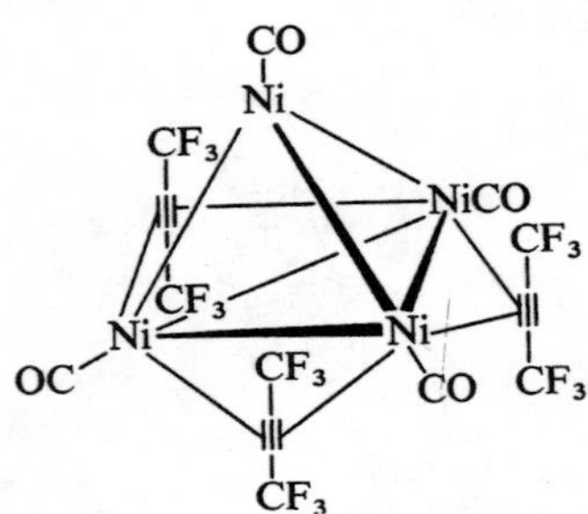

M 832.905

Deep red-violet air-sensitive cryst. Mp 119-21° dec.

Davidson, J.L. *et al*, *J. Chem. Soc., Dalton Trans.*, 1979, 506 (*synth, ir, struct*)

$C_{16}H_{12}Ni_2$ **Ni-00140**

Bis[(1,2,3,3*a*,6*a*-η:3*a*,4,5,6,6*a*-η)pentalene]dinickel, 9CI

[37279-19-9]

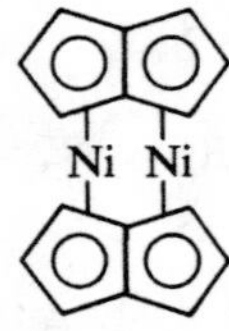

M 321.651

Red-brown solid, stable in air for several hours. Sl. sol. CS_2, THF, toluene, Et_2O, Me_2CO. Mp >315°.

Katz, T.J. *et al*, *J. Am. Chem. Soc.*, 1972, **94**, 3281 (*synth, ir, ms, pmr*)

$C_{16}H_{13}ClN_2Ni$ **Ni-00141**

(2,2′-Bipyridine-*N,N′*)chlorophenylnickel, 9CI

Phenyl(2,2′-bipyridine)nickel chloride

[29187-01-7]

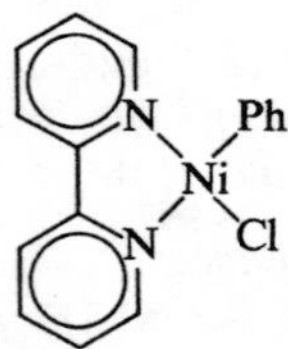

M 327.435

Catalyst for the dimerisation of alkenes. Reddish-brown cryst. +1PhCl (chlorobenzene), dec. in air in a few hours. Solns. in solvs. other than chlorobenzene unstable. Sol. PhCl, THF, Me_2CO, toluene. Dec. at 75.5-75.7°.

Uchino, M. *et al*, *J. Organomet. Chem.*, 1975, **84**, 93 (*synth*)

$C_{16}H_{14}N_4Ni$ **Ni-00142**

(2,2′-Bipyridine-*N,N′*)bis(2-propenenitrile)nickel, 9CI

Bis(acrylonitrile)(2,2′-bipyridine)nickel, 8CI. *(2,2′-Bipyridine-*N,N′*)bis[(1,2-η)-ethenecarbonitrile]nickel*

[38566-75-5]

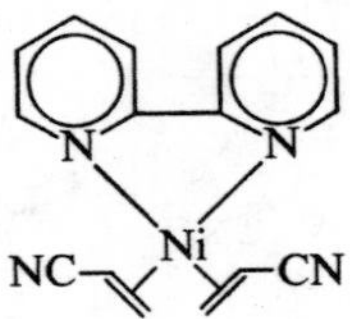

M 321.003

Red cryst. (THF/hexane). Mp 155.5° dec.

Yamamoto, A. *et al*, *J. Am. Chem. Soc.*, 1967, **89**, 5989 (*synth*)

$C_{16}H_{16}Ni$ **Ni-00143**

Bis[(1,2,3,4-η)-1,3,5,7-cyclooctatetraene]nickel, 9CI

[12112-24-2]

M 266.992

Cryst., polymerises >−20°.

Bogdanovic, B. *et al*, *Justus Liebigs Ann. Chem.*, 1966, **699**, 1 (*synth, ir*)

$C_{16}H_{18}N_6Ni$ **Ni-00144**

Bis(*tert*-butylisocyanide)(tetracyanoethylene)nickel, 8CI

[(1,2-η)-Ethenetetracarbonitrile]bis(2-isocyano-2-methylpropane)nickel, 9CI. *Tetracyanoethylenebis(*tert*-butylisonitrile)nickel*

[24917-37-1]

M 353.048

Reddish-brown air stable cryst. (toluene). Mp 164-7° dec.

Stalick, J.K. *et al*, *J. Am. Chem. Soc.*, 1970, **92**, 5333 (*struct*)

Otsuka, S. *et al*, *J. Am. Chem. Soc.*, 1971, **93**, 6462 (*synth, ir, pmr*)

$C_{16}H_{18}Ni$ **Ni-00145**

Bis[(1,2,3-η)-2,4,7-cyclooctatrien-1-yl]nickel, 10CI

[75095-20-4]

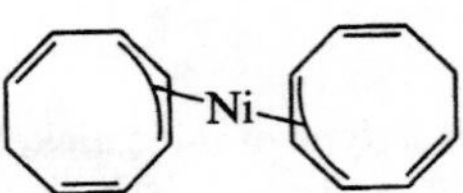

M 269.008

Dark-red cryst. (pentane). Mp 168-70°.

Henc, B. *et al*, *J. Organomet. Chem.*, 1980, **191**, 425 (*synth, pmr, cmr, struct, ir, raman*)

$C_{16}H_{18}Ni_2$ Ni-00146

[μ-[η³:η³-2,3-Bis(methylene)-1,4-butanediyl-]]bis[(1,2,3-η)-2,4-cyclopentadien-1-yl]dinickel, 9CI
Di-π-Cyclopentadienyl[μ-(π₂-2,3-dimethylethylenetetramethylene)]dinickel, 8CI
[35914-81-9]

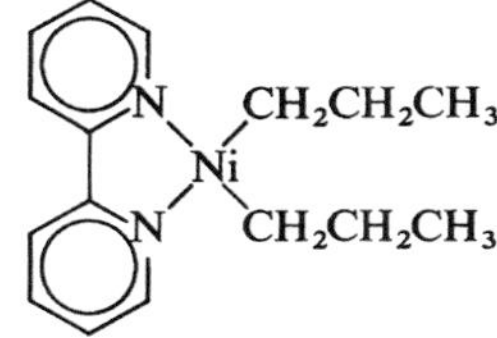

M 327.698
Deep-red cryst.

Keim, W., *Angew. Chem., Int. Ed. Engl.*, 1968, **7**, 879 (*synth*)
Smith, A.E., *Inorg. Chem.*, 1972, **11**, 165 (*struct*)

$C_{16}H_{22}N_2Ni$ Ni-00147

(2,2'-Bipyridine-*N,N'*)dipropylnickel, 9CI
Dipropyl(2,2'-bipyridine)nickel
[33340-22-6]

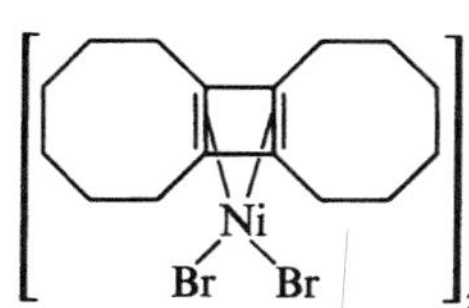

M 301.053
Sol. C_6H_6, DMF. Phys. props. assumed to be similar to diethyl deriv., i.e. green air-sensitive cryst.

Yamamoto, A. *et al*, *J. Am. Chem. Soc.*, 1971, **93**, 3350 (*synth*)
Yamamoto, T. *et al*, *Bull. Chem. Soc. Jpn.*, 1976, **49**, 191 (*nmr*)

$C_{16}H_{24}Br_2Ni$ Ni-00148

Dibromo(1,2,3,4,5,6,7,8,9,10,11,12-dodecahydrocyclobuta[1,2:3,4]dicyclooctenenickel, 8CI
[12308-54-2]

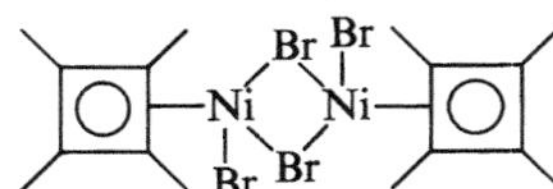

M 434.864
Dimeric, probably *via* 2μ-Br.
Dimer:
$C_{32}H_{48}Br_4Ni_2$ M 869.727
Cryst. (C_6H_6/pet. ether). Dec. >300°.

Wittig, G. *et al*, *Justus Liebigs Ann. Chem.*, 1968, **712**, 79 (*synth*)

$C_{16}H_{24}Br_4Ni_2$ Ni-00149

Di-μ-bromodibromobis[(1,2,3,4-η)-1,2,3,4-tetramethyl-1,3-cyclobutadiene]dinickel, 10CI
Tetrabromobis(tetramethylcyclobutadiene)dinickel
[71078-13-2]

M 653.362
Bridged dimer. Red-violet cryst.
Monomer: Dibromo(tetramethylcyclobutadiene)nickel.
$C_8H_{12}Br_2Ni$ M 326.681
Unknown.

Thewalt, U. *et al*, *Z. Naturforsch., B*, 1979, **34**, 859 (*synth, struct*)

$C_{16}H_{24}Cl_4Ni_2$ Ni-00150

Di-μ-chlorodichlorobis[(1,2,3,4-η)-1,2,3,4-tetramethyl-1,3-cyclobutadiene]dinickel, 10CI
Bis(tetramethylcyclobutadienyl)dinickel tetrachloride
[33112-02-6]

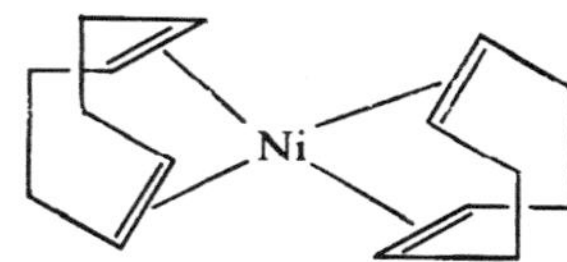

M 475.558
Catalyst for polymerisation of hydrocarbons. Red-violet cryst. (butanol/$CHCl_3$).
Monomer: Dichloro(tetramethylcyclobutadiene)nickel. (Tetramethylcyclobutadienyl)nickel dichloride.
$C_8H_{12}Cl_2Ni$ M 237.779
Unknown.

Criegee, R. *et al*, *Angew. Chem.*, 1959, **71**, 70 (*synth*)
Dunitz, J.D. *et al*, *Helv. Chim. Acta*, 1962, **45**, 647 (*struct*)
Onsager, O.-T. *et al*, *Helv. Chim. Acta*, 1969, **52**, 187 (*synth*)

$C_{16}H_{24}Ni$ Ni-00151

Bis[(1,2,5,6-η)-1,5-cyclooctadiene]nickel, 9CI
Bis(1,5-cyclooctadiene)nickel, 8CI
[1295-35-8]

M 275.056
Catalyst for isomerisation and hydrosilylation of unsaturated compds. Co-catalyst for oligomerisation, cyclooligomerisation, or polymerisation of alkenes, butadiene. Yellow cryst. Mp 140-2°. Air-sensitive.

Wilke, G. *et al*, *Angew. Chem.*, 1960, **72**, 581 (*synth*)
Fr. Pat., 1 320 729, (*1963*); *CA*, **59**, 14026 (*synth*)
Wilke, G. *et al*, *Justus Liebigs Ann. Chem.*, 1966, **699**, 1 (*synth*)
Müller, J. *et al*, *Angew. Chem., Int. Ed. Engl.*, 1967, **6**, 304 (*synth, ir, pmr, ms*)
Nesmeyanov, A.N. *et al*, *Dokl. Akad. Nauk. SSSR*, 1974, **216**, 816; *CA*, **81**, 70680 (*cmr*)

$C_{16}H_{26}Ni$ Ni-00152

Bis[(1,2,3-η)-2-cycloocten-1-yl]nickel, 10CI
[65106-71-0]

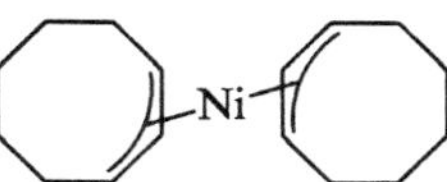

M 277.071
Yellow cryst. (pentane).

Henc, B. *et al*, *J. Organomet. Chem.*, 1980, **191**, 425 (*synth, pmr, cmr, ir, raman*)

$C_{16}H_{26}NiSi_2$ Ni-00153

1,1′-Bis(trimethylsilyl)nickelocene, 9CI
Bis(π-trimethylsilylcyclopentadienyl)nickel
[60975-31-7]

M 333.242

Tolstikov, G.A. *et al*, *Zh. Obsch. Khim.*, 1976, **46**, 1178 (*synth*)
Sultanov, A.Sh. *et al*, *Zh. Obsch. Khim.*, 1977, **47**, 1336 (*ms*)

$C_{16}H_{29}NNiP^{\oplus}$ Ni-00154

(η⁵-2,4-Cyclopentadien-1-yl)(2-isocyano-2-methylpropane)-(triethylphosphine)nickel(1+), 9CI
(tert-*Butylisonitrile*)(*π-cyclopentadienyl*)(*triethylphosphine*)*nickel*(*1*+), 8CI. (*π-Cyclopentadienyl*)(tert-*butylisonitrile*)(*triethylphosphine*)*nickel*(*1*+)

M 325.076 (ion)
Iodide:
$C_{16}H_{29}INNiP$ M 451.980
Mp 117-9° dec.

Yamamoto, Y. *et al*, *J. Organomet. Chem.*, 1969, **18**, 189 (*synth*)

$C_{16}H_{37}NiO_6P_2^{\oplus}$ Ni-00155

[(1,2,3-η)-2-Buten-1-yl]bis[(triethyl phosphite)-*P*]nickel(1+), 9CI
1-Methyl-π-allylbis(*phosphorous acid*)*nickel*(*1*+) *hexamethyl ester*, 8CI. *1-Methylallylbis*(*triethyl phosphite*)*nickel*(*1*+)

M 446.102 (ion)
Hexafluorophosphate: [32678-25-4].
$C_{16}H_{37}F_6NiO_6P_3$ M 591.066
Butadiene polymerisation catalyst. Yellow cryst. Sol. MeOH. Mp 63-5°. Air-sensitive.

Tolman, C.A., *J. Am. Chem. Soc.*, 1970, **92**, 6777 (*synth*, *pmr*, *ir*)
Tolman, C.A. *et al*, *Inorg. Chem.*, 1973, **12**, 2770 (*pe*)

$C_{17}H_{14}N_2Ni$ Ni-00156

η⁵-2,4-Cyclopentadien-1-yl[2-(phenylazo)phenyl]nickel, 10CI, 9CI
[53361-87-8]

M 305.001
Deep-blue cryst. (pet. ether). Mp 118-20°.

Kleiman, J.P. *et al*, *J. Am. Chem. Soc.*, 1963, **85**, 1544 (*synth*, *pmr*)
Ustynyuk, Yu.A. *et al*, *Dokl. Akad. Nauk SSSR*, 1969, **187**, 112; *CA*, **71**, 70710 (*pmr*)
Ustynyuk, Yu. A. *et al*, *J. Organomet. Chem.*, 1970, **23**, 551 (*synth*)
Cross, R.J. *et al*, *J. Organomet. Chem.*, 1974, **72**, 21 (*synth*)

$C_{17}H_{15}Ni_3O_2$ Ni-00157

Dicarbonyltricyclopentadienyldinickel
Di-μ₃-carbonyltris(*η⁵-2,4-cyclopentadien-1-yl*)*trinickel*, 9CI. *Dicarbonyltri-π-cyclopentadienyltrinickel*, 8CI
[12194-69-3]

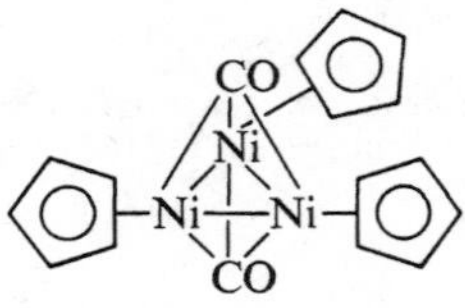

M 427.374

Fischer, E.O. *et al*, *Chem. Ber.*, 1958, **91**, 1725 (*synth*)
Byers, L.R. *et al*, *J. Am. Chem. Soc.*, 1981, **103**, 1942 (*struct*)

$C_{17}H_{29}NiP$ Ni-00158

Bis(bicyclo[2.2.1]hept-2-ene)(trimethylphosphine)nickel
Bis(*norbornene*)(*trimethylphosphine*)*nickel*

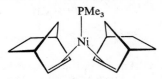

M 323.080
No phys. details recorded. Mixt. of two rotational *exo,exo*-isomers present in soln. at −34° as shown by cmr.

Hoffmann, E.G. *et al*, *Z. Naturforsh*, *B*, 1976, **31**, 1712 (*nmr*)

$C_{17}H_{32}ClNiP$ Ni-00159

Chloro(η⁵-2,4-cyclopentadien-1-yl)(tributylphosphine)nickel, 9CI
(*π-Cyclopentadienyl*)*chloro*(*tributylphosphine*)*nickel*. (*Tributylphosphine*)*chloro*(*π-cyclopentadienyl*)*nickel*
[1298-65-3]

M 361.557
Dark-brown solid, stable in air. Sol. C_6H_6, THF, aliphatic solvs. Mp 59-59.5°.

Yamazaki, H. *et al*, *J. Organomet. Chem.*, 1966, **6**, 86 (*synth*)

$C_{18}H_{14}Ni$ Ni-00160

Bis[(1,2,3-η)-1*H*-inden-1-yl]nickel, 9CI
Diindenylnickel
[52409-46-8]

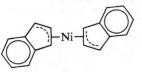

M 288.999
The compound named Bis(1,2,3,3*a*,7*a*-η)-1*H*-inden-1-ylnickel is probably identical. Catalyses oxidn. of phosphines to phosphites. Cryst. (hexane). Subl. at 70-80° *in vacuo*.

Fritz, H.P. *et al*, *J. Organomet. Chem.*, 1969, **19**, 449 (*synth, ms, ir*)
Koehler, F.H., *Chem. Ber.*, 1974, **107**, 570 (*nmr*)
Japan. Pat., 74 24 900, (*1974*); *CA*, **82**, 86404 (*use*)

$C_{18}H_{15}Ni^{\ominus\ominus\ominus}$ Ni-00161

Triphenylnickelate(3−)

$[NiPh_3]^{\ominus\ominus\ominus}$

M 290.007 (ion)

Tri-Li salt: [73464-03-6].
$C_{18}H_{15}Li_3Ni$ M 310.830
Extremely air- and moisture-sensitive dark-brown cryst. + 3THF(THF). Sol. Et_2O, THF, C_6H_6, spar. sol. hexane. Gives intensely dark-red solns. Dec. at 115°.

Taube, R. *et al*, *Z. Chem.*, 1979, **19**, 412 (*synth*)

$C_{18}H_{20}N_2Ni$ Ni-00162

(2,2′-Bipyridine-*N,N′*)[(1,2,5,6-η)-1,5-cyclooctadiene]nickel, 9CI

(1,5-Cyclooctadiene)(2,2′-bipyridine)nickel

[55425-72-4]

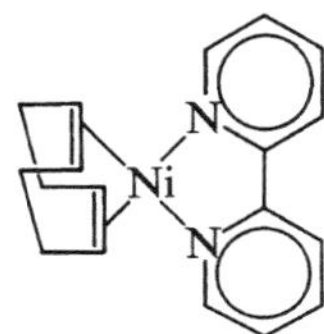

M 323.059

Catalyst for methylacetylene polymerisation, hydrosilylation of olefins, condensation of sulfinyl aniline, and graft polymerisation of polyols with styrene and/or methyl methacrylate. Blue-violet prisms.

Japan. Pat., 70 28 574, (*1970*); *CA*, **74**, 3729 (*synth*)
Nefedov, V.I. *et al*, *Koord. Khim.*, 1979, **5**, 1524; *CA*, **91**, 219894 (*struct, pe*)
Dinjus, E. *et al*, *J. Organomet. Chem.*, 1982, **236**, 123 (*struct*)

$C_{18}H_{20}N_2Ni$ Ni-00163

(2,2′-Bipyridine-*N,N′*)[(1,2,3,4-η)-1,2,3,4-tetramethyl-1,3-cyclobutadiene]nickel, 9CI

(Tetramethylcyclobutadiene)(2,2′-bipyridine)nickel

[68457-36-3]

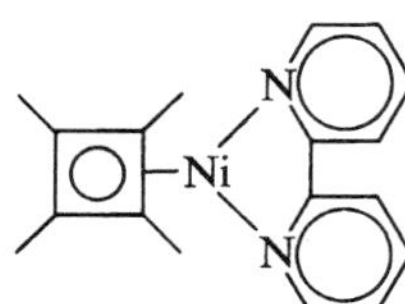

M 323.059

Copper-coloured cryst. Sol. C_6H_6 → intense blue soln. Mp 225° dec. $Bp_{0.001}$ 130° subl.

Griesbsch, U. *et al*, *Angew. Chem., Int. Ed. Engl.*, 1978, **17**, 950 (*synth, ms, ir, pmr, cmr*)

$C_{18}H_{22}Ni$ Ni-00164

Bis[(1,2,3,3a,7a-η)-4,5,6,7-tetrahydro-1*H*-inden-1-yl]nickel, 9CI

[58569-57-6]

M 297.062

Oxygen-sensitive clear liq., changing to yellow-brown in a few minutes. $Bp_{0.7}$ 100-20°.

Scroggins, W.T. *et al*, *Inorg. Chem.*, 1976, **15**, 1381 (*synth*)

$C_{18}H_{22}Ni$ Ni-00165

Bis(2,4,6-trimethylphenyl)nickel

Dimesitylnickel

M 297.062

Compound not isol. as solid. Sol. THF.

Tsutsui, M. *et al*, *J. Am. Chem. Soc.*, 1960, **82**, 6255 (*synth*)

$C_{18}H_{24}NiO_2$ Ni-00166

(1,5-Cyclooctadiene)(2,3,5,6-tetramethyl-*p*-benzoquinone)-nickel, 8CI

[(1,2,5,6-η)-1,5-Cyclooctadiene][(2,3-η-)-2,3,5,6-tetramethyl-2,5-cyclohexadiene-1,4-dione]-nickel, 10CI. (1,5-Cyclooctadiene)duroquinonenickel

[61037-54-5]

M 331.076

η^2-bonding, η^4-bonding, and *O*-bonding have been claimed for the duroquinone. Catalyst for synth. of $\alpha\beta$-unsaturated organosilicon compds. Cryst. (Et_2O). Mp 205° (201°) dec.

Schrauzer, G.N. *et al*, *Z. Naturforsch., B*, 1962, **17**, 73 (*synth*)
Pidcock, A. *et al*, *J. Chem. Soc. (A)*, 1970, 2922 (*ir*)
Nesmeyanov, A.N. *et al*, *CA*, 1976, **85**, 201403 (*synth*)
Nesmeyanov, A.N. *et al*, *J. Organomet. Chem.*, 1979, **172**, 185 (*synth, ms, nmr*)

$C_{18}H_{30}BrF_5NiP_2$ Ni-00167

Bromo(pentafluorophenyl)bis(triethylphosphine)nickel, 9CI

Pentafluorophenylbromobis(triethylphosphine)nickel

M 541.969

trans-form [15703-00-1]

Yellow-orange air-stable cryst. (MeOH). Mp 130-1°.

Phillips, J.R. *et al*, *J. Organomet. Chem.*, 1964, **2**, 455 (*synth*)

Goggin, P.L. *et al*, *J. Chem. Soc.* (*A*), 1966, 1462 (*ir*)
Fahey, D.R., *J. Am. Chem. Soc.*, 1970, **92**, 402 (*synth*)

$C_{18}H_{33}NiP$ Ni-00168

(1,5,9-Cyclododecatriene)(triethylphosphine)nickel, 8CI
Triethylphosphinecyclododecatrienenickel
[12113-51-8]

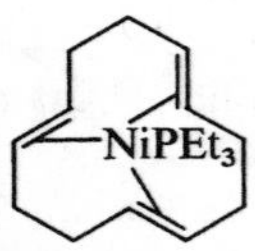

M 339.122
Red cryst. Mp 100°.

Wilke, G. *et al*, *Angew. Chem.*, 1961, **73**, 755 (*synth*)
Bogdanović, B. *et al*, *Justus Liebigs Ann. Chem.*, 1966, **699**, 1 (*synth*)
Bogdanović, B. *et al*, *Justus Liebigs Ann. Chem.*, 1969, **727**, 143.

$C_{18}H_{35}BrNiP_2$ Ni-00169

Bromo(phenyl)bis(triethylphosphine)nickel, 9CI
Phenylbromobis(triethylphosphine)nickel

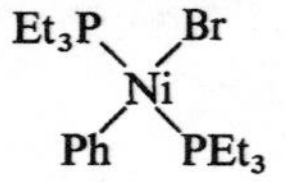

M 452.016

trans-form
Air-sensitive yellow cryst. Mp 82-3° dec.

Smith, G. *et al*, *J. Organomet. Chem.*, 1980, **198**, 199 (*synth, pmr, nmr*)

$C_{18}H_{35}NiP$ Ni-00170

η^5-Cyclopentadienyl(methyl)(tributylphosphine)nickel
Methyl(cyclopentadienyl)(tributylphosphine)nickel

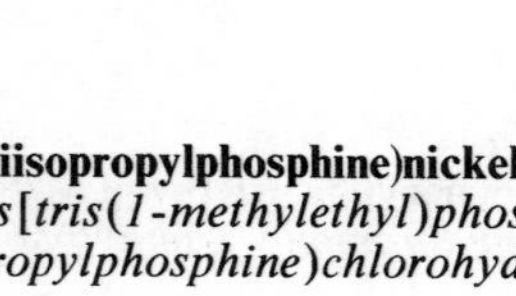

M 341.138
Green-brown cryst. (hexane). Sol. most org. solvs. Mp 29-30°.

Yamazaki, H. *et al*, *J. Organomet. Chem.*, 1966, **6**, 86 (*synth*)

$C_{18}H_{43}ClNiP_2$ Ni-00171

Chlorohydrobis(triisopropylphosphine)nickel, 8CI
Chlorohydrobis[tris(1-methylethyl)phosphine]nickel, 9CI. *Bis(triisopropylphosphine)chlorohydridonickel*
[52021-75-7]

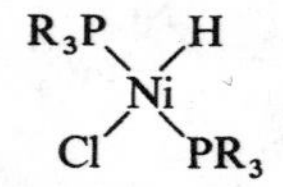

R = $(H_3C)_2CH$–

M 415.628

trans-form [30376-85-3]
Brown cryst. Air-sensitive. Sol. C_6H_6, THF, Et_2O, pet. ether. Mp 65-6°. Reacts with CCl_4, $CHCl_3$ or CS_2.

Green, M.L.H. *et al*, *J. Chem. Soc.* (*A*), 1971, 152 (*synth*)
Inorg. Synth., 1977, **17**, 83 (*synth, ir, pmr*)

$C_{18}Ni_9O_{18}^{\ominus\ominus}$ Ni-00172

Octadecacarbonylnonanickelate(2–)
Nona-μ-carbonylnonacarbonylnonanickelate(2–), 9CI
[60475-87-8]

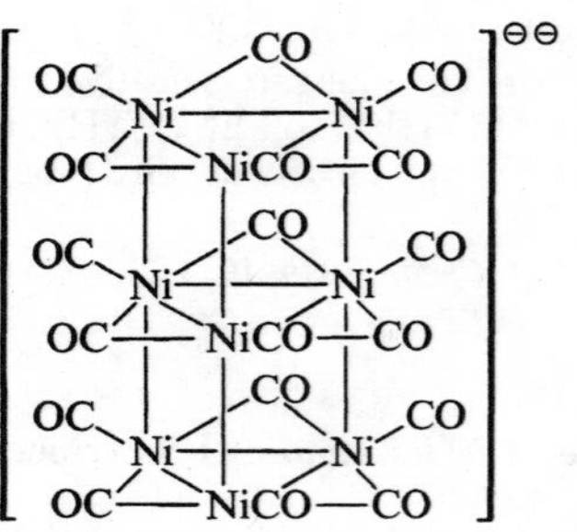

M 1032.397 (ion)
Struct. resembles the platinum analogue. Rapidly degraded by CO to Dodecacarbonylpentanickelate(2–), Ni-00101 and Nickel carbonyl, Ni-00014 .
Bis(tetraphenylphosphonium) salt: [60512-63-2]. $C_{66}H_{40}Ni_9O_{18}P_2$ M 1711.189
Dark-prisms (Me_2CO/2-propanol). Sol. Me_2CO, MeCN, THF, spar. sol. EtOH, insol. H_2O, toluene. Air-sensitive in solid state and soln.
Bis(benzyltrimethylammonium) salt: [60512-62-1]. $C_{38}H_{32}N_2Ni_9O_{18}$ M 1332.883
Red-brown solid (MeOH). Sol. THF, Me_2CO, MeCN. Air-sensitive.

Longoni, G. *et al*, *Inorg. Chem.*, 1976, **15**, 3029 (*synth, ir*)

$C_{19}H_8F_{10}Ni$ Ni-00173

[(1,2,3,4,5,6-η)-Methylbenzene]bis(pentafluorophenyl)nickel, 10CI
π-Toluenebis(pentafluorophenyl)nickel. Bis(pentafluorophenyl)(η^6-toluene)nickel
[66197-14-6]

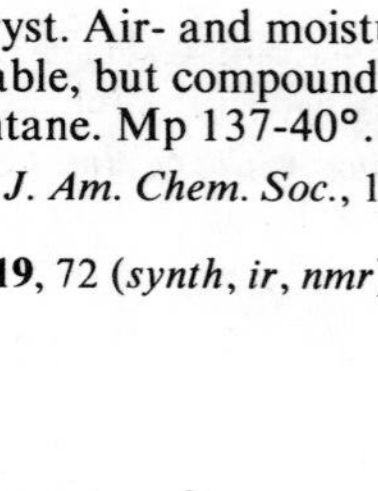

M 484.946
Dark red-brown cryst. Air- and moisture-sensitive. Toluene soln. stable, but compound dec. in pentane. Sol. toluene, pentane. Mp 137-40°. Darkens at 125°.

Klabunde, K.J. *et al*, *J. Am. Chem. Soc.*, 1978, **100**, 1313 (*synth*)
Inorg. Synth., 1979, **19**, 72 (*synth, ir, nmr*)

$C_{19}H_{18}N_2Ni$ Ni-00174

(η^5-2,4-Cyclopentadien-1-yl)[5-methyl-2-[(4-methylphenyl)-azo]phenyl]nickel, 9CI

*(η^5-2,4-Cyclopentadien-1-yl)[6-(4-methylphenylazo)-3-methylphenyl]nickel. Cyclopentadienyl[6-(*p-*tolylazo)-*m-*tolyl]nickel, 8CI*

[38882-45-0]

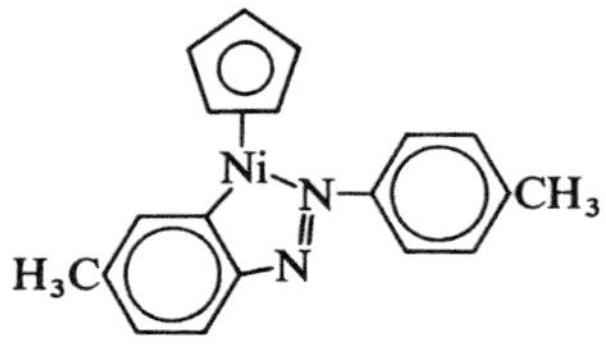

M 333.055

Dark-violet cryst.

Ustynyuk, Y.A. *et al*, *Dokl. Akad. Nauk SSSR, Ser. Sci. Khim.*, 1969, **187**, 112 (*synth, pmr, ir, uv*)
Semion, V.A. *et al*, *Zh. Strukt. Khim.*, 1972, **13**, 543 (*struct*)

$C_{19}H_{24}NNi_3$ Ni-00175

Tris(π-cyclopentadienyl)(μ_3-*tert*-butylaminato)trinickel

Tris(η^5-2,4-cyclopentadien-1-yl)[μ_3-[2-methyl-2-propanaminato(2−)]]trinickel, 9CI

[39450-84-5]

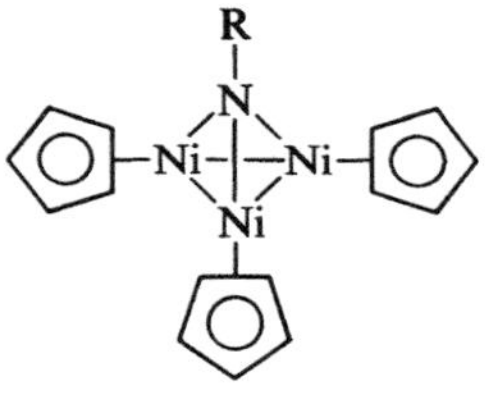

R = $(H_3C)_3C$—

M 442.475

Black cryst. (C_6H_6/heptane). Subl. at 230° without melting (sealed tube under N_2).

Otsuka, S. *et al*, *Inorg. Chem.*, 1968, **7**, 261 (*synth*)
Mueller, J. *et al*, *Chem. Ber.*, 1973, **106**, 1122 (*synth*)
Kamijyo, N. *et al*, *Bull. Chem. Soc. Jpn.*, 1974, **47**, 373 (*struct*)

$C_{19}H_{35}NNiP_2$ Ni-00176

(Cyano-*C*)phenylbis(triethylphosphine)nickel, 9CI

Phenylcyanobis(triethylphosphine)nickel

[41685-72-7]

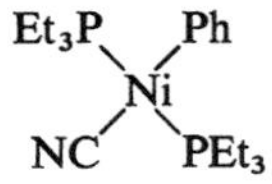

M 398.130

***trans*-form** [58769-90-7]

Air-sensitive cryst. (hexane).

Tolman, C.A. *et al*, *Inorg. Chem.*, 1973, **12**, 2770 (*pe*)
Parshall, G.W., *J. Am. Chem. Soc.*, 1974, **96**, 2360 (*synth*)
Favero, G. *et al*, *J. Organomet. Chem.*, 1976, **105**, 389 (*ir*)
Favero, G. *et al*, *J. Organomet. Chem.*, 1978, **162**, 99.

$C_{19}H_{37}BrNiP_2$ Ni-00177

Bromo(2-methylphenyl)bis(triethylphosphine)nickel, 9CI

*Bromo-*o*-tolylbis(triethylphosphine)nickel, 8CI*

[33808-30-9]

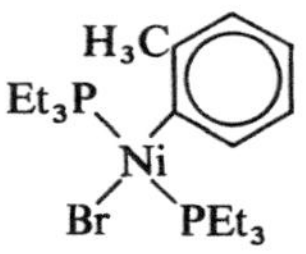

M 466.043

***trans*-form** [26521-33-5]

Orange-brown cryst. (EtOH). Mp 102-3° dec.

Chatt, J. *et al*, *J. Chem. Soc.*, 1960, 1718 (*synth*)
Miller, R.G. *et al*, *J. Am. Chem. Soc.*, 1970, **92**, 1511 (*pmr*)
Smith, G. *et al*, *J. Organomet. Chem.*, 1980, **198**, 199 (*synth*)

$C_{19}H_{38}NiP_2$ Ni-00178

Methylphenylbis(triethylphosphine)nickel, 9CI

Phenyl(methyl)bis(triethylphosphine)nickel

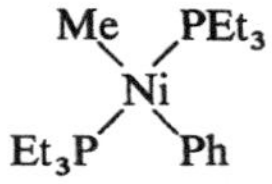

M 387.147

***trans*-form** [57811-74-2]

Yellow-brown cryst. (hexane). Highly air-sensitive. Mp 71.5-72°.

Morrell, D.G. *et al*, *J. Am. Chem. Soc.*, 1975, **97**, 7262 (*synth*)

$C_{19}H_{45}BrNiP_2$ Ni-00179

Bromo(methyl)bis(triisopropylphosphine)nickel, 8CI

Bromo(methyl)bis[tris(1-methylethyl)phosphine]nickel. Methylbromobis(triisopropylphosphine)nickel

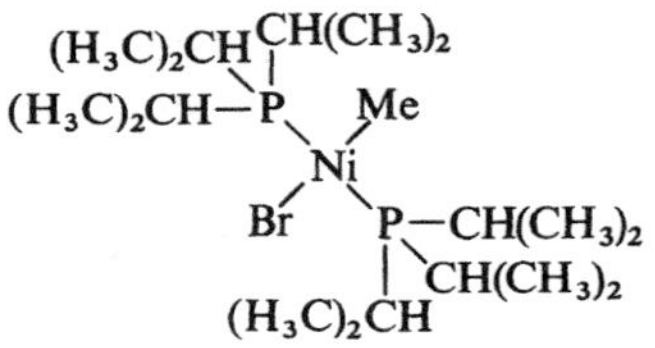

trans-form

M 474.106

***trans*-form** [31387-20-9]

Good catalyst for acetylene polymerisation. Yellow cryst. (Et_2O at −78°). Mp 82° dec. Solns. are v. air-sensitive.

Green, M.L. *et al*, *J. Chem. Soc. (A)*, 1971, 639 (*synth, pmr*)

$C_{20}H_{12}F_{18}Ni$ Ni-00180

[(1,2,5,6-η)-1,5-Cyclooctadiene][hexakis(trifluoromethyl)benzene]nickel, 9CI

[Hexakis(trifluoromethyl)benzene](1,5-cyclooctadiene)nickel

[11068-15-8]

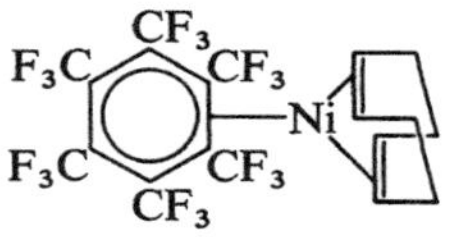

M 652.976

Purple-red cryst. Mp 161-2° dec.

Stone, F.G.A. *et al*, *J. Chem. Soc. (A)*, 1971, 448 (*synth, ir, pmr*)

$C_{20}H_{16}N_4Ni$ **Ni-00181**

Bis(2,2′-bipyridine-*N*,*N*′)nickel, 10CI

Bis(bipyridyl)nickel

[15186-68-2]

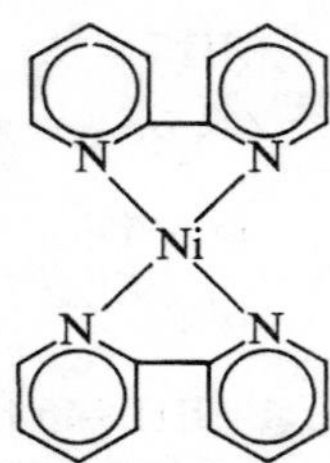

M 371.063

Blue-violet cryst. (Et_2O), air-sensitive. Sol. aromatic solvs. Mp 155°.

Behrens, H. *et al*, *Z. Naturforsch., B*, 1966, **21**, 489 (*synth*)
Inorg. Synth., 1977, **17**, 117 (*synth*)

$C_{20}H_{16}Ni_2$ **Ni-00182**

1,1″:1′,1″-Binickelocene, 10CI

Bis(fulvalene)dinickel

[62518-80-3]

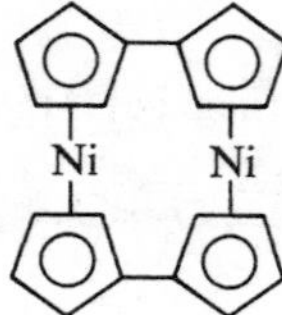

M 373.726

Reddish-brown cryst. (1,3,5-trimethylbenzene).

Smart, J.C. *et al*, *J. Am. Chem. Soc.*, 1977, **99**, 956 (*synth, ir*)
Sharp, P.R. *et al*, *J. Am. Chem. Soc.*, 1981, **103**, 753 (*struct*)

$C_{20}H_{20}Ni_5S_4$ **Ni-00183**

Tetra-π-cyclopentadienyltetra-μ_3-thioxopentanickel, 8CI

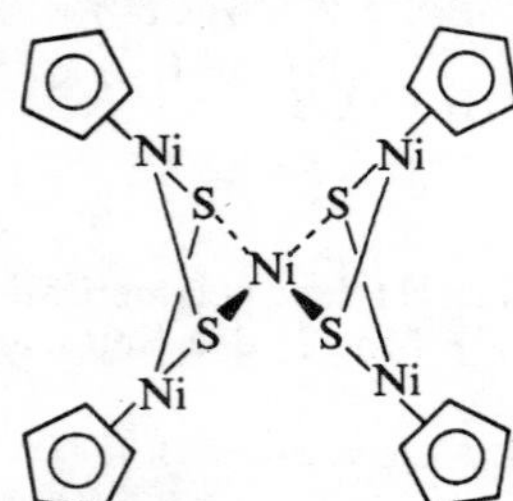

M 682.068

Black cryst. which dec. vigorously on rapid heating. Mp 135°.

Vahrenkamp, H. *et al*, *Angew. Chem., Int. Ed. Engl.*, 1969, **8**, 144 (*synth, struct*)

$C_{20}H_{22}N_2Ni$ **Ni-00184**

Azobenzene(1,5-cyclooctadiene)nickel

[*(1,2,5,6-η)-1,5-Cyclooctadiene*][(N,N′-η)*diphenyldiazene*]*nickel, 10CI*

[66752-80-5]

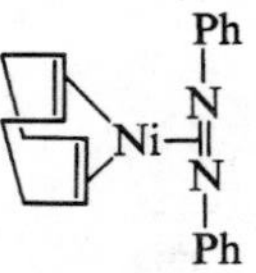

M 349.097

Dark-red cryst.

Muetterties, E.L. *et al*, *J. Am. Chem. Soc.*, 1978, **100**, 2090 (*synth*)

$C_{20}H_{22}Ni^{\ominus\ominus}$ **Ni-00185**

[(1,2,5,6-η)-1,5-Cyclooctadiene]diphenylnickelate(2−), 10CI

Diphenyl(1,5-cyclooctadiene)nickelate(2−)

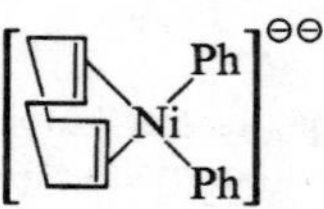

M 321.084 (ion)

Di-Li salt: [67684-22-4].
$C_{20}H_{22}Li_2Ni$ M 334.966
Pale-yellow cryst. + 5THF (THF). V. air-sensitive.

Uhlig, E. *et al*, *Z. Anorg. Allg. Chem.*, 1978, **442**, 11 (*synth, pmr*)

$C_{20}H_{23}Ni_4$ **Ni-00186**

Tetrakis(η^5-2,4-cyclopentadien-1-yl)tri-μ_3-hydrotetranickel, 9CI

Tetrakis(π-cyclopentadienyl)trihydridotetranickel. Tri-μ_3-hydridotetrakis(π-cyclopentadienyl)tetranickel.

[52110-59-5]

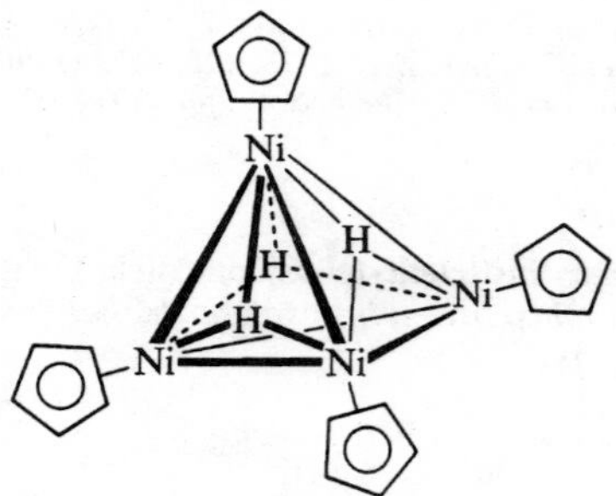

M 498.162

Black-violet cryst. (Et_2O/pentane). Solns. are air-sensitive. Sol. C_6H_6, THF, spar. sol. pentane. Mp >320° (under N_2).

Müller, J. *et al*, *Angew. Chem., Int. Ed. Engl.*, 1973, **12**, 1005 (*synth, ir, ms, struct*)
Köetzle, T.F. *et al*, *Adv. Chem. Ser.*, 1978, **167**, 61 (*struct*)

$C_{20}H_{24}Ni_3$ Ni-00187

Tris(η^5-2,4-cyclopentadien-1-yl)[μ_3-(2,2-dimethylpropylidyne)]trinickel, 10CI

Tris[(π-*cyclopentadienyl*)*nickel*]-tert-*butylmethane*

[71920-09-7]

R = —$C(CH_3)_3$

M 440.480

Black solid. Mp 191-6° dec. Bp_1 191-6° subl.

Booth, B.L. *et al*, *J. Organomet. Chem.*, 1979, **178**, 371 (*synth, ir, pmr*)

$C_{20}H_{30}Ni$ Ni-00188

Bis(η^5-pentamethylcyclopentadienyl)nickel

Decamethylnickelocene, 10CI

[74507-63-4]

M 329.147

Sl. air-sensitive, green-black cryst. Sol. most org. solvs. Mp 283° dec. $Bp_{0.0001}$ 100-10° subl.

Cauletti, C. *et al*, *J. Electron Spectrosc. Relat. Phenom.*, 1980, **19**, 327 (*pe*)

Werner, H. *et al*, *J. Organomet. Chem.*, 1980, **198**, 97 (*synth, ms, ir*)

$C_{20}H_{32}As_4Ni$ Ni-00189

Bis[1,2-phenylenebis[dimethylarsine]-*As,As'*]nickel

Di(o-*phenylenebisdimethylarsine*)*nickel*

M 630.849

Orange cryst. (EtOH). Mp 190-6° dec.

Chatt, J. *et al*, *J. Chem. Soc.*, 1962, 2537 (*synth*)

$C_{20}H_{36}N_4Ni$ Ni-00190

Tetrakis(2-isocyano-2-methylpropane)nickel, 9CI

Tetrakis(tert-*butylisocyanide*)*nickel*, 8CI. *Tetrakis*(tert-*butylisonitrile*)*nickel*

[19068-11-2]

$[(H_3C)_3CNC]_4Ni$ (T_d)

M 391.221

Pale-yellow cryst. (EtOH/Et_2O). V. air-sensitive. Mp 170° dec.

Nakamura, A. *et al*, *J. Am. Chem. Soc.*, 1969, **91**, 6994 (*synth*)

Tolman, C.A. *et al*, *Inorg. Chem.*, 1973, **12**, 2770 (*pe*)

Inorg. Synth., 1977, **17**, 117 (*synth*)

$C_{20}H_{38}Ni_2P^{\ominus}$ Ni-00191

(μ-Dicyclohexylphosphine)tetrakis(ethylene)dinickelate(1−)

(μ-*Dicyclohexylphosphino*)*tetrakis*(η^2-*ethene*)*dinickelate*(1−), 9CI

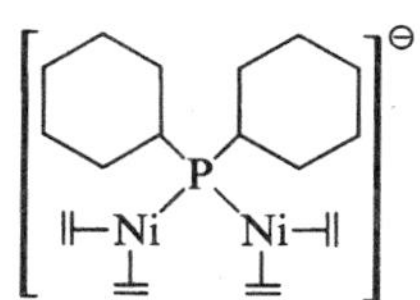

M 426.874 (ion)

Li salt: [60349-40-8].

$C_{20}H_{38}LiNi_2P$ M 433.815

Cryst. + 4THF (THF). Limited stability at r.t.

Jonas, K. *et al*, *Angew. Chem., Int. Ed. Engl.*, 1976, **15**, 622 (*synth, pmr*)

$C_{20}H_{39}NiP$ Ni-00192

Dimethyl(tricyclohexylphosphine)nickel

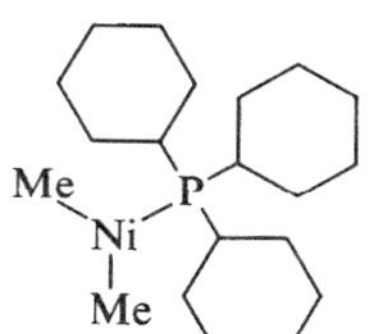

M 369.192

Yellow cryst., stable at r.t.

Bonnemann, H. *et al*, *Organic Chemistry of Nickel*, 1974, Academic Press, New York, 163.

$C_{20}H_{39}NiPS$ Ni-00193

(η^5-2,4-Cyclopentadien-1-yl)(1-propanethiolato)(tributylphosphine)nickel, 9CI

1-*Propanethiolato*(*cyclopentadienyl*)-(*tributylphosphine*)*nickel*

[38467-42-4]

M 401.252

Green solid. Sol. C_6H_6, hexane, pentane, reacts slowly with CH_2Cl_2 and CCl_4. Mp 41-4°.

Sato, M. *et al*, *J. Organomet. Chem.*, 1972, **39**, 389 (*synth, ir, pmr*)

$C_{21}H_{12}F_{10}Ni$ Ni-00194

Bis(pentafluorophenyl)[(1,2,3,4,5,6-η)-1,3,5-trimethylbenzene]nickel, 9CI

Bis(*pentafluorophenyl*)*mesitylenenickel*. (π-*Mesitylene*)-*bis*(*pentafluorophenyl*)*nickel*

[74153-73-4]

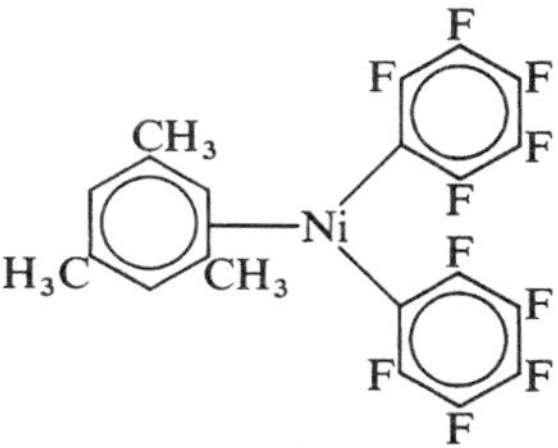

M 513.000

Cryst. The arene group can readily be displaced by other ligands.

Gastinger, R.G. *et al*, *J. Am. Chem. Soc.*, 1980, **102**, 4959 (*synth*, *props*)
Radonovich, L.J. *et al*, *Inorg. Chem.*, 1980, **19**, 3373 (*struct*)

$C_{21}H_{15}Cl_5N_3Ni^{\oplus}$ Ni-00195

Pentachlorophenyltris(pyridine)nickel(1+)
Tris(pyridine)pentachlorophenylnickel(1+)

M 545.325 (ion)
Perchlorate: [78331-77-8].
$C_{21}H_{15}Cl_6N_3NiO_4$ M 644.775
Cryst. (Me_2CO/CH_2Cl_2). Mp 250°. Air-stable.

Coronas, J.M. *et al*, *Inorg. Chim. Acta*, 1981, **48**, 87 (*synth*, *ir*)

$C_{21}H_{15}NiO_3P$ Ni-00196

Tricarbonyl(triphenylphosphine)nickel, 9CI, 8CI
Triphenylphosphinenickel tricarbonyl
[14917-13-6]

$Ni(CO)_3(PPh_3)$ (C_{3v})

M 405.011
Catalyses hydrosilylation of cyclopentadiene, and cyclotrimerisation of acetylene. Mp 126° (123°).

Meriwether, L.S. *et al*, *J. Am. Chem. Soc.*, 1959, **81**, 4200 (*synth*, *ir*)
Meriwether, L.S. *et al*, *J. Am. Chem. Soc.*, 1961, **83**, 3192 (*nmr*)
Bigorgne, M., *J. Inorg. Nucl. Chem.*, 1964, **26**, 107 (*ir*)
Edgell, W.F. *et al*, *Inorg. Chem.*, 1965, **4**, 1629 (*synth*, *ir*)
Haas, H. *et al*, *J. Chem. Phys.*, 1967, **47**, 2996 (*ir*)
Delbecke, F.T. *et al*, *J. Organomet. Chem.*, 1974, **64**, 265 (*synth*, *ir*)
Bodner, G.M., *Inorg. Chem.*, 1975, **14**, 1932 (*synth*, *cmr*)
Vaisarova, V. *et al*, *Collect. Czech. Chem. Commun.*, 1976, **41**, 1906 (*use*)
DuPlessis, J.A.K. *et al*, *S. Afr. J. Chem.*, 1979, **32**, 147; *CA*, **93**, 25811y (*use*)
Bodner, G.M. *et al*, *Inorg. Chem.*, 1980, **19**, 1951 (*cmr*)

$C_{21}H_{20}BrNiP$ Ni-00197

Bromo(η^3-2-propenyl)(triphenylphosphine)nickel, 9CI
Allylbromo(triphenylphosphine)nickel. Bromo-π-allyl-(triphenylphosphine)nickel
[12336-45-7]

X = Br

M 441.957
Red cryst. (C_6H_6/hexane). Mp 140-2°.

Dubini, M. *et al*, *J. Organomet. Chem.*, 1966, **6**, 188 (*synth*)
Walter, D. *et al*, *Angew. Chem., Int. Ed. Engl.*, 1966, **5**, 897 (*pmr*)

$C_{21}H_{20}ClNiP$ Ni-00198

Chloro(η^3-2-propenyl)triphenylphosphinenickel
(π-Allyl)chlorotriphenylphosphinenickel, 8CI
[12247-36-8]
As Bromo(η^3-2-propenyl)(triphenylphosphine)nickel, Ni-00197 with

X = Cl

M 397.506
Catalyst for regular polymerisation of propadiene and alkylpropadienes. Orange cryst. (THF/Et_2O). Dec. at 140-50°. Solid can be handled for short periods in air, but solns. quickly dec.

Heck, R.F. *et al*, *Chem. Ind. (London)*, 1961, 986 (*synth*, *ir*, *pmr*)
Seinosuke, O. *et al*, *Eur. Polym. J.*, 1967, **3**, 73 (*use*)

$C_{21}H_{21}NiP$ Ni-00199

Hydro-η^3-propenyl(triphenylphosphine)nickel
π-Allylhydro(triphenylphosphine)nickel, 8CI. η^3-Propenyl(hydrotriphenylphosphine)nickel. Hydrido(η^3-allyl)(triphenylphosphine)nickel
[31854-76-9]

M 363.061
Red-brown cryst. Stable <−30°.

Boennemann, H., *Angew. Chem., Int. Ed. Engl.*, 1970, **9**, 736 (*synth*, *ir*, *pmr*)

$C_{21}H_{30}Ni$ Ni-00200

Tris[(2,3-η)-bicyclo[2.2.1]hept-2-ene]nickel, 9CI
Tris(norbornene)nickel
[38882-52-9]

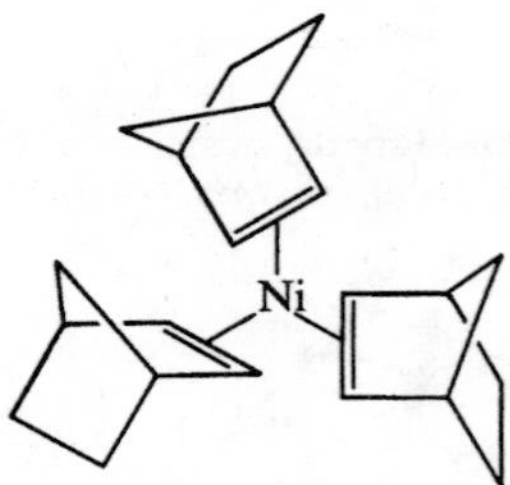

M 341.158
No phys. details published.

Fischer, K. *et al*, *Angew. Chem., Int. Ed. Engl.*, 1973, **12**, 943 (*synth*, *struct*)
Hoffmann, E.G. *et al*, *Z. Naturforsch, B*, 1976, **31**, 1712 (*nmr*)

$C_{21}H_{38}BrNiP$ Ni-00201

Bromo(η^3-2-propenyl)(tricyclohexylphosphine)nickel, 10CI
Allylbromo(tricyclohexylphosphine)nickel
[47315-25-3]

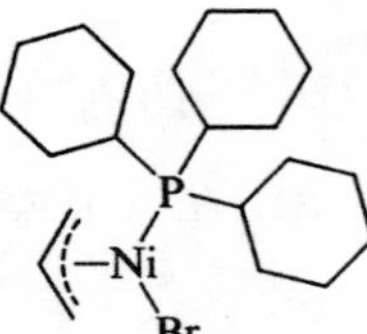

M 460.099

Catalyst for dimerisation of propylene. Yellow-brown solid.

Bogdanović, B. *et al*, *Angew. Chem., Int. Ed. Engl.*, 1980, **19**, 622 (*use*)

$C_{22}H_{15}BrNiO$ Ni-00202

Bromo(carbonyl)(η^3-1,2,3-triphenyl-2-cyclopropen-1-yl)nickel

Carbonylbromo(triphenylcyclopropenyl)nickel

X = Br

M 433.954

Brick-red cryst. Solid dec. v. slowly in air, solns. instantaneously. Indefinitely stable *in vacuo*. Spar. sol. MeOH, THF. Dec. ~120° *in vacuo* without subliming.

Gowling, E.W. *et al*, *Inorg. Chem.*, 1964, **3**, 604 (*synth, ir*)

$C_{22}H_{15}ClNiO$ Ni-00203

Carbonylchloro(η^3-1,2,3-triphenyl-2-cyclopropen-1-yl)nickel, 10CI

Chlorocarbonyl(triphenylcyclopropenyl)nickel

[69120-62-3]

As Bromo(carbonyl)(η^3-1,2,3-triphenyl-2-cyclopropen-1-yl)nickel, Ni-00202 with

X = Cl

M 389.503

Catalyses isomerisation of quadricyclane to norbornadiene. No phys. details recorded.

Gowling, E.W. *et al*, *Inorg. Chem.*, 1964, **3**, 604 (*synth*)

$C_{22}H_{20}Ni_2S_2$ Ni-00204

Bis(η^5-2,4-cyclopentadien-1-yl)bis(μ-phenylthiolato)dinickel

Bis(μ-benzenethiolato)di-π-cyclopentadienyldinickel, 8CI. *Bis(π-cyclopentadienyl)di[μ-(phenylthiolato)]-dinickel*

M 465.900

Bridged dimer. Air-stable black cryst. (Et_2O or hexane). Mod. thermally stable. V. sol. org. solvs. Mp 125°.

Monomer: (Cyclopentadienyl)(phenylthiolato)nickel. (Benzenethiolato)(cyclopentadienyl)nickel.

$C_{11}H_{10}NiS$ M 232.950

Unknown.

Schropp, W.K., *J. Inorg. Nucl. Chem.*, 1962, **24**, 1688 (*synth, ir*)

Elgen, P.C., *Inorg. Chem.*, 1971, **10**, 980.

Hirabayashi, T., *J. Organomet. Chem.*, 1972, **39**, C85 (*synth*)

$C_{22}H_{20}Ni_3$ Ni-00205

Tris(η^5-2,4-cyclopentadien-1-yl)[μ_3-(phenylmethylidyne)]trinickel, 9CI

[12715-82-1]

As Tris(cyclopentadienyl)(μ_3-2,2-dimethylpropylidyne)-trinickel, Ni-00187 with

R = Ph

M 460.470

Black solid. Mp 158-60°.

Voevodskaya, T.I. *et al*, *J. Organomet. Chem.*, 1972, **37**, 187 (*synth, struct*)

Booth, B.L. *et al*, *J. Organomet. Chem.*, 1979, **178**, 371 (*synth*)

$C_{22}H_{22}ClNiP$ Ni-00206

[(1,2,3-η)-2-Butenyl]chloro(triphenylphosphine)nickel, 9CI

Chloro(1-methylallyl)(triphenylphosphine)nickel. (1-Methylallyl)chloro(triphenylphosphine)nickel

[53426-50-9]

M 411.533

Catalyst for oligomerisation of olefins. Red-brown cryst.

Vitulli, G. *et al*, *J. Organomet. Chem.*, 1975, **84**, 399 (*synth, pmr*)

D'Aniello, M.J. *et al*, *J. Am. Chem. Soc.*, 1978, **100**, 1474 (*synth, use*)

$C_{22}H_{22}Ni$ Ni-00207

(1,5-Cyclooctadiene)(diphenylacetylene)nickel

Diphenylethyne(1,5-cyclooctadiene)nickel

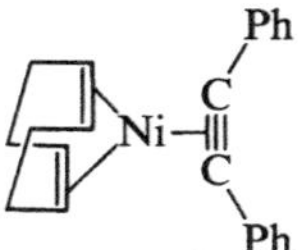

M 345.106

Compd. not isol. Exists in soln. in equilibrium with PhC≡CPh and $[(C_8H_{12})Ni]_2(PhC{\equiv}CPh)$.

Muetterties, E.L. *et al*, *J. Am. Chem. Soc.*, 1978, **100**, 2090 (*synth*)

$C_{22}H_{23}NiP$ Ni-00208

Methyl(η^3-2-propenyl)(triphenylphosphine)nickel

Allyl(methyl)(triphenylphosphine)nickel

M 377.087

Yellow-ochre cryst. Stable at r.t. Sol. C_6H_6. Dec. >40° in soln.

Bogdanovic, B. *et al*, *Angew. Chem., Int. Ed. Engl.*, 1966, **5**, 582 (*synth*)

$C_{22}H_{25}NiO_2P$ Ni-00209

Cyclooctenyl[(diphenylphosphino)acetato-*O,P*]nickel

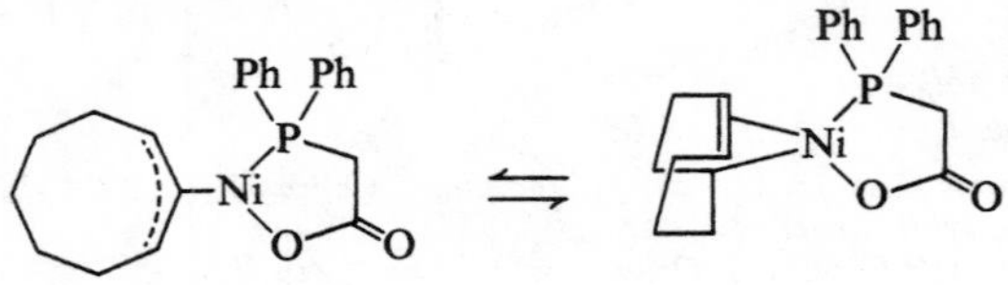

η^3-Allyl-*form* 4-enyl-*form*

M 411.102

Ethylene oligomerisation catalyst: SHOP reaction. Burgundy-red solvated cryst. (hexane/octane). Mp 214-6°.

η*³-*Allyl-form [84099-45-6]

[(*1,2,3-η*)-*2-Cycloocten-1-yl*][(*diphenylphosphino*)*acetato*-O,P]*nickel*, 10CI

In equilibrium with 4-enyl-form in soln.

4-enyl-form [84108-24-7]

[(*1,4,5-η*)-*4-Cycloocten-1-yl*][(*diphenylphosphino*)*acetato*-O,P]*nickel*, 10CI

In rapid equilibrium with η^3-allyl-form in soln.

Peuckert, M. *et al*, *Organometallics*, 1983, **2**, 594 (*synth, nmr, use*)

$C_{22}H_{28}N_4Ni$ Ni-00210

(Azobenzene)bis(*tert*-butylisocyanide)nickel, 8CI

(*Diphenyldiazene*-N,N′)*bis*(*2-isocyano-2-methylpropane*)*nickel*, 9CI. *Bis*(tert-*butylisonitrile*)(*azobenzene*)-*nickel*

[32714-19-5]

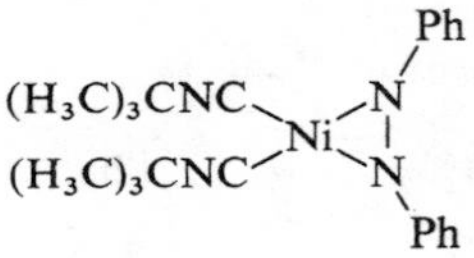

M 407.180

Red cryst. (Et_2O). Mp 163-4°.

Otsuka, S. *et al*, *J. Am. Chem. Soc.*, 1971, **93**, 6462 (*synth, ir, pmr*)
Dickson, R.S. *et al*, *J. Am. Chem. Soc.*, 1972, **94**, 2988 (*struct*)
Ittel, S.D., *Inorg. Chem.*, 1977, **16**, 2589 (*ir*)
Inorg. Synth., 1977, **17**, 117 (*synth*)

$C_{22}H_{30}Ni_2O_2$ Ni-00211

Di-*μ*-carbonylbis[(1,2,3,4,5-*η*)-1,2,3,4,5-pentamethyl-2,4-cyclopentadien-1-yl]dinickel, 10CI

[69239-93-6]

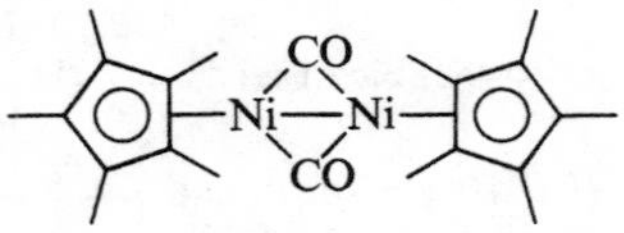

M 443.858

Purple-red cryst. Mp 162-3° (under Ar). $Bp_{0.1}$ 120° subl.

Mise, T. *et al*, *J. Organomet. Chem.*, 1978, **164**, 391 (*synth, pmr, ir, uv*)

$C_{22}H_{33}NiP$ Ni-00212

Bisethylene(triphenylphosphine)nickel, 8CI

Bisethene(*triphenylphosphine*)*nickel*

[33042-32-9]

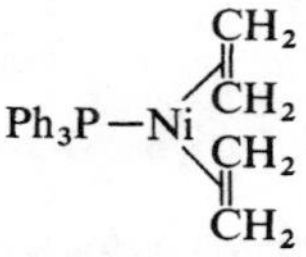

M 387.166

Jolly, P.W. *et al*, *Angew. Chem., Int. Ed. Engl.*, 1971, **10**, 328 (*synth*)

$C_{22}H_{36}NiP_2$ Ni-00213

(3-Methylphenyl)(2,4,6-trimethylphenyl)bis(trimethylphosphine)nickel, 10CI

Mesityl(m-*tolyl*)*bis*(*trimethylphosphine*)*nickel*. m-*Tolyl*(*mesityl*)*bis*(*trimethylphosphine*)*nickel*

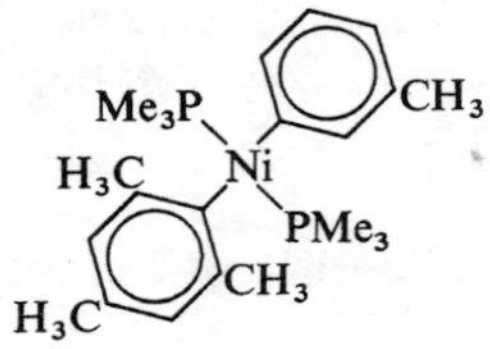

M 421.164

trans-form [77170-52-6]

Solid. Mp 151-2°.

Wada, M. *et al*, *J. Chem. Soc., Dalton Trans.*, 1981, 240 (*synth*)

$C_{22}H_{41}NiP$ Ni-00214

Bis(ethylene)tricyclohexylphosphinenickel, 8CI

Bis(η^2-*ethene*)*tricyclohexylphosphinenickel*, 9CI

[33152-09-9]

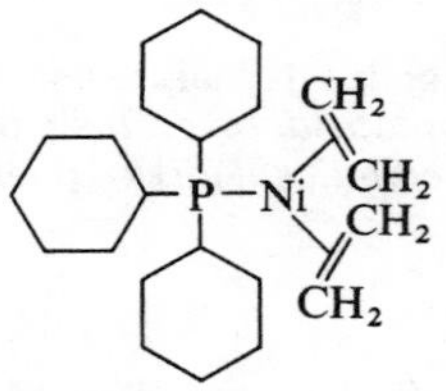

M 395.230

Almost white solid. Insol. Et_2O.

Jolly, P.W. *et al*, *Angew. Chem., Int. Ed. Engl.*, 1971, **10**, 328 (*synth*)
Krueger, C. *et al*, *J. Organomet. Chem.*, 1972, **34**, 387 (*struct*)

$C_{23}H_{20}BrNiP$ Ni-00215

Bromo(η^5-2,4-cyclopentadien-1-yl)(triphenylphosphine)nickel, 9CI

π-Cyclopentadienylbromo(*triphenylphosphine*)*nickel*

[1298-79-9]

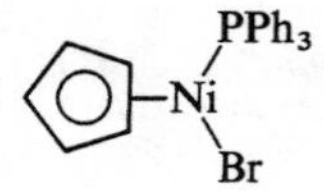

M 465.979

Red cryst. (cyclohexane). Air stable as solid and soln. Sol. C_6H_6, THF, less sol. aliphatic hydrocarbons. Mp 118-20° dec.

Yamazaki, H. *et al*, *J. Organomet. Chem.*, 1966, **6**, 86 (*synth*)
van den Akker, M. *et al*, *Recl. Trav. Chim. Pays-Bas*, 1967, **86**, 897 (*synth, uv, ir, pmr*)
Thomson, J. *et al*, *Can. J. Chem.*, 1973, **51**, 1179 (*nmr, uv*)

$C_{23}H_{20}ClNiP$ **Ni-00216**

Chloro(η^5-2,4-cyclopentadien-1-yl)triphenylphosphinenickel, 10CI, 9CI

Cyclopentadienyl(triphenylphosphine)chloronickel. Triphenylphosphinecyclopentadienylnickel chloride

[31904-79-7]

M 421.528

Dark red. Mp 138-9° (in air), 166-8° dec. (in N_2).

Yamazaki, H. *et al*, *J. Organomet. Chem.*, 1966, **6**, 86.
Barnett, K.W., *J. Chem. Educ.*, 1974, **51**, 422 (*synth*)
Gmelin's Handbuch der Anorg. Chem., 8th Ed., 1974, Suppl., 17, 46.

$C_{23}H_{20}Cl_3GeNiP$ **Ni-00217**

(η^5-2,4-Cyclopentadien-1-yl)(trichlorogermyl)(triphenylphosphine)nickel, 9CI

(Trichlorogermyl)(π-cyclopentadienyl)(triphenylphosphine)nickel. (Triphenylphosphine)(π-cyclopentadienyl)(trichlorogermyl)nickel

[41509-20-0]

M 565.024

Dark-green cryst. + $\frac{1}{2}C_6H_6$ (C_6H_6/hexane). Air-stable as solid, but slowly oxidised by air in soln.

Glockling, F. *et al*, *J. Inorg. Nucl. Chem.*, 1970, **32**, 3103 (*synth, struct*)

$C_{23}H_{20}Cl_3NiPSn$ **Ni-00218**

(η^5-2,4-Cyclopentadien-1-yl)(trichlorostannyl)(triphenylphosphine)nickel, 9CI

(π-Cyclopentadienyl)(trichlorotin)(triphenylphosphine)nickel. (Triphenylphosphine)(π-cyclopentadienyl)(trichlorostannyl)nickel. (Trichlorostannyl)(π-cyclopentadienyl)(triphenylphosphine)nickel

[12283-56-6]

M 611.124

Yellow solid, dec. slowly in air and above 135°. Sol. polar org. solvs., insol. nonpolar solvs.

van der Akker, M. *et al*, *J. Organomet. Chem.*, 1967, **10**, P37 (*synth, pmr*)
Thomson, J. *et al*, *Can. J. Chem.*, 1973, **51**, 1179 (*uv, nmr*)
Bancroft, G.M. *et al*, *Can. J. Chem.*, 1975, **53**, 307 (*mössbauer*)

$C_{23}H_{23}NiO_2P$ **Ni-00219**

(Acetato-*O*)(η^3-2-propenyl)(triphenylphosphine)nickel, 10CI

Acetato(π-allyl)triphenylphosphinenickel, 8CI. (π-Allyl)triphenylphosphinenickel acetate. (η-2-Propenyl)ethanoato(triphenylphosphine)nickel

[79361-71-0]

M 421.097

Deep-red cryst. (THF/Et_2O). Mp 125-8° dec.

Yamamoto, A., *J. Am. Chem. Soc.*, 1981, **103**, 6863 (*synth, ir, pmr*)

$C_{23}H_{28}B_9NiP$ **Ni-00220**

[Decahydro-7-methyl-π-7-phospha-10-carbaundecaborato(1–)](triphenyl-π-cyclopropenyl)nickel, 8CI

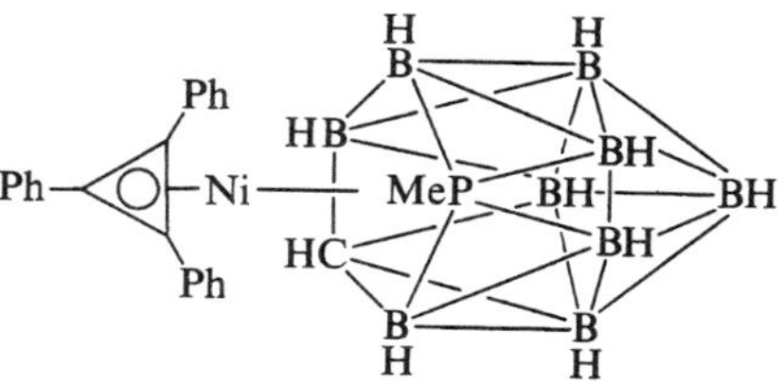

M 491.428

Red cryst. (heptane/C_6H_6). Mp 202-3°.

Welcker, P.S. *et al*, *Inorg. Chem.*, 1970, **9**, 286 (*synth, ir, ms, pmr*)

$C_{23}H_{37}NiO_3P$ **Ni-00221**

Tricarbonyl[1-(tricyclohexylphosphonio)ethyl]nickel, 9CI

Nickel tricarbonyl (tricyclohexylphosphine)methylylid

[39045-48-2]

M 451.207

Yellow cryst.

Heydenreich, F. *et al*, *Isr. J. Chem.*, 1972, **10**, 293 (*synth, ir, ms, pmr*)
Barnett, B.L. *et al*, *J. Cryst. Mol. Struct.*, 1972, **2**, 271 (*struct*)

$C_{23}H_{39}NiP$ **Ni-00222**

(η^5-2,4-Cyclopentadien-1-yl)hydro(tricyclohexylphosphine)nickel

Hydrido(π-cyclopentadienyl)(tricyclohexylphosphine)nickel

M 405.225

Yellow cryst.

Jonas, K. *et al*, *Angew. Chem., Int. Ed. Engl.*, 1969, **8**, 519 (*synth, ir, pmr*)

$C_{24}F_{20}Ni^{\ominus\ominus}$ Ni-00223

Tetrakis(pentafluorophenyl)nickelate(2−), 10CI

$[Ni(C_6F_5)_4]^{\ominus\ominus}$ (D_{4h})

M 726.922 (ion)

Bis(tetrabutylammonium) salt: [66302-98-5].
$C_{40}H_{72}F_{20}N_2Ni$ M 1019.680
Solid. Sol. Me_2CO. Mp 175°. Light and air stable at r.t., both as solid and in soln.

Uson, R. *et al*, *J. Chem. Soc., Chem. Commun.*, 1977, 789 (*synth*)

$C_{24}H_{16}N_4Ni$ Ni-00224

Bis[1,10-phenanthroline-N^1,N^{10}]nickel

[10170-11-3]

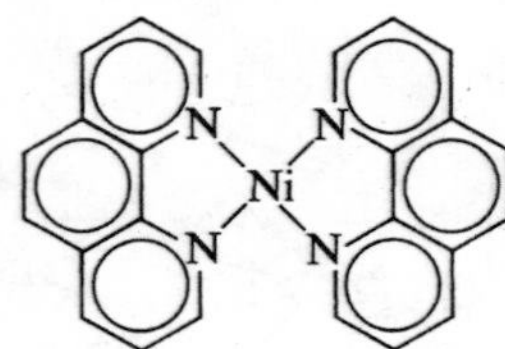

M 419.107

Blue-black solid (Et_2O). Mp 280°.

Inorg. Synth., 1977, **17**, 117 (*synth*)

$C_{24}H_{18}N_2Ni$ Ni-00225

(2,2′-Bipyridine)(diphenylacetylene)nickel

(2,2′-Bipyridine-N,N′)[1,1′-(1,2-ethynediyl)bis[benzene]]nickel, 10CI

[75507-31-2]

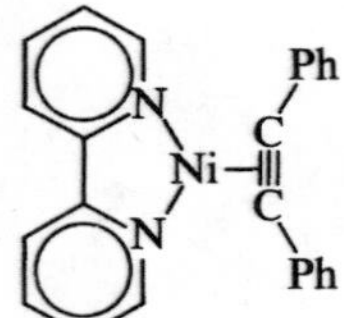

M 393.110

No phys. details given.

Hoberg, H. *et al*, *Angew. Chem.*, 1980, **92**, 951 (*synth*)

$C_{24}H_{20}N_2Ni_2$ Ni-00226

Bis(η^5-2,4-cyclopentadien-1-yl)bis[μ-phenylisonitrile]dinickel

Dicyclopentadienylbis(phenylisocyanide)dinickel

CNPh
Ni—Ni
CNPh

M 453.815

Deep-red cryst. (pentane). Mp 91°.

Pauson, P.L. *et al*, *Angew. Chem.*, 1962, **74**, 466 (*synth*)

$C_{24}H_{20}Ni^{\ominus\ominus}$ Ni-00227

Tetraphenylnickelate(2−), 9CI

$NiPh_4^{\ominus\ominus}$ (D_{4h})

M 367.112 (ion)

Di-Li salt: [54688-82-3].
$C_{24}H_{20}Li_2Ni$ M 380.994
Yellowish cryst. + 4THF (THF). Mod. sol. THF. Dec. at 102-3°.

Taube, R. *et al*, *Angew. Chem., Int. Ed. Engl.*, 1975, **14**, 261 (*synth*)

$C_{24}H_{20}Ni_2$ Ni-00228

Di-π-cyclopentadienyl(μ-diphenylacetylene)dinickel, 8CI

Bis(η^5-2,4-cyclopentadien-1-yl)[μ-[1,1′-(η^2:η^2-1,2-ethynediyl)bis[benzene]]]dinickel, 9CI. *(μ-Diphenylacetylene)bis(π-cyclopentadienylnickel)*

[35828-66-1]

PhC≡CPh
Ni—Ni

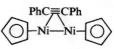

M 425.802

Mills, O.S. *et al*, *Acta Crystallogr.*, 1965, **18**, 562 (*struct*)
Dessy, R.E. *et al*, *J. Am. Chem. Soc.*, 1968, **90**, 1995 (*polarog*)
Randall, E.W. *et al*, *J. Organomet. Chem.*, 1974, **64**, 271 (*synth, spectra*)
Rossetti, R. *et al*, *Inorg. Chim. Acta*, 1975, **15**, 149 (*ms*)

$C_{24}H_{21}N_2NiP$ Ni-00229

Bis[(1,2-η)-2-propenenitrile]triphenylphosphinenickel

Bis(acrylonitrile)triphenylphosphinenickel, 8CI. *Bis[(1,2-η)-ethenecarbonitrile]triphenylphosphinenickel. Bis(cyanoethylene)triphenylphosphinenickel*

$Ni(CH_2{=}CHCN)_2(PPh_3)$

M 427.107

Catalyses polymerisation of butadiene to cyclooctadiene and cyclododecatriene; catalyses hydrosilylation of butadiene. Yellow cryst. Dec. at 185°.

▷Pyrophoric

Schrauzer, G.N., *J. Am. Chem. Soc.*, 1959, **81**, 5310 (*synth, ir*)
Ono, I. *et al*, *Hydrocarbon Process.*, 1967, **46**, 147 (*use*)

$C_{24}H_{23}NiP$ Ni-00230

(η^5-2,4-Cyclopentadien-1-yl)methyl(triphenylphosphine)nickel, 9CI

Methyl(π-cyclopentadienyl)(triphenylphosphine)nickel

[1298-85-7]

R
Ni
PPh_3

R = Me

M 401.109

Green cryst. (hexane). May be handled in air, especially in solid state. Sol. most org. solvs. Mp 126-9° (under N_2).

Yamazaki, H. *et al*, *J. Organomet. Chem.*, 1966, **6**, 86 (*synth*)
Thomson, J. *et al*, *Can. J. Chem.*, 1973, **51**, 1179 (*nmr, uv*)

$C_{24}H_{24}Ni$ Ni-00231

Tris(η^2-phenylethylene)nickel

Tris(η^2-ethenylbenzene)nickel, 10CI. *Tris(styrene)nickel*

[62054-32-4]

$(PhCH{=}CH_2)_3Ni$

M 371.144

Red-brown cryst., dec. >20°.

Blackborrow, J.R. *et al*, *J. Organomet. Chem.*, 1976, **120**, C49 (*synth*)

$C_{24}H_{25}NiO_2P$ Ni-00232

Methyl(2,4-pentanedionato-*O,O'*)(triphenylphosphine)nickel, 9CI

Acetylacetonato(methyl)(triphenylphosphine)nickel

[60146-61-4]

As Methyl(2,4-pentanedionato-*O,O'*)-(trimethylphosphine)nickel, Ni-00066 with

L = Me, R = Ph

M 435.124

Yellow-brown cryst. (toluene/hexane or toluene/MeCN). Stable as solid, solns. are v. air-sensitive. Sol. aromatic and ethereal solvs., insol. hydrocarbons.

Huggins, J.M. *et al*, *J. Am. Chem. Soc.*, 1981, **103**, 3002 (*synth*)

$C_{24}H_{28}N_2Ni$ Ni-00233

Di(*tert*-butylisocyanide)diphenylacetylenenickel

[1,1'-(η^2-1,2-Ethynediyl)bis[benzene]]bis(2-isocyano-2-methylpropane)nickel, 9CI. *(Diphenylacetylene)bis(t-*ert*-butyl isocyanide)nickel*

[32802-08-7]

M 403.189

Yellow cryst. (hexane). Mp 125° dec.

Otsuka, S. *et al*, *J. Am. Chem. Soc.*, 1971, **93**, 6462 (*synth*)
Dickson, R.S. *et al*, *J. Organomet. Chem.*, 1972, **36**, 191 (*struct*)
Inorg. Synth., 1977, **17**, 117 (*synth*)

$C_{24}H_{28}Ni^{\ominus\ominus}$ Ni-00234

Cyclododecatrienediphenylnickelate(2−)

Diphenyl(cyclododecatriene)nickelate(2−)

M 375.175 (ion)

Cyclododecatriene ligand readily displaced by other unsaturated molecules.

Di-Li salt, tetrakis(THF) complex:
$C_{40}H_{60}Li_2NiO_4$ M 677.484
Cryst.

Di-Li salt, bis(TMEDA) complex:
$C_{36}H_{60}Li_2N_4Ni$ M 621.469
Cryst.

Jonas, K. *et al*, *Angew. Chem., Int. Ed. Engl.*, 1980, **19**, 520 (*synth*)

$C_{24}H_{36}Ni^{\oplus\oplus}$ Ni-00235

Bis[(1,2,3,4,5,6-η)hexamethylbenzene]nickel(2+), 9CI

M 383.238 (ion)

Hexachloroplatinate: [12313-05-2].
$C_{24}H_{36}Cl_6NiPt$ M 791.036
Brownish-yellow solid. Insol. all org. solvs.

Lindner, H.H. *et al*, *J. Organomet. Chem.*, 1968, **12**, P18 (*synth*)
Anderson, S.E. *et al*, *J. Am. Chem. Soc.*, 1970, **92**, 4244 (*synth*)
Anderson, S.E., *J. Organomet. Chem.*, 1974, **71**, 263 (*pmr*)

$C_{24}H_{40}N_2NiP_2$ Ni-00236

(Azobenzene)bis(triethylphosphine)nickel

[(N,N'-η)-Diphenyldiazene]bis(triethylphosphine)nickel, 10CI

[54325-35-8]

M 477.231

Red solid (Et_2O). Mp 140° dec.

Ittel, S.D. *et al*, *Inorg. Chem.*, 1975, **14**, 1183 (*synth, ir, pmr*)
Inorg. Synth., 1977, **17**, 117 (*synth*)

$C_{24}H_{40}NiP_2$ Ni-00237

Diphenylbis(triethylphosphine)nickel, 10CI

Bis(triethylphosphine)diphenylnickel

[72151-11-2]

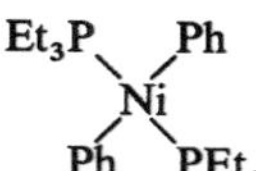

M 449.218

trans-form

Catalyst for cyclooligomerisation of butadiene. Pale-yellow cryst. Sol. org. solvs. Mp 128-34°. Dec. v. rapidly in EtOH soln.

Chatt, J. *et al*, *J. Chem. Soc.*, 1960, 1718 (*synth*)

$C_{24}H_{43}NiO_2P$ Ni-00238

Methyl(2,4-pentanedionato-*O,O'*)tricyclohexylphosphinenickel, 9CI

(Acetylacetonato)methyltricyclohexylphosphinenickel. Methyltricyclohexylphosphinenickel acetylacetonate

[36427-01-7]

As Methyl(2,4-pentanedionato-*O,O'*)-(trimethylphosphine)nickel, Ni-00066 with

L = Me, R = cyclohexyl

M 453.266

Yellow cryst. (Et_2O/pentane). Sol. Et_2O, aromatic solvs., spar. sol. hydrocarbons.

Jolly, P.W. *et al*, *J. Organomet. Chem.*, 1971, **33**, 109 (*synth*)
Barnett, B.A. *et al*, *J. Organomet. Chem.*, 1972, **42**, 169 (*struct*)

$C_{24}H_{60}NiO_{12}P_4$ Ni-00239

Tetrakis(triethylphosphite-*P*)nickel, 9CI

Tetrakis(phosphorous acid)nickel dodecaethyl ester, 8CI

[14839-39-5]

$[(EtO)_3P]_4Ni$ (T_d)

M 723.316

Air-sensitive white cryst. Insol. H_2O, v. sol. nonpolar org. solvs. Mp 108°.

Vinal, R.S. *et al*, *Inorg. Chem.*, 1964, **3**, 1062 (*synth*)
Cassoux, P. *et al*, *J. Chem. Phys.*, 1967, **64**, 1813 (*nmr*)
Myers, V.G. *et al*, *Inorg. Chem.*, 1969, **8**, 1204 (*ir*)
Keiter, R.L. *et al*, *Inorg. Chem.*, 1970, **9**, 404 (*ir, pmr*)
Inorg. Synth., 1971, **13**, 112 (*synth*)
Tolman, C.A. *et al*, *Inorg. Chem.*, 1973, **12**, 2770 (*pe*)

$C_{24}H_{60}NiP_4$ Ni-00240

Tetrakis(triethylphosphine)nickel, 9CI, 8CI

[51320-65-1]

$(Et_3P)_4Ni$ (T_d)

M 531.323

Light-yellow cryst. (pentane), dec. at 93-4°. Mp 42°. Stable at −20°, becomes violet at r.t. but will reverse if cooled promptly. If left at r.t. for a long time becomes irreversibly violet.

▷Spontaneously inflammable in air

Aresta, M. *et al*, *Inorg. Chim. Acta*, 1975, **12**, 165 (*synth*)
Inorg. Synth., 1977, **17**, 117.

$C_{24}H_{61}NiO_{12}P_4^{\oplus}$ Ni-00241

Hydrotetrakis(triethylphosphite-*P*)nickel(1+), 9CI

Hydridotetrakis(triethylphosphite)nickel(1+). Tetrakis(triethyl phosphite)hydridonickel(1+)

[31306-07-7]

$[NiH[P(OEt)_3]_4]^{\oplus}$

M 724.324 (ion)

Catalyst for coupling of butadiene and ethylene to form hexadienes. Cation obt. only as pale-yellow soln., extremely air-sensitive and dec. at r.t. Sol. C_6H_6, Me_2CO, $CHCl_3$.

Drinkard, W.C. *et al*, *Inorg. Chem.*, 1970, **9**, 392 (*synth*)
Tolman, C.A., *Inorg. Chem.*, 1972, **11**, 3128 (*pmr*)

$C_{25}H_{21}NiP$ Ni-00242

(η^5-2,4-Cyclopentadien-1-yl)ethynyl(triphenylphosphine)nickel, 10CI

Ethynyl(π-cyclopentadienyl)(triphenylphosphine)nickel

[1298-86-8]

C≡CH
Ni
PPh_3

M 411.105

Green cryst. (hexane). Sol. most org. solvs. Mp 111.5-112.5° dec.

Yamazaki, H. *et al*, *J. Organomet. Chem.*, 1966, **6**, 86 (*synth, ir, pmr*)
Sonogashira, K. *et al*, *J. Chem. Soc., Chem. Commun.*, 1977, 291 (*synth*)

$C_{25}H_{25}NiP$ Ni-00243

(η^5-2,4-Cyclopentadien-1-yl)ethyl(triphenylphosphine)nickel, 9CI

Ethyl(π-cyclopentadienyl)(triphenylphosphine)nickel. (Triphenylphosphine)(π-cyclopentadienyl)ethylnickel

[1298-87-9]

Et
Ni
Ph_3P

M 415.136

Green cryst. Sol. most org. solvs. Mp 118-20° (under N_2).

Yamazaki, H. *et al*, *J. Organomet. Chem.*, 1966, **6**, 86 (*synth*)
Thomson, J. *et al*, *J. Organomet. Chem.*, 1972, **40**, 205 (*pmr*)
Thomson, J. *et al*, *Can. J. Chem.*, 1973, **51**, 1179 (*nmr, uv*)

$C_{25}H_{28}NiO_2P$ Ni-00244

Ethyl(2,4-pentanedionato-*O,O'*)triphenylphosphinenickel, 9CI

(Triphenylphosphine)ethylnickel acetylacetonate. (Acetylacetonato)ethyl(triphenylphosphine)nickel

[41970-28-9]

H_3C O Et
Ni
O PPh_3
H_3C

M 450.159

Yellow cryst. (toluene, C_6H_6, Me_2CO or Et_2O). Mp 93°.

Yamamoto, A. *et al*, *J. Am. Chem. Soc.*, 1973, **95**, 4073 (*synth*)
Cotton, F.A. *et al*, *J. Am. Chem. Soc.*, 1974, **96**, 4820 (*nmr, cryst struct*)
Nesmeyanov, A.N. *et al*, *J. Organomet. Chem.*, 1977, **129**, 421 (*props*)

$C_{26}H_{20}Ni$ Ni-00245

(η^5-2,4-Cyclopentadien-1-yl)[(1,2,3-η)-1,2,3-triphenyl-2-cyclopropen-1-yl]nickel

(Triphenylcyclopropenyl)cyclopentadienylnickel

[31832-92-5]

Ph
Ni Ph
Ph

M 391.134

Deep orange-red cryst. (heptane). Air-stable. Mp 137-8°.

Rausch, M.D. *et al*, *J. Am. Chem. Soc.*, 1970, **92**, 4981 (*synth, ir, ms*)
Weaver, D.L. *et al*, *Inorg. Chem.*, 1971, **10**, 1504 (*struct*)

$C_{26}H_{24}Cl_2NiP_2$ Ni-00246

Dichloro[1,2-ethanediylbis(diphenylphosphine)-*P*,*P'*]nickel, 9CI

Dichloro[ethylenebis(diphenylphosphine)]nickel, 8CI. *[1,2-bis(diphenylphosphino)ethane]nickel dichloride*

[38754-20-0]

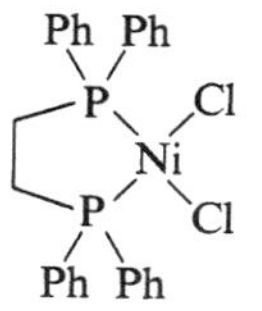

M 528.019

Orange, feathery needles or glistening, yellow-brown platelets.

Booth, G. *et al*, *J. Chem. Soc.*, 1965, 3238 (*synth*)
v. Hecke, G.R. *et al*, *Inorg. Chem.*, 1966, **5**, 1968 (*ir*, *pmr*)

$C_{26}H_{27}NiP$ Ni-00247

(π-Cyclopentadienyl)isopropyl(triphenylphosphine)nickel, 8CI

(η^5-2,4-Cyclopentadien-1-yl)(1-methylethyl)(triphenylphosphine)nickel, 9CI. *Isopropyl(π-cyclopentadienyl)-(triphenylphosphine)nickel. Triphenylphosphine(π-cyclopentadienyl)isopropylnickel*

[32627-07-9]

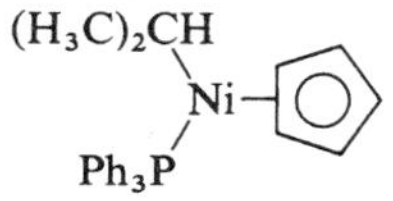

M 429.163

V. air-sensitive solid. Mp 97-9°.

Thomson, J. *et al*, *Can. J. Chem.*, 1970, **48**, 3443 (*synth*, *ir*)
Thomson, J. *et al*, *J. Organomet. Chem.*, 1972, **40**, 205 (*pmr*)
Thomson, J. *et al*, *Can. J. Chem.*, 1973, **51**, 1179 (*nmr*, *uv*)

$C_{26}H_{27}NiP$ Ni-00248

(η^5-2,4-Cyclopentadien-1-yl)propyl(triphenylphosphine)nickel, 9CI

Propyl(π-cyclopentadienyl)(triphenylphosphine)nickel. Triphenylphosphine(π-cyclopentadienyl)propylnickel

[1298-90-4]

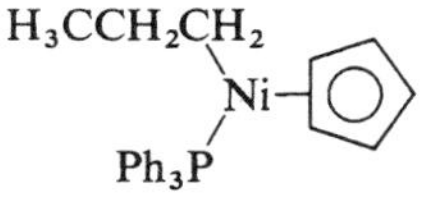

M 429.163

Green cryst. Sol. most org. solvs. Mp 75-7° (under N_2).

Yamazaki, H. *et al*, *J. Organomet. Chem.*, 1966, **6**, 86 (*synth*)
Thomson, J. *et al*, *J. Organomet. Chem.*, 1972, **40**, 205 (*pmr*)
Thomson, J. *et al*, *Can. J. Chem.*, 1973, **51**, 1179 (*nmr*, *uv*)

$C_{26}H_{27}NiP$ Ni-00249

[(1,2,3,6,7,8-η)-2,6-Octadiene-1,8-diyl](triphenylphosphine)nickel, 9CI

[41600-73-1]

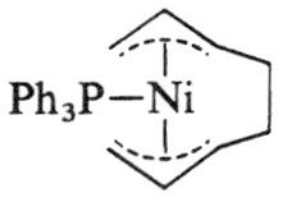

M 429.163

Catalyses oligomerisation reactions of butadiene. No physical details recorded.

Buessmeier, B. *et al*, *J. Am. Chem. Soc.*, 1974, **96**, 4726 (*synth*)

$C_{26}H_{39}NiP_3$ Ni-00250

Tris(dimethylphenylphosphine)dimethylnickel, 9CI

Dimethyltris(dimethylphenylphosphine)nickel

[54808-95-6]

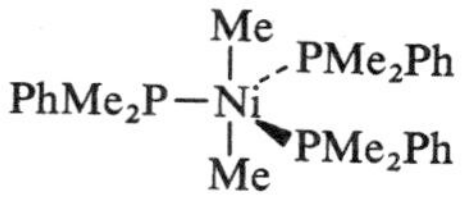

M 503.205

Cryst. (Et_2O). Unstable >60°. Can be stored in a deep freeze for several months. Readily loses PMe_2Ph in dilute soln. to yield *trans*-$[NiMe_2(PMe_2Ph)_2]$.

Jeffery, E.A., *Aust. J. Chem.*, 1973, **26**, 219 (*synth*, *pmr*, *ir*)

$C_{26}H_{45}NiP$ Ni-00251

[(1,2,3,8-η)-2,6-Octadiene-1,8-diyl](tricyclohexylphosphine)nickel, 9CI

[36656-76-5]

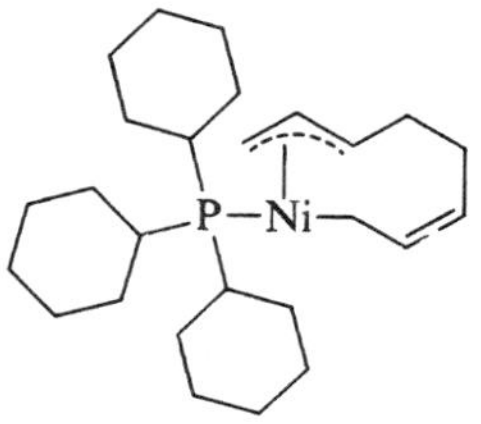

M 447.305

Yellow cryst. (toluene/isopentane). Unstable in air and in benzene soln. Stable in an inert atmosphere at −5°. Dec. at ca. 100°.

Brown, J.M. *et al*, *J. Chem. Soc., Dalton Trans.*, 1971, 1240 (*synth*, *spectra*)
Jolly, P.W. *et al*, *Angew. Chem., Int. Ed. Engl.*, 1971, **10**, 328 (*synth*)

$C_{26}H_{54}Br_2Ni_2P_2$ Ni-00252

Dibromo(2,6-octadiene-1,8-diyl)bis(triisopropylphosphine)dinickel

Dibromo[μ-[(1,2,3-η:6,7,8-η)-2,6-octadiene-1,8-diyl]]bis[tris(1-methylethyl)phosphine]dinickel, 9CI

[39014-88-5]

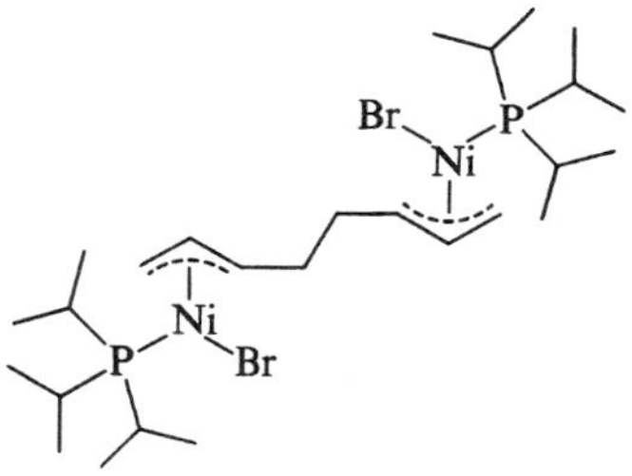

M 705.848

Yellow-brown cryst.

Cameron, T.S. *et al*, *J. Coord. Chem.*, 1972, **2**, 43 (*synth*, *struct*)
Cameron, T.S. *et al*, *Acta Crystallogr., Sect. B*, 1972, **28**, 2021 (*struct*)

$C_{27}H_{29}NiP$ Ni-00253

Butyl(η^5-2,4-cyclopentadien-1-yl)(triphenylphosphine)nickel, 9CI

(π-Cyclopentadienyl)butyl(triphenylphosphine)nickel

[1298-93-7]

As (η^5-2,4-Cyclopentadien-1-yl)-methyl(triphenylphosphine)nickel, Ni-00230 with

R = $H_3C(CH_2)_3$–

M 443.190

Green cryst. (hexane). Solns. sensitive to air. Sol. most org. solvs. Mp 88-91° (under N_2).

Yamazaki, H. *et al*, *J. Organomet. Chem.*, 1966, **6**, 86 (*synth*)
Thomson, J. *et al*, *Can. J. Chem.*, 1973, **51**, 1179 (*uv,nmr*)

$C_{27}H_{35}NiP_2$ Ni-00254

Bis(dimethylphenylphosphine)ethynyl(2,4,6-trimethylphenyl)-nickel, 10CI

Ethynylmesitylbis(dimethylphenylphosphine)nickel

[72110-76-0]

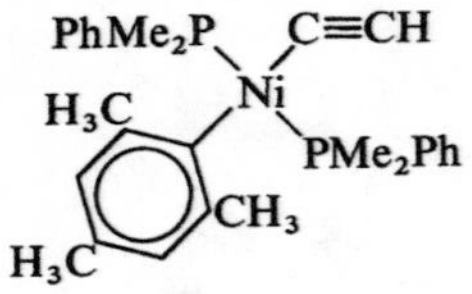

M 480.211

Yellow cryst. (MeOH). Sol. Me_2CO. Mp 115-7° dec.

Wada, M. *et al*, *J. Organomet. Chem.*, 1979, **178**, 261 (*synth*)

$C_{27}H_{45}NiP$ Ni-00255

(Tricyclohexylphosphine)[(1,2,2',5,5',6-η)-2,3,5-tris(methylene)-1,6-hexanediyl]nickel, 9CI

[35744-03-7]

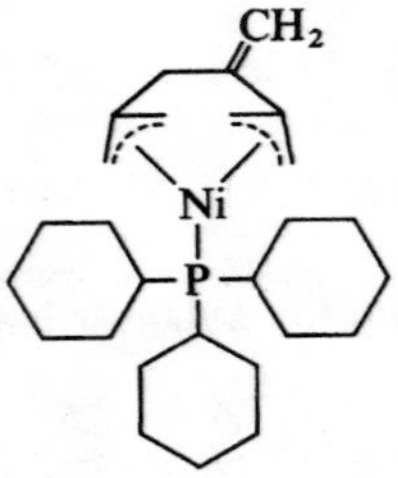

M 459.316

Englert, M. *et al*, *Angew. Chem., Int. Ed. Engl.*, 1972, **11**, 136 (*synth, pmr*)
Barnett, B.L. *et al*, *Angew. Chem., Int. Ed. Engl.*, 1972, **11**, 137 (*struct*)

$C_{28}H_{20}Br_2Ni$ Ni-00256

(Tetraphenylcyclobutadienyl)dibromonickel

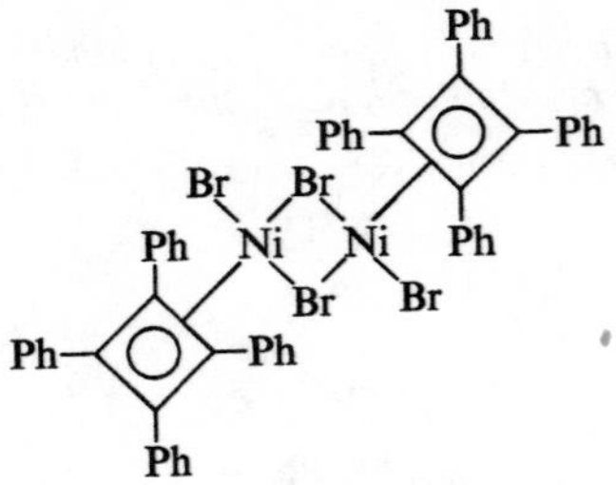

M 574.964

Almost certainly dimeric.

Dimer: Di-μ-bromodibromobis(1,2,3,4-tetraphenyl-1,3-cyclobutadiene)dinickel. Bis(tetraphenylcyclobutadienyl)dinickel tetrabromide.

$C_{56}H_{40}Br_4Ni_2$ M 1149.928

Blue-black air-stable cryst. (PhBr). V. sl. sol. org. solvs. Dec. at 317°.

Freedman, H.H., *J. Am. Chem. Soc.*, 1961, **83**, 2194 (*synth*)
Maitlis, P.M. *et al*, *J. Am. Chem. Soc.*, 1963, **85**, 1887 (*synth*)
Pollock, D.F. *et al*, *Can. J. Chem.*, 1966, **44**, 2673 (*synth*)

$C_{28}H_{20}Ni_2O_4P_2$ Ni-00257

Tetracarbonylbis[μ-(diphenylphosphino)]dinickel, 10CI, 8CI

[15350-17-1]

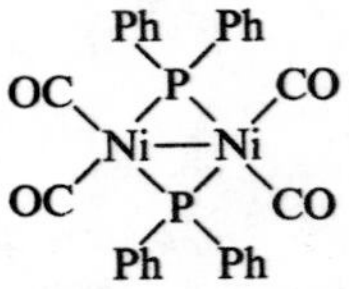

M 599.791

Hayter, R.G., *Inorg. Chem.*, 1964, **3**, 711 (*synth*)
Jarvis, J.A.J. *et al*, *J. Chem. Soc. (A)*, 1970, 1867 (*struct*)

$C_{28}H_{24}As_2NiO_2$ Ni-00258

Dicarbonyl[1,2-ethanediylbis[diphenylarsine]]nickel, 10CI

Dicarbonyl[ethylenebis[diphenylarsine]]nickel. [Ethylenebis[diphenylarsine]]nickel dicarbonyl

[69204-58-6]

As Dicarbonyl[1,2-ethanediylbis[dimethylarsine]]nickel, Ni-00056 with

R = Ph

M 601.030

Cream cryst. (DMF/MeOH). Mp 140-4° (*in vacuo*).

Chatt, J. *et al*, *J. Chem. Soc.*, 1960, 1378 (*synth, ir*)
Plankey, B.J. *et al*, *Inorg. Chem.*, 1979, **18**, 957 (*ir*)

$C_{28}H_{24}F_5INiP_2$ Ni-00259

[1,2-Ethanediylbis(diphenylphosphine)-*P,P'*]iodopentafluoroethylnickel

(Bisdiphenylphosphinoethane)iodopentafluoroethylnickel. Iodo(pentafluoroethyl)(bisdiphenylphosphinoethane)nickel. Iodo[ethylenebis(diphenylphosphine)]-pentafluoroethylnickel

Ph Ph / P / CF_2CF_3 / Ni / P / I / Ph Ph

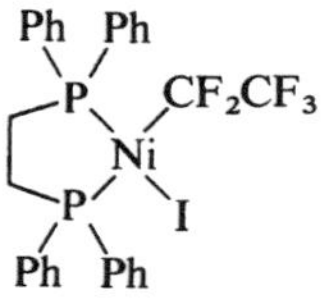

M 703.032

Reddish-brown cryst. (C_6H_6), dec. >260°.

McBride, D.W. *et al*, *J. Chem. Soc.*, 1963, 723 (*synth*)

$C_{28}H_{24}NiO_2P_2$ Ni-00260

Dicarbonyl[ethylenebis[diphenylphosphine]]nickel, 8CI

Dicarbonyl[1,2-ethanediylbis[diphenylphosphine]nickel, 9CI

[15793-01-8]

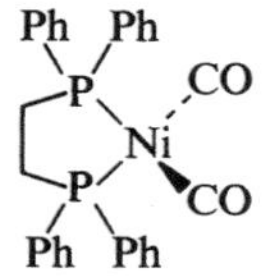

Ph Ph / P / CO / Ni / P / CO / Ph Ph

M 513.134

Cryst. (EtOH). Mp 138-40°.

Chatt, J. *et al*, *J. Chem. Soc.*, 1960, 1378 (*synth*)
Bodner, G.M., *Inorg. Chem.*, 1975, **14**, 1932 (*nmr*)

$C_{28}H_{26}NiO_2P_2$ Ni-00261

Dicarbonylbis(methyldiphenylphosphine)nickel, 9CI

Bis(methyldiphenylphosphine)dicarbonylnickel

[53540-37-7]

$Ni(CO)_2(PMePh_2)_2$

M 515.150

Yellow cryst. (C_6H_6/Et_2O). Mp 105-7°.

Cenini, S. *et al*, *Gazz. Chim. Ital.*, 1974, **104**, 1161 (*synth*)
Tanaka, K. *et al*, *Chem. Lett.*, 1974, 831 (*synth*)

$C_{28}H_{29}NNiP^{\oplus}$ Ni-00262

(η^5-2,4-Cyclopentadien-1-yl)(2-isocyano-2-methylpropane)-(triphenylphosphine)nickel(1+), 9CI

(tert-*Butylisocyanide*)-*π-cyclopentadienyl(triphenylphosphine)nickel(1+), 8CI. (π-Cyclopentadienyl)(triphenylphosphine)*(tert-*butylisonitrile)nickel(1+)*

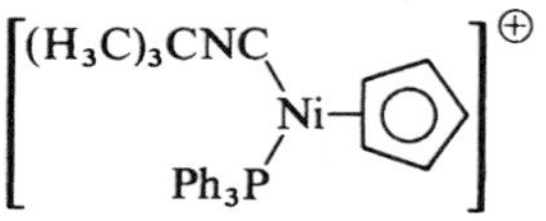

$[(H_3C)_3CNC$ / Ni–Cp / $Ph_3P]^{\oplus}$

M 469.208 (ion)

Iodide:
$C_{28}H_{29}INNiP$ M 596.112
Mp 137-9° dec.

Tetraphenylborate:
$C_{52}H_{49}BNNiP$ M 788.440
Mp 161-2° dec.

Yamamoto, Y. *et al*, *J. Organomet. Chem.*, 1969, **18**, 189 (*synth*)

$C_{28}H_{30}BrNiP$ Ni-00263

Bromo[(1,2,3,4,5-η)-1,2,3,4,5-pentamethyl-2,4-cyclopentadien-1-yl](triphenylphosphine)nickel, 10CI

(π-Pentamethylcyclopentadienyl)bromo(triphenylphosphine)nickel

[69239-97-0]

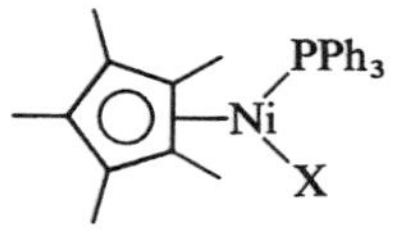

PPh_3 / Ni / X

X = Br

M 536.113

Red cryst. (C_6H_6/hexane). Air-stable in the solid state. Mp 209-11° dec.

Mise, T. *et al*, *J. Organomet. Chem.*, 1978, **164**, 391 (*synth, pmr*)

$C_{28}H_{30}INiP$ Ni-00264

Iodo[(1,2,3,4,5-η)-1,2,3,4,5-pentamethyl-2,4-cyclopentadien-1-yl](triphenylphosphine)nickel, 10CI

(π-Pentamethylcyclopentadienyl)iodo(triphenylphosphine)nickel

[69239-94-7]

As Bromo[(1,2,3,4,5-η)-1,2,3,4,5-pentamethyl-2,4-cyclopentadien-1-yl](triphenylphosphine)nickel, Ni-00263 with

X = I

M 583.113

Brown-red cryst. (C_6H_6/hexane). Air-stable in the solid state. Mp 196-8° dec.

Mise, T. *et al*, *J. Organomet. Chem.*, 1978, **164**, 391 (*synth, pmr*)

$C_{28}H_{39}NiOP_2^{\oplus}$ Ni-00265

Bis(dimethylphenylphosphine)(1-methoxyethylidene)(2,4,6-trimethylphenyl)nickel(1+), 9CI

Mesityl[methoxy(methyl)carbene]bis(dimethylphenylphosphine)nickel(1+). [Methoxy(methyl)carbene]mesitylbis(dimethylphenylphosphine)nickel(1+)

CH_3 / $PhMe_2P$ / C–OMe / H_3C / Ni / PMe_2Ph / CH_3 / H_3C $]^{\oplus}$

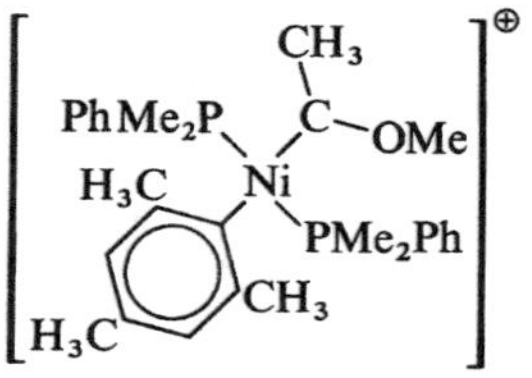

M 512.253 (ion)

Carbene complex.

***trans*-form**

Perchlorate: [72110-82-8].
$C_{28}H_{39}ClNiO_5P_2$ M 611.704
Cryst. (MeOH). Mp 150-4° dec. Stable in soln., even in air.

Wada, M. *et al*, *J. Organomet. Chem.*, 1979, **178**, 261 (*synth, nmr*)

$C_{28}H_{40}NiP_2$ Ni-00266

Bis(phenylethynyl)bis(triethylphosphine)nickel, 9CI

Bis(phenylacetylenyl)bis(triethylphosphine)nickel

[18533-63-6]

$Ni(C{\equiv}CPh)_2(PEt_3)_2$

M 497.262

Yellow-orange cryst. Mp 106-8°.

Chatt, J. *et al*, *J. Chem. Soc.*, 1960, 1718 (*synth*)
Fahey, D.R. *et al*, *Inorg. Chim. Acta*, 1979, **36**, 269 (*pe*)

$C_{28}H_{49}NiP$ Ni-00267

[(1,2,3,8-η)-2,6-dimethyl-2,6-octadiene-1,8-diyl]tricyclohexylphosphinenickel, 9CI

[38979-77-0]

M 475.359

Yellow plates (Et_2O).

Barnett, B. *et al*, *Tetrahedron Lett.*, 1972, 1457 (*synth, struct*)

$C_{28}H_{52}N_4Ni$ Ni-00268

Tetrakis(isocyanocyclohexane)nickel

Tetrakis(cyclohexylisocyanide)nickel, 8CI. *Tetrakis(cyclohexylisonitrile)nickel*

[24917-34-8]

$(C_6H_{11}NC)_4Ni$ (T_d)

M 503.436

Pale-yellow cryst. (hexane). V. air-sensitive. Mp 75° dec.

Nakamura, A. *et al*, *J. Am. Chem. Soc.*, 1969, **91**, 6994 (*synth*)
Inorg. Synth., 1977, **17**, 117 (*synth*)

$C_{28}H_{52}Ni_2P_2$ Ni-00269

Bis[μ-(dicyclohexylphosphino)]bis(η^2-ethene)dinickel, 9CI

Bisethylenebis-μ-dicyclohexylphosphinedinickel

[41232-31-9]

M 568.046

Cryst. No other phys. data recorded.

Barnett, B.L. *et al*, *Cryst. Struct. Commun.*, 1973, **2**, 85 (*struct*)

$C_{28}H_{56}NiP_2$ Ni-00270

Diethynylbis(tributylphosphine)nickel, 10CI

Bis(tributylphosphine)diethynylnickel

M 513.388

trans-form [73701-79-8]

Yellow oil. Can be stored for a long time at 4°. Mp <25°.

Sonogashira, K. *et al*, *J. Organomet. Chem.*, 1980, **188**, 237 (*synth*)

$C_{29}H_{20}F_5NiP$ Ni-00271

(η^5-2,4-Cyclopentadien-1-yl)(pentafluorophenyl)(triphenylphosphine)nickel, 10CI

Pentafluorophenyl(cyclopentadienyl)(triphenylphosphine)nickel

[12321-01-6]

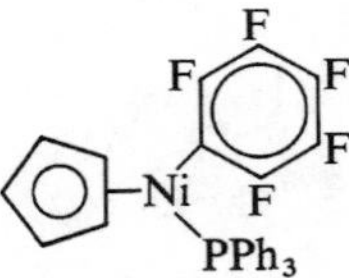

M 553.133

Dark-green needles (hexane). Mp 214-5° dec.

Churchill, M.R. *et al*, *J. Chem. Soc. (A)*, 1968, 2970 (*struct*)
Rausch, M.D. *et al*, *Inorg. Chem.*, 1969, **8**, 1355 (*synth*)
Gastinger, R.G. *et al*, *J. Am. Chem. Soc.*, 1980, **102**, 4959 (*spectra*)

$C_{29}H_{25}NiP$ Ni-00272

(η^5-2,4-Cyclopentadien-1-yl)phenyl(triphenylphosphine)nickel, 9CI

Phenyl(π-cyclopentadienyl)(triphenylphosphine)nickel

[1298-98-2]

As (η^5-2,4-Cyclopentadien-1-yl)methyl(triphenylphosphine)nickel, Ni-00230 with

R = Ph

M 463.180

Dark-green cryst. (hexane). Sol. most org. solvs. Mp 137-9° dec. (under N_2).

Yamazaki, H. *et al*, *J. Organomet. Chem.*, 1966, **6**, 86 (*synth*)
Churchill, M.A. *et al*, *J. Chem. Soc. (A)*, 1969, 266 (*struct*)
Thomson, J. *et al*, *Can. J. Chem.*, 1973, **51**, 1179 (*nmr, uv*)

$C_{29}H_{27}NiO_2P$ Ni-00273

(2,4-Pentanedionato-*O,O'*)phenyl(triphenylphosphine)nickel, 9CI

(Triphenylphosphine)phenylnickel acetylacetonate. (Acetylacetonato)phenyl(triphenylphosphine)nickel

[56664-78-9]

As Methyl(2,4-pentanedionato-*O,O'*)-(trimethylphosphine)nickel, Ni-00066 with

L = R = Ph

M 497.195
Yellow cryst. (toluene/Et_2O or Et_2O/THF). Sol. THF, C_6H_6, $CHCl_3$, toluene. Mp 148-149.5° dec. Solns. dec. rapidly in air.

Maruyama, K. *et al*, *J. Organomet. Chem.*, 1978, **155**, 359 (*synth, nmr*)
Huggins, J.M. *et al*, *J. Am. Chem. Soc.*, 1981, **103**, 3002 (*synth*)

$C_{29}H_{33}NiP$ Ni-00274

Methyl[(1,2,3,4,5-η)-1,2,3,4,5-pentamethyl-2,4-cyclopentadien-1-yl](triphenylphosphine)nickel, 10CI
(Pentamethylcyclopentadienyl)methyl(triphenylphosphine)nickel
[69239-92-5]

M 471.243
Air-sensitive, dark-green cryst. (hexane). Sol. C_6H_6. Dec. at 130°.

Mise, T. *et al*, *J. Organomet. Chem.*, 1978, **164**, 391 (*synth, pmr*)

$C_{30}H_{20}Ni_2O_6P_2$ Ni-00275

Hexacarbonylbis[μ-(diphenylphosphino)]dinickel, 8CI
Bis(diphenylphosphino)hexacarbonyldinickel, 9CI
[19664-27-8]

M 655.812
Yellow cryst. (C_6H_6), dec. above 100°. Mp 190-200°.

Hayter, R.G., *Inorg. Chem.*, 1964, **3**, 711 (*synth, ir, pmr*)
Mais, R.H.B. *et al*, *J. Chem. Soc. (A)*, 1967, 1744 (*struct*)

$C_{30}H_{27}NiO_3P$ Ni-00277

Benzoyl(2,4-pentanedionato-*O,O'*)(triphenylphosphine)nickel, 10CI
Acetylacetonato(benzoyl)(triphenylphosphine)nickel
As Methyl(2,4-pentanedionato-*O,O'*)-(trimethylphosphine)nickel, Ni-00066 with

L = COPh, R = Ph

M 525.205
Deep-yellow solid. Solns. decarbonylate rapidly. Rather insensitive to air. Thermally stable in the solid state. Sol. Me_2CO, C_6H_6. Mp 106-10°.

Maruyama, K. *et al*, *J. Organomet. Chem.*, 1978, **157**, 463 (*synth, ir, pmr*)

$C_{30}H_{30}Ni_6$ Ni-00278

Hexakis(η^5-2,4-cyclopentadien-1-yl)hexanickel, 10CI
[75349-30-3]

Struct. resembles Ni-00279 (neutral molecule)

M 742.707
Black amorph. solid or black cryst. (CH_2Cl_2/CS_2). Cryst. form mod. air-stable, amorph. form air-sensitive. Mod. sol. THF, CH_2Cl_2, spar. sol. C_6H_6, Me_2CO, insol. hexane.

Paquette, M. *et al*, *J. Am. Chem. Soc.*, 1980, **102**, 6621 (*synth, struct*)

$C_{30}H_{30}Ni_6^{\oplus}$ Ni-00279

Hexakis(η^5-2,4-cyclopentadien-1-yl)hexanickel(1+), 10CI

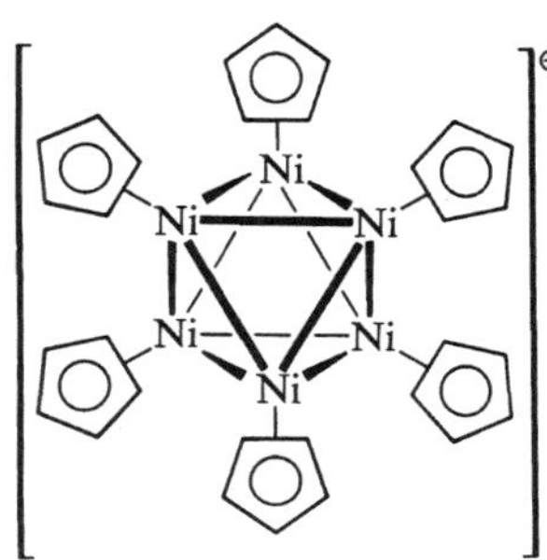

M 742.707 (ion)
Hexafluorophosphate: [76119-25-0].
$C_{30}H_{30}F_6Ni_6P$ M 887.671
Brown solid. Sol. Me_2CO.

Paquette, M. *et al*, *J. Am. Chem. Soc.*, 1980, **102**, 6621 (*synth, struct*)

$C_{30}H_{31}BrNiP_2$ Ni-00280

Bromo[ethane-1,2-diylbis[diphenylphosphine]](η^3-2-methyl-2-propenyl)nickel
Bromo[ethylenebis(diphenylphosphine)](2-methyl-π-allyl)nickel, 8CI
[12304-08-4]

M 592.116
Deep-red cryst., air-stable for indefinite periods.

Churchill, M.R. *et al*, *J. Chem. Soc. (A)*, 1970, 206 (*synth, struct*)

$C_{30}H_{31}NNiP^{\oplus}$ Ni-00281

(η^5-2,4-Cyclopentadien-1-yl)(isocyanocyclohexane)(triphenylphosphine)nickel(1+), 8CI

(Cyclohexylisonitrile)(π-cyclopentadienyl)(triphenylphosphine)nickel(1+), 8CI. *(Cyclohexylisocyanide)(η^5-2,4-cyclopentadien-1-yl)(triphenylphosphine)-nickel(1+)*

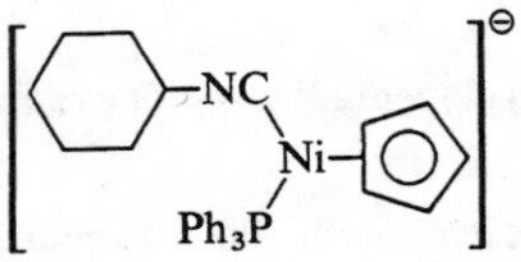

M 495.245 (ion)

Iodide:

$C_{30}H_{31}INNiP$ M 622.150

Mp 138-41° dec.

Tetraphenylborate:

$C_{54}H_{51}BNNiP$ M 814.477

Mp 98-101° dec.

Trichlorogermanate: [41365-09-7].

$C_{30}H_{31}Cl_3GeNNiP$ M 674.194

Brown solid. Mp 60°.

Yamamoto, Y. *et al*, *J. Organomet. Chem.*, 1969, **18**, 189 (*synth*)
Glockling, F. *et al*, *J. Inorg. Nucl. Chem.*, 1973, **35**, 1481 (*synth, pmr*)

$C_{30}H_{33}NiP$ Ni-00282

[(1,2,5,6,9,10-η)-1,5,9-Cyclododecatriene](triphenylphosphine)nickel, 9CI

[12123-87-4]

As [(1,2,5,6,9,10-η)-1,5,9-Cyclododecatriene](trimethylphosphine)nickel, Ni-00136 with

R = Ph

M 483.254

Yellow cryst. (pentane). Mp 80-90° dec.

Bogdanovic, B. *et al*, *Justus Liebigs Ann. Chem.*, 1969, **727**, 143 (*synth*)

$C_{30}H_{34}NiP_2$ Ni-00283

[1,2-Ethanediylbis[diphenylphosphine]-*P,P'*]diethylnickel, 9CI

[Ethylenebis[diphenylphosphine]]diethylnickel. Diethyl[1,2-bis(diphenylphosphino)ethane]nickel

[60542-89-4]

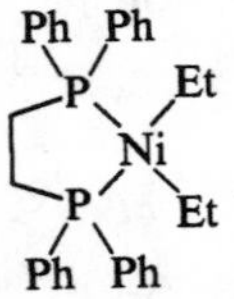

M 515.236

Catalyst for insertion reaction between CO, Grignard reagents and aryl halides to give ketones and tertiary alcohols. No phys. details recorded.

Yamamoto, A., *Organotransition-Met. Chem., Proc. Jpn.-Am. Semin., 1st*, , 1974, Plenum, New York, 281 (*synth*)
Yamamoto, T. *et al*, *Chem. Lett.*, 1976, 1217 (*use*)

$C_{30}H_{34}Ni_2$ Ni-00284

Bis(cyclooctadiene)(μ-diphenylacetylene)dinickel

Bis[(1,2,5,6-η)-1,5-cyclooctadiene][μ-[1,1'-(η^2:η^2-1,2-ethynediyl)bis[benzene]]]dinickel, 10CI. *(μ-Diphenylacetylene)-bis(cyclooctadienenickel)*

[61458-99-9]

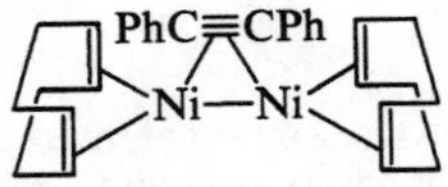

M 511.979

Dark-red cryst. Mp 173-5°.

Day, V.W. *et al*, *J. Am. Chem. Soc.*, 1976, **98**, 8289 (*struct*)
Muetterties, E.L. *et al*, *J. Am. Chem. Soc.*, 1978, **100**, 2090 (*synth*)

$C_{30}H_{36}NiP_2$ Ni-00285

Bis(dimethylphenylphosphine)bis(2-methylphenyl)nickel

Bis(dimethylphenylphosphine)di-o-tolylnickel, 8CI

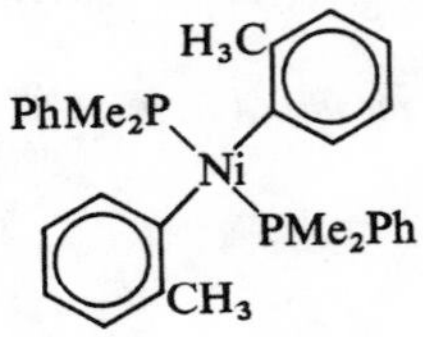

M 517.252

trans-form [15526-03-1]

Pale-yellow cryst. (EtOH). Mp 148-51°.

Moss, J.R. *et al*, *J. Chem. Soc. (A)*, 1966, 1793 (*synth, pmr*)

$C_{31}H_{25}ClN_2Ni$ Ni-00286

Chlorobis(pyridine)[(1,2,3-η)-1,2,3-triphenyl-2-cyclopropen-1-yl]nickel, 9CI

(Triphenyl-π-cyclopropenyl)chlorobis(pyridine)nickel

[36351-87-8]

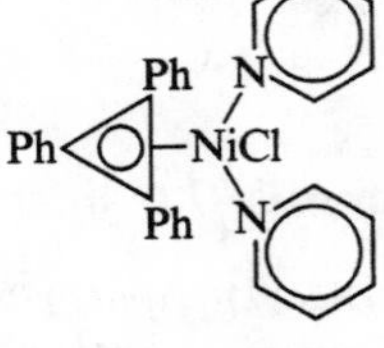

M 519.695

Maroon cryst. + 1Py (pyridine).

Weaver, D.L. *et al*, *J. Am. Chem. Soc.*, 1969, **91**, 6506 (*synth, ir, struct*)

$C_{31}H_{29}NiP_2^{\oplus}$ Ni-00287

(π-Cyclopentadienyl)[ethylenebis[diphenylphosphine]]nickel(1+)

(η⁵-2,4-Cyclopentadien-1-yl)[1,2-ethanediylbis(diphenylphosphine)-P,P′]nickel(1+), 9CI

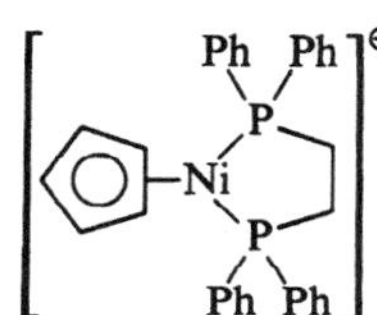

M 522.208 (ion)

Iodide: [41517-40-2].
$C_{31}H_{29}INiP_2$ M 649.112
Green cryst. Mp 133° dec.

Hexafluorophosphate: [41517-41-3].
$C_{31}H_{29}F_6NiP_3$ M 667.172
Green cryst. Mp 203°.

Tetrabromonickelate: [41517-23-1].
$C_{31}H_{29}Br_4Ni_2P_2$ M 900.514
Green cryst. Mp 220° dec.

Tetrachloronickelate: [41517-22-0].
$C_{31}H_{29}Cl_4Ni_2P_2$ M 722.710
Green cryst. Mp 122° dec.

Salzer, A. *et al*, *Synth. Inorg. Met.-Org. Chem.*, 1972, **2**, 249 (*ir*)
Kaempfe, L.A. *et al*, *Inorg. Chem.*, 1973, **12**, 2578 (*synth*)
Bancroft, G.M. *et al*, *Can. J. Chem.*, 1975, **53**, 307 (*mössbauer*)

$C_{32}H_{20}Ni^{\ominus\ominus}$ Ni-00288

Tetrakis(phenylethynyl)nickelate(2−), 9CI

Tetrakis(phenylacetylenyl)nickelate(2−)

$[Ni(C{\equiv}CPh)_4]^{\ominus\ominus}$ (D_{4h})

M 463.200 (ion)

Di-Li salt: [54712-91-3].
$C_{32}H_{20}Li_2Ni$ M 477.082
Beige cryst. + 4THF. Sol. THF. Dec. with dark discolouration >90°.

Taube, R. *et al*, *Angew. Chem., Int. Ed. Engl.*, 1975, **14**, 261 (*synth*)

$C_{32}H_{20}Ni^{\ominus\ominus\ominus\ominus}$ Ni-00289

Tetrakis(phenylethynyl)nickelate(4−)

Tetrakis(phenylacetylenyl)nickelate(4−)

$[Ni(C{\equiv}CPh)_4]^{\ominus\ominus\ominus\ominus}$ (T_d)

M 463.200 (ion)

Tetra-K salt:
$C_{32}H_{20}K_4Ni$ M 619.593
Orange-brown solid.

▷Highly pyrophoric

Nast, R., *Z. Naturforsch., B*, 1953, **8**, 381 (*synth*)

$C_{32}H_{40}NiP_2$ Ni-00290

Bis(4-phenyl-1,3-butadiynyl)bis(triethylphosphine)nickel, 8CI

[31386-94-4]

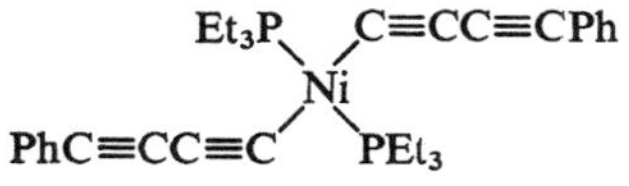

Et_3P, $C{\equiv}CC{\equiv}CPh$, Ni, $PhC{\equiv}CC{\equiv}C$, PEt_3

M 545.306
Solid. Dec. at 130°.

Masai, H. *et al*, *J. Organomet. Chem.*, 1971, **26**, 271 (*synth, ir*)

$C_{32}H_{44}NiP_4$ Ni-00291

Tetrakis(dimethylphenylphosphine)nickel, 10CI

[61994-77-2]

$(Me_2PhP)_4Ni$ (T_d)

M 611.285

Tolman, C.A. *et al*, *J. Organomet. Chem.*, 1976, **117**, C30 (*synth*)

$C_{32}H_{60}NiP_2$ Ni-00292

[(2,3-η)-2,3-Dimethyl-2-butene][1,2-ethanediylbis(dicyclohexylphosphine)-*P,P′*]nickel, 9CI

(η²-Tetramethylethylene)[1,2-bis(dicyclohexylphosphino)ethane]nickel

[54102-18-0]

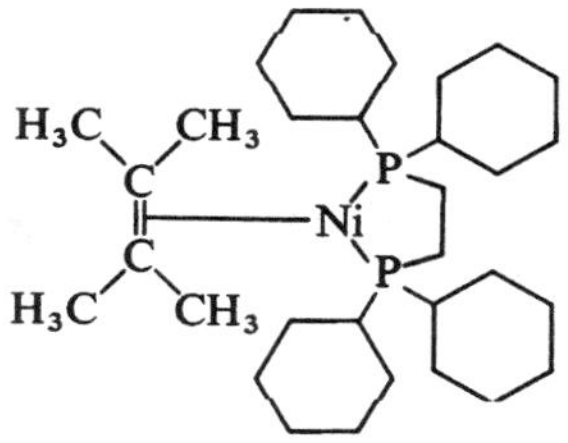

M 565.464
Cryst.

Brauer, D.J. *et al*, *J. Organomet. Chem.*, 1974, **77**, 423 (*struct*)

$C_{32}H_{66}NiP_2$ Ni-00293

[(1,2,5,6-η)-1,5-Cyclooctadiene]bis(tributylphosphine)nickel, 9CI

Bis(tributylphosphine)(1,5-cyclooctadiene)nickel

[51266-28-5]

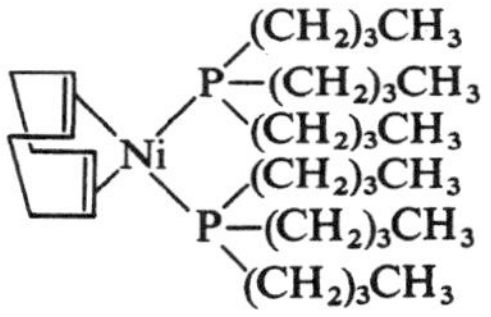

M 571.511
Yellow cryst. Sol. pet. ether. Mp 102-4°.

▷Pyrophoric

Cundy, C.S., *J. Organomet. Chem.*, 1974, **69**, 305 (*synth, ir, pmr*)

$C_{33}H_{25}Ni^{\oplus}$ Ni-00294

(η⁵-2,4-Cyclopentadien-1-yl)(1,2,3,4-tetraphenyl-1,3-cyclobutadiene)nickel(1+)

(π-Tetraphenylcyclobutadienyl)(π-cyclopentadienyl)nickel(1+)

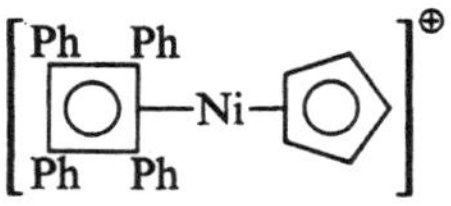

M 480.251 (ion)

Bromide:
$C_{33}H_{25}BrNi$ M 560.155
Orange-yellow cryst. (CH_2Cl_2/pet. ether). Mp 187° dec.

Maitlis, P.M. *et al*, *J. Am. Chem. Soc.*, 1965, **87**, 719 (*synth, pmr*)

$C_{34}H_{30}Ni_2P_2$ Ni-00295

Bis(η^5-2,4-cyclopentadien-1-yl)bis[μ-(diphenylphosphino)]-dinickel, 9CI

Di-π-cyclopentadienylbis[μ-(diphenylphosphino)]dinickel, 8CI

[1299-11-2]

M 617.939

Dark-brown cryst. (toluene). Mp 264-5°.

Hayter, R.G., *Inorg. Chem.*, 1963, **2**, 1031 (*synth*)
Coleman, J.M. *et al*, *J. Am. Chem. Soc.*, 1967, **89**, 542 (*struct*)

$C_{34}H_{39}NiP$ Ni-00296

Bis[(1,2,5,6-η)-1,5-cyclooctadiene]triphenylphosphinenickel, 10CI

(Triphenylphosphine)bis(1,5-cyclooctadiene)nickel

[61684-26-2]

M 537.346

Catalyst in polymerisation of dienes. Compd. not isol.

Inorg. Synth., 1974, **15**, 5 (*synth*)
Murakami, M. *et al*, *Chem. Lett.*, 1979, 931 (*use*)

$C_{34}H_{57}NiP$ Ni-00297

(Tricyclohexylphosphine)bis(3-vinylcyclohexene)nickel, 8CI

Bis(3-ethenylcyclohexene)(tricyclohexylphosphine)nickel

[33042-30-7]

M 555.488

White powder, extremely air-sensitive. Olefins displaced by CO, even at −78°.

Jolly, P.W. *et al*, *Angew. Chem., Int. Ed. Engl.*, 1971, **10**, 328 (*synth*)

$C_{34}H_{66}NiO_2P_2$ Ni-00298

(2,3,5,6-Tetramethyl-2,5-cyclohexadiene-1,4-dione)bis(tributylphosphine)nickel

(2,3,5,6-Tetramethyl-p-benzoquinone)bis(tributylphosphine)nickel, 8CI. *Duroquinonebis(tributylphosphine)nickel*

[12577-39-8]

M 627.532

Solid. Mp 76-80°.

Pidcock, A. *et al*, *J. Chem. Soc. (A)*, 1970, 2922 (*synth*)

$C_{35}H_{63}N_7Ni_4$ Ni-00299

Heptakis(2-isocyano-2-methylpropane)tetranickel, 9CI

Heptakis(tert-butylisonitrile)tetranickel. Heptakis(tert-butylisocyanide)tetranickel

[73377-49-8]

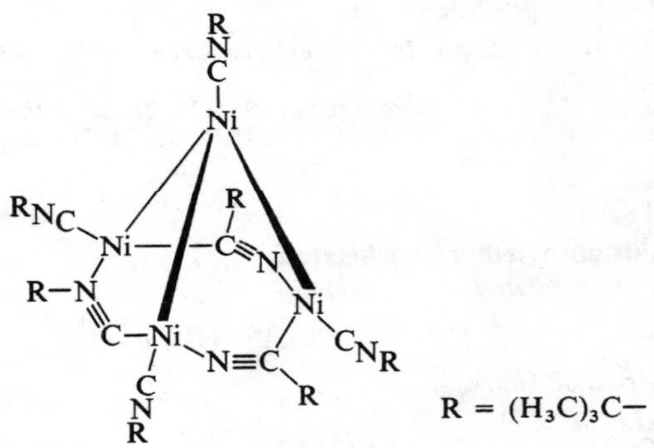

M 816.690

Catalyst for selective hydrogenation of acetylenes to *cis* olefins, and for hydrogenation of isocyanides and nitriles. Red-brown cryst. (Et_2O). Highly air-sensitive. Insol. pentane. Forms complex with C_6H_6, most acetylenes and dienes.

Inorg. Synth., 1977, **17**, 117 (*synth, ir*)
Thomas, M.G. *et al*, *J. Am. Chem. Soc.*, 1977, **99**, 743 (*synth, pmr*)
Muetterties, E.L. *et al*, *Inorg. Chem.*, 1980, **19**, 1552 (*struct*)

$C_{36}H_{28}Ni$ Ni-00300

(Cyclooctatetraene)(η^4-1,2,3,4-tetraphenylcyclobutadiene)-nickel

[1,1′,1″,1‴-(η^4-1,3-Cyclobutadiene-1,2,3,4-tetrayl)tetrakis[benzene]][(1,2,5,6-η)-1,3,5,7-cyclooctatetraene]nickel, 10CI

[72845-23-9]

M 519.307

Green cryst. Sol. C_6H_6, toluene, THF, slowly dec. in chlorinated hydrocarbons. Mp 260° dec.

Hoberg, H., *Angew. Chem., Int. Ed. Engl.*, 1980, **19**, 145 (*synth*)

$C_{36}H_{30}Br_2NiP_2$ Ni-00301

Dibromobis(triphenylphosphine)nickel, 9CI
Bis(triphenylphosphine)nickel bromide
[14126-37-5]

$(Ph_3P)_2NiBr_2$ (T_d)

M 743.079
Catalyst for hydrogenation of unsatd. molecules, oligomerisation of terminal alkynes, dehalogenation reactions, butadiene dimerisation, and cross-coupling reactions. Dark-green cryst. Mp 222-5°. Paramagmetic with two unpaired electrons μ_{eff} = 2.97 BM. Dipole moment 5.9D.

Venanzi, L.M., *J. Chem. Soc.*, 1958, 719 (*synth*)
Jarvis, J.A.J. *et al*, *J. Chem. Soc.* (*A*), 1968, 1473 (*struct*)
Winzer, A. *et al*, *Z. Chem.*, 1970, **10**, 438 (*synth*)
Matienzo, J. *et al*, *Inorg. Chem.*, 1973, **12**, 2762.
Que, L. *et al*, *Inorg. Chem.*, 1973, **12**, 156 (*uv*)
Allen, E.A. *et al*, *Spectrochim. Acta, Part A*, 1974, **30**, 1219 (*ir*)
Fieser, M. *et al*, *Reagents for Organic Synthesis*, Wiley, 1967-83, **6**, 58.

$C_{36}H_{30}Cl_2NiP_2$ Ni-00302

Dichlorobis(triphenylphosphine)nickel, 10CI, 9CI
Bis(triphenylphosphine)nickel dichloride
[14264-16-5]

$(Ph_3P)_2NiCl_2$

M 654.177
Catalyst for cross-coupling of Grignard reagents, hydrosilylations and hydrogenation, oligomerisation and polymerisation of many unsatd. species. Purple cryst. Mp 205-6° (247-50° dec.).
▷QR6170000.
Tetrahedral-form [39716-73-9]
Paramagnetic.
Trans-square-planar-form [53996-95-5]
Diamagnetic.

Venanzi, L.M., *J. Chem. Soc.*, 1958, 719 (*synth*)
Garton, J. *et al*, *J. Chem. Soc.*, 1963, 3625 (*cryst struct*)
Gmelins Handbuch der Anorg. Chem., Syst. No. 57, Part C, 2nd Suppl., 1969, 1046 (*rev*)
Makienzo, L.J. *et al*, *Inorg. Nucl. Chem. Lett.*, 1972, **8**, 1085.
Barnett, K.W., *J. Chem. Educ.*, 1974, **51**, 422 (*synth*)
Felkin, H. *et al*, *Tetrahedron*, 1975, **31**, 2735 (*use*)
Fieser, M. *et al*, *Reagents for Organic Synthesis*, Wiley, 1967-83, **6**, 59.

$C_{36}H_{32}Ni$ Ni-00303

(1,5-Cyclooctadiene)(η^4-1,2,3,4-tetraphenylcyclobutadiene)-nickel
[1,1′,1″,1‴-(η^4-1,3-Cyclobutadiene-1,2,3,4-tetrayl)tetrakis[benzene]][(1,2,5,6-η)-1,5-cyclooctadiene]nickel, 10CI
[72827-41-9]

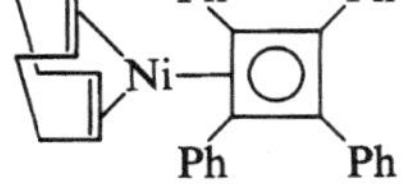

Ph Ph
Ni
Ph Ph

M 523.339
Green cryst. Sol. C_6H_6, toluene, THF. Slowly dec. in chlorinated hydrocarbons. Mp 220° dec.

Hoberg, H., *Angew. Chem., Int. Ed. Engl.*, 1980, **19**, 145 (*synth*)

$C_{36}H_{40}NiP_2$ Ni-00304

Methyl(2,4,6-trimethylphenyl)bis(methyldiphenylphosphine)-nickel
Mesitylmethylbis(methyldiphenylphosphine)nickel, 8CI

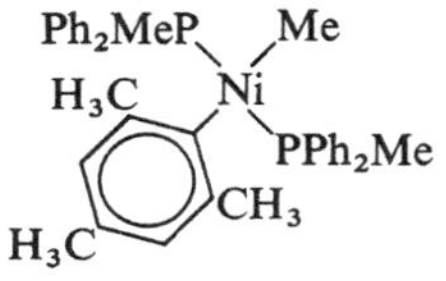

Ph_2MeP Me
H_3C Ni
PPh_2Me
CH_3
H_3C

M 593.350
trans-form [26025-12-7]
Air-stable yellow cryst. (hexane). Mp 118.5-120° dec.

Rausch, M.D. *et al*, *Inorg. Chem.*, 1970, **9**, 512 (*synth*, *nmr*)

$C_{36}H_{67}ClNiP_2$ Ni-00305

Chlorohydrobis(tricyclohexylphosphine)nickel, 9CI, 8CI
Hydridochlorobis(tricyclohexylphosphine)nickel
[25703-57-5]
As Chlorohydrobis(triisopropylphosphine)nickel, Ni-00171 with

R = cyclohexyl

M 656.016
trans-form [22829-35-2]
Yellow-brown cryst. (pet. ether). Stable in air for several hours. V. sol. C_6H_6, THF, CH_2Cl_2. Reacts with CCl_4, $CHCl_3$ and CS_2. Solns. dec. within minutes: cryst. dec. at 150° under argon.

Green, M.L.H. *et al*, *J. Chem. Soc., Chem. Commun.*, 1969, 208 (*synth*, *ir*, *pmr*)
Clark, H.C. *et al*, *Can. J. Chem.*, 1975, **53**, 3462 (*props*)
Inorg. Synth., 1977, **17**, 84 (*synth*)

$C_{36}H_{68}Ni_2P_4$ Ni-00306

Di-μ-*o*-phenylenetetrakis(triethylphosphine)dinickel, 8CI
Di(μ-phenylene)tetrakis(triethylphosphine)dinickel
[32841-78-4]

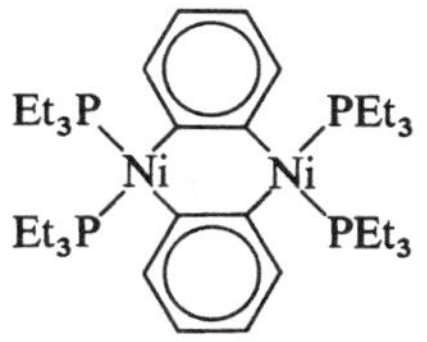

Et_3P PEt_3
Ni Ni
Et_3P PEt_3

M 742.208
Bright-yellow cryst. Extremely air-sensitive. Can be stored for months at −78°, slowly dec. at r.t. Solns. are stable for hours at 0°.

Dobson, J. *et al*, *J. Am. Chem. Soc.*, 1971, **93**, 554 (*synth*)

$C_{36}H_{71}BNiP_2$ Ni-00307

Hydro[tetrahydroborato(1−)-*H,H'*]bis(tricyclohexylphosphine)nickel, 9CI

Hydridobis(tricyclohexylphosphine)nickel tetrahydroborate. Bis(tricyclohexylphosphine)hydridonickel borohydride

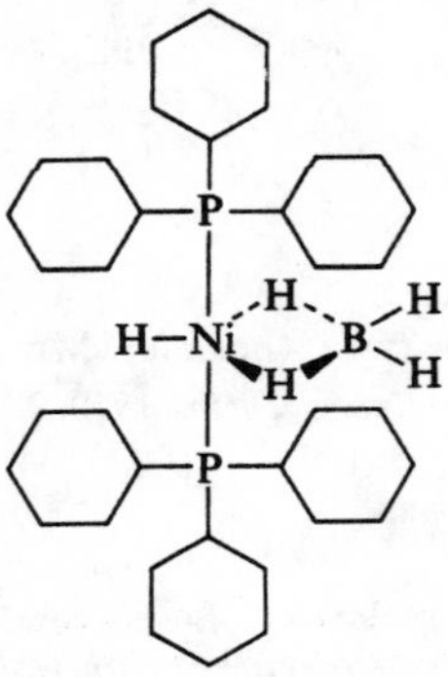

M 635.404

trans-form [24899-12-5]

Bright-yellow cryst., stable at r.t. Fairly stable in air, but soln. dec. in a few minutes. Sol. C_6H_6. Mp 121-5° dec.

Green, M.L.H. *et al*, *J. Chem. Soc., Dalton Trans.*, 1969, 1287 (*synth, ir, pmr*)
Inorg. Synth., 1977, **17**, 88 (*synth, ir, nmr*)
Saito, T. *et al*, *J. Chem. Soc., Dalton Trans.*, 1978, 482 (*struct*)

$C_{36}H_{84}NiO_{12}P_4$ Ni-00308

Tetrakis(triisopropylphosphite)nickel

*Tetrakis[tris(1-methylethyl)phosphite-*P*)nickel,* 9CI. *Tetrakis(phosphorous acid)nickel dodecaisopropyl ester,* 8CI

[14040-52-9]

$[[(H_3C)_2CHO]_3P_4Ni$ (T_d)

M 891.637

Cryst. (pentane). V. sol. org. solvs., almost insol. H_2O. Mp 187°.

Jensen, K.A. *et al*, *Acta Chem. Scand.*, 1965, **19**, 768 (*synth*)
Inorg. Synth., 1977, **17**, 117 (*synth*)

$C_{37}H_{66}NiO_2P_2$ Ni-00309

[(*C,O*-η)-Carbon dioxide]bis(tricyclohexylphosphine)nickel, 9CI

[57307-01-4]

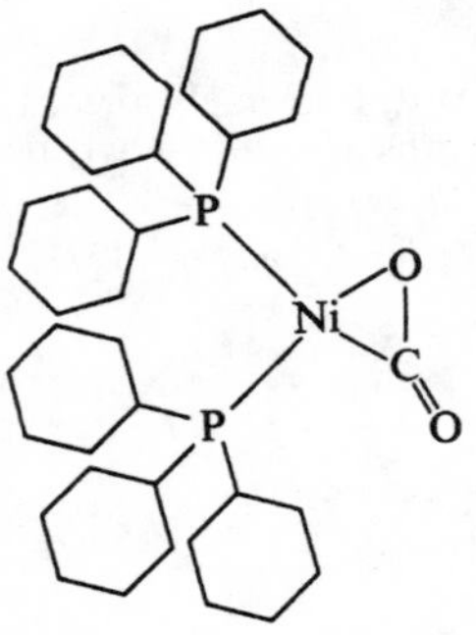

M 663.565

Red-orange cryst. + $\frac{3}{4}$toluene (toluene). Air-stable for a few hours.

Aresta, M. *et al*, *J. Chem. Soc., Chem. Commun.*, 1975, 636 (*synth, props, struct*)

$C_{38}H_{26}Cl_5F_5NiP_2$ Ni-00310

Bis(methyldiphenylphosphine)(pentachlorophenyl)(pentafluorophenyl)nickel, 9CI, 8CI

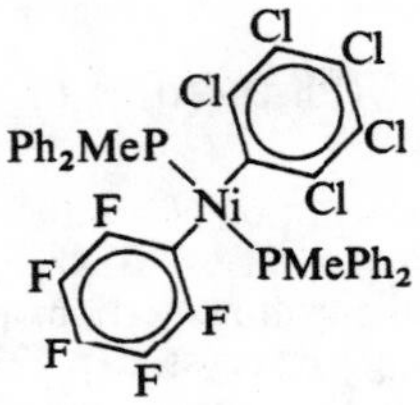

M 875.518

trans-form [26025-18-3]

Light-yellow cryst. (hexane). Can be stored in air at r.t. indefinitely. Solns. can be stored in air for weeks without change. Mp 187.5-189° (under N_2).

Rausch, M.D. *et al*, *Inorg. Chem.*, 1970, **9**, 512 (*synth, pmr*)
Churchill, M.R. *et al*, *J. Chem. Soc. (A)*, 1971, 3463 (*struct*)

$C_{38}H_{26}F_{10}NiP_2$ Ni-00311

Bis(methyldiphenylphosphine)bis(pentafluorophenyl)nickel, 9CI

Bis(pentafluorophenyl)bis(methyldiphenylphosphine)-nickel

[26025-10-5]

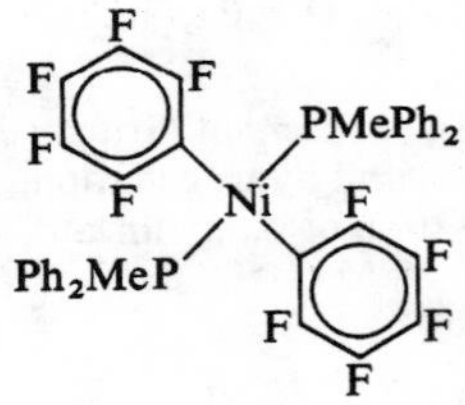

M 793.245

Air-stable lemon-yellow cryst. (hexane/C_6H_6). Mp 192-3°. Solns. in org. solvs. stable for several weeks without change.

Rausch, M.D. *et al*, *Inorg. Chem.*, 1970, **9**, 512 (*synth, pmr*)
Churchill, M.R. *et al*, *J. Chem. Soc., Dalton Trans.*, 1972, 670 (*struct*)

$C_{38}H_{30}As_2NiO_2$ Ni-00312

Dicarbonylbis(triphenylarsine)nickel, 9CI, 8CI

[15709-52-1]

$(Ph_3As)_2Ni(CO)_2$ (C_{2v})

M 727.187

Pale-yellow platelets. Sl. sol. org. solvs.

Bouquet, G. *et al*, *Bull. Soc. Chim. Fr.*, 1962, 433 (*synth, ir*)

$C_{38}H_{30}NiO_2P_2$ Ni-00313

Dicarbonylbis(triphenylphosphine)nickel, 10CI, 9CI, 8CI

Bis(triphenylphosphine)nickel dicarbonyl. Bis(triphenylphosphine)dicarbonylnickel

[13007-90-4]

$Ni(PPh_3)_2(CO)_2$

M 639.291

Catalyst for carbonylations, hydrosilylations, alkene oligomerisation or polymerisation, butadiene cyclooligomerisation, acetylene cyclotrimerisation, and alkene hydroformylation. Pale-cream solid. Mp 210-5°.

Reppe, W. *et al*, *Justus Liebigs Ann. Chem.*, 1948, **560**, 104 (*synth*)
Rose, J.D. *et al*, *J. Chem. Soc.*, 1950, 69 (*synth, ir*)
Meriwether, L.S. *et al*, *J. Am. Chem. Soc.*, 1959, **81**, 4200 (*synth, ir*)
Tanaka, K. *et al*, *Chem. Lett.*, 1974, 813; *CA*, **81**, 72007 (*synth*)
Bodner, G. *et al*, *Inorg. Chem.*, 1975, **14**, 1932 (*cmr*)
Fieser, M. *et al*, *Reagents for Organic Synthesis*, Wiley, 1967-83, **7**, 94; **8**, 147.

$C_{38}H_{30}NiO_2Sb_2$ Ni-00314

Dicarbonylbis(triphenylstibine)nickel, 9CI, 8CI
Bis(triphenylantimony)dicarbonylnickel
[28042-59-3]

$(Ph_3Sb)_2Ni(CO)_2$ (C_{2V})

M 820.844
Butadiene oligomerisation catalyst. No physical details recorded.

Benlian, D. *et al*, *Bull. Soc. Chim. Fr.*, 1963, 1583 (*synth*)

$C_{38}H_{30}NiO_5P_2$ Ni-00315

Dicarbonyl(triphenylphosphine)(triphenylphosphite-*P*)nickel, 9CI
[55333-49-8]

$[(PhO)_3P]Ni(CO)_2PPh_3$

M 687.290
Compd. not isol.

Bodner, G.M., *Inorg. Chem.*, 1975, **14**, 1932 (*nmr*)

$C_{38}H_{30}NiO_8P_2$ Ni-00316

Dicarbonylbis(triphenylphosphite-*P*)nickel, 9CI
Dicarbonylbis(phosphorous acid)nickel hexaphenyl ester, 8CI
[14653-44-2]

$[(PhO)_3P]_2Ni(CO)_2$ (C_{2v})

M 735.288
Catalyses oligomerisation and cyclooligomerisation of butadiene, allene and acetylene. Cryst. Mp 95°.

Bigorgne, M. *et al*, *CA*, 1967, **67**, 59211 (*ir, raman*)
Tolman, C.A., *J. Am. Chem. Soc.*, 1970, **92**, 2956 (*pmr*)
Olechowski, J.R., *J. Organomet. Chem.*, 1971, **32**, 269 (*synth*)
Bodner, G.M., *Inorg. Chem.*, 1975, **14**, 1932 (*nmr*)

$C_{38}H_{32}F_2NiP_2$ Ni-00317

(1,1-Difluoroethylene)bis(triphenylphosphine)nickel, 8CI
[(1,2-η)-1,1-Difluoroethene]bis(triphenylphosphine)nickel, 10CI
[25397-20-0]

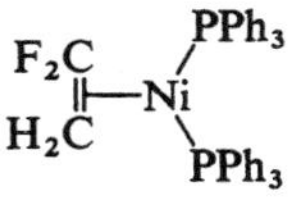

F_2C=H_2C → Ni(PPh_3)$_2$

M 647.305
Yellow cryst. Mp 110° dec.

Ashley-Smith, J. *et al*, *J. Chem. Soc. (A)*, 1969, 3019 (*synth*)

$C_{38}H_{34}NiP_2$ Ni-00318

Ethylenebis(triphenylphosphine)nickel, 8CI
(η^2-Ethene)bis(triphenylphosphine)nickel, 9CI
[23777-40-4]

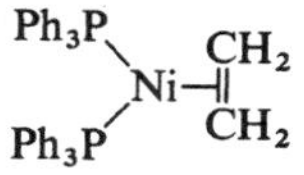

(Ph_3P)$_2$Ni–(CH_2=CH_2)

M 611.324
Yellow cryst.

Wilke, G. *et al*, *Angew. Chem., Int. Ed. Engl.*, 1962, **1**, 549 (*synth*)
Tolman, C.A. *et al*, *Inorg. Chem.*, 1973, **12**, 2770 (*pe*)
Schramm, K. *et al*, *Inorg. Chem.*, 1980, **19**, 2441 (*synth*)
Dreissig, W. *et al*, *Acta Crystallogr., Sect. B*, 1981, **37**, 931 (*struct*)

$C_{38}H_{35}ClNiP_2$ Ni-00319

Chloro(ethyl)bis(triphenylphosphine)nickel, 10CI
Ethylchlorobis(triphenylphosphine)nickel
[62965-83-7]

$NiClEt(PPh_3)_2$

M 647.785
Orange cryst. Extremely unstable. Cannot be recryst. Sol. C_6H_6. Mp 60° dec.

Nesmeyanov, A.N. *et al*, *J. Organomet. Chem.*, 1977, **129**, 421 (*synth*)

$C_{38}H_{66}NiO_2P_2$ Ni-00320

Dicarbonylbis(tricyclohexylphosphine)nickel, 9CI, 8CI
Bis(tricyclohexylphosphine)dicarbonylnickel
[28796-12-5]

$Ni(CO)_2[P(C_6H_{11})_3]_2$

M 675.576
Catalyst for oligomererization of alkenes and the hydrocyanation of butadiene and pentenenitrile. Formed as soln. in toluene.

Tolman, C.A., *J. Am. Chem. Soc.*, 1970, **92**, 2956 (*pmr, ir*)
B.P., 1 417 554, (*1975*); *CA*, **84**, 76501 (*use*)

$C_{38}H_{70}NiP_2$ Ni-00321

Ethylenebis(tricyclohexylphosphine)nickel
(η^2-Ethene)bis(tricyclohexylphosphine)nickel, 10CI
[41685-59-0]

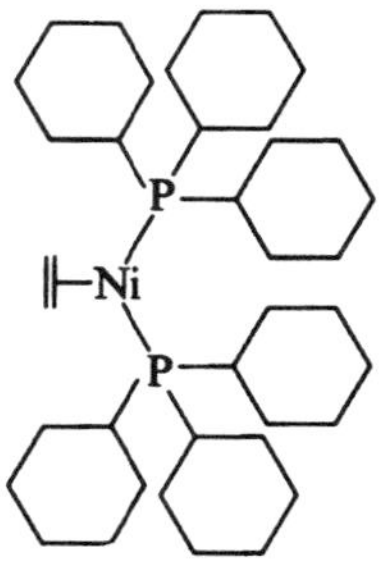

M 647.609
Bright-yellow, extremely air-sensitive solid.

Inorg. Synth., 1974, **15**, 30 (*synth*)

$C_{39}H_{30}F_6NiOP_2$ Ni-00322

[Oxy[trifluoro-1-(trifluoromethyl)ethylidene]]bis(triphenylphosphine)nickel, 8CI

[(O,2-η)-1,1,1,3,3,3-Hexafluoro-2-propanone]bis(triphenylphosphine)nickel, 9CI. π-Hexafluoroacetonebis(triphenylphosphine)nickel. Bis(triphenylphosphine)nickel(hexafluoroacetone)

[50864-88-5]

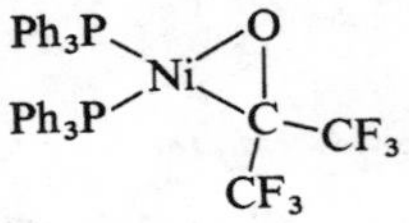

M 749.293

Deep-orange cryst. (C_6H_6). Mp 234-5°.

Browning, J. *et al*, *J. Chem. Soc., Chem. Commun.*, 1968, 929 (*synth*)
Ashley-Smith, J. *et al*, *J. Chem. Soc. (A)*, 1969, 3019 (*synth*)
Countryman, R. *et al*, *J. Cryst. Mol. Struct.*, 1972, **2**, 281 (*struct*)

$C_{39}H_{30}F_6NiP_2S$ Ni-00323

[Thio[trifluoro-1-(trifluoromethyl)ethylidene]]bis(triphenylphosphine)nickel, 8CI

Bis(triphenylphosphine)nickel(hexafluorothioacetone). π-Hexafluorothioacetonebis(triphenylphosphine)nickel

[21219-66-9]

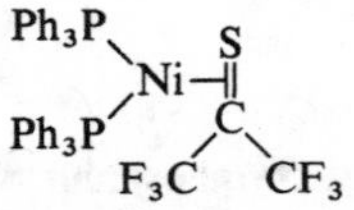

M 765.354

Yellowish cryst. Mp 209-11°.

Browning, J. *et al*, *J. Chem. Soc. (A)*, 1969, 20 (*synth*)

$C_{39}H_{33}NNiP_2$ Ni-00324

[(2,3-η)-2-Propenenitrile]bis(triphenylphosphine)nickel, 10CI

Acrylonitrilebis(triphenylphosphine)nickel

[63688-68-6]

$Ni(CH_2{=}CHCN)(PPh_3)_2$

M 636.334

No phys. details recorded.

Ittel, S.D., *Inorg. Chem.*, 1977, **16**, 2589 (*ir*)

$C_{40}H_{28}N_2Ni$ Ni-00325

(1,10-Phenanthroline)(η⁴-1,2,3,4-tetraphenylcyclobutadiene)nickel

[1,1′,1″,1‴-(η⁴-1,3-Cyclobutadiene-1,2,3,4-tetrayl)tetrakis[benzene]](1,10-phenanthroline-N¹,N¹⁰)nickel, 10CI

[72827-43-1]

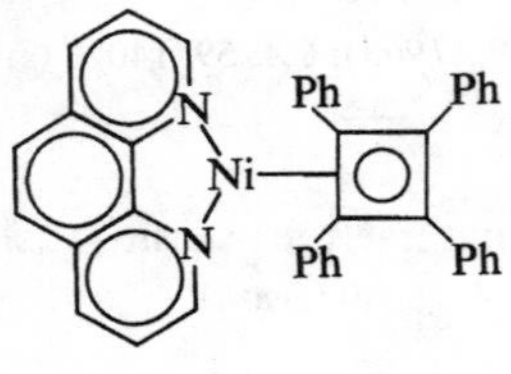

M 595.365

No phys. details recorded.

Hoberg, H. *et al*, *Angew. Chem.*, 1980, **92**, 131 (*synth*)

$C_{40}H_{30}F_8NiP_2$ Ni-00326

(Octafluoro-1,4-butanediyl)bis(triphenylphosphine)nickel

(Octafluorotetramethylene)bis(triphenylphosphine)nickel, 8CI

[27661-80-9]

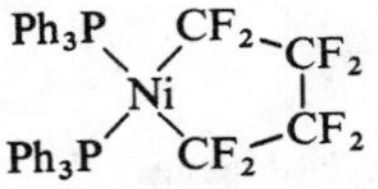

M 783.302

Yellow cryst. Mp 182-3°.

Cundy, C.S. *et al*, *J. Chem. Soc. (A)*, 1970, 1647 (*synth*)

$C_{40}H_{36}NiP_2$ Ni-00327

[(2,3-η)-2-Butyne]bis(triphenylphosphine)nickel

(Dimethylacetylene)bis(triphenylphosphine)nickel. Bis(triphenylphosphine)(η²-2-butyne)nickel

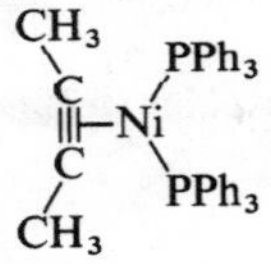

M 637.362

Yellow cryst. + $1C_6H_6$.

Wilke, G. *et al*, *Angew. Chem., Int. Ed. Engl.*, 1962, **1**, 549 (*synth*)

$C_{40}H_{60}NiO_8P_4$ Ni-00328

Tetrakis(diethyl phenylphosphonite-*P*)nickel, 9CI

Tetrakis(phenylphosphonous acid)nickel octaethyl ester, 8CI

[22655-01-2]

$[Ph(EtO)_2P]_4Ni$ (T_d)

M 851.494

White cryst.

Orio, A.A. *et al*, *Inorg. Chim. Acta*, 1969, **3**, 8 (*synth, uv*)
Inorg. Synth., 1971, **13**, 117 (*synth*)
Tolman, C.A. *et al*, *Inorg. Chem.*, 1973, **12**, 2770 (*pe*)

$C_{40}H_{60}NiP_4$ Ni-00329

Tetrakis(diethylphenylphosphine)nickel, 9CI

[55293-69-1]

$(Et_2PhP)_4Ni$

M 723.499

Light-yellow cryst. becoming red at 61° under N_2. Mp 83-6° (under N_2).

Aresta, M. *et al*, *Inorg. Chim. Acta*, 1975, **12**, 167 (*synth*)
Inorg. Synth., 1977, **17**, 117 (*synth*)

$C_{40}H_{74}NiP_2$ Ni-00330

[(2,3-η)-2-Butene]bis(tricyclohexylphosphine)nickel, 9CI
[36180-73-1]

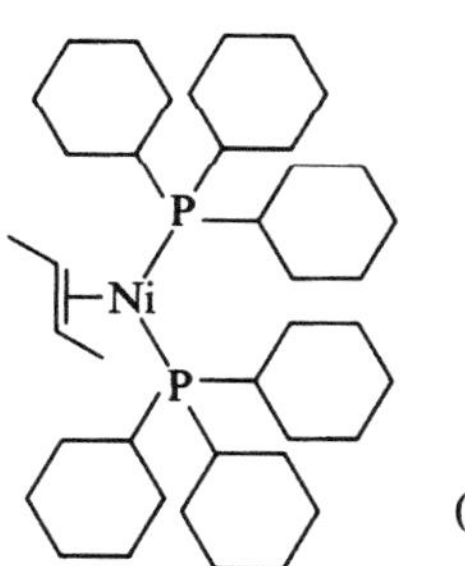

(*E*)-*form*

M 675.662

(E)-form
Orange-yellow cryst.

(Z)-form
Yellow cryst.

Jolly, P.W. *et al*, *J. Organomet. Chem.*, 1971, **33**, 109 (*synth*)

$C_{41}H_{35}NiP_2^{\oplus}$ Ni-00331

(η⁵-2,4-Cyclopentadien-1-yl)bis(triphenylphosphine)nickel(1+), 9CI

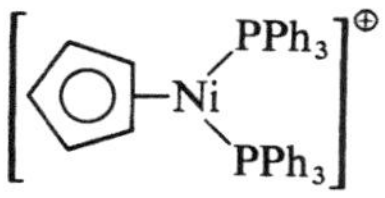

$[(\eta^5\text{-}C_5H_5)Ni(PPh_3)_2]^{\oplus}$

M 648.365 (ion)

Iodide: [67409-71-6].
$C_{41}H_{35}INiP_2$ M 775.270
Green cryst. Mp 90° dec.

Trichlorostannate: [55642-26-7].
$C_{41}H_{35}Cl_3NiP_2Sn$ M 873.414
Brown-black cryst. + $1CH_2Cl_2$ (CH_2Cl_2).

van den Akker, M. *et al*, *J. Organomet. Chem.*, 1967, **10**, P37 (*synth*)
Salzer, A. *et al*, *Synth. Inorg. Met.-Org. Chem.*, 1972, **2**, 249 (*ir*)
Thomson, J. *et al*, *Can. J. Chem.*, 1973, **51**, 1179 (*uv, nmr*)
Bancroft, G.M. *et al*, *Can. J. Chem.*, 1975, **53**, 307 (*mössbauer*)
Olsson, T. *et al*, *Acta Chem. Scand., Ser. B*, 1978, **32**, 293 (*synth*)

$C_{42}H_{30}Br_2Ni_2$ Ni-00332

Di-μ-bromobis[(1,2,3-η)-1,2,3-triphenyl-2-cyclopropen-1-yl]dinickel, 9CI
[12151-05-2]

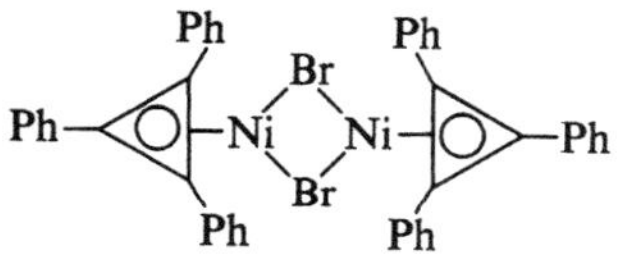

$[(Ph_3C_3)Ni(\mu\text{-}Br)]_2$

M 811.887

Bridged dimer. Olefin isomerization catalyst. Red cryst. (toluene).

Monomer: Bromo(η³-triphenyl-2-cyclopropen-1-yl)nickel.
$C_{21}H_{15}BrNi$ M 405.944
Unknown.

Netherlands Pat., 6 409 178, (*1965*); *CA*, **63**, 5276 (*synth*)

$C_{42}H_{30}ClF_5NiP_2$ Ni-00333

Chloro(pentafluorophenyl)bis(triphenylphosphine)nickel, 9CI, 8CI
Pentafluorophenylchlorobis(triphenylphosphine)nickel
[25037-28-9]

$NiCl(C_6F_5)(PPh_3)_2$

M 785.782

Yellow cryst. (CH_2Cl_2/hexane). Sol. C_6H_6, Me_2CO, $CHCl_3$. Insol. Et_2O, hexane. Mp 210°.

Ashley-Smith, J. *et al*, *J. Chem. Soc. (A)*, 1969, 3019 (*synth, ir*)
Caballero, F. *et al*, *Synth. React. Inorg., Metal-Org. Chem.*, 1977, **7**, 531 (*synth, ir, uv*)

$C_{42}H_{35}BrNiP_2$ Ni-00334

Bromo(phenyl)bis(triphenylphosphine)nickel, 9CI, 8CI
Phenyl(bromo)bis(triphenylphosphine)nickel
[41798-98-5]

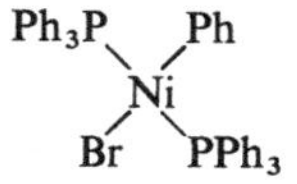

$trans\text{-}NiBr(Ph)(PPh_3)_2$

M 740.280

trans-form [33571-44-7]
Catalyst in the dimerization of propene. Yellow-brown cryst. Mp 124-5° dec.

Hidai, M. *et al*, *J. Organomet. Chem.*, 1971, **30**, 279 (*synth*)

$C_{42}H_{35}ClNiP_2$ Ni-00335

Chlorophenylbis(triphenylphosphine)nickel, 8CI
Bis(triphenylphosphine)chlorophenylnickel. Phenylchlorobis(triphenylphosphine)nickel
[38413-93-3]

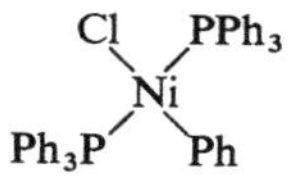

$trans\text{-}NiCl(Ph)(PPh_3)_2$

M 695.829

trans-form [33571-43-6]
Brownish-yellow cryst. Mod. air-stable. Sol. toluene, chlorobenzene, insol. pet. ether. Mp 122-3°.

Hidao, M. *et al*, *J. Organomet. Chem.*, 1971, **30**, 279 (*synth*)
Hidao, M. *et al*, *Organotransition-Met. Chem., Proc. Jpn.-Am. Semin., 1st*, 1974 (*Pub. 1975*), 269-71, Plenum, New York (*pmr, ir*)

$C_{42}H_{36}Ni$ Ni-00336

Tris[(1,2-η)-1,2-diphenylethene]nickel
Tris(stilbene)nickel. Tris(ethenediylbisbenzene)nickel

$(PhCH{=}CHPh)_3Ni$

M 599.436

Brown cryst.

Fr. Pat., 1 320 729, (*1963*); *CA*, **59**, 14026 (*synth*)

$C_{42}H_{38}NiO_4P_2$ **Ni-00337**

[(2,3-η)-Dimethyl-2-butenedioate]bis(triphenylphosphine)nickel, 9CI

M 727.397

(E)-form [36351-96-9]

(Dimethyl fumarate)bis(triphenylphosphine)nickel, 8CI

Ital. Pat., 795 312, (*1967*); *CA*, **76**, 113378 (*synth*)
Dubini, M. *et al*, *Chim. Ind. (Milan)*, 1967, **49**, 1283 (*synth*)
Ittel, S.D., *Inorg. Chem.*, 1977, **16**, 2589 (*synth*)

$C_{42}H_{42}NNiP_3$ **Ni-00338**

[Tris(2-diphenylphosphinoethyl)amine]nickel

[2-(Diphenylphosphino)-N,N-bis[2-(diphenylphosphino)ethyl]ethanamine-N,P,P′,P″]nickel, 9CI

[52633-73-5]

M 712.412

Red cryst. Mod. stable in air but unstable in soln. even under N_2. Sol. THF, CH_2Cl_2.

Sacconi, L. *et al*, *Inorg. Chem.*, 1975, **14**, 1380 (*synth, struct*)
Stoppioni, P. *et al*, *J. Organomet. Chem.*, 1982, **236**, 119 (*props*)

$C_{42}H_{48}N_{12}Ni_4O_6P_4$ **Ni-00339**

Hexacarbonyltetrakis(3,3′,3″-phosphinidynetripropionitrile)-tetranickel, 8CI

Hexacarbonyltetrakis[tris(2-cyanoethyl)phosphine]tetranickel

[20393-28-6]

M 1175.573

Orange cryst. Mp 160° dec. Original report (Meriwether, L.S. *et al*, 1959) has incorrect formula.

Bennett, M.J. *et al*, *J. Am. Chem. Soc.*, 1967, **89**, 5366 (*synth, ir, struct*)

$C_{42}H_{72}NiP_2$ **Ni-00340**

Hydrido(phenyl)bis(tricyclohexylphosphine)nickel, 8CI

Hydro(phenyl)bis(tricyclohexylphosphine)nickel. Phenylhydridobis(tricyclohexylphosphine)nickel

[25703-61-1]

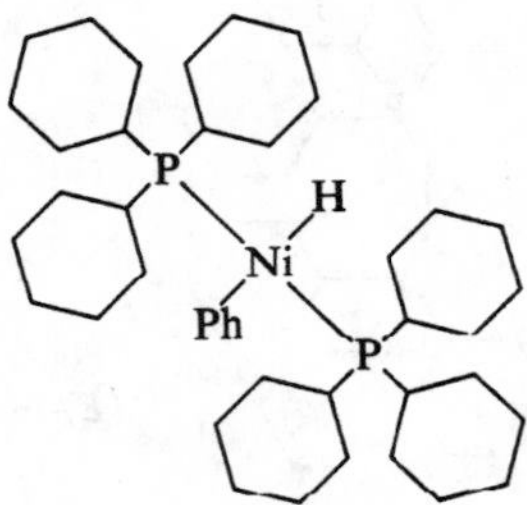

M 697.668

trans-(?)-form

Yellow cryst., stable at r.t.

Jonas, K. *et al*, *Angew. Chem., Int. Ed. Engl.*, 1969, **8**, 519 (*synth, ir, pmr*)

$C_{43}H_{35}ClNiOP_2$ **Ni-00341**

Benzoylchlorobis(triphenylphosphine)nickel, 8CI

Chloro(benzoyl)bis(triphenylphosphine)nickel

[61335-49-7]

$NiCl(COPh)(PPh_3)_2$

M 723.839

Yellow cryst. Intermed. in insertion reaction between $Ni(PPh_3)_4$, CO and aryl halides to give esters.

Hidai, M. *et al*, *Organotransition Met. Chem., Proc. Jpn.-Am. Semin., 1st*, 1974, Plenum, New York, 265 (*synth, ir*)

$C_{44}H_{30}Ni_8O_8P_6$ **Ni-00342**

Octacarbonylhexakis[μ_4-(phenylphosphinidine)]octanickel, 9CI

[60650-12-6]

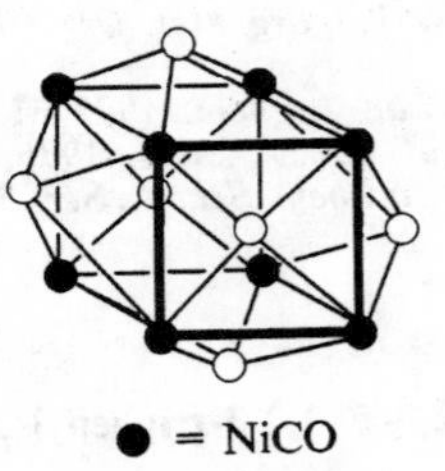

M 1342.079

Black cryst. (hexane).

Lower, L.D. *et al*, *J. Am. Chem. Soc.*, 1976, **98**, 5046 (*synth, struct, ir, pmr*)

$C_{44}H_{36}NiOP_2$ **Ni-00343**

[α-[(Diphenylphosphinomethylene)]benzenemethanolato-*O,P*]phenyl(triphenylphosphine)nickel, 10CI

[66674-76-8]

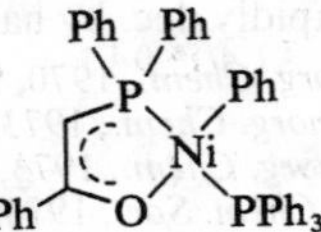

M 701.405

Cryst.

Keim, W. *et al*, *Angew. Chem., Int. Ed. Engl.*, 1978, **17**, 466 (*synth*)

$C_{44}H_{38}NiP_2$ Ni-00344

Styrenebis(triphenylphosphine)nickel

Phenylethenebis(triphenylphosphine)nickel

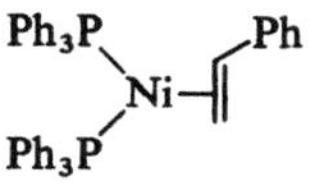

M 687.422

Yellow-orange cryst.

Wilke, G. *et al*, *Angew. Chem., Int. Ed. Engl.*, 1962, **1**, 549 (*synth*)

$C_{44}H_{42}NiP_2$ Ni-00345

[(1,2,5,6-η)-1,5-Cyclooctadiene]bis(triphenylphosphine)nickel, 9CI

Bis(triphenylphosphine)(1,5-cyclooctadiene)nickel

[12151-13-2]

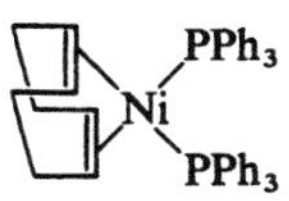

M 691.453

Catalyst for di- or trimerization of 1,3-diolefins, graft copolymerisation of polyols with methyl methacrylate and polymerisation of methylacetylene. Red-brown cryst.

Wilke, G., *Angew. Chem.*, 1961, **73**, 33 (*synth*)
Ger. Pat., 1 191 375, (*1965*); *CA*, **63**, 7045 (*use*)
Fahey, D.R. *et al*, *J. Mol. Catal.*, 1978, **3**, 447 (*use*)

$C_{44}H_{46}NiO_6P_2$ Ni-00346

(η^2-Ethene)bis[tris(2-methylphenyl)phosphite-*P*]nickel, 9CI

Ethylenebis(tri-o-tolylphosphite)nickel. Ethylenebis-(phosphorous acid)nickel hexa-o-tolyl ester, 8CI

[31666-47-4]

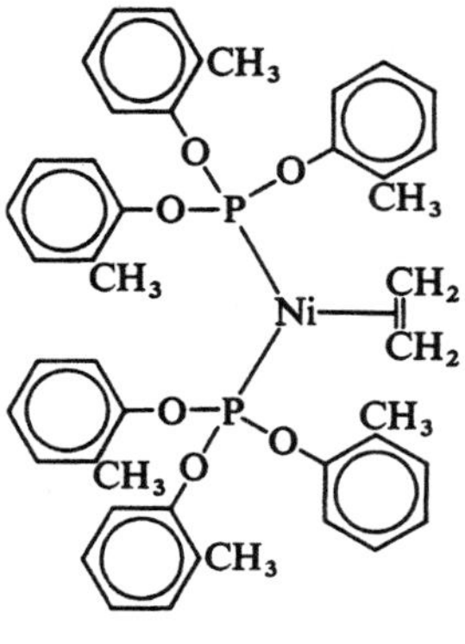

M 791.481

Yellow cryst. (C_6H_6/MeOH). Dec. at 118-20°. Sol. C_6H_6, toluene, rapidly dec. by halogenated solvs.

Seidel, W.C. *et al*, *Inorg. Chem.*, 1970, **9**, 2354 (*synth, ir, pmr*)
Guggenberger, L.J., *Inorg. Chem.*, 1973, **12**, 499 (*struct*)
Tolman, C.A. *et al*, *Inorg. Chem.*, 1973, **12**, 2770 (*pe*)
Tolman, C.A., *J. Am. Chem. Soc.*, 1974, **96**, 2780 (*uv*)
Tolman, C.A. *et al*, *Inorg. Chem.*, 1975, **14**, 2353 (*nmr*)

$C_{46}H_{35}BrNiP$ Ni-00347

Bromo(η^4-1,2,3,4-tetraphenylcyclobutadiene)(triphenylphosphine)nickel

Bromo[1,1′,1″,1‴-(η^4-1,3-cyclobutadiene-1,2,3,4-tetrayl)tetrakis[benzene]](triphenylphosphine)nickel, 10CI

[79061-13-5]

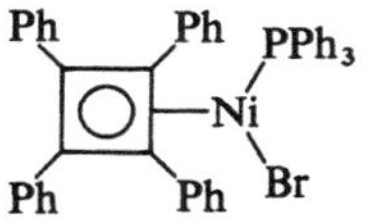

M 757.350

V. air-sensitive, violet cryst. Mp 192° dec.

Hoberg, H. *et al*, *J. Organomet. Chem.*, 1981, **213**, C49 (*synth, ir, ms*)

$C_{48}H_{30}Cl_{12}Ni_2P_2$ Ni-00348

Di-μ-chlorobis(pentachlorophenyl)bis(triphenylphosphine)dinickel, 10CI

Bis(triphenylphosphine)dichlorobis(pentachlorophenyl)-dinickel. Bis(pentachlorophenyl)di-μ-chlorobis(triphenylphosphine)dinickel

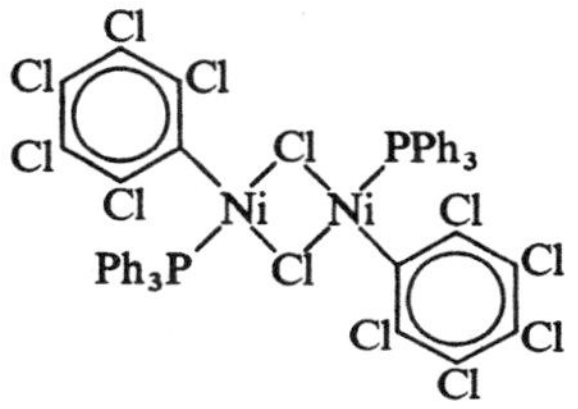

trans-form

M 1211.529

Bridged dimer.

trans-form

Peach-pink solid. Mp 242° dec. Dec. in soln.

Monomer: [21609-02-9]. *Chloro(pentachlorophenyl)-(triphenylphosphine)nickel.*
$C_{24}H_{15}Cl_6NiP$ M 605.764
Unknown.

Mackinnon, K.P. *et al*, *Aust. J. Chem.*, 1968, **21**, 2801 (*synth*)
Coronas, J.M. *et al*, *J. Organomet. Chem.*, 1980, **184**, 263.

$C_{48}H_{30}F_{18}NiP_2$ Ni-00349

[Hexatris(trifluoromethyl)benzene]bis(triphenylphosphine)-nickel, 8CI

Bis(triphenylphosphine)[hexakis(trifluoromethyl)benzene]nickel

[32697-44-2]

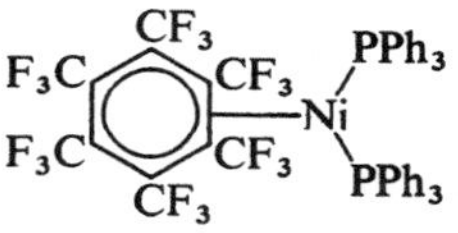

M 1069.374

Purple cryst. Mp 135-7° dec.

Stone, F.G.A. *et al*, *J. Chem. Soc. (A)*, 1971, 448 (*synth*)

$C_{48}H_{40}N_2NiP_2$ **Ni-00350**

(Azobenzene)bis(triphenylphosphine)nickel, 8CI

(Diphenyldiazene-N,N')bis(triphenylphosphine)nickel

[32015-52-4]

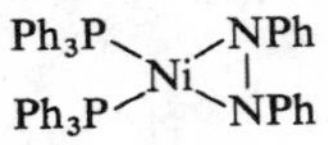

Ph_3P, Ph_3P / Ni / NPh, NPh

M 765.495

Dark-red solid (pentane). Mp 205°.

Klein, H.F. *et al*, *J. Chem. Soc., Chem. Commun.*, 1971, 42 (*synth*)
Inorg. Synth., 1977, **17**, 117 (*synth*)

$C_{48}H_{40}NiP_2^{\ominus\ominus}$ **Ni-00351**

Diphenylbis(triphenylphosphine)nickelate(2−)

Bis(triphenylphosphine)diphenylnickelate(2−)

$[NiPh_2(PPh_3)_2]^{\ominus\ominus}$

M 737.482 (ion)

Di-Li salt:

$C_{48}H_{40}Li_2NiP_2$ M 751.364

Light-brown solid + $3Et_2O$ (Et_2O).

Uhlig, E. *et al*, *Z. Chem.*, 1977, **17**, 272 (*synth*)

$C_{48}H_{47}As_3NNi^{\oplus}$ **Ni-00352**

[Tris(2-diphenylarsinoethyl)amine]phenylnickel(1+)

[2-(Diphenylarsino)-N,N-bis[2-(diphenylarsino)ethyl]-ethanamine-As,As',As'',N]phenylnickel(1+), 9CI

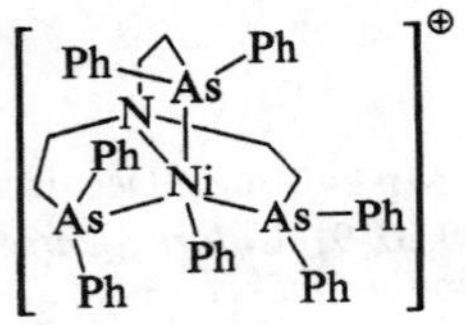

M 921.361 (ion)

Tetraphenylborate: [53450-18-3].

$C_{72}H_{67}As_3BNNi$ M 1240.593

Cherry-red cryst. (CH_2Cl_2/butanol).

Dapporto, P. *et al*, *Inorg. Chim. Acta*, 1974, **9**, L2 (*struct*)
Sacconi, L. *et al*, *Inorg. Chem.*, 1976, **15**, 325 (*synth, uv, struct*)

$C_{48}H_{108}NiP_3$ **Ni-00353**

Tetrakis(tributylphosphine)nickel, 9CI

[28101-79-3]

$[(H_3CCH_2CH_2CH_2)_3P]_4Ni$

M 836.992

Ivory needles becoming red at 44° under N_2. Mp 52-5° (under N_2).

Aresta, M. *et al*, *Inorg. Chim. Acta*, 1975, **12**, 167 (*synth*)
Inorg. Synth., 1977, **17**, 117 (*synth*)

$C_{49}H_{77}N_7Ni_4$ **Ni-00354**

Heptakis(isocyanocyclohexane)tetranickel, 10CI

Heptakis(cyclohexylisonitrile)tetranickel

[73377-51-2]

As Heptakis(2-isocyano-2-methylpropane)tetranickel, Ni-00299 with

R = cyclohexyl

M 998.954

Red-brown cryst. (pentane).

Muetterties, E.L. *et al*, *Inorg. Chem.*, 1980, **19**, 1552 (*synth, pmr, ir*)

$C_{50}H_{42}NiP_2$ **Ni-00355**

Diphenylethylenebis(triphenylphosphine)nickel

[1,1'-(η^2-1,2-Ethenediyl)bis(benzene)]bis(triphenylphosphine)nickel, 9CI. *Stilbenebis(triphenylphosphine)-nickel*, 8CI. *[(1,2-η)-1,2-Bisphenylethene]bistriphenylphosphinenickel*

[12151-25-6]

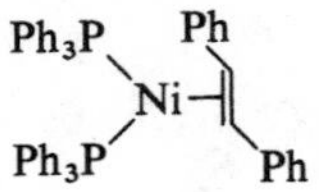

M 763.519

***(E)*-form** [53586-21-3]

Dark-red solid (pentane). Mod. air-sensitive. Mp 205-8° dec.

Wilke, G. *et al*, *Angew. Chem.*, 1962, **74**, 693 (*synth*)
Ittel, S.D. *et al*, *J. Organomet. Chem.*, 1974, **74**, 121 (*synth*)

$C_{52}H_{48}NiP_4$ **Ni-00356**

Bis[1,2-bis(diphenylphosphino)ethane]nickel

Bis[1,2-ethanediylbis(diphenylphosphine)-P,P']nickel, 9CI. *Bis[ethylenebis(diphenylphosphine)]nickel*

[15628-25-8]

As Bis[1,2-bis(dimethylphosphino)ethane]nickel, Ni-00097 with

R = Ph

M 855.536

Orange cryst. (C_6H_6/MeOH), mod. air-sensitive. Sol. aromatic solvs. Mp 253-6°.

Chatt, J. *et al*, *J. Chem. Soc.*, 1962, 2537 (*synth*)
Tolman, C.A. *et al*, *Inorg. Chem.*, 1973, **12**, 2770 (*pe*)
Inorg. Synth., 1977, **17**, 117 (*synth*)

$C_{52}H_{49}NiP_4^{\oplus}$ **Ni-00357**

Bis[1,2-ethanediylbis[diphenylphosphine]-*P,P'*]hydronickel(1+), 9CI

Bis[1,2-bis(diphenylphosphino)ethane]-hydridonickel(1+)

$[NiH(Ph_2PCH_2CH_2PPh_2)_2]^{\oplus}$

M 856.544 (ion)

Hexafluorophosphate: [52666-94-1].

$C_{52}H_{49}F_6NiP_5$ M 1001.508

Orange cryst.

Perchlorate: [55147-09-6].

$C_{52}H_{49}ClNiO_4P_4$ M 955.995

Yellow cryst. Insol. nonpolar solvs., dec. by H_2O or other polar solvs. Mp 180°.

Trichlorosiliconate:

$C_{52}H_{49}Cl_3NiP_4Si$ M 990.989

Brick-red or yellow cryst. Mp 130-5°.

Green, M.L.H. *et al*, *J. Chem. Soc., Dalton Trans.*, 1974, 269 (*synth, pmr, ir*)
Lappert, M.F. *et al*, *J. Organomet. Chem.*, 1974, **80**, 329 (*synth*)

$C_{52}H_{52}NiO_4P_4$ **Ni-00358**

Tetrakis(methyldiphenylphosphinite-*P*)nickel, 9CI

Tetrakis(diphenylphosphinous acid)nickel tetramethyl ester, 8CI

[41685-57-8]

$Ni[P(OMe)Ph_2]_4$ (T_d)

M 923.565

Yellow cryst. (pentane). Mp 185°.

Tolman, C.A. *et al*, *Inorg. Chem.*, 1973, **12**, 2770 (*pe*)
Inorg. Synth., 1977, **17**, 117 (*synth*)

$C_{52}H_{52}NiP_4$ Ni-00359

Tetrakis(methyldiphenylphosphine)nickel, 10CI, 9CI

[25037-29-0]

$Ni(PMePh_2)_4$

M 859.568

Orange cryst. Mp 168-70° dec.

Browning, J. *et al*, *J. Chem. Soc. (A)*, 1969, 20 (*synth, ir*)
Tolman, C.A. *et al*, *J. Am. Chem. Soc.*, 1974, **96**, 53 (*synth*)

$C_{54}H_{44}NiP_2$ Ni-00360

[Ethylenebis[diphenylphosphine]](η^4-1,2,3,4-tetraphenylcyclobutadiene)nickel

[1,1′,1″,1‴-(η^4-1,3-Cyclobutadiene-1,2,3,4-tetrayl)tetrakis[benzene]][1,2-ethanediylbis[diphenylphosphine]-P,P′]nickel, 10CI. *[1,2-Bis(diphenylphosphino)ethane]tetraphenylcyclobutadienenickel*

[72827-44-2]

M 813.579

Solid. Mp 215° dec. Diamagnetic.

Hoberg, H. *et al*, *J. Organomet. Chem.*, 1980, **195**, 355 (*synth, pmr, raman, ms*)

$C_{54}H_{45}NiP_3$ Ni-00361

Tris(triphenylphosphine)nickel

[25136-46-3]

$(Ph_3P)_3Ni$

M 845.561

Reagent for olefin purification. Catalyst for organic halide coupling and cyanation of halides. Red-brown powder. Mp 124-6°. V. sensitive to O_2, usually prepd. *in situ*.

Tolman, C.A. *et al*, *J. Am. Chem. Soc.*, 1972, **94**, 2669 (*synth, nmr*)
Kende, A.S. *et al*, *Tetrahedron Lett.*, 1975, 3375 (*synth, use*)
Fieser, M. *et al*, *Reagents for Organic Synthesis*, Wiley, 1967-83, **8**, 523.

$C_{54}H_{45}NiSi_3^{\ominus\ominus\ominus}$ Ni-00362

Tris(triphenylsilyl)nickelate(3–)

$[Ni(SiPh_3)_3]^{\ominus\ominus\ominus}$

M 836.896 (ion)

Tri-K salt: [67699-36-9].
$C_{54}H_{45}K_3NiSi_3$ M 954.191
Fine, red-brown cryst. +3THF (THF). V. sol. THF, mod. sol. C_6H_6. Thermally unstable.

Dinjus, E. *et al*, *Z. Chem.*, 1975, **15**, 31 (*synth*)
Uhlig, E. *et al*, *Z. Anorg. Allg. Chem.*, 1978, **442**, 11 (*synth, pmr, nmr*)

$C_{54}H_{46}BrNiP_2$ Ni-00363

Bromohydrotris(triphenylphosphine)nickel, 9CI

Hydridotris(triphenylphosphine)nickel bromide. Bromohydridotris(triphenylphosphine)nickel

[57584-08-4]

$NiBrH(PPh_3)_3$

M 895.499

Nesmeyanov, A.N. *et al*, *Dokl. Akad. Nauk SSSR, Ser. Sci. Khim.*, 1975, **223**, 1140.

$C_{54}H_{102}Ni_2P_4$ Ni-00364

Di-μ-hydrobis[1,3-propanediylbis[dicyclohexylphosphine]-*P,P′*]dinickel, 9CI

Di-μ-hydrobis[trimethylenebis[dicyclohexylphosphine]]dinickel, 8CI. *Di-μ-hydridobis[1,3-(dicyclohexylphosphino)propane]dinickel*

[27121-63-7]

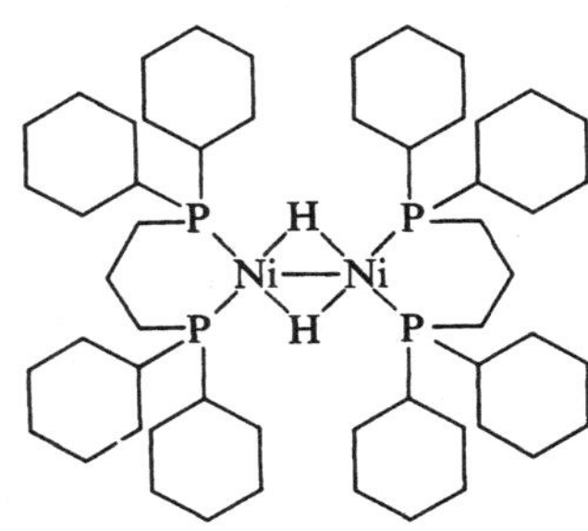

M 992.675

Deep-red, thermally stable cryst.

Jonas, K. *et al*, *Angew. Chem., Int. Ed. Engl.*, 1970, **9**, 312 (*synth*)
Barnett, B.L. *et al*, *Chem. Ber.*, 1977, **110**, 3900 (*struct*)

$C_{55}H_{45}NiOP_3$ Ni-00365

Carbonyltris(triphenylphosphine)nickel, 9CI, 8CI

Tris(triphenylphosphine)carbonylnickel

[15376-83-7]

$[Ni(CO)(PPh_3)_3]$ (C_{3v})

M 873.571

Haas, H. *et al*, *J. Chem. Phys.*, 1967, **47**, 2996 (*ir*)
Inoue, Y. *et al*, *Chem. Lett.*, 1972, 1119 (*synth, ir*)

$C_{55}H_{45}NiO_{10}P_3$ Ni-00366

Carbonyltris(triphenylphosphite-*P*)nickel, 9CI

Carbonyltris(phosphorous acid)nickel nonaphenyl ester, 8CI. *Tris(triphenylphosphite)nickel monocarbonyl*

[14552-96-6]

$Ni(CO)[P(OPh)_3]_3$

M 1017.566

Catalyses olefin cyclization and polymerization. Cryst. (hexane). Mp 98-9°.

Fr. Pat., 1 321 454, (*1963*); *CA*, **59**, 11293h (*use*)
U.S.P., 3 187 062, (*1965*); *CA*, **63**, 6886c (*use*)
Olechowski, J.R., *J. Organomet. Chem.*, 1971, **32**, 269 (*synth, ir*)

U.S.P., 3 661 882, (*1972*); *CA*, **77**, 49813w (*use*)

$C_{56}H_{40}Ni$ Ni-00367

Bis(η^4-1,2,3,4-tetraphenylcyclobutadiene)nickel

Bis[1,1',1'',1'''-(η^4-1,3-cyclobutadiene-1,2,3,4-tetrayl)-tetrakis[benzene]]nickel, 10CI

[61483-84-9]

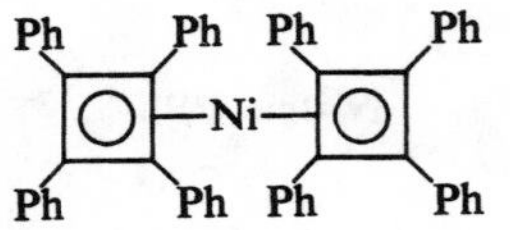

M 771.622

Blue cryst. Mp 404° dec.

Hoberg, H. *et al*, *Angew. Chem., Int. Ed. Engl.*, 1978, **17**, 123 (*synth*)
Hoberg, H. *et al*, *J. Organomet. Chem.*, 1979, **168**, C52 (*synth*)

$C_{56}H_{49}NNiP_3^{\oplus}$ Ni-00368

Acetonitrilehydrotris(triphenylphosphine)nickel(1+)

Hydro(methylcarbonitrile)tris(triphenylphosphine)nickel(1+), 10CI. *Hydrido(acetonitrile)-tris(triphenylphosphine)nickel(1+)*

$[NiH(CH_3CN)(PPh_3)_3]^{\oplus}$

M 887.621 (ion)

Tetrafluoroborate: [75627-85-9].
$C_{56}H_{49}BF_4NNiP_3$ M 974.425
Orange cryst. (Me_2CO). Sol. polar solvs., insol. pentane, Et_2O. Dec. at 191-5°. Air-sensitive.

Nesmeyanov, A.N. *et al*, *J. Organomet. Chem.*, 1980, **195**, C13 (*synth, nmr, raman*)

$C_{57}H_{45}NiP_2^{\oplus}$ Ni-00369

[(1,2,3-η)-1,2,3-Triphenyl-2-cyclopropen-1-yl]bis(triphenylphosphine)nickel(1+), 9CI

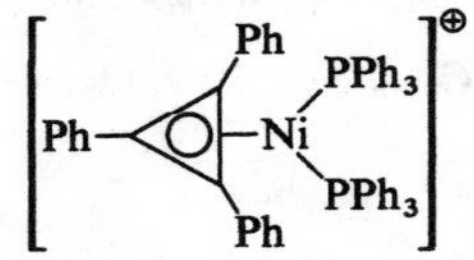

M 850.620 (ion)

Hexafluorophosphate: [75507-34-5].
$C_{57}H_{45}F_6NiP_3$ M 995.584
Red cryst.

Perchlorate: [77598-41-5].
$C_{57}H_{45}ClNiO_4P_2$ M 950.071

Mealli, C. *et al*, *Angew. Chem., Int. Ed. Engl.*, 1980, **92**, 967 (*synth*)
Mealli, C. *et al*, *J. Organomet. Chem.*, 1981, **205**, 273 (*synth*)

$C_{58}H_{40}NiO_2$ Ni-00370

Bis[(2,3,4,5-η)-2,3,4,5-tetraphenyl-2,4-cyclopentadien-1-one]nickel, 9CI

Bis(tetracyclone)nickel

[52336-61-5]

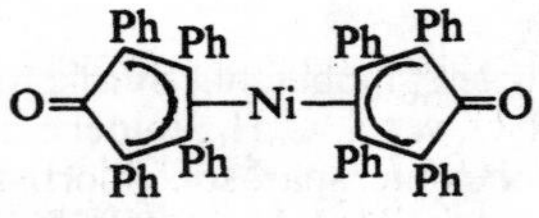

M 827.643

Brown powder (C_6H_6/pet. ether). Mp ca. 245° dec.

Weiss, E. *et al*, *J. Inorg. Nucl. Chem.*, 1959, **11**, 42 (*synth*)
Bird, C.W. *et al*, *J. Organomet. Chem.*, 1974, **69**, 311 (*synth*)
Nesmeyanov, A.N. *et al*, *J. Organomet. Chem.*, 1979, **172**, 185 (*synth, ir, nmr, ms*)

$C_{60}H_{45}F_5NiP_3^{\oplus}$ Ni-00371

Pentafluorophenyltris(triphenylphosphine)nickel(1+)

Tris(triphenylphosphine)pentafluorophenylnickel(1+)

$[Ni(C_6F_5)(PPh_3)_3]^{\oplus}$

M 1012.619 (ion)

Perchlorate: [64848-96-0].
$C_{60}H_{45}ClF_5NiO_4P_3$ M 1112.069
Yellow cryst. ($CHCl_3$/EtOH). Mp 195°. Stable as solid.

Caballero, F. *et al*, *J. Organomet. Chem.*, 1977, **137**, 229 (*synth, uv, ir*)

$C_{60}H_{60}Br_2Ni_2P_4$ Ni-00372

Dibromobis[1,2-ethanediylbis(diphenylphosphine)-*P*,*P'*][μ-[(1,2,3-η:6,7,8-η)-2,6-octadiene-1,8-diyl]dinickel, 9CI

[38980-25-5]

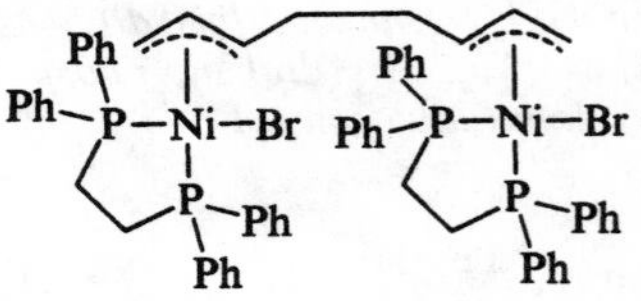

M 1182.217

Orange-red cryst. + 1$CHCl_3$ ($CHCl_3$).

Cameron, T.S. *et al*, *J. Coord. Chem.*, 1972, **2**, 43 (*synth, struct*)
Green, M.I. *et al*, *J. Chem. Soc., Dalton Trans.*, 1974, 269 (*synth*)

$C_{63}H_{63}NiO_9P_3$ Ni-00373

Tris[tris(2-methylphenyl)phosphite-*P*]nickel, 9CI

Tris(phosphorous acid)nickel nona-o-tolylester, 8CI. *Tris(tri-o-tolylphosphite)nickel*

[28829-00-7]

$Ni[P(OC_6H_4CH_3)_3]_3$

M 1115.797

Catalyses isomerization of dienes and of 1,8-bishomocubane. Red solid (hexane). Mp 125-50° dec.

Gosser, L.W. *et al*, *Inorg. Chem.*, 1970, **9**, 2350 (*synth, ir, pmr*)
Gosser, L.W. *et al*, *Tetrahedron Lett.*, 1971, 2555 (*use*)
Tolman, C.A. *et al*, *Inorg. Chem.*, 1973, **12**, 2770.
Inorg. Synth., 1974, **15**, 9 (*synth*)
Noyori, R. *et al*, *J. Am. Chem. Soc.*, 1976, **98**, 1471 (*use*)
Corain, B. *et al*, *Inorg. Chim. Acta*, 1978, **26**, 37 (*synth*)

$C_{63}H_{63}NiP_3$ Ni-00374

Tris[tris(4-methylphenyl)phosphine]nickel, 9CI

*Tris(tri-*p*-tolylphosphine)nickel*

[54806-28-9]

M 971.802

Catalyses cyanation of aryl halides.

Cassar, L. *et al*, *Adv. Chem. Ser.*, 1974, **132**, 252 (*use*)

$C_{64}H_{48}Ni_2$ Ni-00375

μ-Cyclooctatetraenebis[η^4-1,2,3,4-tetraphenylcyclobutadiene]dinickel

Bis[1,1′,1″,1‴-(η^4-1,3-cyclobutadiene-1,2,3,4-tetrayl)-tetrakis[benzene]][μ-[(1,2-η:5,6-η)-1,3,5,7-cyclooctatetraene]]dinickel, 10CI

[77208-31-2]

M 934.463

Brown cryst. + 1 toluene (toluene). Spar. sol. toluene, THF. Mp 275° dec. Intense red solns. in toluene and THF. Has considerable stability to water and acids at 20°.

Froehlich, C. *et al*, *J. Organomet. Chem.*, 1981, **204**, 131 (*synth, ir, uv, ms, pmr*)

$C_{72}H_{60}As_4Ni$ Ni-00376

Tetrakis(triphenylarsine)nickel, 10CI

[14564-53-5]

$(Ph_3As)_4Ni$ (T_d)

M 1283.642

Orange-yellow cryst. (Et_2O). Thermally unstable and mod. air-sensitive. Sol. aromatic solvs. Mp 107°.

Behrens, H. *et al*, *Z. Anorg. Allg. Chem.*, 1965, **341**, 124 (*synth*)
Inorg. Synth., 1977, **17**, 117 (*synth*)

$C_{72}H_{60}NiO_{12}P_4$ Ni-00377

Tetrakis(triphenyl phosphite-*P*)nickel, 10CI, 9CI

Tetrakis(phosphorous acid)nickel dodecaphenyl ester, 8CI

[14221-00-2]

$Ni[P(OPh)_3]_4$

M 1299.844

Initiator for polymerisation reactions, catalyst for alkene additions. Cryst. ($MeOH/C_6H_6$). Mp 151-2°.

Inorg. Synth., 1967, **9**, 181 (*synth*)

Levison, J.J. *et al*, *J. Chem. Soc. (A)*, 1970, 96 (*synth, nmr*)
Fieser, M. *et al*, *Reagents for Organic Synthesis*, Wiley, 1967-83, **7**, 354.

$C_{72}H_{60}NiP_4$ Ni-00378

Tetrakis(triphenylphosphine)nickel, 10CI, 9CI

[15133-82-1]

$Ni(PPh_3)_4$ (T_d)

M 1107.851

Catalyst for hydrosilylation and cross-coupling reacns. Red-brown solid (C_6H_6/heptane). Mp 122-4°.

Inorg. Synth., 1971, **13**, 124; 1977, **17**, 120 (*synth*)

$C_{84}H_{60}Ni_2$ Ni-00379

(π-Pentaphenylcyclopentadienyl)(π-tetraphenylcyclobutadiene)(μ-π-triphenylpropenyl)dinickel

[1,1′,1″,1‴-(η^4-1,3-Cyclobutadiene-1,2,3,4-tetrayl)tetrakis[benzene][(1,2,3,4,5-η)-1,2,3,4,5-pentaphenyl-2,4-cyclopentadien-1-yl][μ-(1,2,3-η:1,3-η)-1,2,3-triphenyl-1-propen-1-yl-2-ylidene]]dinickel, 10CI

[61483-83-8]

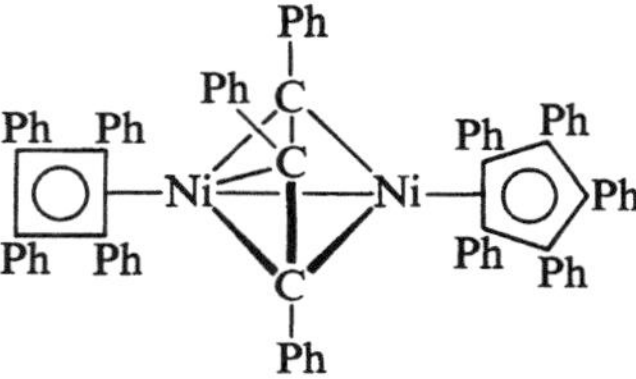

M 1186.778

Deep-violet cryst. Mp 270° dec.

Hoberg, H. *et al*, *Angew. Chem., Int. Ed. Engl.*, 1977, **16**, 183 (*synth, struct, ms*)

$Cl_{12}NiP_4$ Ni-00380

Tetrakis(phosphorous trichloride)nickel, 9CI

Tetrakis(trichlorophosphine)nickel

[36421-86-0]

$Ni(PCl_3)_4$ (T_d)

M 608.021

Light-yellow air-stable hexagonal cryst. (pentane). Sol. org. solvs. Pale-yellow at r.t., becoming white at −30°; slowly dec. in soln. or solid state at r.t. Stable to water.

Irvine, J.W. *et al*, *Science*, 1951, **113**, 742 (*synth, props*)
Mathieu, R. *et al*, *Inorg. Chem.*, 1970, **9**, 2030 (*nmr*)
Bishop, J.K.B. *et al*, *Can. J. Chem.*, 1971, **49**, 3910 (*nqr*)

$F_{12}NiP_4$ Ni-00381

Tetrakis(phosphorous trifluoride)nickel, 9CI

Tetrakis(trifluorophosphine)nickel

[13859-65-9]

$Ni(PF_3)_4$ (T_d)

M 410.566

Colourless, odourless, mobile liq. Stable to water in the cold. Insol. H_2O, v. sol. C_6H_6, toluene, mod. sol. pentane, cyclohexane, spar. sol. chlorinated hydrocarbons. d_{25} 1.800. Mp −55°. Bp 70.7°. n_D^{27} 1.3352.

Wilkinson, G., *J. Am. Chem. Soc.*, 1951, **73**, 5501 (*synth*)
Kiser, R.W., *J. Am. Chem. Soc.*, 1967, **89**, 3653 (*ms*)
Edwards, H.G.M. *et al*, *Spectrochim. Acta, Part A*, 1970, **26**, 897 (*ir*, *raman*)
Lynden-Bell, R.M. *et al*, *J. Chem. Soc. (A)*, 1970, 565 (*nmr*)
Marriott, J.C. *et al*, *J. Chem. Soc., Dalton Trans.*, 1970, 595 (*struct*)
Mathieu, R. *et al*, *Inorg. Chem.*, 1970, **9**, 2030 (*nmr*)
Timms, P.L., *J. Chem. Soc. (A)*, 1970, 2526 (*synth*)
Bassett, P.J. *et al*, *J. Chem. Soc., Dalton Trans.*, 1974, 2316 (*pe*)

Pd Palladium

R. J. Cross

Palladium (Fr., Ger.), Paladio (Sp.), Palladio (Ital.), Палладий (Palladii) (Russ.), パラジウム (Japan.)

Atomic Number. 46

Atomic Weight. 106.4. The greater than usual geological isotopic variation found for this element means that the uncertainty in its atomic weight may exceed that implied even by the figure given. This in turn limits the accuracy of the molecular weights quoted for entries to the first decimal place or less.

Electronic Configuration. [Kr] $4d^{10}$.

Oxidation States. The most common oxidation levels are +2 (d^8) and 0 (d^{10}), with +4 being accessible (d^6). Pd(IV) compounds tend to be 18-electron species, but both 16- and 18-electron molecules are common for Pd(0) and Pd(II).

Coordination Number. Conventional (η^1) ligands generally form complexes which are 4-coordinate tetrahedral (Pd(0)), 4-coordinate square-planar (Pd(II)), or 6-coordinate octahedral (Pd(IV)).

Colour. Variable.

Availability. $PdCl_2$ and Na_2PdCl_4 are common starting materials. Palladium is relatively expensive and prices tend to fluctuate somewhat on the world market.

Handling. Most of the organopalladium compounds described in this section are air and thermally stable as pure compounds. Sensitivity to air and moisture and probably thermal degradation are often heightened in solution, however, so handling time is best kept to a minimum, and protection by an inert atmosphere is desirable.

Toxicity. Palladium is not especially toxic.

Isotopic Abundance. ^{102}Pd, 1.0%; ^{104}Pd, 11.0%; ^{105}Pd, 22.2%; ^{106}Pd, 27.3%; ^{108}Pd, 26.7%; ^{110}Pd, 11.8%.

Spectroscopy. ^{105}Pd has $I = \frac{5}{2}$, and nmr signals can be obtained, but sensitivity is very low and little use of this nucleus has been made. Most compounds are diamagnetic, however, and use of other nuclei (^{1}H, ^{13}C, ^{31}P) can yield valuable data.

Analysis. Palladium can be determined gravimetrically as the bis(dimethylglyoximate), or as palladium metal. Compounds are digested by HNO_3 and solutions neutralised by Na_2CO_3. Conversion to the yellow dimethylglyoximate is by adding dimethylglyoxime. Alternatively, precipitation with KI followed by conversion to Pd (heat) can be used.

Atomic absorption spectroscopy can be used in the range 0–15 ppm, with a sensitivity of 0.25 μg cm^{-3}.

References. Many palladium compounds have uses in selective organic syntheses and as homogenous catalysts for organic reactions. Easy transitions between 18- and 16-electron molecules are often involved.

As well as references cited in the introduction to the *Sourcebook*, general information and background material may be obtained from:

Maitlis, P. M., *The Organic Chemistry of Palladium*, Academic Press, New York, 1971, Vols. 1 and 2.

Hartley, F. R., *The Chemistry of Platinum and Palladium*, Applied Science, 1973.

$[PdBr_3CO]^{\ominus}$

Pd-00001

$[PdCl_3(CO)]^{\ominus}$

Pd-00002

$[PdCl(SnCl_3)_2(CO)]^{\ominus}$

Pd-00003

$[PdI(CF_3)]_n$

Pd-00004

$[PdCl_2H(CO)]^{\ominus}$

Pd-00005

$PdCl_2(CO)_2$

Pd-00006

$[PdCl_3(H_2C{=}CH_2)]^{\ominus}$

Pd-00007

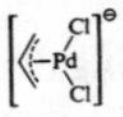

Pd-00008

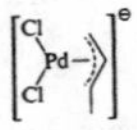

Pd-00009

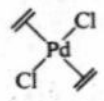

Pd-00010

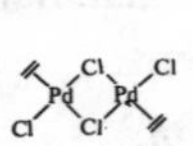

trans-form

Pd-00011

$[Pd(CN)_4]^{\ominus\ominus\ominus\ominus}$ (T_d)

Pd-00012

$Pd(CO)_4$

Pd-00013

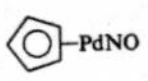

Pd-00014

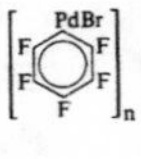

Pd-00015

$[PdCl(C_6F_5)]_n$

Pd-00016

$Pd(CO)_2(F_3CC{\equiv}CCF_3)$

Pd-00017

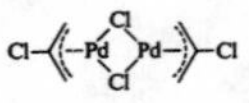

Pd-00018

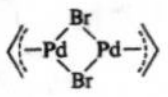

Pd-00019

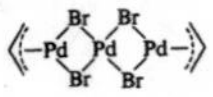

Pd-00020

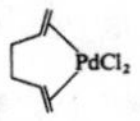

Pd-00021

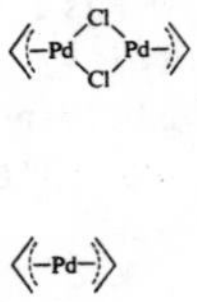

Pd-00022

Pd-00023

$Pd(H_2C{=}CH_2)_3$

Pd-00024

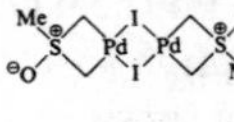

Pd-00025

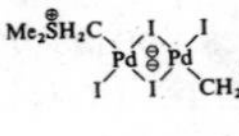

Pd-00026

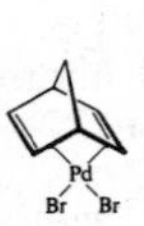

Pd-00027

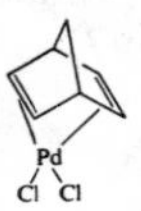

Pd-00028

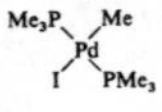

Pd-00029

$Pd(C{\equiv}CH)_4^{\ominus\ominus}$ (D_{4h})

Pd-00030

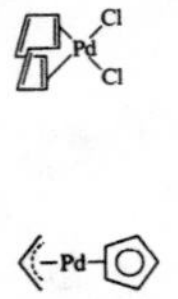

Pd-00031

Pd-00032

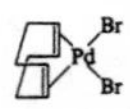

Pd-00033

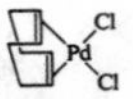

Pd-00034

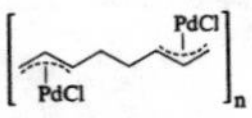

Pd-00035

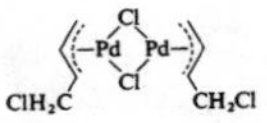

Pd-00036

$[Pd(NCCH_3)_4]^{\oplus\oplus}$ (D_{4h})

Pd-00037

$[Pd(CNMe)_4]^{\oplus\oplus}$ (D_{4h})

Pd-00038

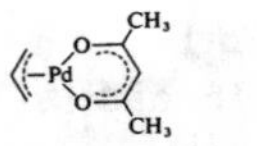

Pd-00039

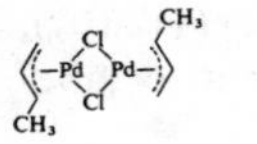

Pd-00040

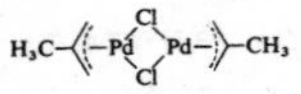

Pd-00041

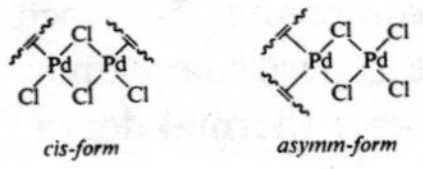

cis-form *asymm-form*

Pd-00042

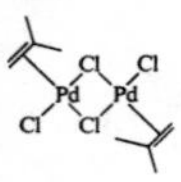

Pd-00043

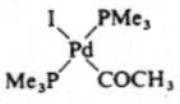

Pd-00044

$[Pd(CN)_3(C_6F_5)]^{\ominus\ominus}$

Pd-00045

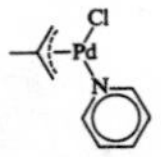

Pd-00046

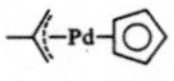

Pd-00047

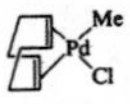

Pd-00048

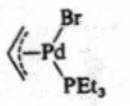

Pd-00049

$[PdH(PMe_3)_3]^{\oplus}$

Pd-00050

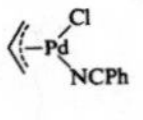

Pd-00051

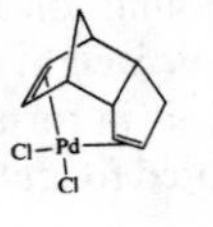

Pd-00052

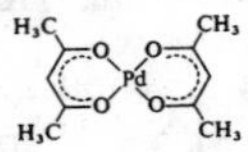

Pd-00053

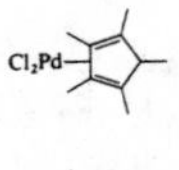

Pd-00054

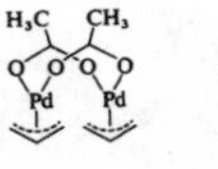

Pd-00055

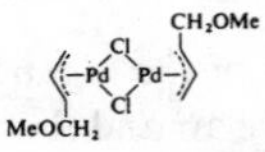

Pd-00056

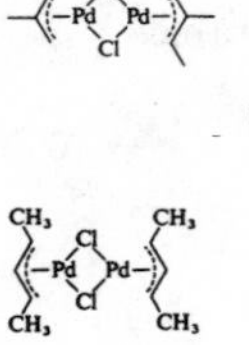

Pd-00057

Pd-00058

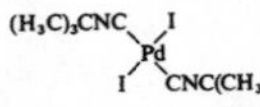

Pd-00059

$Pd(O_2)[(H_3C)_3CNC]_2$

Pd-00060

$Pd[CNC(CH_3)_3]_2$

Pd-00061

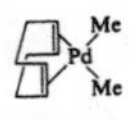

Pd-00062

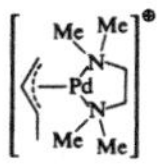

Pd-00063

$[PdMe(PMe_3)_3]^{\oplus}$

Pd-00064

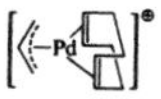

Pd-00065

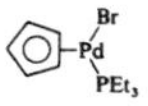

Pd-00066

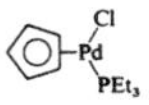

Pd-00067

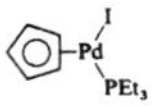

Pd-00068

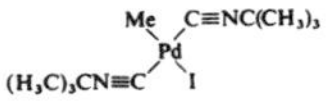

Pd-00069

$[Pd(COCH_3)(PMe_3)_3]^{\oplus}$

Pd-00070

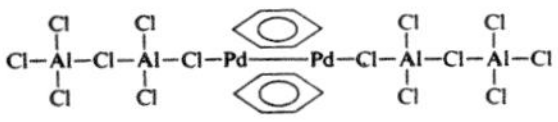

Pd-00071

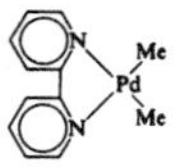

Pd-00072

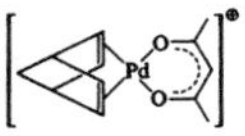

Pd-00073

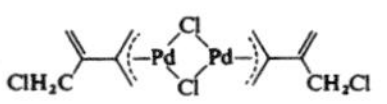

Pd-00074

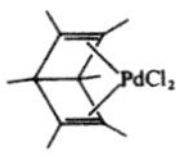

Pd-00075

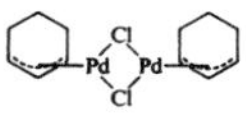

Pd-00076

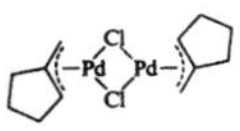

Pd-00077

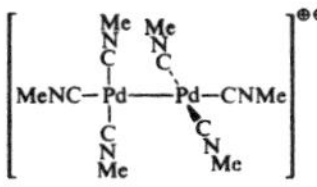

Pd-00078

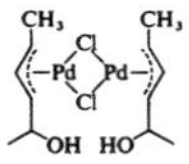

Pd-00079

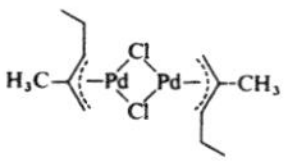

Pd-00080

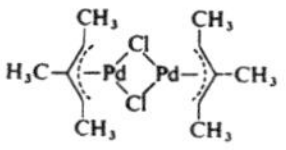

Pd-00081

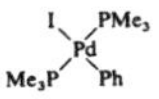

Pd-00082

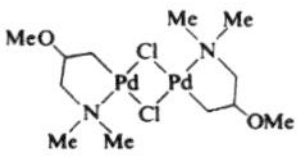

Pd-00083

$PdHCl(PEt_3)_2$ (C_{2v})

Pd-00084

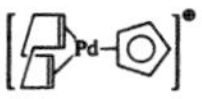

Pd-00085

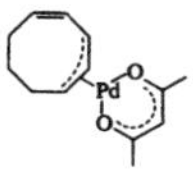

Pd-00086

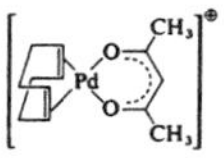

Pd-00087

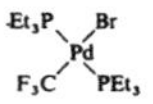

Pd-00088

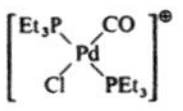

Pd-00089

$PdBrMe(PEt_3)_2$

Pd-00090

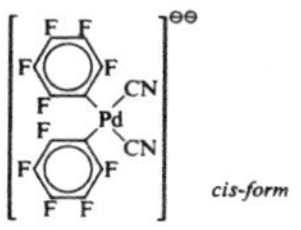

cis-form

Pd-00091

$[(H_2NCH_2CH_2NH_2)PdCl_2(C_6F_5)_2]$ (O_h)

Pd-00092

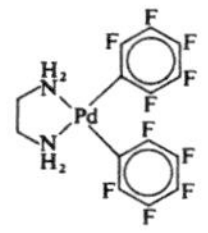

Pd-00093

$(PhCN)_2PdCl_2$

Pd-00094

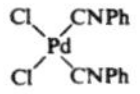

Pd-00095

$Pd(CNPh)_2$

Pd-00096

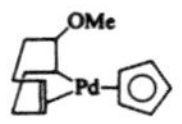

Pd-00097

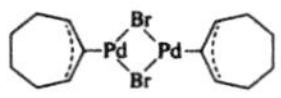

Pd-00098

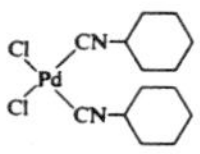

Pd-00099

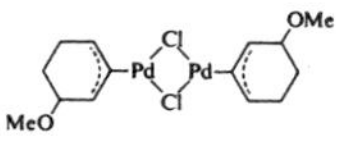

Pd-00100

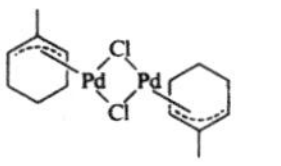

Pd-00101

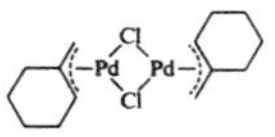

Pd-00102

$[Pd(CNC_6H_{11})_2]$

Pd-00103

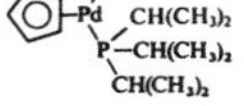

Pd-00104

$[PdCl(MeNC)(AsEt_3)_2]^{\oplus}$

Pd-00105

$[PdCl(MeNC)(PEt_3)_2]^{\oplus}$

Pd-00106

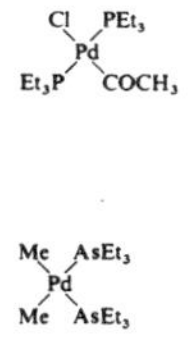

Pd-00107

Pd-00108

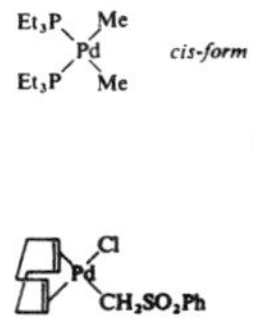

cis-form

Pd-00109

Pd-00110

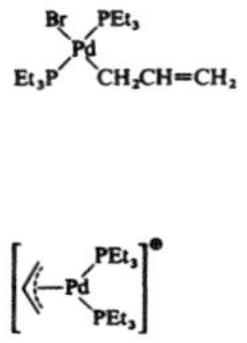

Pd-00111

Pd-00112

$Pd_4(CO)_4(F_3CC{\equiv}CCF_3)_3$

Pd-00113

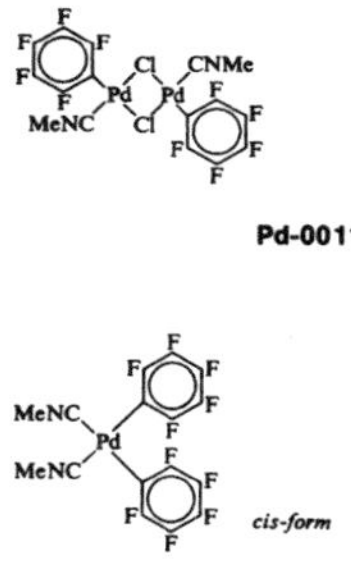

Pd-00114

cis-form

Pd-00115

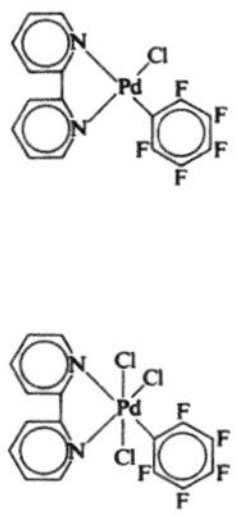

Pd-00116

Pd-00117

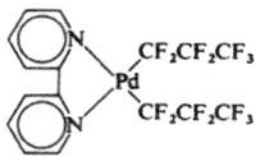

Pd-00118

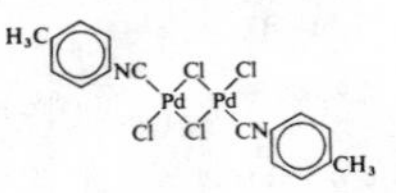

Pd-00119

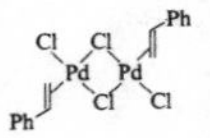

Pd-00120

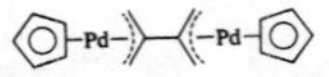

Pd-00121

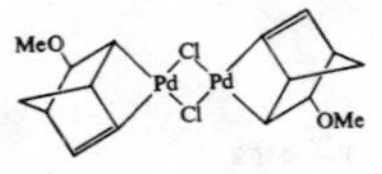

Pd-00122

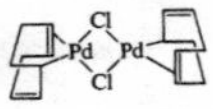

Pd-00123

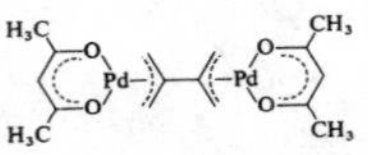

Pd-00124

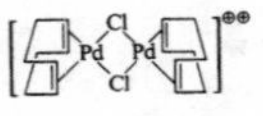

Pd-00125

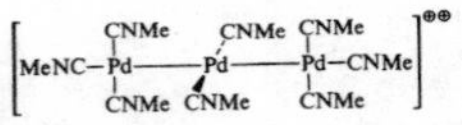

Pd-00126

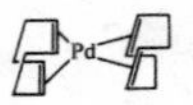

Pd-00127

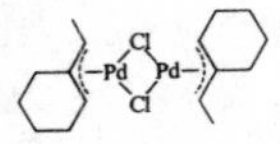

Pd-00128

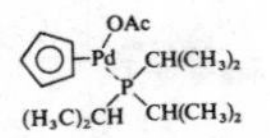

Pd-00129

$(Me_3P)_3PdCOPh^{\oplus}$

Pd-00130

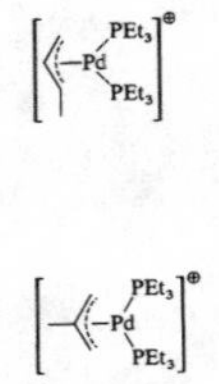

Pd-00131

Pd-00132

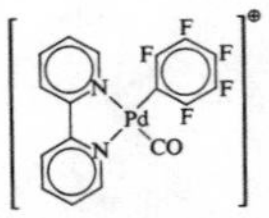

Pd-00133

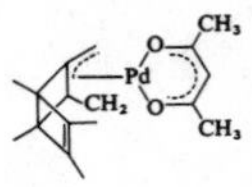

Pd-00134

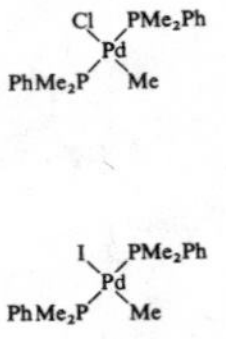

Pd-00135

Pd-00136

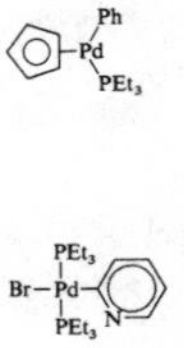

Pd-00137

Pd-00138

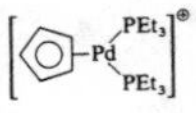

Pd-00141

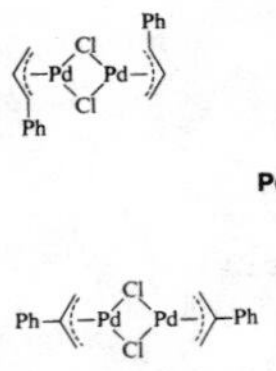

Pd-00142

Pd-00143

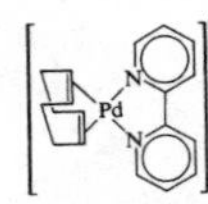

Pd-00144

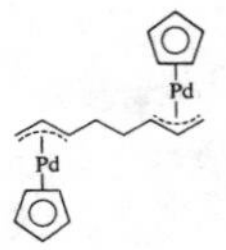

Pd-00145

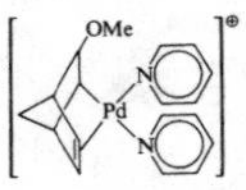

Pd-00146

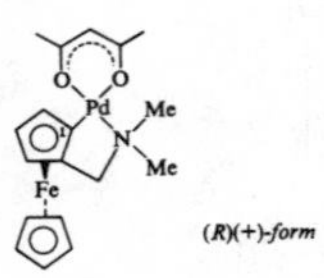

(R)(+)-form

Pd-00147

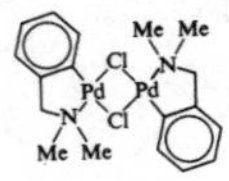

Pd-00148

cis-form

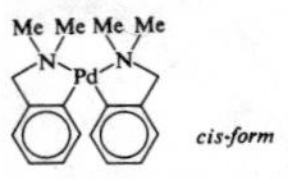

Pd-00149

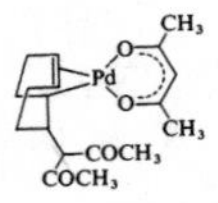

Pd-00150

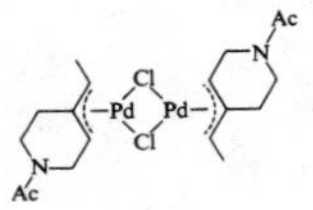

Pd-00151

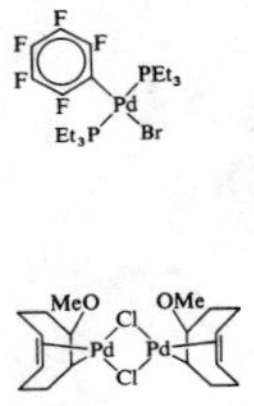

Pd-00152

Pd-00153

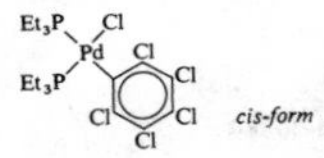

cis-form

Pd-00154

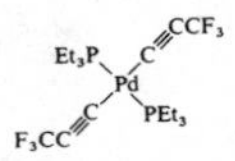

Pd-00155

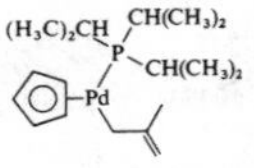

Pd-00156

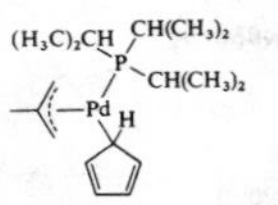

Pd-00157

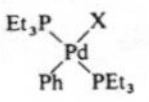

X = Br

Pd-00158

As Pd-00158 with
X = Cl

Pd-00159

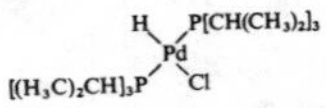

Pd-00160

$[PdCN(C_6F_5)_3]^{\ominus\ominus}$

Pd-00161

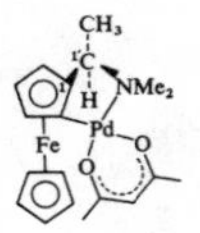

Pd-00162

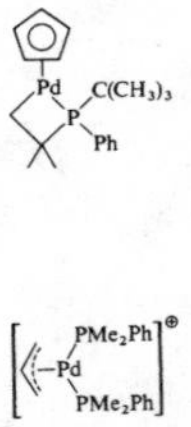

Pd-00163

Pd-00164

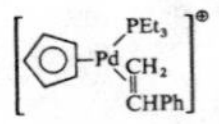

Pd-00165

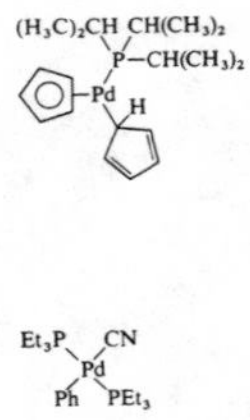

Pd-00166

Pd-00167

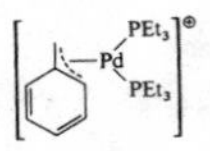

Pd-00168

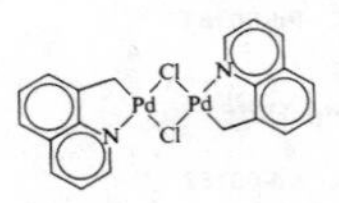

Pd-00169

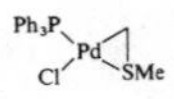

Pd-00170

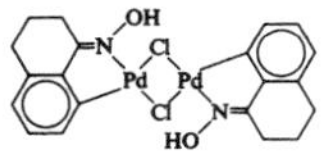

Pd-00171

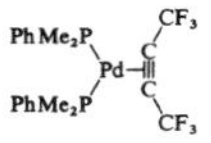

Pd-00172

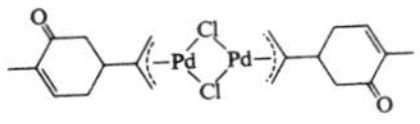

Pd-00173

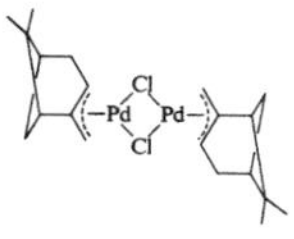

Pd-00174

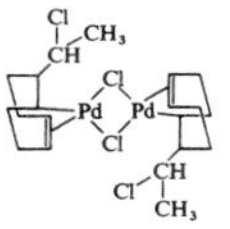

Pd-00175

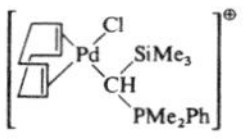

Pd-00176

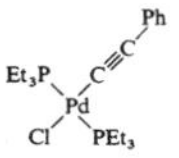

Pd-00177

$[[(H_3C)_3CNC]_2PdCl]_2$

Pd-00178

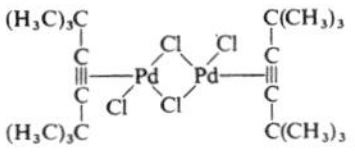

Pd-00179

$[Pd(C_6F_5)(C_5H_5N)_3]^{\oplus}$

Pd-00180

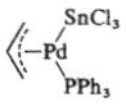

Pd-00181

$PdCl_2(C_6F_5)_2(bipy)$

Pd-00182

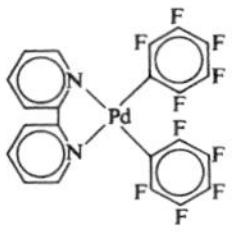

Pd-00183

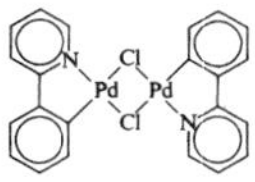

Pd-00184

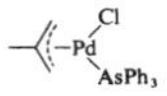

Pd-00185

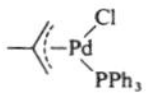

Pd-00186

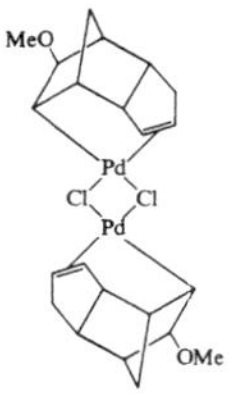

Pd-00187

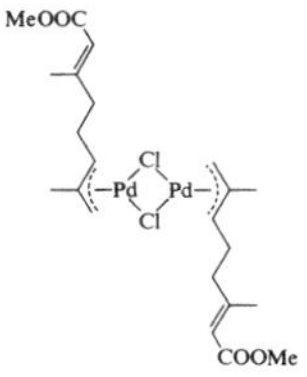

Pd-00188

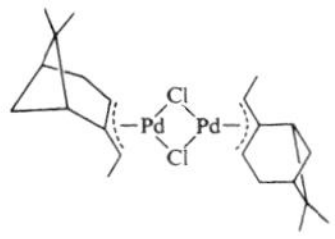

Pd-00189

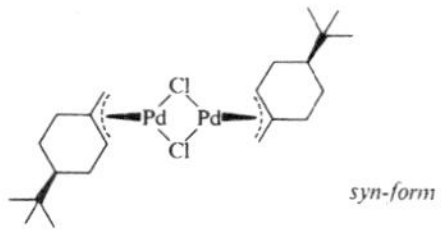

syn-form

Pd-00190

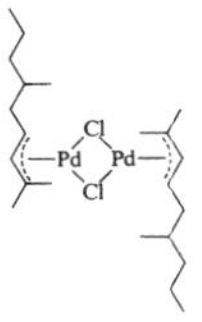

Pd-00191

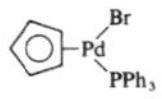

Pd-00192

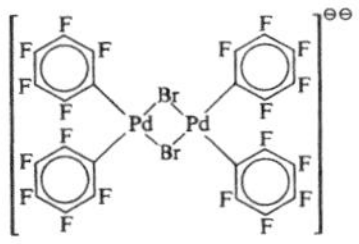

Pd-00193

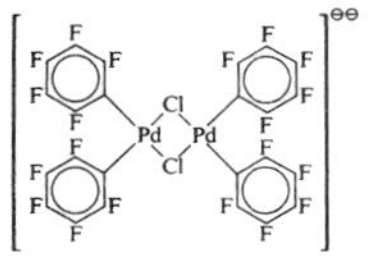

Pd-00194

$[Pd(C_6F_5)_4]^{\ominus\ominus}$ (D_{4h})

Pd-00195

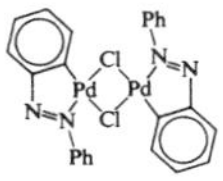

Pd-00196

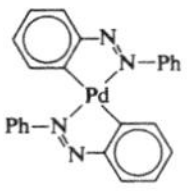

Pd-00197

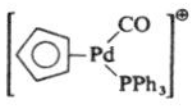

Pd-00198

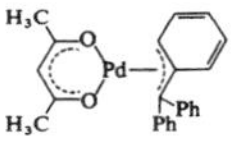

Pd-00199

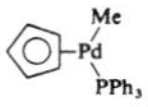

Pd-00200

$Pd(C_6Cl_5)(C_6F_5)(PEt_3)_2$

Pd-00201

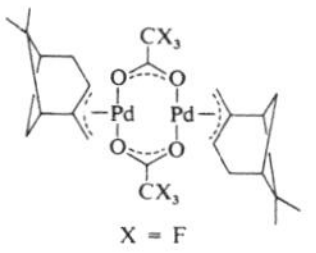

X = F

Pd-00202

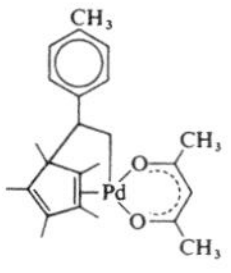

Pd-00203

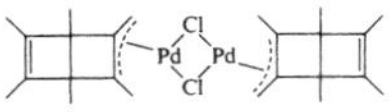

Pd-00204

As Pd-00202 with
X = H

Pd-00205

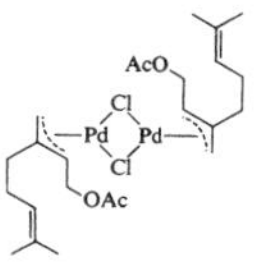

Pd-00206

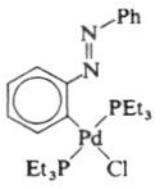

Pd-00207

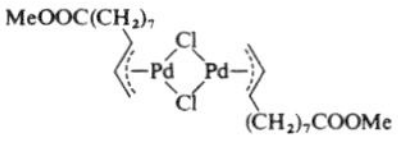

Pd-00208

$[Pd(C_6F_5)(PEt_3)_3]^{\oplus}$

Pd-00209

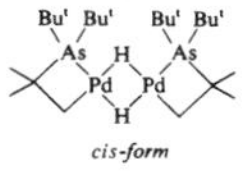

cis-form

Pd-00210

$[(H_3C)_3C]_3PPdP[C(CH_3)_3]_3$

Pd-00211

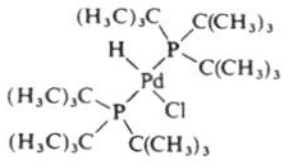

Pd-00212

$Pd[P(OEt)_3]_4$ (T_d)

Pd-00213

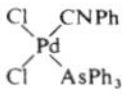

Pd-00214

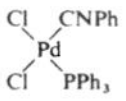

Pd-00215

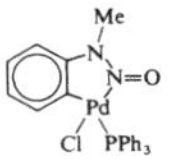

Pd-00216

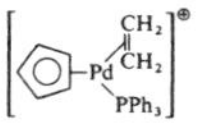

Pd-00217

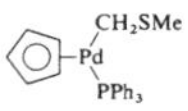

Pd-00218

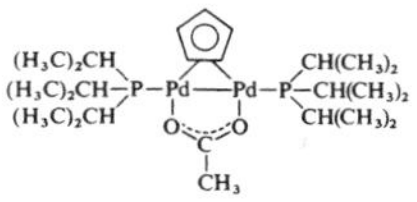

Pd-00219

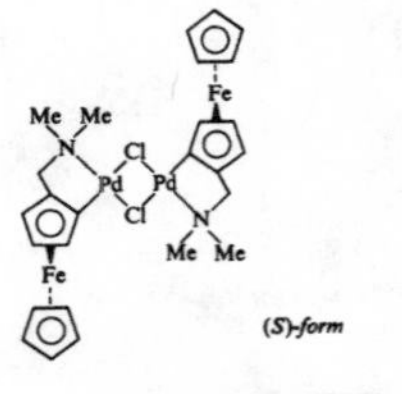

(*S*)-form

Pd-00220

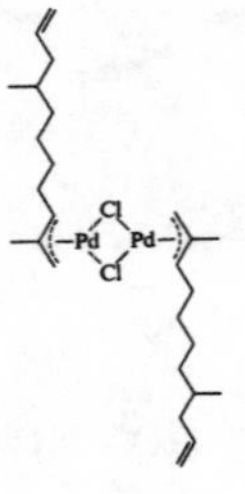

Pd-00221

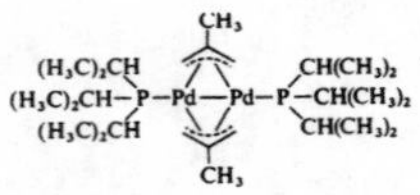

Pd-00222

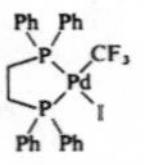

Pd-00223

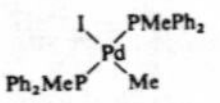

Pd-00224

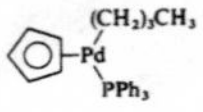

Pd-00225

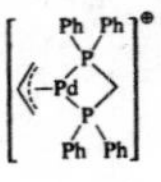

Pd-00226

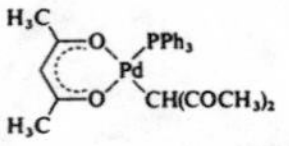

Pd-00227

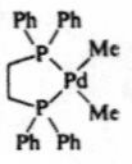

Pd-00228

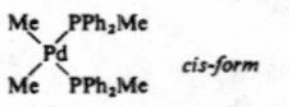

cis-form

Pd-00229

$[Pd(C{\equiv}CPh)_2(PEt_3)_2]$ (D_{2h})

Pd-00230

$[(H_3C)_3C]_2PPhPdPPh[C(CH_3)_3]_2$

Pd-00231

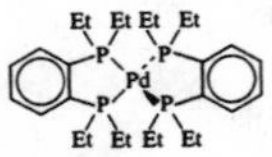

Pd-00232

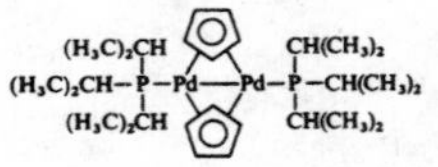

Pd-00233

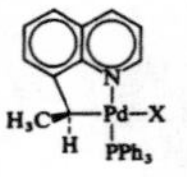

X = Br

Pd-00234

As Pd-00234 with X = Cl

Pd-00235

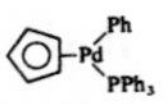

Pd-00236

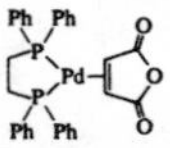

Pd-00237

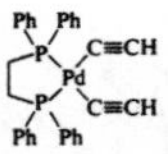

Pd-00238

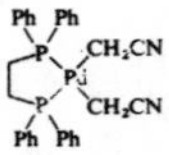

Pd-00239

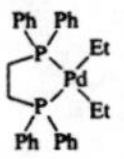

Pd-00240

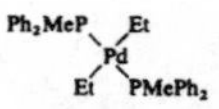

Pd-00241

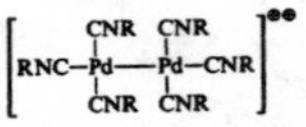

R = $(H_3C)_3C$–

Pd-00242

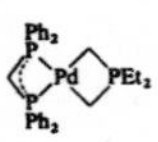

Pd-00243

$Pd(C{\equiv}CPh)_4^{\ominus\ominus}$ (D_{4h})

Pd-00244

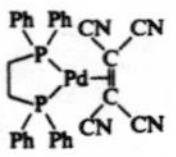

Pd-00245

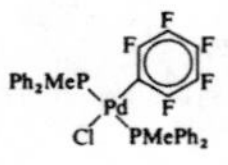

Pd-00246

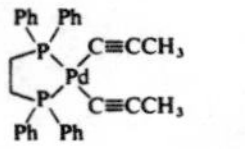

Pd-00247

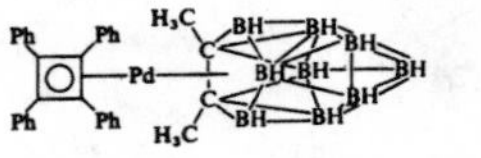

Pd-00248

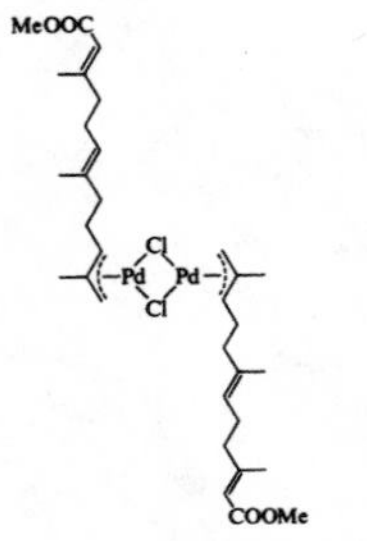

Pd-00249

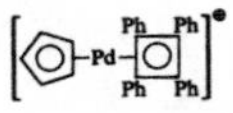

Pd-00250

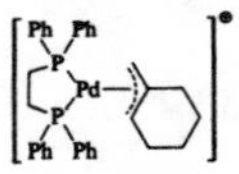

Pd-00251

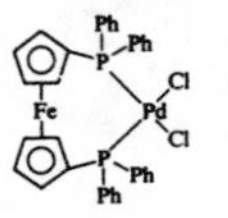

Pd-00252

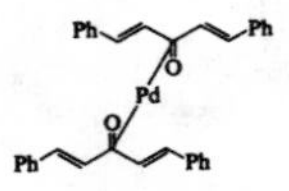

Pd-00253

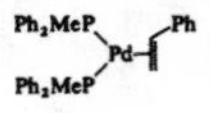

Pd-00254

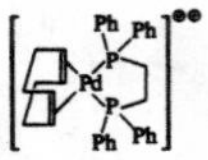

Pd-00255

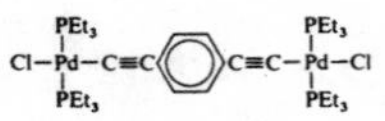

Pd-00256

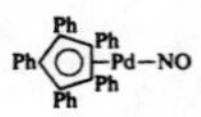

Pd-00257

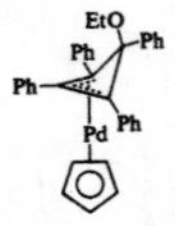

Pd-00258

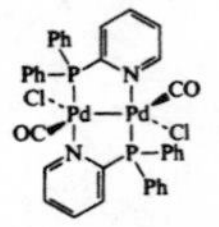

Pd-00259

$Pd(PPh_3)_2Cl_2$

Pd-00260

$(NO)(PPh_3)_2Pd{-}Pd(PPh_3)_2(NO)$

Pd-00261

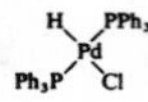

Pd-00262

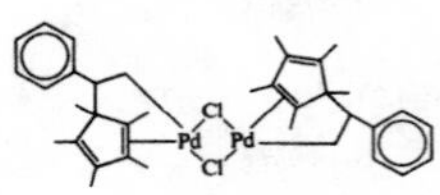

Pd-00263

$[(C_6H_{11})_3P]_2PdClH$

Pd-00264

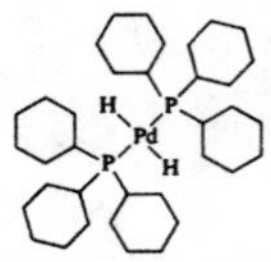

Pd-00265

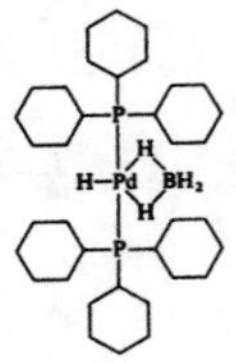

Pd-00266

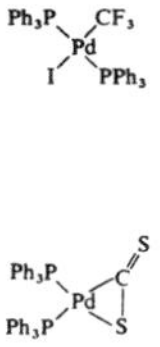

Pd-00267

Pd-00268

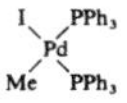

cis-form

Pd-00269

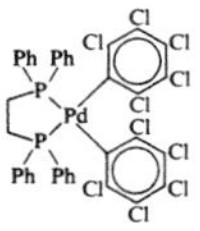

Pd-00270

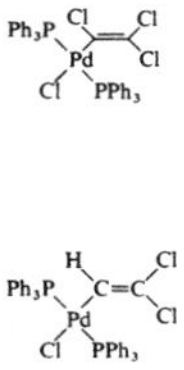

Pd-00271

Pd-00272

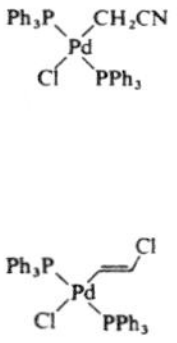

Pd-00273

(E)-trans-form

Pd-00274

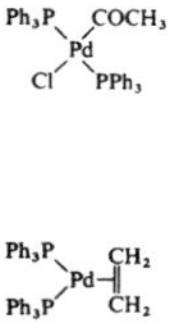

Pd-00275

Pd-00276

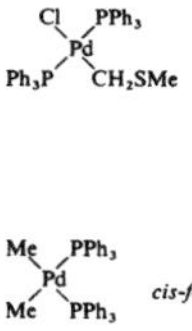

Pd-00277

cis-form

Pd-00278

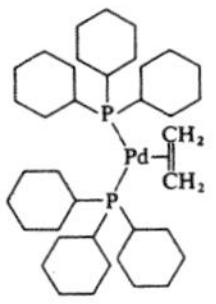

Pd-00279

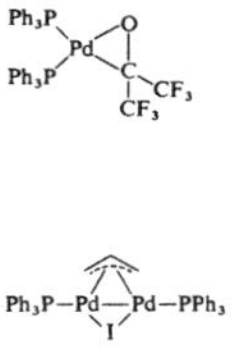

Pd-00280

Pd-00281

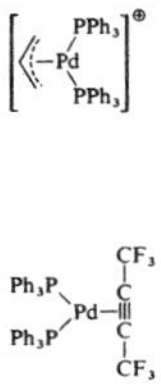

Pd-00282

Pd-00283

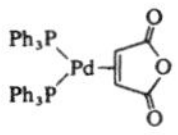

Pd-00284

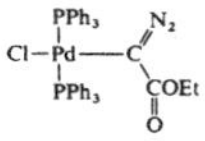

Pd-00285

$Pd(OAc)_2(PPh_3)_2$

Pd-00286

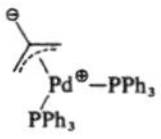

Pd-00287

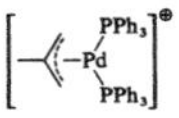

Pd-00288

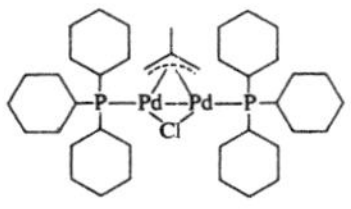

Pd-00289

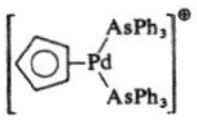

Pd-00290

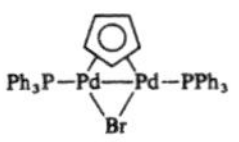

Pd-00291

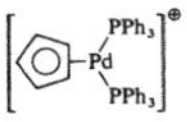

Pd-00292

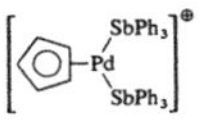

Pd-00293

$[PdBr(C_6F_5)(AsPh_3)_2]$

Pd-00294

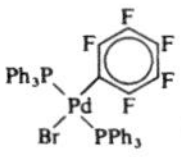

trans-form

Pd-00295

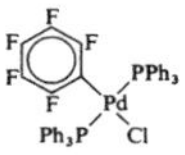

Pd-00296

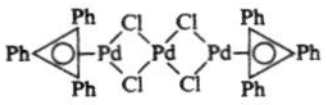

Pd-00297

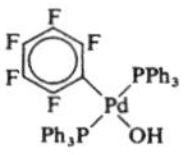

Pd-00298

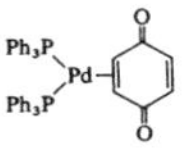

Pd-00299

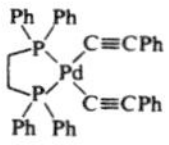

Pd-00300

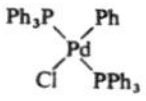

Pd-00301

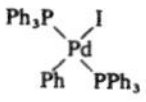

Pd-00302

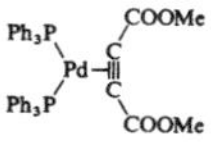

Pd-00303

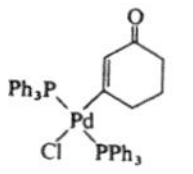

Pd-00304

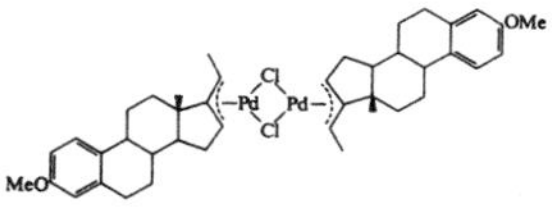

Pd-00305

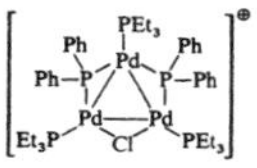

Pd-00306

$[Pd(CO)(C_6F_5)(PPh_3)_2]^{\oplus}$

Pd-00307

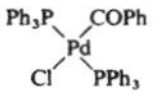

Pd-00308

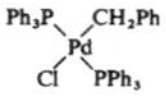

Pd-00309

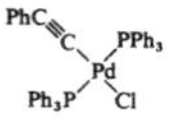

Pd-00310

$(Ph_3P)_2PdH(C{\equiv}CPh)$

Pd-00311

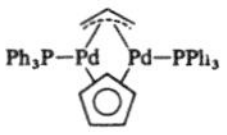

Pd-00312

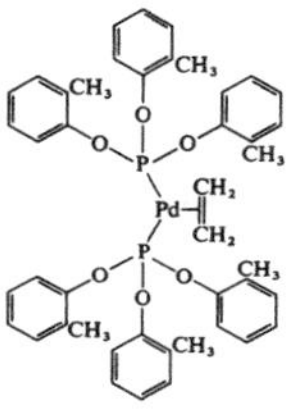

Pd-00313

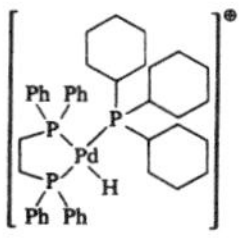

Pd-00314

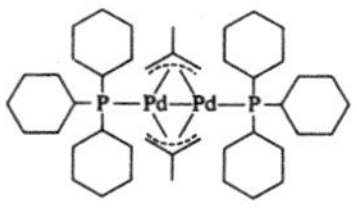

Pd-00315

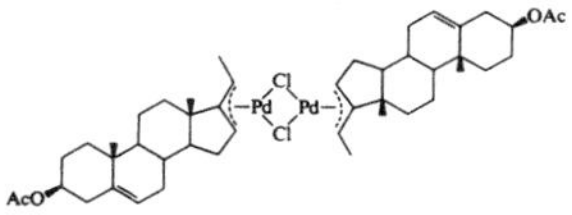

Pd-00316

$[Pd(C_6Cl_5)(C_5H_5N)(PPh_3)_2]^{\oplus}$

Pd-00317

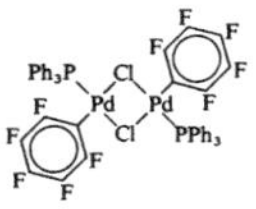

Pd-00318

$Pd(GePh_3)_2(PEt_3)_2$

Pd-00319

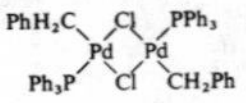

Pd-00320

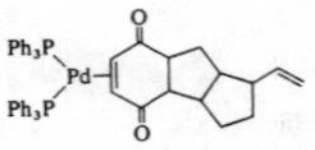

Pd-00321

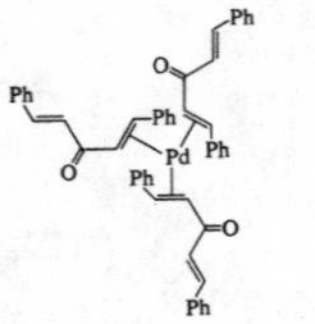

Pd-00322

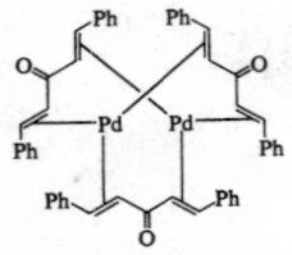

Pd-00323

$Pd(C{\equiv}CPh)_2(PPh_3)_2$

Pd-00324

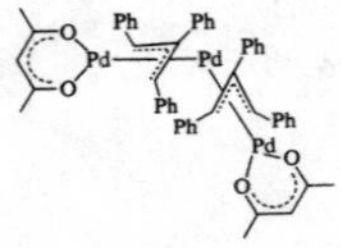

Pd-00325

$Pd_4(CO)_5[P(CH_2CH_2CH_2CH_3)_3]_4$

Pd-00326

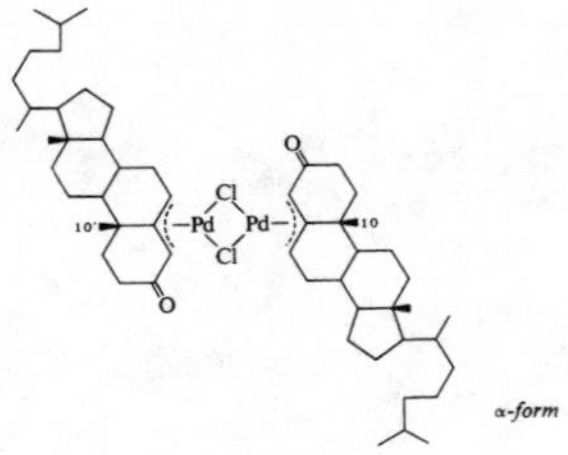

α-form

Pd-00327

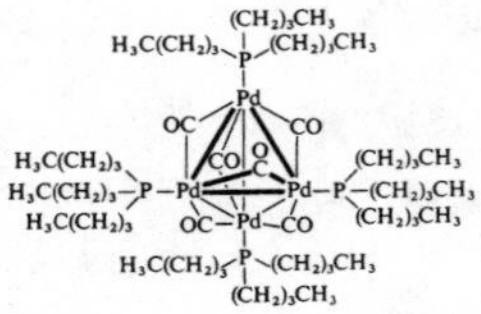

Pd-00328

$PdCO(PPh_3)_3$ (C_{3v})

Pd-00329

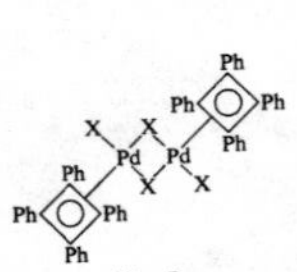

X = Br

Pd-00330

As Pd-00330 with
X = Cl

Pd-00331

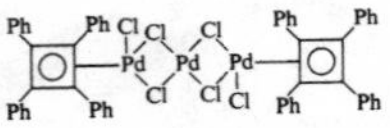

Pd-00332

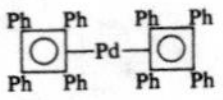

Pd-00333

$Pd_3(CO)_3(PPh_3)_3$

Pd-00334

$[Pd(C_6F_5)(AsPh_3)_3]^{\oplus}$

Pd-00335

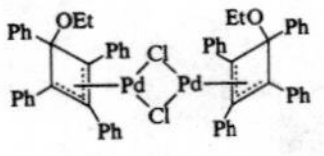

Pd-00336

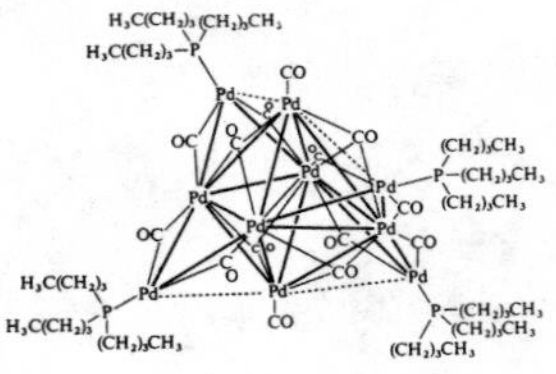

Pd-00337

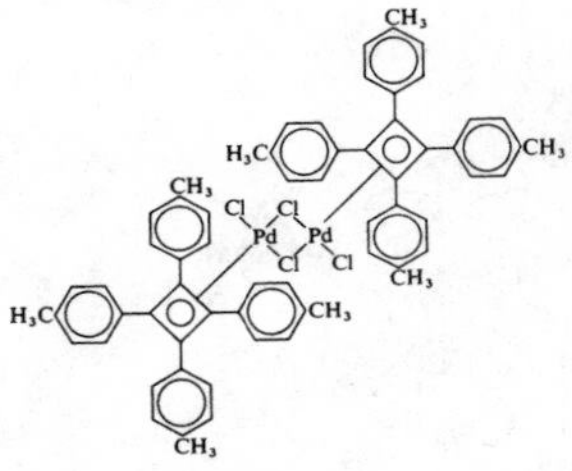

Pd-00338

$Pd(AsPh_3)_4$ (T_d)

Pd-00339

$Pd(PbPh_3)_2(PPh_3)_2$

Pd-00340

$Pd(PPh_3)_4$ (T_d)

Pd-00341

$Pd(SbPh_3)_4$ (T_d)

Pd-00342

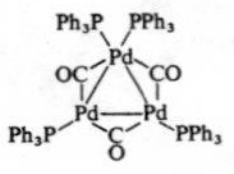

Pd-00343

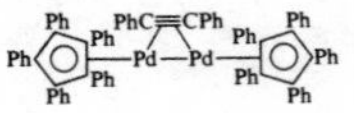

Pd-00344

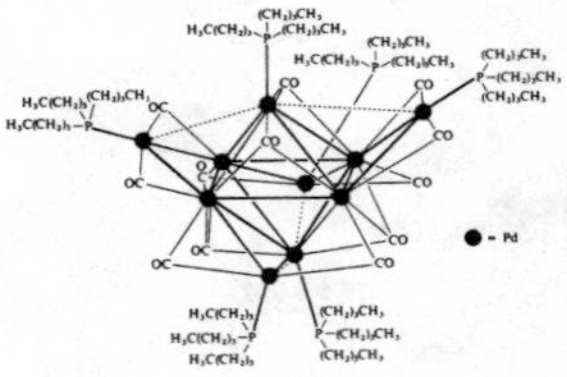

Pd-00345

$Pd(PF_3)_4$ (T_d)

Pd-00346

$CBr_3OPd^{\ominus}$ Pd-00001

Tribromocarbonylpalladate(1–), 9CI
Carbonyltribromopalladate(1–)
[66213-28-3]

$[PdBr_3CO]^{\ominus}$

M 374.142 (ion)
K salt:
CBr_3KOPd M 413.241
Yellow-green solid.
Tetrabutylammonium salt: [66213-29-4].
$C_{17}H_{36}Br_3NOPd$ M 616.610
Catalyses carbonylation of aromatic nitro compounds.
Red cryst. (Et_2O). Mp 120° dec.

Kutyukov, G.G. *et al*, *Zh. Neorg. Khim.*, 1968, **13**, 1542; *Russ. J. Inorg. Chem. (Engl. Transl.)*, **13**, 809 (*synth*)
Browning, J. *et al*, *J. Chem. Soc., Dalton Trans.*, 1977, 2061 (*synth, ir, pmr, raman*)
Tietz, H. *et al*, *Z. Chem.*, 1980, **20**, 295 (*use*)

$CCl_3OPd^{\ominus}$ Pd-00002

Carbonyltrichloropalladate(1–), 9CI
Trichlorocarbonylpalladate(1–)
[44252-60-0]

$[PdCl_3(CO)]^{\ominus}$

M 240.789 (ion)
Diethylammonium salt: [75934-65-5].
$C_5H_{12}Cl_3NOPd$ M 314.935
Solid (heptane).
Tetrabutylammonium salt: [19508-35-1].
$C_{17}H_{36}Cl_3NOPd$ M 483.257
Catalyses carbonylation of aromatic nitro compounds.
Orange cryst. (Me_2CO/Et_2O). Mp 95° dec.

Browning, J. *et al*, *J. Chem. Soc., Dalton Trans.*, 1977, 2061 (*synth, ir, raman, pmr*)
Tietz, H. *et al*, *Z. Chem.*, 1980, **20**, 295 (*use*)
Calderazzo, F. *et al*, *Inorg. Chem.*, 1981, **20**, 1310 (*synth, ir*)

$CCl_7OPdSn_2^{\ominus}$ Pd-00003

Carbonylchlorobis(trichlorostannyl)palladate(1–), 9CI

$[PdCl(SnCl_3)_2(CO)]^{\ominus}$

M 619.981 (ion)
Tetraethylammonium salt: [26221-09-0].
$C_9H_{20}Cl_7NOPdSn_2$ M 750.234
Orange solid. Anion geometry not specified.

Kingston, J.V. *et al*, *J. Chem. Soc. (A)*, 1971, 3765 (*synth, ir*)

CF_3IPd Pd-00004

Iodo(trifluoromethyl)palladium
(Trifluoromethyl)iodopalladium
[54056-39-2]

$[PdI(CF_3)]_n$

M 302.331
Polymeric. Amber cryst. (toluene/pentane). Mp 83-90° dec.

Klabunde, K.J. *et al*, *J. Am. Chem. Soc.*, 1974, **96**, 7674 (*synth, ir*)
Klabunde, K.J. *et al*, *Inorg. Chem.*, 1980, **19**, 3719 (*synth, ir, nmr*)

$CHCl_2OPd^{\ominus}$ Pd-00005

(Carbonyl)dichlorohydropalladate(1–)
Dichloro(carbonyl)palladate(1–) hydride. Hydridocarbonyldichloropalladate(1–)

$[PdCl_2H(CO)]^{\ominus}$

M 206.344 (ion)
Catalyses synth. of long-chained nitro compounds.
Pyridinium salt: [25792-40-9].
$C_6H_7Cl_2NOPd$ M 286.453
Yellow solid, air-sensitive.
Tetraphenylarsonium salt: [25792-41-0].
$C_{25}H_{21}AsCl_2OPd$ M 589.688
Brown solid.
Quinolinium salt: [25870-10-4].
$C_{10}H_9Cl_2NOPd$ M 336.513
Yellow-green solid, air-sensitive.

Kingston, J.V. *et al*, *J. Chem. Soc., Chem. Commun.*, 1969, 455 (*synth, ir*)

$C_2Cl_2O_2Pd$ Pd-00006

Dicarbonyldichloropalladium, 9CI
Dicarbonylpalladium dichloride
[13682-72-9]

$PdCl_2(CO)_2$

M 233.347
Prepd. from CO and $PdCl_2(NCPh)_2$. Catalyses conversion of aromatic nitro compds. by CO to isocyanates. No phys. details available.

Yamahara, T. *et al*, *CA*, 1974, **80**, 120518y (*synth, use*)

$C_2H_4Cl_3Pd^{\ominus}$ Pd-00007

Trichloro(ethylene)palladate(1–), 8CI
Trichloro(η^2-ethene)palladate(1–), 9CI. Ethenetrichloropalladate(1–). Ethylenetrichloropalladate(1–)
[34664-23-8]

$[PdCl_3(H_2C{=}CH_2)]^{\ominus}$

M 240.833 (ion)
Tetrabutylammonium salt:
$C_{18}H_{40}Cl_3NPd$ M 483.300
Yellow solid (Et_2O); unstable at r.t.

Goodfellow, R.J. *et al*, *J. Chem. Soc. (A)*, 1968, 504 (*synth, ir*)

$C_3H_5Cl_2Pd^{\ominus}$ Pd-00008

Dichloro(η^3-2-propenyl)palladate(1–), 9CI
(π-Allyl)dichloropalladate(1–). (Enyl)-dichloropalladate(1–)
[35428-96-7]

$[(\eta^3\text{-}C_3H_5)PdCl_2]^{\ominus}$

M 218.399 (ion)
Cocatalyst in synth. of unsaturated tertiary amines.
Tetraphenylphosphonium salt:
$C_{27}H_{25}Cl_2PPd$ M 557.794
Yellow cryst. Mp 200° dec.
π-Allylbipyridylpalladium salt:

$C_{16}H_{18}Cl_2N_2Pd_2$ M 522.078
Cryst. (nitrobenzene); air-stable. Mp 198° dec.
Hexadecyltrimethylammonium salt:
$C_{22}H_{47}Cl_2NPd$ M 502.946
Pale-yellow cryst. Mp 101° dec.

Paiaro, G. *et al*, *Tetrahedron Lett.*, 1965, 1583 (*synth*, *ir*)
Goodfellow, R.J. *et al*, *J. Chem. Soc. (A)*, 1966, 784 (*synth*, *pmr*, *ir*)

$C_4H_7Cl_2Pd^{\ominus}$ Pd-00009

Dichloro(η^3-2-butenyl)palladate(1−)
Dichloro(1-methylallyl)palladate(1−)

M 232.425 (ion)
(η^3-2-Butenyl)(N,N,N′,N′-tetramethylethylenediamine)palladium(1+) salt:
$C_{10}H_{33}Cl_2N_2Pd_2$ M 465.130
Yellow solid. Mp 90-2° dec.

Hegedus, L.S. *et al*, *J. Am. Chem. Soc.*, 1982, **104**, 697 (*synth*, *struct*, *pmr*, *ir*)

$C_4H_8Cl_2Pd$ Pd-00010

Dichlorobis(ethylene)palladium
Dichlorobis(η^2-ethene)palladium, 9CI
[41820-43-3]

M 233.433
Cocatalyst for acrylate dimerisations. Yellow solid, stable only under C_2H_4 at pressure. Synth. is accompanied by butene formn.

Ketley, A.D. *et al*, *Inorg. Chem.*, 1967, **6**, 657 (*synth*)

$C_4H_8Cl_4Pd_2$ Pd-00011

Di-μ-chlorodichlorobis(ethylene)dipalladium
Di-μ-chlorodichlorobis(η^2-ethene)dipalladium, 9CI. *Tetrachlorobis(ethylene)dipalladium*, 8CI. *Bis(ethylene)-dichloro-μ-dichloropalladium*
[12122-75-7]

trans-form

M 410.759
Catalyses vinylation, vinyl ether synthesis and olefin isomerisation.
cis-form [12287-18-2]
Brown-red cryst., unstable in moist air.
trans-form
Catalyses carbonylation of ethylene. Cryst., unstable in moist air.

Kharasch, M.S. *et al*, *J. Am. Chem. Soc.*, 1938, **60**, 882 (*synth*)
Holden, J.R. *et al*, *J. Am. Chem. Soc.*, 1955, **77**, 4987 (*struct*)
Stern, E.W. *et al*, *Proc. Chem. Soc., London*, 1961, 370 (*use*)
Sparke, M.B. *et al*, *J. Catal.*, 1965, **4**, 332 (*use*)
Goodfellow, R.J. *et al*, *J. Chem. Soc. (A)*, 1967, 1897 (*ir*)
Grogan, M.J. *et al*, *J. Am. Chem. Soc.*, 1968, **90**, 918 (*ir*, *struct*)
Ketley, A.D. *et al*, *J. Organomet. Chem.*, 1968, **13**, 243 (*use*)
Wakatsuki, Y. *et al*, *Bull. Chem. Soc. Jpn.*, 1971, **44**, 786 (*ir*)
Pregaglia, G.F. *et al*, *J. Organomet. Chem.*, 1973, **47**, 165 (*ir*, *raman*)
Partenheimer, W. *et al*, *Inorg. Nucl. Chem. Lett.*, 1974, **10**, 1143 (*ir*)
Stille, J.K. *et al*, *J. Organomet. Chem.*, 1979, **169**, 239 (*use*)

$C_4N_4Pd^{\ominus\ominus\ominus\ominus}$ Pd-00012

Tetracyanopalladate(4−)

$[Pd(CN)_4]^{\ominus\ominus\ominus\ominus}$ (T_d)

M 210.491 (ion)
Tetra-K salt:
$C_4K_4N_4Pd$ M 366.884
Yellowish-white cryst.; stable in liq. ammonia for 2 hr. at r.t.

Burbage, J.J. *et al*, *J. Am. Chem. Soc.*, 1943, **65**, 1484 (*synth*)

C_4O_4Pd Pd-00013

Tetracarbonylpalladium
Palladium carbonyl, 9CI. *Palladium tetracarbonyl*
[36344-80-6]

$Pd(CO)_4$

M 218.462
No physical data available, obt. by matrix isoln.

Darling, J.H. *et al*, *J. Chem. Soc., Dalton Trans.*, 1973, 1079 (*synth*, *ir*)

C_5H_5NOPd Pd-00014

(η^5-2,4-Cyclopentadien-1-yl)nitrosylpalladium
Nitrosyl(cyclopentadienyl)palladium

M 201.521
Red-brown oil.

Fischer, E.O. *et al*, *Z. Naturforsch., B*, 1963, **18**, 771 (*synth*, *ir*, *pmr*)

C_6BrF_5Pd Pd-00015

Bromo(pentafluorophenyl)palladium
(Pentafluorophenyl)bromopalladium
[48133-13-7]

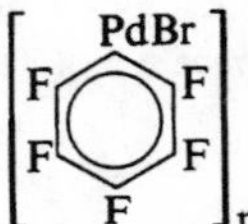

M 353.382
Polymeric. Orange-brown powder (Me_2CO/C_6H_6/pentane) Dec. in arene solvs. (over several hours). Mp 105° dec.

Klabunde, K.J. *et al*, *J. Am. Chem. Soc.*, 1974, **96**, 7674 (*synth*, *ir*)
Klabunde, K.J. *et al*, *Inorg. Chem.*, 1980, **19**, 3719 (*synth*, *ir*, *nmr*)

C_6ClF_5Pd Pd-00016

Chloro(pentafluorophenyl)palladium, 9CI
(Pentafluorophenyl)palladium chloride. (Perfluorophenyl)chloropalladium

[54056-35-8]

$[PdCl(C_6F_5)]_n$

M 308.931

Polymeric. Solid; thermally stable to about 25°.

Klabunde, K.J. *et al*, *Angew. Chem., Int. Ed. Engl.*, 1975, **14**, 287 (*synth*)

$C_6F_6O_2Pd$ Pd-00017

Dicarbonyl(hexafluoro-2-butyne)palladium

(Hexafluoro-2-butyne)palladium dicarbonyl

$Pd(CO)_2(F_3CC{\equiv}CCF_3)$

M 324.475

Isol. only as volatile complex which spontaneously forms (*in vacuo*) nonvolatile $Pd_4(CO)_4(C_4F_6)_3$.

Klabunde, K.J. *et al*, *J. Am. Chem. Soc.*, 1978, **100**, 4437.

$C_6H_8Cl_4Pd_2$ Pd-00018

Di-μ-chlorobis(η³-2-chloro-2-propenyl]dipalladium, 9CI

Di-μ-chlorobis(2-chloroallyl)dipalladium, 8CI. *Di-μ-chlorodi-π-(β-chloroallyl)dipalladium*

[12012-87-2]

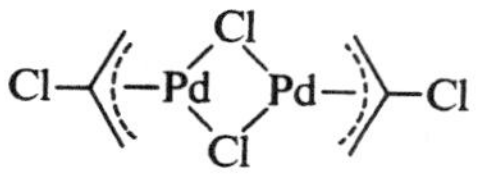

M 434.781

Possible use as oil additive, antioxidant. Yellow cryst. (CH_2Cl_2 or C_6H_6/heptane).

Monomer: Chloro(2-chloro-2-propenyl)palladium. Chloro(2-chloroallyl)palladium. (2-Chloroallyl)palladium chloride.

$C_3H_4Cl_2Pd$ M 217.391

Unknown.

Schultz, R.G., *Tetrahedron*, 1964, **20**, 2809 (*synth, pmr*)
Lupin, M.S. *et al*, *J. Chem. Soc. (A)*, 1966, 1687 (*synth, pmr*)

$C_6H_{10}Br_2Pd_2$ Pd-00019

Di-μ-bromobis(η³-2-propenyl)dipalladium, 9CI

Di-π-allyldi-μ-bromodipalladium, 8CI. *Bisallyldi-μ-bromodipalladium. Di-μ-bromobis(π-allyl)dipalladium*

[12077-82-6]

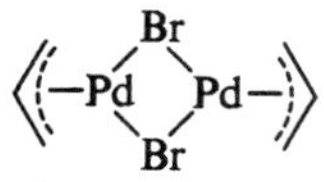

M 454.793

Cocatalyst in polymerisation of butadiene. Shows inhibitory effect on rat liver mitochondrial respiration and ATPase activity, and on respiration by bovine heart submitochondrial fractions. Solid ($CHCl_3$). Mp 145° dec.

Monomer: Bromo(2-propenyl)palladium. Allylbromopalladium. π-Allylpalladium bromide.

C_3H_5BrPd M 227.397

Unknown.

Sakakibara, M. *et al*, *J. Chem. Soc., Chem. Commun.*, 1969, 396 (*synth*)
Lammens, H. *et al*, *Org. Mass Spectrom.*, 1971, **5**, 335 (*ms*)
Lobaneva, O.A. *et al*, *Zh. Neorg. Khim.*, 1972, **17**, 3011; *Russ. J. Inorg. Chem. (Engl. Transl.)*, 1972, **17**, 1583 (*uv*)
Mann, B.E. *et al*, *J. Chem. Soc., Dalton Trans.*, 1973, 2390 (*cmr*)
Chenskaya, T.B. *et al*, *J. Organomet. Chem.*, 1978, **148**, 85 (*ir, raman*)
Kolesova, G.M. *et al*, *Vopr. Med. Khim.*, 1979, **25**, 537; *CA*, **91**, 204224q (*pharmacol*)

$C_6H_{10}Br_4Pd_3$ Pd-00020

Tetra-μ-bromobis(η³-2-propenyl)tripalladium, 9CI

Di-π-allyltetra-μ-bromotripalladium, 8CI. *Bis(π-allyl)-tetra-μ-bromotripalladium*

[12294-63-2]

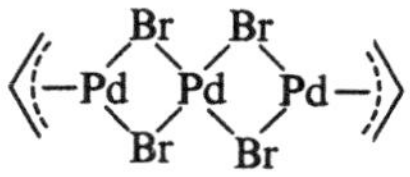

M 721.021

Dark-brown solid (H_2O). Mp 145-60° dec.

Moiseev, I.I. *et al*, *Izv. Akad. Nauk SSSR, Ser. Khim.*, 1964, 775; *Bull Acad. Sci. USSR, Div. Chem. Sci.*, *1964*, *727* (*synth*)
Zaitsev, L.M. *et al*, *Zh. Neorg. Khim.*, 1967, **12**, 396; *Russ. J. Inorg. Chem. (Engl. Transl.)*, 1967, **12**, 203 (*synth*)

$C_6H_{10}Cl_2Pd$ Pd-00021

Dichloro[(1,2,5,6-η)-1,5-hexadiene]palladium, 9CI

[12106-22-8]

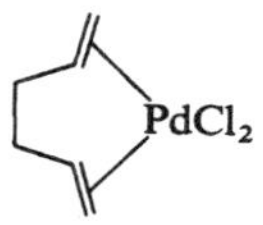

M 259.471

Hendra, P.J. *et al*, *Spectrochim. Acta*, 1961, **17**, 909 (*ir*)
Zakharova, I.A. *et al*, *Russ. J. Inorg. Chem. (Engl. Transl.)*, 1966 **11**, 1364 (*synth, struct*)
Zakharova, I.A. *et al*, *J. Organomet. Chem.*, 1974, **72**, 283 (*ir*)

$C_6H_{10}Cl_2Pd_2$ Pd-00022

Di-μ-chlorobis(η³-2-propenyl)dipalladium, 10CI, 9CI

Di-π-allyldi-μ-chlorodipalladium, 8CI. *Bis(allylchloropalladium)*

[12012-95-2]

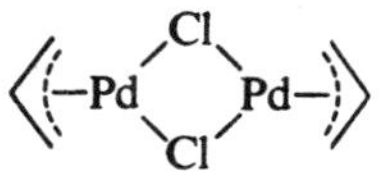

M 365.891

Bridged dimer. Hydrosilylation catalyst. Pale-yellow cryst. (C_6H_6). Mp 160°.

▷RT3510000.

Monomer: Chloro(η³-2-propenyl)palladium. Allylchloropalladium.

C_3H_5ClPd M 182.946

Unknown.

Smidt, J. *et al*, *Angew. Chem.*, 1959, **71**, 284 (*synth*)
Dehm, H.C. *et al*, *J. Am. Chem. Soc.*, 1960, **82**, 4429 (*pmr*)
Levdik, V.F. *et al*, *Zh. Strukt. Khim.*, 1962, **3**, 472 (*struct*)
Dent, W.T. *et al*, *J. Chem. Soc.*, 1964, 1585 (*synth, ir*)
Lupin, M.S. *et al*, *J. Chem. Soc. (A)*, 1968, 3095 (*ms*)
Shaw, B.L. *et al*, *J. Chem. Soc., Chem. Commun.*, 1971, 790 (*cmr*)

$C_6H_{10}Pd$ Pd-00023

Bis(η^3-2-propenyl)palladium, 9CI

Di-π-allylpalladium, 8CI. *Bisallylpalladium*

[12240-87-8]

⟨(–Pd–)⟩

M 188.565

Exists in soln. as *syn* and *anti* stereoisomers. Catalyses hydrogenation of dienes to alkenes. Light-yellow cryst. (pentane).

Belg. Pat., 631 127, (*1963*); *CA*, **61**, 690 (*synth*)
Wilke, G., *Angew. Chem., Int. Ed. Engl.*, 1963, **2**, 105.
Job, B.E. *et al*, *J. Chem. Soc. (A)*, 1967, 423 (*synth, pmr, ms*)
Nesmeyanov, A.N. *et al*, *Dokl. Akad. Nauk. SSSR*, 1974, **216**, 816; *CA*, **81**, 70680 (*cmr*)
Henc, B. *et al*, *J. Organomet. Chem.*, 1980, **191**, 425 (*pmr, cmr, raman*)

$C_6H_{12}Pd$ Pd-00024

Tris(ethylene)palladium

Tris(η^2-ethene)palladium, 9CI

[57158-85-7]

$Pd(H_2C{=}CH_2)_3$

M 190.581

Cryst. (butane).

Green, M. *et al*, *J. Chem. Soc., Dalton Trans.*, 1977, 271 (*synth, ir, pmr, cmr*)

$C_6H_{14}I_2O_2Pd_2S_2$ Pd-00025

Di-μ-iodobis[(methylsulfoxoniumylidene)bis(methylene)]dipalladium, 9CI

[62465-46-7]

M 648.944

Yellow cryst. (DMSO aq.). Mp 200° dec.

Bravo, P. *et al*, *J. Organomet. Chem.*, 1976, **118**, C78 (*synth, ir, pmr*)

$C_6H_{16}I_4Pd_2S_2$ Pd-00026

Bis(dimethylsulfonium-η-methylide)di-μ-iododiiododipalladium, 9CI

[53564-90-2]

M 872.770

Brown solid (DMSO aq.). Mp 204°.

Bravo, P. *et al*, *J. Organomet. Chem.*, 1974, **74**, 143 (*synth, ir, pmr*)

> *Having problems with locating a compound? Have you checked the indexes?*

$C_7H_8Br_2Pd$ Pd-00027

[(2,3,5,6-η)-Bicyclo[2.2.1]hepta-2,5-diene]dibromopalladium, 9CI

Dibromo(norbornadiene)palladium. Norbornadienedibromopalladium

[42765-77-5]

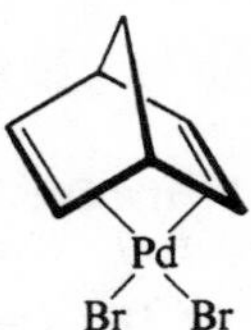

M 358.368

Orange cryst. (CH_2Cl_2). Inhibits rat liver mitochondria and rat liver ATPase.

Alexander, R.A. *et al*, *J. Am. Chem. Soc.*, 1960, **82**, 535 (*synth, ir, struct*)
Adams, D.M. *et al*, *Inorg. Chim. Acta*, 1973, **7**, 277 (*ir*)
Zakharova, I.A. *et al*, *J. Organomet. Chem.*, 1975, **102**, 227 (*ir*)
Kolesova, G.M. *et al*, *Vapr. Med. Khim.*, 1979, **25**, 537; *CA*, **91**, 204224q (*pharmacol*)

$C_7H_8Cl_2Pd$ Pd-00028

[(2,3,5,6-η)-Bicyclo[2.2.1]hepta-2,5-diene]dichloropalladium, 9CI

Dichloro(2,5-norbornadiene)palladium, 8CI. *Norbornadienedichloropalladium. Bicyclo[2.2.1]hepta-2,5-dienepalladium dichloride*

[12317-46-3]

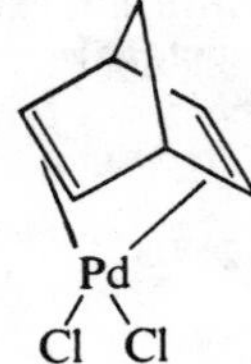

M 269.466

Needles (CH_2Cl_2). Mp 190-200° dec.

Bennett, M.A. *et al*, *J. Chem. Soc.*, 1959, 3178 (*synth, ir*)
Alexander, R.A. *et al*, *J. Am. Chem. Soc.*, 1960, **82**, 535 (*synth*)

$C_7H_{21}IP_2Pd$ Pd-00029

Iodomethylbis(trimethylphosphine)palladium, 9CI

Methylbis(trimethylphosphine)palladium iodide

[42582-39-8]

M 400.515

Bright-yellow solid (CH_2Cl_2/Et_2O). Mp 124° dec.

Yamamoto, Y. *et al*, *Inorg. Chem.*, 1974, **13**, 438.
Werner, H. *et al*, *J. Chem. Res. (M)*, 1978, 2720; *J. Chem. Res. (S)*, 1978, 201 (*synth, ms, pmr, nmr*)
Werner, H. *et al*, *Chem. Ber.*, 1980, **113**, 267.

$C_8H_4Pd^{\ominus\ominus}$ Pd-00030

Tetrakis(ethynyl)palladate(2−)

Tetra(acetylenide)palladate(2−)

$Pd(C{\equiv}CH)_4^{\ominus\ominus}$ (D_{4h})

M 206.540 (ion)

Di-K salt:

$C_8H_4K_2Pd$ M 284.736
Solid.

Nast, R. *et al*, *Chem. Ber.*, 1978, **111**, 1627 (*synth*)

$C_8H_8Cl_2Pd$ Pd-00031

Dichloro[(1,2,5,6-η)-1,3,5,7-cyclooctatetraene]palladium, 9CI
Cyclooctatetraenepalladium dichloride
[33504-97-1]

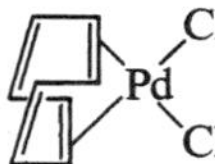

M 281.477
Red cryst.; air-sensitive.

Baenziger, N.C. *et al*, *Acta Crystallogr., Sect. B*, 1978, **34**, 1340 (*struct*)

$C_8H_{10}Pd$ Pd-00032

(η^5-2,4-Cyclopentadien-1-yl)(η^3-2-propenyl)palladium, 10CI, 9CI
π-Allyl-π-cyclopentadienylpalladium, 8CI.
Cyclopentadienylallylpalladium
[1271-03-0]

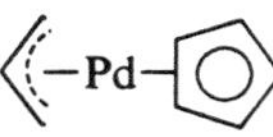

M 212.587
Red needles (pet. ether). Mp 63-63.5°. Subl. readily.

Shaw, B.L., *Proc. Chem. Soc., London*, 1960, 247 (*synth*)
Minasyan, M.K. *et al*, *Zh. Strukt. Khim.*, 1966, **7**, 906; *CA*, **66**, 906 (*struct*)
King, R.B. *et al*, *Appl. Spectrosc.*, 1969, **23**, 148 (*ms*)
Mann, B.E. *et al*, *J. Chem. Soc., Chem. Commun.*, 1971, 790 (*cmr*)
Mann, B.E. *et al*, *J. Chem. Soc., Dalton Trans.*, 1973, 2390 (*pmr*)

$C_8H_{12}Br_2Pd$ Pd-00033

Dibromo[(1,2,5,6-η)-1,5-cyclooctadiene]palladium, 9CI
(1,5-Cyclooctadiene)dibromopalladium
[12145-47-0]

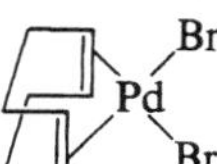

M 374.411
Orange-red solid (AcOH). Mp 213° dec.

Chatt, J. *et al*, *J. Chem. Soc.*, 1957, 3413 (*synth*)

$C_8H_{12}Cl_2Pd$ Pd-00034

Dichloro[(1,2,5,6-η)-1,5-cyclooctadiene]palladium, 10CI, 9CI
1,5-Cyclooctadienepalladium dichloride
[12107-56-1]

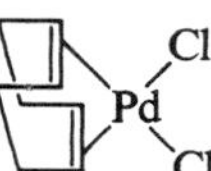

M 285.509
Pale-yellow needles (AcOH). Sol. C_6H_6, $CHCl_3$. Mp 205-10° dec.

Chatt, J. *et al*, *J. Chem. Soc.*, 1957, 3413 (*synth, ir*)
Fischer, E.O. *et al*, *Chem. Ber.*, 1960, **93**, 2075 (*synth, ir*)
Heimbach, P., *J. Organomet. Chem.*, 1973, **49**, 483 (*pmr*)
Rettig, M.F. *et al*, *J. Am. Chem. Soc.*, 1981, **103**, 2980 (*struct*)

$C_8H_{12}Cl_2Pd_2$ Pd-00035

Dichloro(μ-2,6-octadienediyl)dipalladium
Dichloro[μ-[(1,2,3-η:6,7,8-η)-2,6-octadien-1,8-diyl-]]dipalladium, 9CI.
μ-1-3-η:6-8-η-Octadienato(2-)-bis(chloropalladium)
[61926-82-7]

[PdCl ... PdCl]n

M 391.929
Chloride bridged polymer. Catalyses additive dimerisation of butadiene with diethylamine. Yellow solid. Insol. nondonor solvents.

Lazutkin, A.M. *et al*, *Zh. Obshch. Khim.*, 1976, **46**, 2625 (*synth*)
White, D.A., *J. Chem. Res. (S)*, 1977, 226; *J. Chem. Res. (M)*, 1977, 2401 (*synth, use*)

$C_8H_{12}Cl_4Pd_2$ Pd-00036

Di-μ-chlorobis[(1,2,3-η)-4-chloro-2-buten-1-yl]dipalladium
Di-μ-chlorobis(1-chloromethylallyl)dipalladium

Cl, Pd, Pd, Cl, ClH_2C, CH_2Cl

M 462.835
Was originally formulated as dichloro(1,3-butadiene)-palladium, $[PdCl_2(C_4H_6)]$.

Shaw, B.L., *Chem. Ind. (London)*, 1962, 1190 (*pmr, struct*)

$C_8H_{12}N_4Pd^{\oplus\oplus}$ Pd-00037

Tetrakis(acetonitrile)palladium(2+), 8CI
Tetrakis(methyl cyanide)palladium(2+)

$[Pd(NCCH_3)_4]^{\oplus\oplus}$ (D_{4h})

M 270.630 (ion)

Bis(tetrafluoroborate): [21797-13-7].
$C_8H_{12}B_2F_8N_4Pd$ M 444.237
Catalyses polymerisation of styrene. Yellow cryst. ($MeCN/Et_2O$).

Bistrifluoromethanesulfonate: [68569-14-2].
$C_{10}H_{12}F_6N_4O_6PdS_2$ M 568.758
Catalyses prepn. of unsaturated amines. No physical data available.

Bis(hexachloroantimonate): [17500-34-4].
$C_8H_{12}Cl_{12}N_4PdSb_2$ M 939.566
No physical data available.

Bis(tetrachlorothallate): [21374-01-6].
$C_8H_{12}Cl_8N_4PdTl_2$ M 963.020
Mp 83-6° dec.

Reedijk, J. *et al*, *Recl. Trav. Chim. Pays-Bas*, 1967, **86**, 1127 (*ir*)
Reedijk, J. *et al*, *Recl. Trav. Chim. Pays-Bas*, 1968, **87**, 513 (*synth*)
Schrann, R.F. *et al*, *J. Chem. Soc., Chem. Commun.*, 1968, 898 (*synth, ir*)
Sen, A. *et al*, *J. Am. Chem. Soc.*, 1981, **103**, 4627 (*use*)

$C_8H_{12}N_4Pd^{\oplus\oplus}$ Pd-00038

Tetrakis(isocyanomethane)palladium(2+), 9CI

Tetrakis(methylisonitrile)palladium(2+). Tetrakis(methyl isocyanide)palladium(2+)

$[Pd(CNMe)_4]^{\oplus\oplus}$ (D_{4h})

M 270.630 (ion)

Bis(hexafluorophosphate): [38317-62-3].
$C_8H_{12}F_{12}N_4P_2Pd$ M 560.558
Cryst. (MeCN).

Miller, J.S. *et al*, *Inorg. Chem.*, 1972, **11**, 2069 (*synth, ir, pmr*)
Garciafigueroa, E. *et al*, *Nouv. J. Chim.*, 1978, **2**, 593 (*ir, raman, struct*)

$C_8H_{12}O_2Pd$ Pd-00039

(2,4-Pentanedionato-*O,O'*)(η^3-2-propenyl)palladium, 9CI

π-Allyl(2,4-pentanedionato)palladium, 8CI. (Acetylacetonato)(allyl)palladium

[12145-53-8]

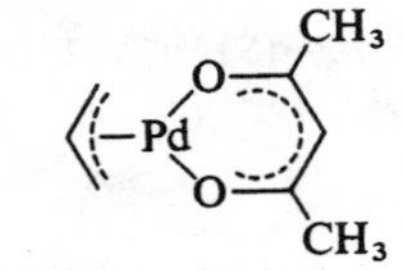

M 246.602

Catalyses linear trimerisation of butadiene and dimerisation of isoprene. Yellow cryst. (pet. ether) dec. on standing at r.t. Mp 72-3°.

Imamura, S. *et al*, *Bull. Chem. Soc. Jpn.*, 1969, **42**, 805 (*synth*)
Astrakhova, A.S. *et al*, *Izv. Akad. Nauk SSSR, Ser. Khim.*, 1971, 1362; *CA*, **75**, 97887d (*use*)
Razuvaev, G.A. *et al*, *J. Organomet. Chem.*, 1971, **32**, 113 (*synth*)
Shaw, B.L. *et al*, *J. Chem. Soc., Chem. Commun.*, 1971, 790 (*cmr*)
Mann, B.E. *et al*, *J. Chem. Soc., Dalton Trans.*, 1973, 2390 (*pmr, cmr*)
Jackson, W.R. *et al*, *Aust. J. Chem.*, 1978, **31**, 1073 (*synth*)

$C_8H_{14}Cl_2Pd_2$ Pd-00040

Bis[(1,2,3-η)-2-butenyl]di-μ-chlorodipalladium, 9CI

Di-μ-chlorobis(1-methyl-π-allyl)dipalladium, 8CI. Di-μ-chlorobis[(1,2,3-η)-2-buten-1-yl]dipalladium. Bis(π-crotylpalladium chloride)

[62662-13-9]

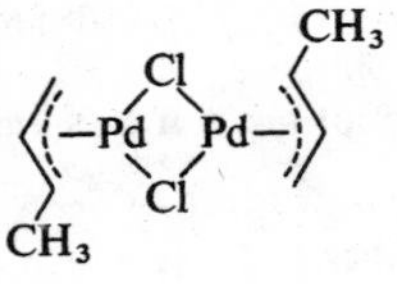

M 393.945

Cryst. ($CHCl_3$). Mp 136-7°.

Monomer: (2-Butenyl)chloropalladium. Chloro(1-methyl-π-allyl)palladium. Crotylpalladium chloride.
C_4H_7ClPd M 196.972
Unknown.

Huttel, R. *et al*, *Angew. Chem.*, 1959, **71**, 258 (*synth*)
Hegarty, B.F. *et al*, *J. Organomet. Chem.*, 1966, **6**, 578 (*uv*)
Ketley, A.D. *et al*, *J. Chem. Soc., Chem. Commun.*, 1968, 169 (*synth, pmr*)
Sakakibara, M. *et al*, *J. Chem. Soc., Chem. Commun.*, 1969, 396 (*synth*)
Lammens, H. *et al*, *Org. Mass Spectrom.*, 1971, **5**, 335 (*ms*)
Sokolov, V.N. *et al*, *J. Organomet. Chem.*, 1971, **29**, 313 (*pmr*)
Sokolov, V.N. *et al*, *J. Organomet. Chem.*, 1973, **54**, 361 (*cmr*)
Leites, L.A. *et al*, *Dokl. Akad. Nauk SSSR, Ser. Sci. Khim.*, 1974, **215**, 634; *CA*, **81**, 12684m (*ir, raman*)

$C_8H_{14}Cl_2Pd_2$ Pd-00041

Di-μ-chlorobis[(1,2,3-η)-2-methyl-2-propenyl]dipalladium, 10CI, 9CI

Bis[(2-methylallyl)chloropalladium]

[12081-18-4]

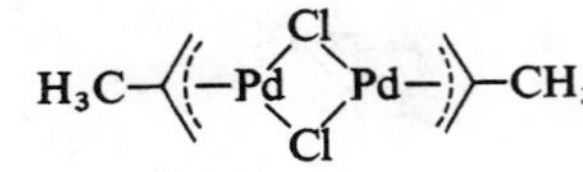

M 393.945

Bridged dimer. Yellow solid. Mp 166-8° dec.

Monomer: Chloro(2-methyl-2-propenyl)palladium. Chloro(2-methylallyl)palladium.
C_4H_7ClPd M 196.972
Unknown.

Hüttel, R. *et al*, *Angew. Chem., Int. Ed. Engl.*, 1959, **71**, 456 (*synth*)
Hüttel, R. *et al*, *Chem. Ber.*, 1961, **94**, 766 (*synth*)
Robinson, J.C. *et al*, *J. Chem. Soc.*, 1963, 4806 (*uv, pmr*)
Lupin, M.S. *et al*, *J. Chem. Soc. (A)*, 1966, **10**, 1410 (*ir*)
Lammens, H. *et al*, *Org. Mass Spectrom.*, 1971, **5**, 335 (*ms*)
Mann, B.E. *et al*, *J. Chem. Soc., Chem. Commun.*, 1971, 790 (*cmr*)
Bandoli, G. *et al*, *Acta Crystallogr., Sect. B*, 1981, **37**, 490 (*struct*)

$C_8H_{16}Cl_4Pd_2$ Pd-00042

Bis[(2,3-η)-2-butene]tetrachlorodipalladium

Di-μ-chlorodichlorobis(2-butene)dipalladium

[53275-27-7]

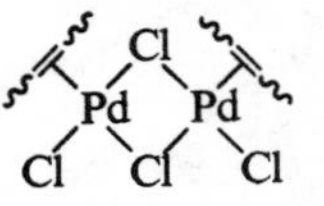

cis-form 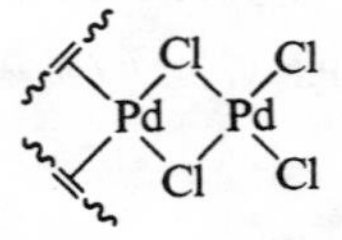 *asymm-form*

M 466.866

3 Isomers known, each theoretically capable of further (*E,Z*)-isomerism, which has not been characterised. Catalyses ethylene dimerisation. Catalytic activity slowly decays due to conversion to inactive allyl complex.

cis-form

Red cryst. Sol. org. solvs. Readily isom. to *trans*-form, which precipitates.

trans-form

Yellow-brown solid. Spar. sol. org. solvs. Mp 50-100° dec. Slowly converts to *cis*-isomer if held at 50° in $CHCl_3$. Can be prepd. from (*E*)- or (*Z*)-2-butene, but characteristics of the individual isomers not recorded.

asymm-form

Red solid. Sol. most. org. solvs. Treatment with PhCN releases butene. Does not readily convert to the other isomers.

Pregaglia, G. *et al*, *Chem. Ind. (London)*, 1966, 1923 (*synth*)
Ketley, A.D. *et al*, *Inorg. Chem.*, 1967, **6**, 657 (*synth, pmr*)
Partenheimer, W. *et al*, *Inorg. Nucl. Chem. Lett.*, 1974, **10**, 1143 (*ir*)
Partenheimer, W. *et al*, *J. Am. Chem. Soc.*, 1974, **96**, 3800 (*ir, pmr*)

$C_8H_{16}Cl_4Pd_2$ Pd-00043

Di-μ-chlorodichlorobis(2-methylpropene)dipalladium, 8CI
Tetrachlorodiisobutenedipalladium

M 466.866
Catalyses dimerisation of α-olefins. Extremely unstable red cryst. Mp 180-90° dec.
Monomer: Dichloro(2-methylpropene)palladium.
$C_4H_8Cl_2Pd$ M 233.433
Unknown.

Kharasch, M.S. *et al, J. Am. Chem. Soc.*, 1938, **60**, 882.
Hüttel, R. *et al, Chem. Ber.*, 1961, **94**, 766 (*synth*)
Fr. Pat., 1 499 833, (*1967*); *CA*, **69**, 76596u (*use*)

$C_8H_{21}IOP_2Pd$ Pd-00044

Acetyliodobis(trimethylphosphine)palladium, 9CI
Iodo(acetyl)bis(trimethylphosphine)palladium

M 428.525
trans-form [68391-83-3]
Pale-yellow cryst. (CH_2Cl_2/Et_2O). Mp 115° dec.

Werner, H. *et al, Chem. Ber.*, 1980, **113**, 267.
Werner, H. *et al, J. Chem. Res. (M)*, 1978, 2720 (*synth, ir, pmr, nmr, ms*)

$C_9F_5N_3Pd^{\ominus\ominus}$ Pd-00045

Tricyano(pentafluorophenyl)palladate(2−)
Tris(cyano-C)(pentafluorophenyl)palladate, 10CI

$[Pd(CN)_3(C_6F_5)]^{\ominus\ominus}$

M 351.531 (ion)
Bis(tetrabutylammonium) salt: [76083-10-8].
$C_{41}H_{72}F_5N_5Pd$ M 836.465
Oil (hexane/Et_2O).

Uson, R. *et al, J. Organomet. Chem.*, 1980, **199**, 111 (*synth, ir*)

$C_9H_{12}ClNPd$ Pd-00046

Chloro[(1,2,3-η)-2-methyl-2-propenyl](pyridine)palladium, 9CI
Chloro(2-methylallyl)pyridinepalladium. [2-Methyl(enyl)]chloro(pyridine)palladium
[50497-55-7]

M 276.074
Yellow cryst. (Et_2O). Mp 122-4°.

Hüttel, R. *et al, J. Organomet. Chem.*, 1977, **139**, 89 (*synth*)

$C_9H_{12}Pd$ Pd-00047

(η^5-2,4-Cyclopentadien-1-yl)(η^3-2-methyl-2-propenyl)palladium, 9CI
(π-Cyclopentadienyl)(2-methylallyl)palladium. (2-Methylallyl)(cyclopentadienyl)palladium. [2-Methyl(enyl)]cyclopentadienylpalladium
[33593-95-2]

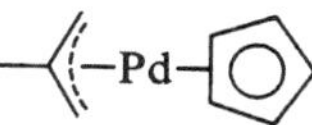

M 226.614
Air-sensitive red cryst. Sol. all org. solvs. Mp 34°. $Bp_{0.1}$ 25° subl.

Mann, B.E. *et al, J. Chem. Soc., Dalton Trans.*, 1973, 2390 (*pmr, cmr*)
Parker, G. *et al, Helv. Chim. Acta*, 1973, **56**, 2819 (*synth*)
Werner, H. *et al, Z. Anorg. Allg. Chem.*, 1981, **479**, 134 (*use, synth*)

$C_9H_{15}ClPd$ Pd-00048

Chloro[(1,2,5,6-η)-1,5-cyclooctadiene]methylpalladium, 9CI
Methylchloro(1,5-cyclooctadiene)palladium
[63936-85-6]

M 265.091
Alkylates styrene. Cryst. (CH_2Cl_2/pentane). Mp >70° dec.

Rudler-Chauvin, M. *et al, J. Organomet. Chem.*, 1977, **134**, 115 (*synth, pmr, use*)

$C_9H_{20}BrPPd$ Pd-00049

Bromo(η^3-2-propenyl)(triethylphosphine)palladium
(π-Allyl)bromo(triethylphosphine)palladium. π-Enyl(bromo)(triethylphosphine)palladium

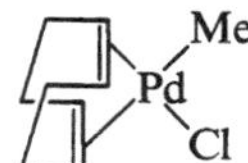

M 345.555
Yellow cryst. (cyclohexane). Mp 45-8°.

Rieke, R.D. *et al, J. Org. Chem.*, 1979, **44**, 3069 (*synth*)

$C_9H_{28}P_3Pd^{\oplus}$ Pd-00050

Hydrotris(trimethylphosphine)palladium(1+)
Hydridotris(trimethylphosphine)palladium(1+)

$[PdH(PMe_3)_3]^{\oplus}$

M 335.661 (ion)
Tetraphenylborate: [68391-94-6].
$C_{33}H_{48}BP_3Pd$ M 654.893
Cryst. (THF/EtOH).

Werner, H. *et al, J. Chem. Res. (M)*, 1978, 2720; *J. Chem. Res. (S)*, 1978, 201 (*synth, ir, pmr, nmr*)
Werner, H. *et al, Chem. Ber.*, 1980, **113**, 267.
Werner, H. *et al, Inorg. Chim. Acta*, 1980, **43**, 199.

$C_{10}H_{10}ClNPd$ Pd-00051

Benzonitrile(chloro)-2-propenylpalladium

Chloro(cyanobenzene)(η^3-2-propenyl)palladium. Allylchloro(benzonitrile)palladium

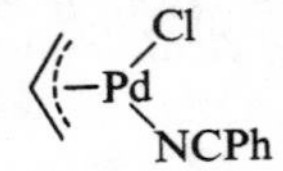

M 286.069

Yellow solid (pet. ether). Mp 115-35° dec.

Klimenko, N.M. *et al*, *Izv. Akad. Nauk SSSR, Ser. Khim.*, 1961, 1355; *CA*, **56**, 4792i (*synth*)

$C_{10}H_{12}Cl_2Pd$ Pd-00052

Dichloro(dicyclopentadiene)palladium

Dichloro[(2,3,5,6-η)-3a,4,7,7a-tetrahydro-4,7-methano-1H-indene]palladium, 9CI. *Dichloro[tricyclo[5.2.1.0^{2,6}]deca-3,8-diene]palladium. Dicyclopentadienedichloropalladium*

[12294-98-3]

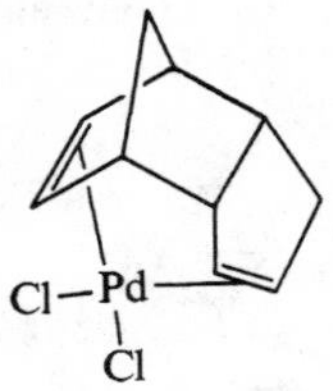

M 309.531

Golden-yellow cryst. (CH_2Cl_2). Mp 165-70° dec.

Chatt, J. *et al*, *J. Chem. Soc.*, 1957, 3413 (*synth*)
Wright, L.L. *et al*, *J. Am. Chem. Soc.*, 1982, **104**, 610 (*struct, stereochem*)

$C_{10}H_{14}O_4Pd$ Pd-00053

Bis(2,4-pentanedionato-*O,O'*)palladium, 9CI

Bis(acetylacetonato)palladium

[14024-61-4]

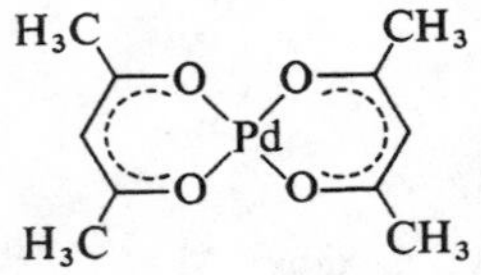

M 304.638

Catalyses dimerisation of isoprene, carbonylation telomerisation and oligomerisation of dienes, vinylation of benzene derivs., dehydrogenation of chromanones and flavones, and carbonylation of epoxyalkenes; produces wet-proof Pd metal deposit on carbon-containing electrodes. Orange/yellow cryst. (benzene). Mp 132-205° dec.

McCarthy, P.J. *et al*, *Inorg. Chem.*, 1967, **6**, 781 (*synth, pmr*)
Sasaki, S. *et al*, *Bull. Chem. Soc. Jpn.*, 1967, **40**, 76 (*ms*)
Knyazeva, A.N. *et al*, *Zh. Strukt. Khim.*, 1970, **11**, 938; *J. Struct. Chem.*, 1970, **11**, 875 (*struct*)
Bulkin, B.J. *et al*, *Appl. Spectrosc.*, 1978, **32**, 151 (*ir, raman*)
Wilkie, C.A. *et al*, *J. Inorg. Nucl. Chem.*, 1978, **40**, 195 (*cmr*)
Okeya, S. *et al*, *Bull. Chem. Soc. Jpn.*, 1981, **54**, 1085 (*synth, ir, pmr, cmr*)

$C_{10}H_{16}Cl_2Pd$ Pd-00054

Dichloro[(1,2,3,4-η)-1,2,3,4,5-pentamethylcyclopentadiene]palladium, 10CI

(Pentamethylcyclopentadiene)dichloropalladium

[33479-23-1]

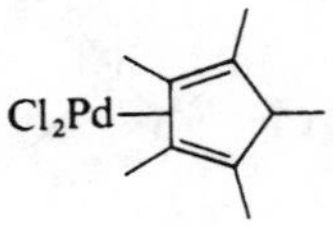

M 313.562

Balakrishnan, P.V. *et al*, *J. Chem. Soc. (A)*, 1971, 1721 (*synth, ir, pmr*)

$C_{10}H_{16}O_4Pd_2$ Pd-00055

Bis[μ-(acetato-*O:O'*)]bis(η^3-2-propenyl)dipalladium, 9CI

Bis(μ-acetato)di-π-allyldipalladium, 8CI. *Di-μ-ethanoatobis(η^3-2-propenyl)dipalladium. Di-μ-acetatobis(allyl)dipalladium*

[12084-71-8]

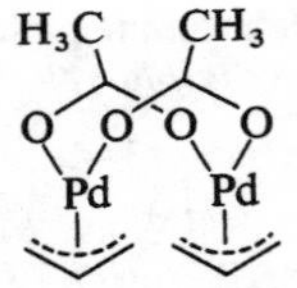

M 413.074

Catalyses dimerization of butadiene and synthesis of unsaturated fatty alcohols. Yellow cryst. (EtOAc). Mp 181-3° (100-30°) dec.

Robinson, S.D. *et al*, *J. Organomet. Chem.*, 1967, **3**, 367 (*synth, pmr*)
Powell, J., *J. Am. Chem. Soc.*, 1969, **91**, 4311 (*pmr*)
Neilan, J.P. *et al*, *J. Org. Chem.*, 1976, **41**, 3455 (*use*)
Brown, R.G. *et al*, *J. Chem. Soc., Dalton Trans.*, 1977, 176 (*cmr, pmr*)
Nesmeyanov, A.N. *et al*, *J. Organomet. Chem.*, 1978, **164**, 259 (*synth*)

$C_{10}H_{18}Cl_2O_2Pd_2$ Pd-00056

Di-μ-chlorobis[(1,2,3-η)-4-methoxy-2-buten-1-yl]dipalladium, 9CI

Di-μ-chlorobis(3-methoxymethylallyl)dipalladium. Di-μ-chlorodi-(4-methoxy-2-buten-1-yl)dipalladium

[31904-80-0]

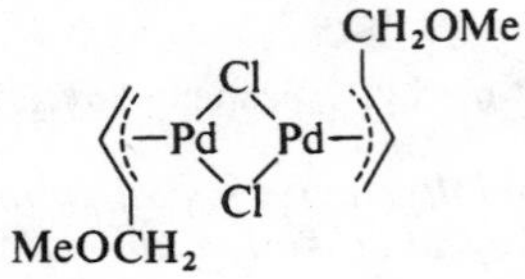

M 453.997

Yellow cryst. (MeOH). Mp 97.5-99.5° dec.

Robinson, S.D. *et al*, *J. Chem. Soc.*, 1963, 4806 (*synth, pmr, uv*)

$C_{10}H_{18}Cl_2Pd_2$ **Pd-00057**

Di-μ-chlorobis[(1,2,3-η)-2-methyl-2-buten-1-yl]dipalladium, 10CI, 9CI

Di-μ-chlorobis(1,2-dimethyl-π-allyl)dipalladium, 8CI

[12301-06-3]

M 421.998

Chloride bridged dimer. Yellow cryst. (CH_2Cl_2/Et_2O). Mp 138°.

Monomer:

C_5H_9ClPd M 210.999

Unknown.

Hüttel, R. *et al*, *Chem. Ber.*, 1963, **96**, 3101; 1964, **97**, 1439 (*synth*)

Hüttel, R. *et al*, *Chem. Ber.*, 1973, **106**, 1789 (*pmr*)

Stakem, F.G. *et al*, *J. Org. Chem.*, 1980, **45**, 3584 (*synth*)

$C_{10}H_{18}Cl_2Pd_2$ **Pd-00058**

Di-μ-chlorobis[(2,3,4-η)-3-penten-2-yl]dipalladium

Di-μ-chlorobis(1,3-dimethyl-π-allyl)dipalladium, 8CI

M 421.998

Yellow cryst. ($CHCl_3$ or C_6H_6). Mp 160° dec.

Monomer: Chloro[(2,3,4-η)-3-penten-2-yl]palladium. π-1,3-Dimethylallylpalladium chloride. Chloro(1,3-dimethylallyl)palladium.

C_5H_9ClPd M 210.999

Unknown.

Davies, G.R. *et al*, *J. Chem. Soc., Chem. Commun.*, 1967, 1151 (*synth, struct, pmr*)

$C_{10}H_{18}I_2N_2Pd$ **Pd-00059**

Diiodobis(2-isocyano-2-methylpropane)palladium, 9CI

Bis(tert-*butylisocyanide*)*diiodopalladium*, 8CI. *Diiodobis*(tert-*butylisonitrile*)*palladium. Bis*(tert-*butylisonitrile*)*diiodopalladium*

[24917-36-0]

M 526.495

***trans*-form** [34710-35-5]

Air-stable orange-red cryst. (hexane). Mp 166°.

Otsuka, S. *et al*, *J. Am. Chem. Soc.*, 1969, **91**, 6994 (*synth, ir, pmr*)

Bailey, N.A. *et al*, *J. Organomet. Chem.*, 1972, **37**, C49 (*struct*)

$C_{10}H_{18}N_2O_2Pd$ **Pd-00060**

Bis(2-isocyano-2-methylpropane)peroxypalladium, 9CI

Bis(tert-*butylisocyanide*)*peroxypalladium*, 8CI. *Bis*(tert-*butylisonitrile*)(*dioxygen*)*palladium. Bis*(*2-isocyano-2-methylpropane*)(*dioxygen*)*palladium*

[21107-86-8]

$Pd(O_2)[(H_3C)_3CNC]_2$

M 304.684

Bluish-grey cryst. Mp 115° (dec., under N_2).

Otsuka, S. *et al*, *J. Am. Chem. Soc.*, 1969, **91**, 6994 (*synth, ir, pmr*)

Nakamura, A. *et al*, *J. Am. Chem. Soc.*, 1971, **93**, 6052 (*ir*)

$C_{10}H_{18}N_2Pd$ **Pd-00061**

Bis[2-isocyano-2-methylpropane]palladium, 9CI

Bis(tert-*butylisonitrile*)*palladium. Bis*(tert-*butylisocyanide*)*palladium*

[24859-25-4]

$Pd[CNC(CH_3)_3]_2$

M 272.686

Catalyses cyclopropanation reaction of diazoalkanes and substituted olefins. Orange cryst. (pentane). Mp 130° dec.

Otsuka, S. *et al*, *J. Am. Chem. Soc.*, 1969, **91**, 6994 (*synth, ir, pmr*)

Nakamura, A. *et al*, *J. Am. Chem. Soc.*, 1977, **99**, 2108 (*use*)

$C_{10}H_{18}Pd$ **Pd-00062**

[(1,2,5,6-η)-1,5-Cyclooctadiene]dimethylpalladium, 9CI

Dimethyl(1,5-cyclooctadiene)palladium

[63936-77-6]

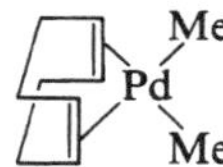

M 244.672

White cryst. (Et_2O). Mp 92° dec.

Rudler-Chauvin, M. *et al*, *J. Organomet. Chem.*, 1977, **134**, 115 (*synth, pmr*)

$C_{10}H_{24}N_2Pd^{\oplus}$ **Pd-00063**

(η^3-2-Butenyl)[1,2-bis(dimethylamino)ethane]palladium(1+)

(1-Methylallyl)(tetramethylethylenediamine)palladium(1+)

M 278.733 (ion)

Tetrafluoroborate:

$C_{10}H_{24}BF_4N_2Pd$ M 365.537

White solid. Mp 128-30° dec.

Dichloro(η^3-2-butenyl)palladium(1−) salt: see Dichloro(η^3-2-butenyl)palladate(1−), Pd-00009

Hegedus, L.S. *et al*, *J. Am. Chem. Soc.*, 1982, **104**, 697 (*synth, struct, pmr, ir*)

$C_{10}H_{30}P_3Pd^{\oplus}$ **Pd-00064**

Methyltris(trimethylphosphine)palladium(1+)

$[PdMe(PMe_3)_3]^{\oplus}$

M 349.688 (ion)

Tetraphenylborate: [68391-96-8].
$C_{34}H_{50}BP_3Pd$ M 668.920
Cryst. (CH_2Cl_2/Et_2O).

Werner, H. *et al*, *J. Chem. Res. (M)*, 1978, 2720; *J. Chem. Res. (S)*, 1978, 201 (*synth, pmr, nmr*)
Werner, H. *et al*, *Chem. Ber.*, 1980, **113**, 267.

$C_{11}H_{17}Pd^{\oplus}$ Pd-00065

[(1,2,5,6-η)-1,5-Cyclooctadiene](η³-2-propenyl)palladium(1+), 9CI
Allyl(1,5-cyclooctadiene)palladium(1+), 8CI

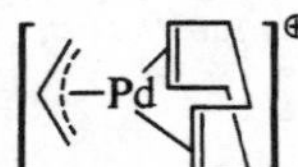

M 255.675 (ion)
Tetrafluoroborate: [32915-11-0].
$C_{11}H_{17}BF_4Pd$ M 342.479
Off-white solid (Et_2O); air-stable.

White, D.A., *Synth. Inorg. Metal-Org. Chem.*, 1971, **1**, 235 (*synth, pmr*)
*I*norg. Synth., 1972, **13**, 55 (*synth, pmr, ir*)

$C_{11}H_{20}BrPPd$ Pd-00066

Bromo(η⁵-2,4-cyclopentadien-1-yl)(triethylphosphine)palladium, 9CI
π-Cyclopentadienyl(triethylphosphine)palladium bromide
[31760-65-3]

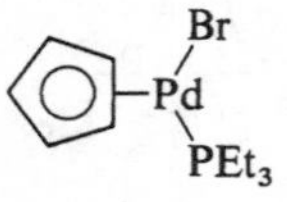

M 369.577
Green cryst. (C_6H_6/hexane). Mp 65-6°.

Cross, R.J. *et al*, *J. Chem. Soc. (A)*, 1971, 2000 (*synth, pmr*)
Kurosawa, H. *et al*, *J. Am. Chem. Soc.*, 1980, 6996.

$C_{11}H_{20}ClPPd$ Pd-00067

Chloro(η⁵-2,4-cyclopentadien-1-yl)(triethylphosphine)palladium, 9CI
π-Cyclopentadienyl(triethylphosphine)palladium chloride
[34854-20-1]

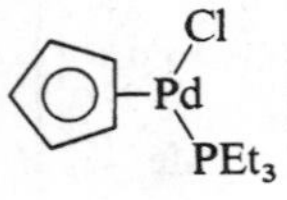

M 325.126
Green cryst. (C_6H_6/hexane). Mp 59-60°.

Cross, R.J. *et al*, *J. Chem. Soc. (A)*, 1971, 2000.

$C_{11}H_{20}IPPd$ Pd-00068

(η⁵-2,4-Cyclopentadien-1-yl)iodo(triethylphosphine)palladium, 9CI
π-Cyclopentadienyl(triethylphosphine)palladium iodide
[34854-21-2]

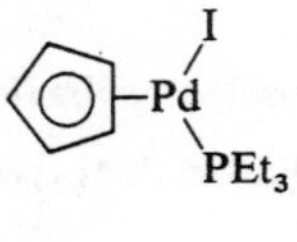

M 416.577
Green cryst. (C_6H_6/hexane). Mp 72-3°.

Cross, R.J. *et al*, *J. Chem. Soc. (A)*, 1971, 2000.

$C_{11}H_{21}IN_2Pd$ Pd-00069

Iodobis(2-isocyano-2-methylpropane)methylpalladium, 9CI
Bis(tert-butylisonitrile)iodomethylpalladium. Bis((tert-butyl isocyanide)iodomethylpalladium, 8CI. Iodo(methyl)bis(2-methyl-2-isocyanopropane)palladium. Methylbis(tert-butylisocyanide)palladium iodide

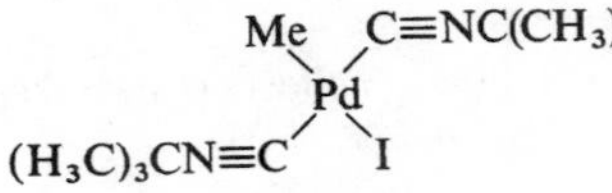

M 414.625
trans-form [25704-93-2]
Cryst. (hexane). Mp 77-8°.

Otsuka, S. *et al*, *J. Am. Chem. Soc.*, 1969, **91**, 7196 (*synth, ir, pmr*)

$C_{11}H_{30}OP_3Pd^{\oplus}$ Pd-00070

Acetyltris(trimethylphosphine)palladium(1+), 9CI

$[Pd(COCH_3)(PMe_3)_3]^{\oplus}$

M 377.699 (ion)
Tetraphenylborate: [68391-98-0].
$C_{35}H_{50}BOP_3Pd$ M 696.931
Cryst. (CH_2Cl_2/Et_2O).

Werner, H. *et al*, *J. Chem. Res. (S)*, 1978, 201; *J. Chem. Res. (M)*, 2720 (*synth, ir, pmr, nmr*)

$C_{12}H_{12}Al_4Cl_{14}Pd_2$ Pd-00071

Bis(benzene)di-μ-chlorobis(μ-chloropentachlorodialuminum-)dipalladium, 9CI
Bis(μ-benzene)tetra-μ-chlorodecachlorotetraaluminumdipalladium, 8CI
[56801-51-5]

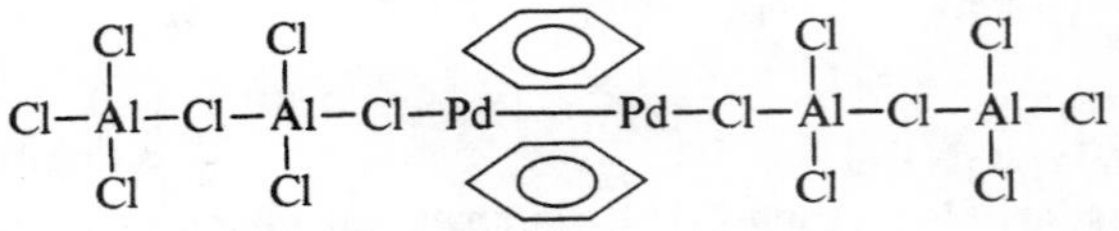

M 973.335
Catalyses dimerisation of ethylene. Deep-brown cryst. (C_6H_6/pentane). Air-sensitive.

Allegra, G. *et al*, *J. Am. Chem. Soc.*, 1970, **92**, 289 (*synth, ir, struct*)
Nardin, G. *et al*, *Gazz. Chim. Ital.*, 1975, **105**, 1047 (*struct*)
Pertici, P. *et al*, *Tetrahedron Lett.*, 1979, 1897 (*use*)

$C_{12}H_{14}N_2Pd$ Pd-00072

(2,2′-Bipyridine-N,N′)dimethylpalladium
Bipyridyl(dimethyl)palladium. Dimethyl(2,2′-bipyridine)palladium

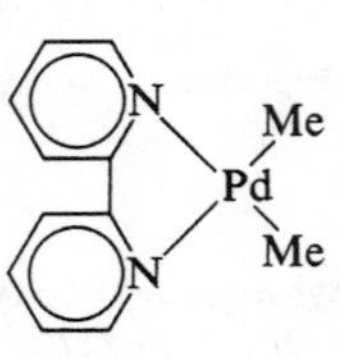

M 292.676
Orange cryst. (Me_2CO). Mp 155° dec.

Calvin, G. *et al*, *J. Chem. Soc.*, 1960, 2008 (*synth, ir*)

$C_{12}H_{15}O_2Pd^{\oplus}$ Pd-00073

[(2,3,5,6-η)-Bicyclo[2.2.1]hepta-2,5-diene][2,4-pentanedionato-*O,O'*]palladium(1+)

*(2,4-Pentanedionato-*O,O'*)[(2,3,5,6-η)-bicyclo-[2.2.1]hepta-2,5-diene]palladium(1+). (Norbornadiene)(acetylacetonato)palladium(1+). (Acetylacetonato)(norbornadiene)palladium(1+)*

M 297.669 (ion)

Tetrafluoroborate:
$C_{12}H_{15}BF_4O_2Pd$ M 384.473
Solid; air-stable.

Inorg. Synth., 1972, **13**, 55 (*synth, pmr*)

$C_{12}H_{16}Cl_4Pd_2$ Pd-00074

Di-μ-chlorobis[η^3-3-(chloromethyl)-2-methylene-3-butenyl-]dipalladium, 9CI

Dichlorobis[2-[1-(chloromethyl)vinyl]-π-allyl]dipalladium. Di-μ-chloro-π-(2-(3-chloro-1-propen-2-yl)-allyl)dipalladium

[12090-04-9]

M 514.910
Yellow-brown cryst. (C_6H_6/heptane). Mp 179-81° dec.

Lupin, M.S. *et al*, *Tetrahedron Lett.*, 1964, 883 (*synth*)
Schultz, R.G., *Tetrahedron*, 1964, **20**, 2809 (*synth, pmr*)

$C_{12}H_{18}Cl_2Pd$ Pd-00075

Dichloro[(2,3,5,6-η)-1,2,3,4,5,6-hexamethylbicyclo-[2.2.0]hexa-2,5-diene]palladium, 9CI

Dichloro[hexamethyl(dewar benzene)]palladium. Dewarhexamethylbenzenepalladium chloride

[12276-69-6]

M 339.600
Yellow cryst. (pet. ether); dec. in $CDCl_3$ after 20 min. at 33°. Mp 81° (79°) dec.

Dietl, H. *et al*, *J. Chem. Soc., Chem. Commun.*, 1967, 759 (*synth, pmr, ir*)
Shaw, B.L. *et al*, *J. Chem. Soc. (A)*, 1969, 602 (*synth, ir, pmr*)

$C_{12}H_{18}Cl_2Pd_2$ Pd-00076

Di-μ-chlorobis[(1,2,3-η)-2-cyclohexen-1-yl]dipalladium

Di-μ-chlorodi-π-2-cyclohexen-1-yldipalladium, 9CI, 8CI

[12090-09-4]

M 446.020
Used in synth. of ketenimine derivs. Yellow cryst. (hexane). Mp 92-5° dec.

Monomer: Chloro(η^3-2-cyclohexenyl)palladium.
C_6H_9ClPd M 223.010
Unknown.

Fischer, E.O. *et al*, *Chem. Ber.*, 1960, **93**, 2075 (*synth*)
Shaw, B.L. *et al*, *Chem. Ind. (London)*, 1961, 517 (*synth, pmr, struct*)
Fischer, E.O. *et al*, *Chem. Ber.*, 1962, **95**, 695 (*synth*)
Hüttell, R. *et al*, *Chem. Ber.*, 1964, **97**, 2037 (*pmr*)
Trost, B.M. *et al*, *Tetrahedron Lett.*, 1974, 2603 (*synth, pmr*)
Ito, Y. *et al*, *Tetrahedron Lett.*, 1977, 1009 (*use*)
Senda, Y. *et al*, *Bull. Chem. Soc. Jpn.*, 1977, **50**, 1608 (*cmr*)
Trost, B.M. *et al*, *J. Am. Chem. Soc.*, 1978, **100**, 3407 (*synth*)

$C_{12}H_{18}Cl_2Pd_2$ Pd-00077

Di-μ-chlorobis(η^3-2-methylenecyclopentyl)dipalladium, 10CI

Di-μ-chlorobis(1,2-trimethylene-π-allyl)dipalladium

[53789-96-1]

M 446.020
Bridged dimer. Yellow solid. Mp 129-30° dec.

Monomer: Chloro(methylenecyclopentyl)palladium.
C_6H_9ClPd M 223.010
Unknown.

Kikukawa, K. *et al*, *J. Organomet. Chem.*, 1974, **77**, 131 (*pmr, synth*)
Trost, B.M. *et al*, *Tetrahedron Lett.*, 1974, 2603 (*pmr*)
Trost, B.M. *et al*, *J. Am. Chem. Soc.*, 1978, **100**, 3407 (*synth*)

$C_{12}H_{18}N_6Pd_2^{\oplus\oplus}$ Pd-00078

Hexakis(isocyanomethane)dipalladium(2+), 9CI

Hexakis(methylisonitrile)dipalladium(2+). Hexakis(methyl isocyanide)dipalladium(2+)

[56116-47-3]

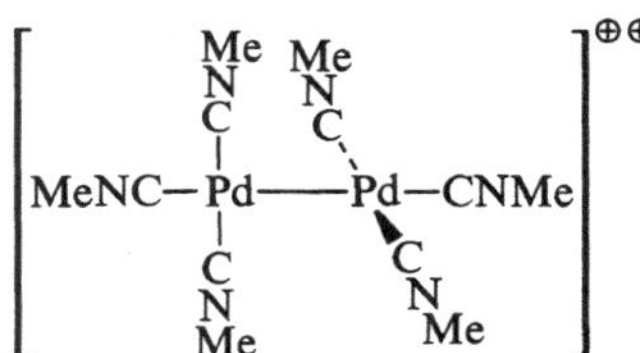

M 459.154 (ion)

Dibromide: [59561-02-3].
$C_{12}H_{18}Br_2N_6Pd_2$ M 618.962
Air-sensitive white powder.

Dichloride: [59561-01-2].
$C_{12}H_{18}Cl_2N_6Pd_2$ M 530.060

White solid.
Bis(hexafluorophosphate): [56116-48-4].
$C_{12}H_{18}F_{12}N_6P_2Pd_2$ M 749.083
Yellow cryst. (Me_2CO/2-propanol or Me_2CO/Et_2O). Forms yellow cryst. 2:1 Me_2CO complex.

Boehm, J.R. *et al*, *J. Am. Chem. Soc.*, 1976, **98**, 4845 (*synth, ir, pmr*)
Goldberg, S.Z. *et al*, *Inorg. Chem.*, 1976, **15**, 535 (*struct*)
Rettig, M.F. *et al*, *J. Organomet. Chem.*, 1976, **111**, 113 (*synth, ir, pmr*)
Garciafigueroa, E. *et al*, *Nouv. J. Chim.*, 1978, **2**, 593 (*ir, raman, struct*)

$C_{12}H_{22}Cl_2O_2Pd_2$ Pd-00079

Di-μ-chlorobis[(1,2,3-η)-4-hydroxy-1-methyl-1-pentenyl]dipalladium, 9CI
Di-μ-chlorobis[(2,3,4-η)-5-hydroxy-3-hexen-2-yl]dipalladium. Di-μ-chlorobis[1-methyl-3-(1-hydroxyethyl)allyl]dipalladium
[41649-55-2]

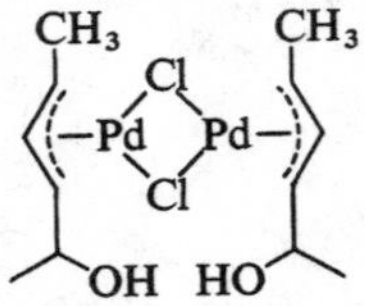

M 482.051
Bridged dimer. Yellow solid (pentane); air-stable.
Monomer: Chloro[(1,2,3-η)-4-hydroxy-1-methyl-1-pentenyl]palladium. 1-(1-Hydroxyethyl)-3-methyl-π-allylpalladium chloride.
$C_6H_{11}ClOPd$ M 241.025
Unknown.

Inorg. Synth., 1974, **15**, 75 (*synth, pmr*)

$C_{12}H_{22}Cl_2Pd_2$ Pd-00080

Di-μ-chlorobis[(1,2,3-η)-2-methyl-2-penten-1-yl]dipalladium, 9CI
Di-μ-chlorobis(1-ethyl-2-methyl-π-allyl)dipalladium, 8CI
[31666-77-0]

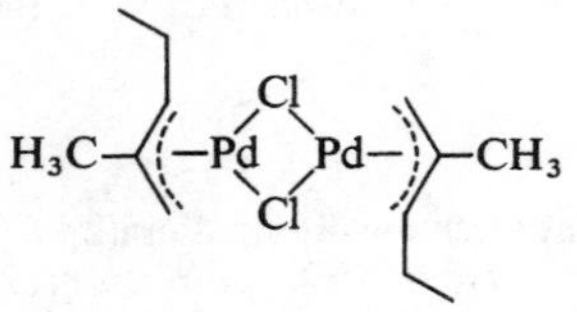

M 450.052
Yellow cryst. (CH_2Cl_2/pentane); air-stable.
Monomer: Chloro(2-methyl-2-penten-1-yl)palladium.
$C_6H_{11}ClPd$ M 225.026
Unknown.

Volger, H.C., *Recl. Trav. Chim. Pays-Bas*, 1969, **88**, 225 (*synth, pmr*)
Inorg. Synth., 1974, **15**, 75 (*synth, pmr*)

$C_{12}H_{22}Cl_2Pd_2$ Pd-00081

Di-μ-chlorobis[(2,3,4-η)-3-methyl-3-penten-2-yl]dipalladium
Di-μ-chlorobis(1,2,3-trimethyl-π-allyl)dipalladium, 8CI
[31666-78-1]

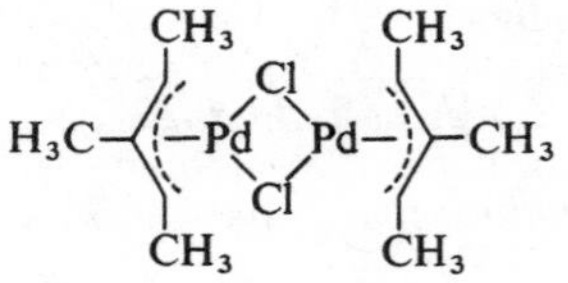

M 450.052
Yellow cryst. (CH_2Cl_2).
Monomer: Chloro(3-methyl-3-penten-2-yl)palladium. Chloro(1,2,3-trimethylallyl)palladium.
$C_6H_{11}ClPd$ M 225.026
Unknown.

Vrieze, K. *et al*, *J. Organomet. Chem.*, 1968, **12**, 533 (*pmr*)
Volger, H.C., *Recl. Trav. Chim. Pays-Bas*, 1969, **88**, 225 (*synth, pmr*)

$C_{12}H_{23}IP_2Pd$ Pd-00082

Iodo(phenyl)bis(trimethylphosphine)palladium, 9CI
Phenyliodobis(trimethylphosphine)palladium. Bis(trimethylphosphine)iodo(phenyl)palladium

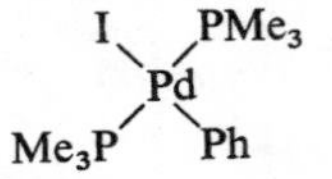

M 462.586
trans-form [68392-03-0]
Cryst. (CH_2Cl_2/Et_2O). Mp 180-3° dec.

Werner, H. *et al*, *J. Chem. Res. (S)*, 1978, 201; *J. Chem. Res. (M)*, 2720 (*synth, pmr, nmr, ms*)

$C_{12}H_{28}Cl_2N_2O_2Pd_2$ Pd-00083

Di-μ-chlorobis[3-(dimethylamino)-2-methoxypropyl]dipalladium, 8CI
Di-μ-chlorobis(2-methoxy-3-N,N-dimethylaminopropyl)dipalladium
[15152-74-6]

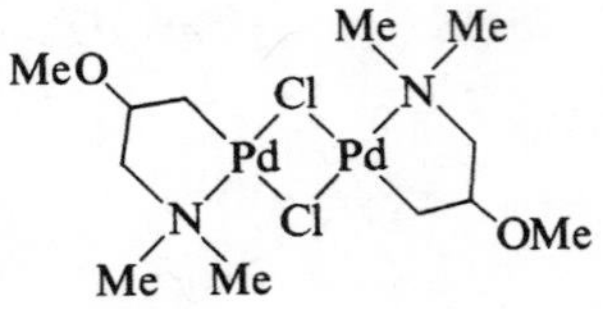

M 516.111
Yellow cryst. (MeOH). Mp 124-6° dec.

Cope, A.C. *et al*, *J. Am. Chem. Soc.*, 1967, **89**, 287 (*synth, nmr*)
Holton, R.A. *et al*, *J. Organomet. Chem.*, 1977, **133**, C5.

$C_{12}H_{31}ClP_2Pd$ Pd-00084

Chlorohydrobis(triethylphosphine)palladium, 9CI, 8CI
Chlorohydridobis(triethylphosphine)palladium. Bistriethylphosphinepalladium hydridochloride. Hydrochlorobis(triethylphosphine)palladium

$PdHCl(PEt_3)_2$ (C_{2v})

M 379.197

trans-form [18117-37-8]

Cryst. Mp 84-7° dec.

Brooks, E.H. *et al*, *J. Chem. Soc. (A)*, 1967, 1030 (*synth, ir, pmr*)
Schneider, M.L. *et al*, *J. Chem. Soc., Dalton Trans.*, 1973, 354 (*struct*)

$C_{13}H_{17}Pd^{\oplus}$ Pd-00085

[(1,2,5,6-η)-1,5-Cyclooctadiene](η⁵-2,4-cyclopentadien-1-yl-)palladium(1+), 9CI

Cyclopentadienyl(1,5-cyclooctadiene)palladium(1+)

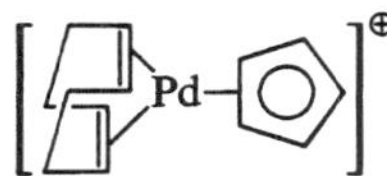

M 279.697 (ion)

Tetrafluoroborate: [35828-71-8].
$C_{13}H_{17}BF_4Pd$ M 366.501
Violet powder; air-stable.

Johnson, B.F.G. *et al*, *J. Chem. Soc. (A)*, 1970, 1738 (*synth, pmr*)
White, D.A., *Synth. Inorg. Metal-Org. Chem.*, 1971, **1**, 133 (*synth, nmr*)
Inorg. Synth., 1972, **13**, 55 (*synth, ir, pmr*)

$C_{13}H_{18}O_2Pd$ Pd-00086

[(1,2,3-η)-2,4-Cyclooctadien-1-yl](2,4-pentanedionato-*O,O'*)palladium, 9CI

Acetylacetonato(2,4-cyclooctadienyl)palladium

[12130-90-4]

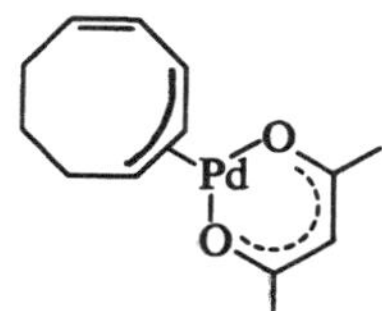

M 312.704

Yellow cryst. (pet. ether). Mp 93-5°.

Robinson, S.D. *et al*, *J. Chem. Soc.*, 1964, 5002 (*synth, pmr, uv*)
Churchill, M.R., *J. Chem. Soc., Chem. Commun.*, 1965, 625 (*struct*)
Mann, B.E. *et al*, *J. Chem. Soc., Dalton Trans.*, 1973, 2390 (*cmr*)

$C_{13}H_{19}O_2Pd^{\oplus}$ Pd-00087

[(1,2,5,6-η)-1,5-Cyclooctadiene](2,4-pentadionato-*O,O'*)palladium(1+), 9CI

(Acetylacetonato)(1,5-cyclooctadiene)palladium(1+). 2,4-Pentanedionato(1,5-cyclooctadiene)palladium(1+)

M 313.712 (ion)

Tetrafluoroborate: [31724-99-9].
$C_{13}H_{19}BF_4O_2Pd$ M 400.516
Deep-yellow cryst. (Et_2O).

Johnson, B.F.G. *et al*, *J. Chem. Soc. (A)*, 1970, 1738 (*synth, ir, pmr*)
White, D.A., *Synth. Inorg. Metal-Org. Chem.*, 1971, **1**, 133 (*synth, pmr*)

$C_{13}H_{30}BrF_3P_2Pd$ Pd-00088

Bromobis(triethylphosphine)(trifluoromethyl)palladium, 9CI

Bis(triethylphosphine)trifluoromethylpalladium bromide. Trifluoromethyl(bromo)bis(triethylphosphine)palladium

M 491.647

trans-form [52518-66-8]

Cryst. (MeOH). Mp 96-7°.

Klabunde, K.J. *et al*, *J. Am. Chem. Soc.*, 1974, **96**, 7674 (*synth, ir, pmr, ms*)

$C_{13}H_{30}ClOP_2Pd^{\oplus}$ Pd-00089

Carbonylchlorobis(triethylphosphine)palladium(1+), 8CI

Chlorocarbonylbis(triethylphosphine)palladium. Carbonylbis(triethylphosphine)palladium(II) chloride

M 406.200 (ion)

trans-form

Tetrafluoroborate: [19644-52-1].
$C_{13}H_{30}BClF_4OP_2Pd$ M 493.004
Yellow cryst. ($CHCl_3$/cyclohexane); very unstable.

Clark, H.C. *et al*, *J. Am. Chem. Soc.*, 1969, **91**, 596 (*synth, ir*)

$C_{13}H_{33}BrP_2Pd$ Pd-00090

Bromomethylbis(triethylphosphine)palladium, 9CI

Bis(triethylphosphine)methylpalladium bromide. Methylbromobis(triethylphosphine)palladium

[29158-92-7]

$PdBrMe(PEt_3)_2$

M 437.675

trans-form

Cryst. (hexane). Mp 73-4° dec.

Calvin, G. *et al*, *J. Chem. Soc.*, 1960, 2008 (*synth, ir*)

$C_{14}F_{10}N_2Pd^{\ominus\ominus}$ Pd-00091

Dicyanobis(pentafluorophenyl)palladate(2−)

Bis(cyano-C)bis(pentafluorophenyl)palladate(2−), 9CI

cis-form

M 492.571 (ion)

cis-form

Bis(tetrabutylammonium) salt: [76109-07-4].
$C_{46}H_{72}F_{10}N_4Pd$ M 977.506

White solid (Me_2CO).

trans-form

Bis(benzyltriphenylphosphonium) salt: [76083-08-4].

$C_{64}H_{44}F_{10}N_2P_2Pd$ M 1199.417

White solid (Et_2O).

Uson, R. *et al*, *J. Organomet. Chem.*, 1980, **199**, 111 (*synth*, *ir*)

$C_{14}H_8Cl_2F_{10}N_2Pd$ Pd-00092

Dichloro(1,2-ethanediamine-*N,N'*)bis(pentafluorophenyl)palladium, 9CI

Dichloro(1,2-diaminoethane)bis(pentafluorophenyl)-palladium

[57204-17-8]

$[(H_2NCH_2CH_2NH_2)PdCl_2(C_6F_5)_2]$ (O_h)

M 571.541

Yellow, air-stable cryst. (Et_2O). Sol. Me_2CO, CH_2Cl_2, $MeNO_2$, sl. sol. C_6H_6, Et_2O, insol. H_2O. Mp 213-5° dec. Stereochem. not specified.

Uson, R. *et al*, *J. Organomet. Chem.*, 1975, **96**, 307 (*synth*, *ir*)

$C_{14}H_8F_{10}N_2Pd$ Pd-00093

(1,2-Ethanediamine-*N,N'*)bis(pentafluorophenyl)palladium, 9CI

(1,2-Diaminoethane)bis(pentafluorophenyl)palladium. (Ethylenediamine)bis(pentafluorophenyl)palladium. Bis(pentafluorophenyl)ethylenediaminepalladium

[54845-68-0]

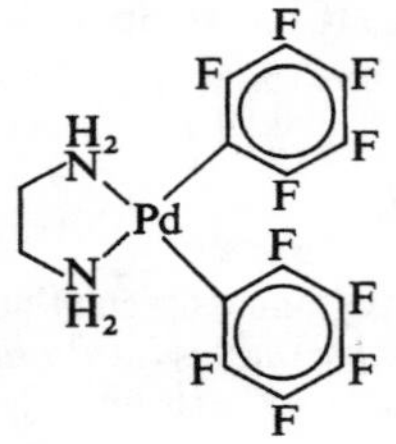

M 500.635

Solid; air-stable. Mp 238° dec.

Usón, R. *et al*, *J. Organomet. Chem.*, 1974, **81**, 115 (*synth*, *ir*)

$C_{14}H_{10}Cl_2N_2Pd$ Pd-00094

Bis(benzonitrile)dichloropalladium, 10CI, 9CI

Dichlorobis(cyanobenzene)palladium. Bis(benzonitrile)-palladium dichloride

[14220-64-5]

$(PhCN)_2PdCl_2$

M 383.572

Source of Pd complexes, catalyst for hydrogenations, hydrosilylations and isomerisations. Light-yellow needles (C_6H_6).

▷ATP-ase inhibitor

cis-form [39958-10-6]

Not separately characterised.

trans-form [15617-18-2]

Not separately characterised.

Kharasch, M.S. *et al*, *J. Am. Chem. Soc.*, 1938, **60**, 882 (*synth*)
Holden, J.R. *et al*, *Acta Crystallogr.*, 1956, **9**, 194 (*struct*)
Inorg. Synth., 1960, **6**, 218 (*synth*)
Walton, R.A., *Spectrochim. Acta*, 1965, **21**, 1795 (*ir*)
Becker, W.D. *et al*, *Z. Naturforsch., B*, 1970, **25**, 1332 (*nmr*)
Dietl, H. *et al*, *J. Am. Chem. Soc.*, 1970, **92**, 2276 (*ir*)
Fieser, M. *et al*, *Reagents for Organic Synthesis*, Wiley, 1967-83, **1**, 56; **5**, 31; **6**, 45.

$C_{14}H_{10}Cl_2N_2Pd$ Pd-00095

Dichlorobis(isocyanobenzene)palladium, 9CI

Dichlorobis(phenyl isocyanide)palladium. Dichlorobis-(phenyl isonitrile)palladium

[41762-42-9]

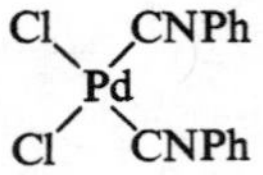

M 383.572

Catalyses reduction of nitrobenzene to aniline, and synthesis of aryl polyisocyanates.

cis-form [40927-17-1]

Yellow solid ($CHCl_3/Et_2O$).

Crociani, B. *et al*, *Inorg. Chem.*, 1970, **9**, 2021 (*synth*, *ir*)
Mondal, T.K. *et al*, *Indian J. Chem., Sect. A*, 1980, **19**, 846 (*use*)

$C_{14}H_{10}N_2Pd$ Pd-00096

Bis(isocyanobenzene)palladium, 9CI

Bis(phenylisocyanide)palladium. Bis(phenylisonitrile)-palladium

[41021-81-2]

$Pd(CNPh)_2$

M 312.666

Dark-brown cryst. (EtOH aq.). Insol. all solvs. except isonitriles, quinoline, Py, $PhNO_2$. Dec. at 170-90°.

Malatesta, L., *J. Chem. Soc.*, 1955, 3924 (*synth*)
Boschi, T. *et al*, *J. Organomet. Chem.*, 1971, **30**, 283 (*ir*)

$C_{14}H_{20}OPd$ Pd-00097

(η^5-2,4-Cyclopentadien-1-yl)[(1,4,5-η)-8-methoxy-4-cyclooc-ten-1-yl]palladium, 9CI

(8-Methoxy-4-cycloocten-1-yl)(π-cyclopentadienyl)-palladium

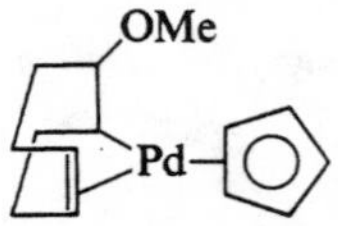

M 310.731

Pale-orange cryst. (pet. ether). Mp 62-4°.

Robinson, S.D. *et al*, *J. Chem. Soc.*, 1964, 5002 (*synth*, *uv*, *pmr*)

$C_{14}H_{22}Br_2Pd_2$ Pd-00098

Di-μ-bromobis[(1,2,3-η)-2-cyclohepten-1-yl]dipalladium, 9CI

Di-μ-bromodi-π-2-cyclohepten-1-yldipalladium, 8CI. Di-μ-bromobis[(1,2,3-η)cycloheptenylpalladium]

[33180-60-8]

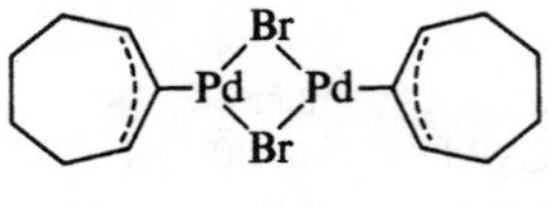

M 562.976

Cryst. ($Et_2O/CHCl_3$). Mp 160-2° dec.

Monomer: Bromo(2-cyclohepten-1-yl)palladium.

$C_7H_{11}BrPd$ M 281.488

Unknown.

Kilbourn, B.T. *et al*, *J. Chem. Soc.*, *Chem. Commun.*, 1968, 1438 (*struct*)
Quinn, H.A. *et al*, *J. Chem. Soc.*, *Dalton Trans.*, 1972, 180 (*synth*, *pmr*)

$C_{14}H_{22}Cl_2N_2Pd$ **Pd-00099**

Dichlorobis(isocyanocyclohexane)palladium, 9CI
Dichlorobis(cyclohexylisocyanide)palladium, 8CI. *Dichlorobis(cyclohexylisonitrile)palladium*
[29827-46-1]

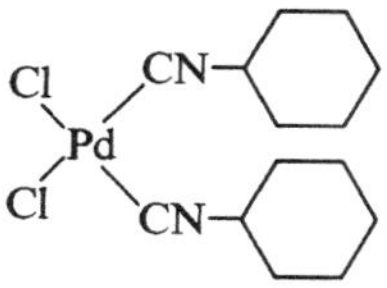

M 395.667

cis-form

Catalyses hydrosilylation of dienes. Yellow cryst. (hexane/C_6H_6). Mp 112-5° (110°).

Crociani, B. *et al*, *Inorg. Chem.*, 1970, **9**, 2021 (*synth*, *ir*)
Fukui, M. *et al*, *Synth. React. Inorg. Metal-Org. Chem.*, 1975, **5**, 207 (*synth*)
Langova, J. *et al*, *Collect. Czech. Chem. Commun.*, 1975, **40**, 432 (*use*)
Vaisarova, V. *et al*, *Collect. Czech. Chem. Commun.*, 1976, **41**, 1906 (*use*)
Kitano, Y. *et al*, *Acta Crystallogr.*, *Sect. B*, 1981, **37**, 1919 (*struct*)

$C_{14}H_{22}Cl_2O_2Pd_2$ **Pd-00100**

Di-μ-chlorobis[(1,2,3-η)-6-methoxy-2-cyclohexen-1-yl]dipalladium
Di-μ-chlorodi-(4-methoxy-2-cyclohexenyl)dipalladium
[12129-98-5]

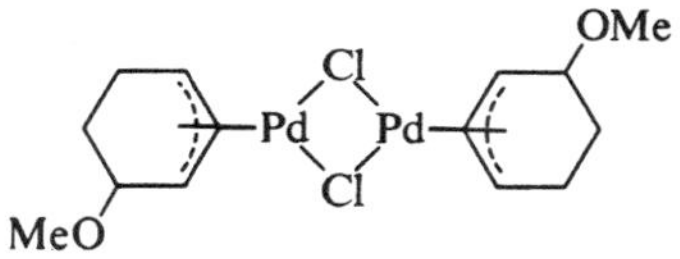

M 506.073
Pale-yellow cryst. (MeOH aq.). Mp 87-91° dec.

Robinson, S.D. *et al*, *J. Chem. Soc.*, 1964, 5002 (*synth*, *ir*, *pmr*, *uv*)

$C_{14}H_{22}Cl_2Pd_2$ **Pd-00101**

Di-μ-chlorobis[(1,2,3-η)-2-methyl-2-cyclohexen-1-yl]dipalladium, 10CI
[32915-13-2]

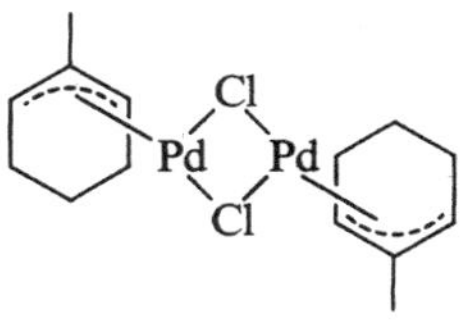

M 474.074
Bridged dimer. Solid. Mp 88-90° dec.
Monomer: Chloro(2-methylcyclohexenyl)palladium.
$C_7H_{11}ClPd$ M 237.037
Unknown.

Huttel, R. *et al*, *Chem. Ber.*, 1964, **97**, 2037 (*synth*, *uv*, *pmr*)
Senda, Y. *et al*, *Bull. Chem. Soc. Jpn.*, 1977, **50**, 1608 (*cmr*)
Trost, B.M. *et al*, *J. Am. Chem. Soc.*, 1978, **100**, 3407 (*synth*, *pmr*)

$C_{14}H_{22}Cl_2Pd_2$ **Pd-00102**

Di-μ-chlorobis(η^3-2-methylenecyclohexyl)dipalladium, 10CI
Di-μ-chlorobis(1,2-tetramethylene-π-allyl)palladium
[53789-97-2]

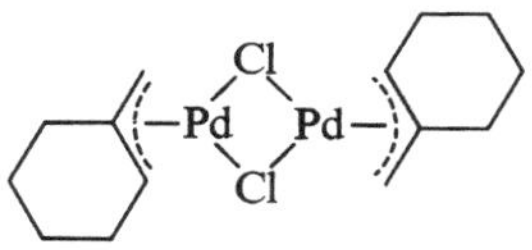

M 474.074
Bridged dimer. Yellow cryst. (hexane). Mp 131-8° dec.
Monomer: Chloro(2-methylenecyclohexyl)palladium.
$C_7H_{11}ClPd$ M 237.037
Unknown.

Senda, Y. *et al*, *Bull. Chem. Soc. Jpn.*, 1977, **50**, 1608 (*cmr*)
Trost, B.M. *et al*, *J. Am. Chem. Soc.*, 1978, **100**, 3407 (*synth*, *pmr*)

$C_{14}H_{22}N_2Pd$ **Pd-00103**

Bis(cyclohexylisonitrile)palladium
Bis(cyclohexyl isocyanide)palladium
[50701-23-0]

$[Pd(CNC_6H_{11})_2]$

M 324.761
Catalyst for polymerisation or cyclisation of unsaturated compds. Yellow cryst. (pentane). Mp 107-10° dec.

Fischer, E.O. *et al*, *Chem. Ber.*, 1962, **95**, 703 (*synth*)

$C_{14}H_{26}BrPPd$ **Pd-00104**

Bromo-π-cyclopentadienyl(triisopropylphosphine)palladium, 8CI
Bromo(η^5-2,4-cyclopentadien-1-yl)[tris-(1-methylethyl)phosphine]palladium, 9CI. *(π-Cyclopentadienyl)-(triisopropylphosphine)palladium bromide*
[34852-80-7]

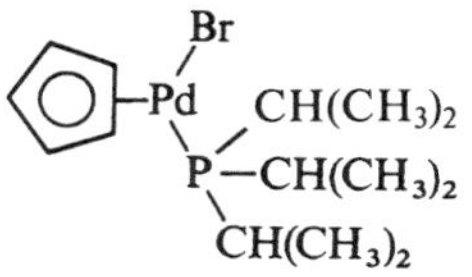

M 411.657
Green solid (C_6H_6/hexane). Mp 111-2°.

Cross, R.J. *et al*, *J. Chem. Soc. (A)*, 1971, 2000 (*synth*, *pmr*, *ir*)
Turner, G.K. *et al*, *J. Organomet. Chem.*, 1976, **121**, C29.
Felkin, H. *et al*, *J. Organomet. Chem.*, 1977, **129**, 429.

$C_{14}H_{33}As_2ClNPd^{\oplus}$ **Pd-00105**

Chloro(isocyanomethane)bis(triethylarsine)palladium(1+), 9CI
Chloro(methylisonitrile)bis(triethylarsine)-palladium(1+). Chloro(methyl isocyanide)bis(triethylarsine)palladium(1+). Isocyanomethanebis(triethylarsine)palladium(1+) chloride

$[PdCl(MeNC)(AsEt_3)_2]^{\oplus}$

M 507.138 (ion)
Hexafluoroantimonate: [37448-33-2].

$C_{14}H_{33}As_2ClF_6NPdSb$ M 742.878
Cryst. (Me_2CO/Et_2O). Mp 110-2°.

Cherwinski, W.J. *et al*, *Inorg. Chem.*, 1972, **11**, 1511 (*synth, ir*)

$C_{14}H_{33}ClNP_2Pd^{\oplus}$ Pd-00106

Chloro(isocyanomethane)bis(triethylphosphine)palladium(1+)
Chloro(methylisonitrile)bis(triethylphosphine)palladium(1+). Chloro(methyl isocyanide)bis(triethylphosphine)palladium(1+)

$[PdCl(MeNC)(PEt_3)_2]^{\oplus}$

M 419.242 (ion)

Tetrafluoroborate:
$C_{14}H_{33}BClF_4NP_2Pd$ M 506.046
Cryst. (CH_2Cl_2/Et_2O). Mp 137-9°.

Cherwinski, W.J. *et al*, *Inorg. Chem.*, 1972, **11**, 1511 (*synth*)

$C_{14}H_{33}ClOP_2Pd$ Pd-00107

Acetylchlorobis(triethylphosphine)palladium
Chloroacetylbis(triethylphosphine)palladium, 8CI

Cl PEt₃ / Pd / Et₃P COCH₃

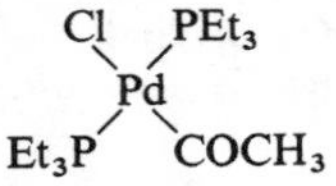

M 421.235

***trans*-form**
Cryst. (pet. ether). Mp 65-7°.

Adams, D.M. *et al*, *J. Chem. Soc.*, 1962, 1112 (*ir*)
Booth, G. *et al*, *J. Chem. Soc. (A)*, 1966, 634 (*synth*)

$C_{14}H_{36}As_2Pd$ Pd-00108

Dimethylbis(triethylarsine)palladium
Bis(triethylarsine)dimethylpalladium

Me AsEt₃ / Pd / Me AsEt₃

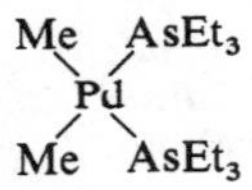

M 460.702

***cis*-form**
Cryst. (hexane/triethylarsine). Mp 49° dec.

Calvin, G. *et al*, *J. Chem. Soc.*, 1960, 2008 (*synth, ir*)

$C_{14}H_{36}P_2Pd$ Pd-00109

Dimethylbis(triethylphosphine)palladium, 9CI
Bis(triethylphosphine)dimethylpalladium
[60933-51-9]

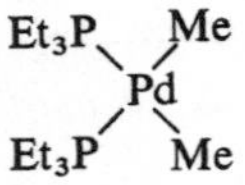

Et₃P Me / Pd / Et₃P Me *cis-form*

M 372.806

***cis*-form**
Cryst. (hexane). Mp 47-9°. Isomerises to *trans*-form over period of several months.

***trans*-form**
Cryst. (hexane). Mp 56-64° (dec. *in vacuo*), 66-7°.

Calvin, G. *et al*, *J. Chem. Soc.*, 1960, 2008 (*synth, ir*)
Ito, T. *et al*, *Bull. Chem. Soc. Jpn.*, 1977, **50**, 1319 (*synth, pmr*)

$C_{15}H_{19}ClO_2PdS$ Pd-00110

Chloro[(1,2,5,6-η)-1,5-cyclooctadiene][(phenylsulfonyl)methyl]palladium, 9CI
(1,5-Cyclooctadiene)phenylsulfonylmethanato)chloropalladium
[55451-36-0]

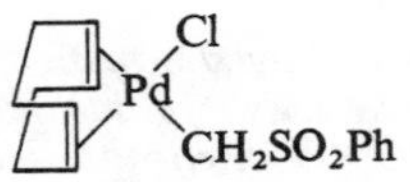

Cl / Pd / CH_2SO_2Ph

M 405.247
Cryst. Dec. at 70° in DMSO.

Julia, M. *et al*, *Tetrahedron Lett.*, 1974, 3443 (*synth*)
Benchekroun, L. *et al*, *J. Organomet. Chem.*, 1977, **128**, 275 (*struct*)

$C_{15}H_{35}BrP_2Pd$ Pd-00111

Bromo(2-propenyl)bis(triethylphosphine)palladium, 9CI
Allyl(bromo)bis(triethylphosphine)palladium. Bromo(enyl)bis(triethylphosphine)palladium
[56960-35-1]

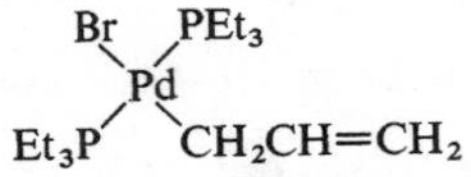

Br PEt₃ / Pd / Et₃P CH₂CH=CH₂

M 463.713

***trans*-form** [70774-42-4]
Cryst. (hexane). Mp 67-9° dec.

Schunn, R.A., *Inorg. Chem.*, 1976, **15**, 208 (*synth*)

$C_{15}H_{35}P_2Pd^{\oplus}$ Pd-00112

(η^3-2-Propenyl)bis(triethylphosphine)palladium(1+), 9CI
π-Allylbis(triethylphosphine)palladium(1+). Enylbis(triethylphosphine)palladium(1+). Bis(triethylphosphine)allylpalladium(1+)

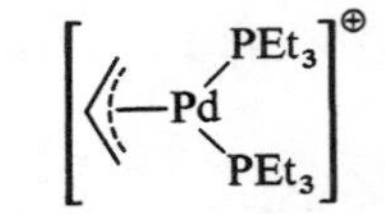

[Pd PEt₃ PEt₃]⊕

M 383.809 (ion)

Chloride: [34675-89-3]. *π-Allylchlorobis(triethylphosphine)palladium, 8CI.*
$C_{15}H_{35}ClP_2Pd$ M 419.262
Catalyses selective hydrogenation of conjugated polyolefins.

Tetraphenylborate: [50723-54-1].
$C_{39}H_{55}BP_2Pd$ M 703.041
Cryst. Mp 108-10°.

Acetate: [79270-06-7].
$C_{17}H_{38}O_2P_2Pd$ M 442.854
No physical data available.

Deeming, A.J. *et al*, *J. Chem. Soc., Dalton Trans.*, 1973, 1848 (*synth, ir, pmr*)
Yamamoto, T. *et al*, *J. Am. Chem. Soc.*, 1981, **103**, 5600 (*synth*)

$C_{16}F_{18}O_4Pd_4$ Pd-00113

Tetracarbonyltris(hexafluoro-2-butyne)tetrapalladium
Tris(hexafluoro-2-butyne)tetracarbonyltetrapalladium

$Pd_4(CO)_4(F_3CC{\equiv}CCF_3)_3$

M 1023.825

Dark red-purple cryst., v. labile hexafluorobutyne ligand. Mp 90-2° (darkens at 80°).

Klabunde, K.J. *et al*, *J. Am. Chem. Soc.*, 1978, **100**, 4437 (*synth, ir, nmr*)

$C_{16}H_6Cl_2F_{10}N_2Pd_2$ Pd-00114

Di-μ-chlorobis(isocyanomethane)bis(pentafluorophenyl)dipalladium

Di-μ-chlorobis(methylisonitrile)bis(pentafluorophenyl-)dipalladium

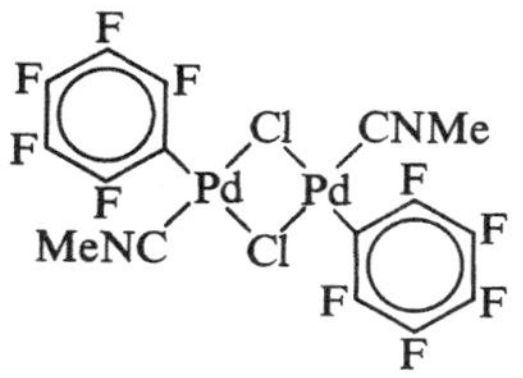

M 699.967

Bridged dimer. Microcrystalline powder (CH_2Cl_2).

Monomer: Chloro(isocyanomethane)-(pentafluorophenyl)palladium.
$C_8H_3ClF_5NPd$ M 349.983
Unknown.

Uson, R. *et al*, *J. Chem. Soc., Dalton Trans.*, 1982, 2389 (*synth, ir*)

$C_{16}H_6F_{10}N_2Pd$ Pd-00115

Bis(isocyanomethane)bis(pentafluorophenyl)palladium

Bis(methylisonitrile)bis(pentafluorophenyl)palladium

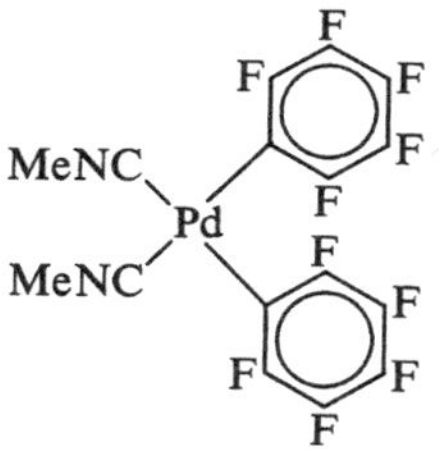

cis-form

M 522.641

Solid. Isomeric configuration not determined.

Uson, R. *et al*, *J. Chem. Soc., Dalton Trans.*, 1982, 2389 (*synth, ir*)

$C_{16}H_8ClF_5N_2Pd$ Pd-00116

(2,2′-Bipyridine-*N,N′*)chloro(pentafluorophenyl)palladium, 9CI

(Pentafluorophenyl)chloro(2,2′-bipyridine)palladium

[60101-93-1]

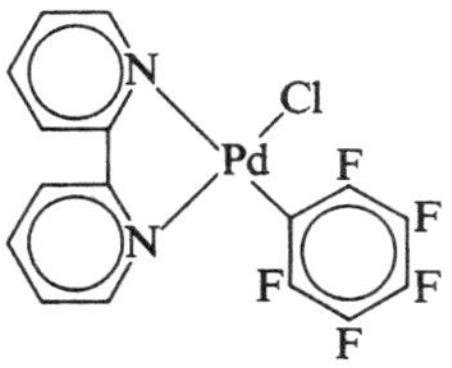

M 465.118

Yellow solid ($CHCl_3$/pet. ether). Mp 285° dec.

Uson, R. *et al*, *Synth. React. Inorg. Met.-Org. Chem.*, 1977, **7**, 235 (*synth, ir*)

$C_{16}H_8Cl_3F_5N_2Pd$ Pd-00117

(2,2′-Bipyridine-*N,N′*)trichloro(pentafluorophenyl)palladium, 9CI

(Pentafluorophenyl)trichloro(2,2′-bypyridine)palladium

[64424-50-6]

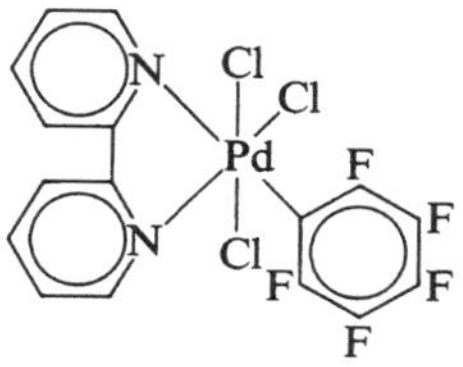

M 536.024

Air-stable, dark-yellow cryst. (C_6H_6). Mp 190° dec.

Uson, R. *et al*, *Synth. React. Inorg. Met.-Org. Chem.*, 1977, **7**, 235 (*synth, ir*)

$C_{16}H_8F_{14}N_2Pd$ Pd-00118

(2,2′-Bipyridine)bis(heptafluoropropyl)palladium

(2,2′-Bipyridine-N,N′)bis(perfluoropropyl)palladium.
Bis(heptafluoropropyl)(2,2′-bipyridine)palladium

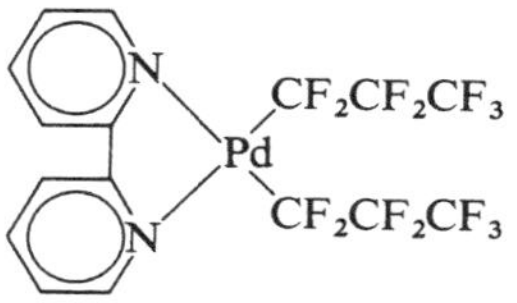

M 600.650

Pale-yellow needles (EtOH). Mp 180-1°.

Maitlis, P.M. *et al*, *Chem. Ind. (London)*, 1962, 1865 (*synth, ir*)

$C_{16}H_{14}Cl_4N_2Pd_2$ Pd-00119

Di-μ-chlorodichlorobis(1-isocyano-4-methylbenzene)dipalladium, 9CI

Di-μ-chlorodichlorobis(p-tolylisonitrile)dipalladium.
Di-μ-chlorodichlorobis(4-methylphenylisonitrile)dipalladium

[54936-74-2]

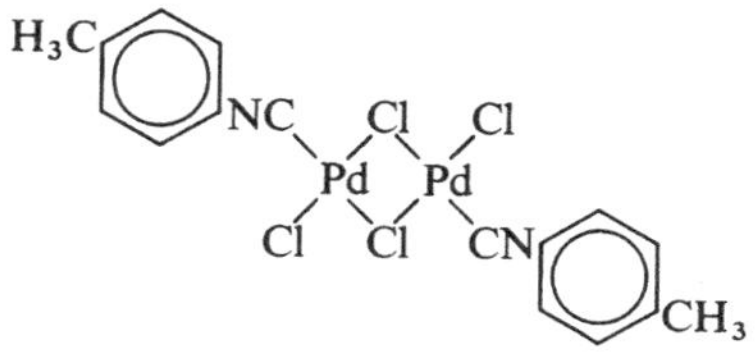

M 588.952

Yellow cryst. (CH_2Cl_2/Et_2O/pet. ether). Mp 236° dec.

Monomer: Dichloro(1-isocyano-4-methylbenzene)-palladium.
$C_8H_7Cl_2NPd$ M 294.476
Unknown.

Boschi, T. *et al*, *Inorg. Chim. Acta*, 1975, **12**, 39 (*synth, ir*)
Calligaro, L. *et al*, *J. Organomet. Chem.*, 1977, **142**, 105.

$C_{16}H_{16}Cl_4Pd_2$ **Pd-00120**

Di-μ-chlorodichlorobis(styrene)dipalladium, 8CI

Di-μ-chlorodichlorobis[(η^2-ethenyl)benzene]dipalladium, 9CI. *Di-μ-chlorodichlorobis(phenylethene)dipalladium*

[12257-72-6]

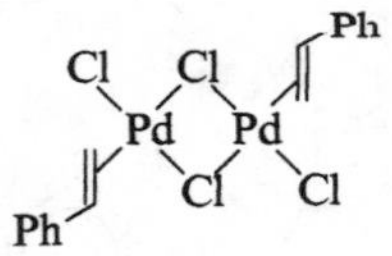

M 562.954

Catalyses conversion of nitromesitylene to mesitylene isonitrile. Red-brown.

Monomer:

$C_8H_8Cl_2Pd$ M 281.477

Unknown.

Kharasch, M.S. *et al*, *J. Am. Chem. Soc.*, 1938, **60**, 882 (*synth*)

Tietz, H. *et al*, *Z. Chem.*, 1980, **20**, 295 (*use*)

$C_{16}H_{18}Pd_2$ **Pd-00121**

[μ-[η^3:η^3-2,3-Bismethylene-1,4-butanediyl]]bis(η^5-2,4-cyclopentadien-1-yl)dipalladium, 9CI

Di-π-cyclopentadienyl[μ-(π_2-2,3-dimethylenetetramethylene)]dipalladium, 8CI

[42161-77-3]

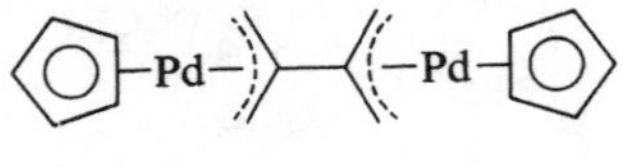

M 423.158

Red needles (pet. ether). Mp 130-50° dec.

Hughes, R.P. *et al*, *J. Organomet. Chem.*, 1973, **54**, 345 (*synth, pmr*)

$C_{16}H_{22}Cl_2O_2Pd_2$ **Pd-00122**

Di-μ-chlorobis[(2,5,6-η)-3-methoxybicyclo[2.2.1]hept-5-en-2-yl]dipalladium, 9CI

Di-μ-chlorobis[methoxynorbornenyl]dipalladium. Di-μ-chlorobis(6-methoxybicyclo[2.2.1]hept-2-ene-5σ,2π-)palladium

[52520-35-1]

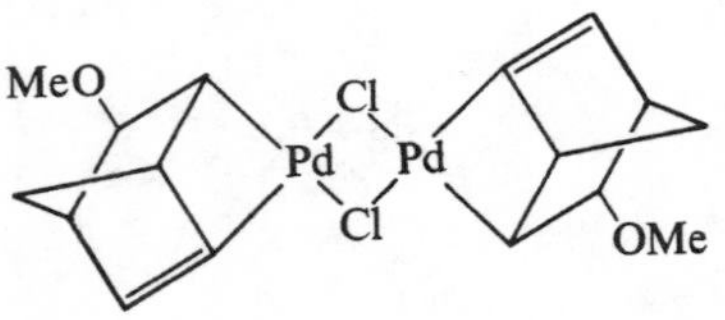

M 530.095

Intermed. in ketenimine synth.; catalyses dimerization of norbornadiene. Pale-yellow solid (Et_2O). Mp 108-11° dec. Undergoes carbonylation to ester.

Monomer:

$C_8H_{11}ClOPd$ M 265.047

Unknown.

Stille, J.K. *et al*, *J. Am. Chem. Soc.*, 1966, **88**, 5135 (*synth, cmr*)

Green, M. *et al*, *J. Chem. Soc. (A)*, 1967, 2054 (*synth, ir, pmr*)

Hines, L.F. *et al*, *J. Am. Chem. Soc.*, 1972, **94**, 485.

Kiji, J. *et al*, *Bull. Chem. Soc. Jpn.*, 1974, **47**, 2523 (*use*)

Parker, G. *et al*, *J. Organomet. Chem.*, 1974, **67**, 131 (*pmr*)

Ito, Y. *et al*, *Tetrahedron Lett.*, 1977, 1009 (*use*)

$C_{16}H_{22}Cl_2Pd_2$ **Pd-00123**

Di-μ-chlorobis[(1,5,6-η)-2,5-cyclooctadien-1-yl]dipalladium, 9CI

Di-μ-chlorodi-π-cyclooctadienyldipalladium, 8CI

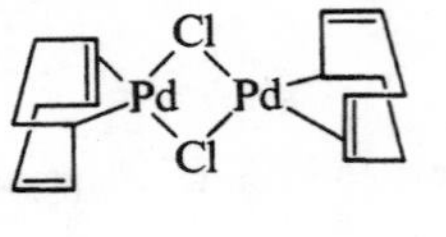

M 498.096

Air-stable cryst.

Dimer: Chloro(2,5-cyclooctadiene)palladium. (2,5-Cyclooctadiene)palladium chloride.

$C_8H_{11}ClPd$ M 249.048

Unknown.

Agami, C. *et al*, *J. Organomet. Chem.*, 1972, **35**, C59 (*synth, ir, raman*)

Dahan, F., *Acta Crystallogr., Sect. B*, 1976, **B32**, 1941 (*struct*)

$C_{16}H_{22}O_4Pd_2$ **Pd-00124**

[μ-[η^3:η^3-2,3-Bismethylene-1,4-butanediyl]]bis(2,4-pentanedionato-*O,O'*)dipalladium, 9CI

[μ-(π_2-2,3-Dimethylenetetramethylene)]bis(2,4-pentanedionato)dipalladium, 8CI

[33012-05-4]

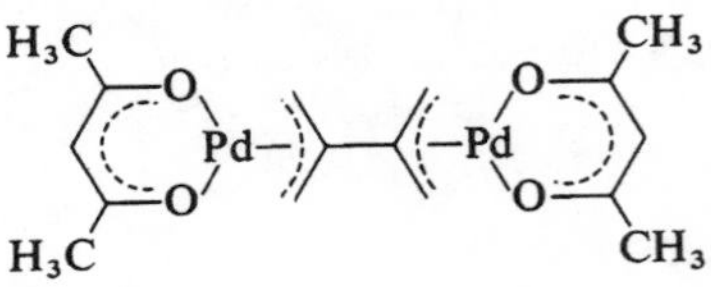

M 491.187

Cryst. ($CHCl_3$/pet. ether). Mp >185° dec.

Hughes, R.P. *et al*, *J. Organomet. Chem.*, 1969, **20**, P17; 1973, **54**, 345 (*synth, pmr*)

$C_{16}H_{24}Cl_2Pd_2^{\oplus\oplus}$ **Pd-00125**

Di-μ-chlorobis[(1,2,5,6-η)-1,5-cyclooctadiene]dipalladium(2+), 9CI

Di-μ-chlorobis[(η-1,5-cyclooctadiene)palladium](2+)

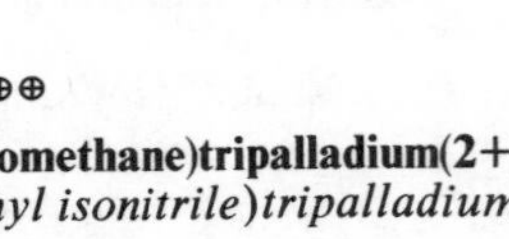

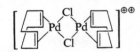

M 500.112 (ion)

Bis(tetrafluoroborate): [59687-80-8].

$C_{16}H_{24}B_2Cl_2F_8Pd_2$ M 673.719

Yellow cryst. (CH_2Cl_2). Mp 128-32° dec.

Eaborn, C. *et al*, *J. Chem. Soc., Dalton Trans.*, 1976, 289 (*synth, ir*)

$C_{16}H_{24}N_8Pd_3^{\oplus\oplus}$ **Pd-00126**

Octakis(isocyanomethane)tripalladium(2+), 9CI

Octakis(methyl isonitrile)tripalladium(2+)

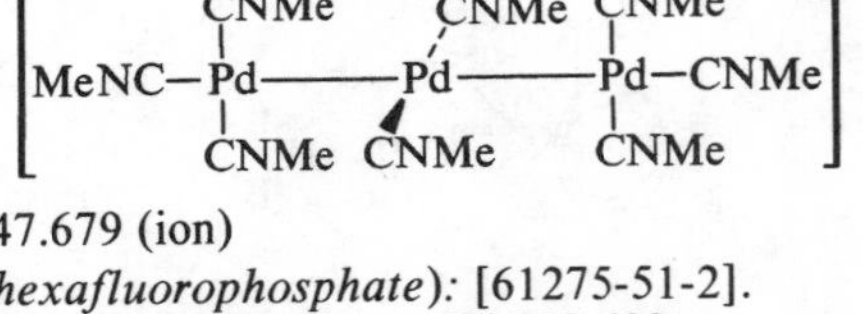

M 647.679 (ion)

Bis(hexafluorophosphate): [61275-51-2].

$C_{16}H_{24}F_{12}N_8P_2Pd_3$ M 937.608

No physical data available.

Balch, A.L. *et al*, *J. Am. Chem. Soc.*, 1976, **98**, 7431 (*synth, ir, pmr*)

Clark, R.J.H. *et al*, *Nouv. J. Chim.*, 1980, **4**, 287 (*ir, raman*)

$C_{16}H_{24}Pd$ Pd-00127

Bis[(1,2,5,6-η)-1,5-cyclooctadiene]palladium, 9CI
[57811-65-1]

M 322.786
Catalyses oligomerisation and telomerisation of butadiene, addition of amines to 1,3-dienes, and cyclooligomerisation of dimethyl cyclopropene. Unstable cryst.

Atkins, R.M. *et al*, *J. Chem. Soc., Chem. Commun.*, 1975, 764 (*synth, ir*)

$C_{16}H_{26}Cl_2Pd_2$ Pd-00128

Di-μ-chlorobis(η³-2-ethylidenecyclohexyl)dipalladium, 10CI
Di-μ-chlorobis(1-methyl-2,3-tetramethylene-π-allyl)dipalladium
[54634-17-2]

M 502.127
Bridged dimer. Yellow cryst. (hexane). Mp 123-9° dec.
Monomer: Chloro(ethylidenecyclohexyl)palladium.
$C_8H_{13}ClPd$ M 251.064
Unknown.

Trost, B.M. *et al*, *Tetrahedron Lett.*, 1974, 2603.
Trost, B.M. *et al*, *J. Am. Chem. Soc.*, 1978, **100**, 3407 (*synth*)

$C_{16}H_{29}O_2PPd$ Pd-00129

Acetato(cyclopentadienyl)triisopropylphosphinepalladium
(Acetato-O)(η⁵-2,4-cyclopentadien-1-yl)[tris(1-methylethyl)phosphine]palladium, 9CI. *(η⁵-2,4-Cyclopentadien-1-yl)(ethanoato)[tris-(1-methylethyl)phosphine]-palladium*
[72981-40-9]

OAc, Pd, CH(CH₃)₂, P, (H₃C)₂CH, CH(CH₃)₂

M 390.798
No physical data available.

Werner, H. *et al*, *J. Chem. Soc., Chem. Commun.*, 1979, 814 (*synth, pmr*)

$C_{16}H_{32}OP_3Pd^{\oplus}$ Pd-00130

Benzoyltris(trimethylphosphine)palladium(1+)

$(Me_3P)_3PdCOPh^{\oplus}$

M 439.769 (ion)
Tetraphenylborate: [68391-71-9].
$C_{40}H_{52}BOP_3Pd$ M 759.001
Cryst. (CH_2Cl_2/Et_2O).

Werner, H. *et al*, *J. Chem. Res. (S)*, 1978, 201; *J. Chem. Res. (M)*, 2720 (*synth, pmr, nmr*)

$C_{16}H_{37}P_2Pd^{\oplus}$ Pd-00131

[(1,2,3-η)-2-Butenyl]bis(triethylphosphine)palladium(1+), 9CI
(1-Methylallyl)bis(triethylphosphine)palladium(1+).
Crotylbis(triethylphosphine)palladium(1+)

M 397.836 (ion)
Tetraphenylborate: [50982-10-0].
$C_{40}H_{57}BP_2Pd$ M 717.068
Cryst. (MeOH). Mp ca. 120° dec.

Deeming, A.J. *et al*, *J. Chem. Soc., Dalton Trans.*, 1973, 1848 (*synth*)

$C_{16}H_{37}P_2Pd^{\oplus}$ Pd-00132

[(1,2,3-η)-2-Methyl-2-propenyl]bis(triethylphosphine)palladium(1+)
(2-Methylallyl)bis(triethylphosphine)palladium(1+).
2-Methylenylbis(triethylphosphine)palladium(1+).
Bis(triethylphosphine)(2-methylallyl)palladium(1+)

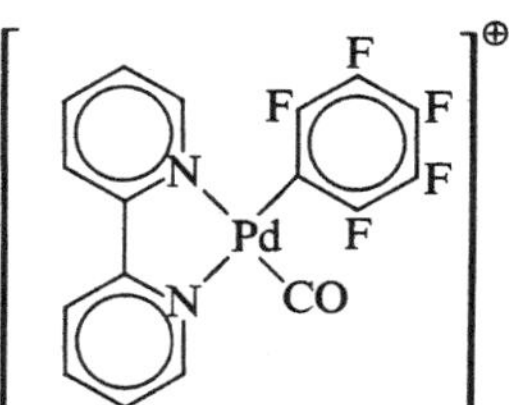

M 397.836 (ion)
Tetrafluoroborate:
$C_{16}H_{37}BF_4P_2Pd$ M 484.639
No physical data available.

Stevens, R.R. *et al*, *J. Organomet. Chem.*, 1970, **21**, 495.

$C_{17}H_8F_5N_2OPd^{\oplus}$ Pd-00133

(2,2′-Bipyridine)carbonyl(pentafluorophenyl)palladium(1+), 9CI
Pentafluorophenyl(carbonyl)(2,2′-bipyridine)palladium(1+)

M 457.675 (ion)
Perchlorate: [60102-03-6].
$C_{17}H_8ClF_5N_2O_5Pd$ M 557.126
Solid, indefinitely stable below −28°.

Usón, R. *et al*, *J. Organomet. Chem.*, 1976, **112**, 105 (*synth, ir*)

$C_{17}H_{24}O_2Pd$ Pd-00134

η³-(1,2,4,5,6-Pentamethyl-3-methylenebicyclo[2.2.0]hex-5-en-2-yl)(2,4-pentanedionato-*O,O'*)palladium

Acetylacetonato-(1,3,4,5,6-pentamethylbicyclo[2.2.0]-hexa-2,5-diene-2-methen-1-yl)palladium

[33218-71-2]

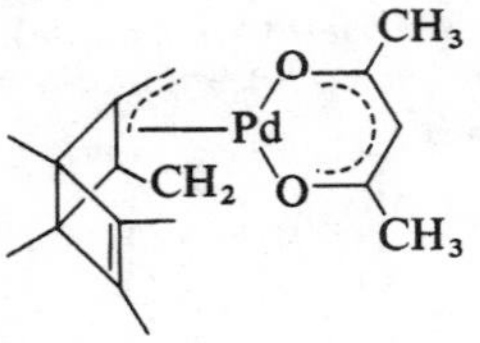

M 366.795

Pale-yellow cryst. (pet. ether). Mp 93-6°.

Shaw, B.L. *et al*, *J. Chem. Soc. (A)*, 1969, 602 (*synth, pmr*)
Malone, J.F. *et al*, *J. Chem. Soc. (A)*, 1970, 3124 (*struct*)

$C_{17}H_{25}ClP_2Pd$ Pd-00135

Chlorobis(dimethylphenylphosphine)methylpalladium, 8CI

Bis(dimethylphenylphosphine)methylpalladium chloride. Methyl(chloro)bis(dimethylphenylphosphine)-palladium

[30179-98-7]

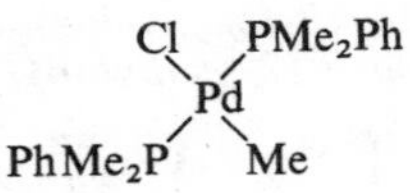

M 433.205

trans-form

Cryst. (MeOH). Mp 129-30° dec. Blackens slowly on storage.

Clark, H.C. *et al*, *Inorg. Chim. Acta*, 1970, **9**, 2670 (*synth, ir, pmr*)

$C_{17}H_{25}IP_2Pd$ Pd-00136

Bis(dimethylphenylphosphine)iodo(methyl)palladium, 9CI

Iodobis(dimethylphenylphosphine)methylpalladium. Methyl(iodo)bis(dimethylphenylphosphine)palladium

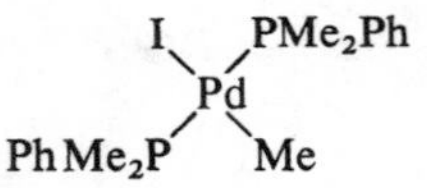

M 524.657

trans-form [42582-38-7]

Cryst. (C_6H_6/hexane). Mp 126-8° dec.

Yamamoto, Y. *et al*, *Inorg. Chem.*, 1974, **13**, 438 (*synth, pmr*)

$C_{17}H_{25}PPd$ Pd-00137

(η⁵-2,4-Cyclopentadien-1-yl)phenyl(triethylphosphine)palladium, 9CI

Phenyl(π-cyclopentadienyl)(triethylphosphine)palladium

[31741-68-1]

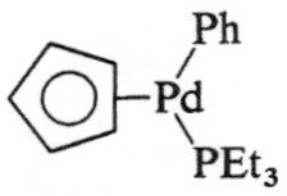

M 366.778

Unstable yellow liq. Pmr δ 5.75ppm J_{PH} 2.0Hz.

Cross, R.J., *J. Chem. Soc. (A)*, 1971, 2000.

$C_{17}H_{34}BrNP_2Pd$ Pd-00138

Bromo(2-pyridinyl)bis(triethylphosphine)palladium

Bromo(2-pyridyl)bis(triethylphosphine)palladium

[73946-35-7]

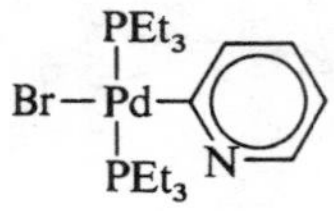

M 500.734

Cryst.

Isobe, K. *et al*, *J. Am. Chem. Soc.*, 1980, **102**, 2475 (*synth, struct, pmr, cmr*)

$C_{17}H_{34}BrNP_2Pd$ Pd-00139

Bromo(3-pyridinyl)bis(triethylphosphine)palladium

Bromo(3-pyridyl)bis(triethylphosphine)palladium

[73946-36-8]

M 500.734

Cryst.

Isobe, K. *et al*, *J. Am. Chem. Soc.*, 1980, **102**, 2475 (*synth, struct, pmr, cmr*)

$C_{17}H_{34}BrNP_2Pd$ Pd-00140

Bromo(4-pyridinyl)bis(triethylphosphine)palladium

Bromo(4-pyridyl)triethylphosphinepalladium

[73946-37-9]

M 500.734

Cryst.

Isobe, K. *et al*, *J. Am. Chem. Soc.*, 1980, **102**, 2475 (*synth, struct, pmr, cmr*)

$C_{17}H_{35}P_2Pd^{\oplus}$ Pd-00141

(η⁵-2,4-Cyclopentadien-1-yl)bis(triethylphosphine)palladium(1+), 9CI

Bis(triethylphosphine)palladium(1+) cyclopentadienyl

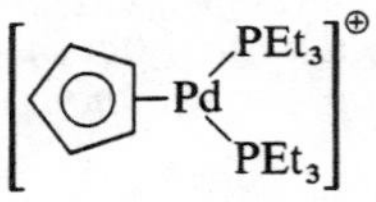

M 407.831 (ion)

Bromide: [34850-19-6].

$C_{13}H_{35}BrP_2Pd$ M 439.691

Red cryst. (CH_2Cl_2/Et_2O). Mp 87-9° dec.

Cross, R.J. *et al*, *J. Chem. Soc. (A)*, 1971, 2000.

$C_{18}H_{18}Cl_2Pd_2$ Pd-00142

Di-μ-chlorobis[(1,2,3-η)-1-phenyl-2-propenyl]dipalladium, 9CI

Di-μ-chlorobis(1-phenyl-π-allyl)dipalladium

[12131-44-1]

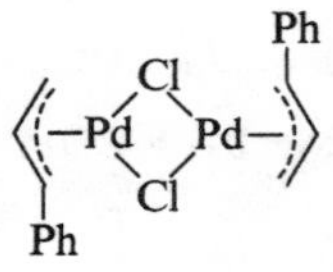

M 518.086

Cryst. ($CHCl_3$/pet. ether). Mp 195-200° (185-6°) dec.

Monomer: π-Phenylallylpalladium chloride.
C_9H_9ClPd M 259.043
Unknown.

Huttel, R., *Chem. Ber.*, 1961, **94**, 766 (*synth*)
Hegarty, B.F. *et al*, *J. Organomet. Chem.*, 1966, **6**, 578 (*uv*)
Ashraf, M.C. *et al*, *Aust. J. Chem.*, 1976, **29**, 2643 (*synth, pmr*)

$C_{18}H_{18}Cl_2Pd_2$ Pd-00143

Di-μ-chlorobis[(1,2,3-η)-2-phenyl-2-propenyl]dipalladium, 9CI
Di-μ-chlorobis(2-phenyl-π-allyl)dipalladium. Bis[μ-chloro-η³-(2-phenylpropenyl)palladium]. Bis[(2-phenyl-π-allyl)palladium chloride]
[31869-34-8]

M 518.086
Catalyses prepn. of allyl amines from primary or secondary amines. Yellow cryst. (C_6H_6). Mp 220-30° (242°) dec.

Monomer: Chloro(2-phenyl-2-propenyl)palladium. (2-Phenylallyl)palladium chloride.
C_9H_9ClPd M 259.043
Unknown.

Huttel, R. *et al*, *Chem. Ber.*, 1961, **94**, 766 (*synth*)
Kuli-Zade, T.S. *et al*, *Zh. Strukt. Khim.*, 1969, **10**, 149; *J. Struct. Chem.*, 1969, **10**, 141 (*struct*)
Volger, H.C., *Recl. Trav. Chim. Pays-Bas*, 1969, **88**, 225 (*synth, pmr*)
Senda, Y. *et al*, *Bull. Chem. Soc. Jpn.*, 1977, **50**, 1608 (*cmr*)
Norman, R.O.C. *et al*, *J. Chem. Soc., Perkin Trans. 2*, 1980, 1099 (*synth*)

$C_{18}H_{20}N_2Pd^{⊕⊕}$ Pd-00144

(2,2′-Bipyridine-*N,N′*)[(1,2,5,6-η)-1,5-cyclooctadiene]palladium(2+), 9CI
(1,5-Cyclooctadiene)(2,2′-bipyridine)palladium(2+)

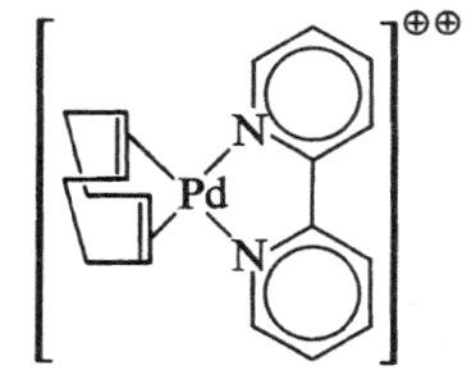

M 370.789 (ion)

Diperchlorate: [59350-31-1].
$C_{18}H_{20}Cl_2N_2O_8Pd$ M 569.691
Green-yellow solid (Me_2CO).

Rotondo, E. *et al*, *Inorg. Chem.*, 1976, **15**, 2102 (*synth, ir*)

$C_{18}H_{20}Pd_2$ Pd-00145

Bis[η⁵-2,4-cyclopentadien-1-yl][μ-[(1,2,3-η:6,7,8-η)-2,6-octadien-1,8-diyl]]dipalladium, 9CI
μ-1-3η:6-8η-Octadienato(2−)bis(η-cyclopentadienatopalladium)
[64756-57-6]

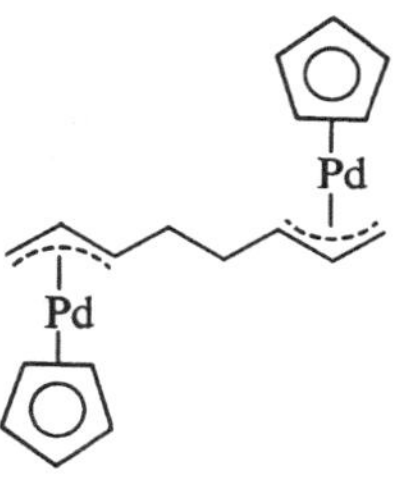

M 449.196
Red-brown cryst. (pentane), air-sensitive and thermally unstable. Reacts with halogenated solvents.

White, D.A., *J. Chem. Res. (S)*, 1977, 226; *J. Chem. Res. (M)*, 1977, 2401

$C_{18}H_{21}N_2OPd^{⊕}$ Pd-00146

[(2,5,6-η)-3-Methoxybicyclo[2.2.1]hept-5-en-2-yl]bis(pyridine)palladium(1+)
(3-Methoxy-5-norbornen-2-yl)bis(pyridine)palladium(1+), 8CI. *(6-Methoxybicyclo[2.2.1]hept-2-ene-5σ,2π)bis(pyridine)palladium(1+)*

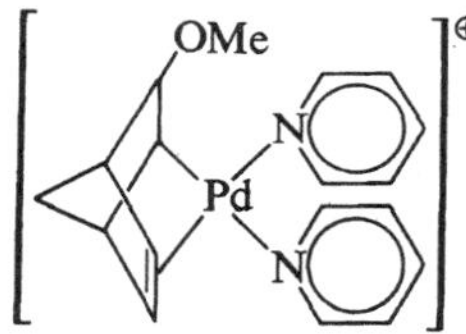

M 387.797 (ion)

Chloride:
$C_{18}H_{21}ClN_2OPd$ M 423.250
Cryst. (Et_2O/EtOH). Mp 120-5° dec.

Green, M. *et al*, *J. Chem. Soc. (A)*, 1967, 2054 (*synth, stereochem*)

$C_{18}H_{23}FeNO_2Pd$ Pd-00147

[2-[(Dimethylamino)methyl]ferrocenyl-*C,N*]-(2,4-pentanedionato-*O,O′*)palladium, 10CI
Acetylacetonato[2-[(dimethylamino)methyl]ferrocenyl]-palladium
[58616-69-6]

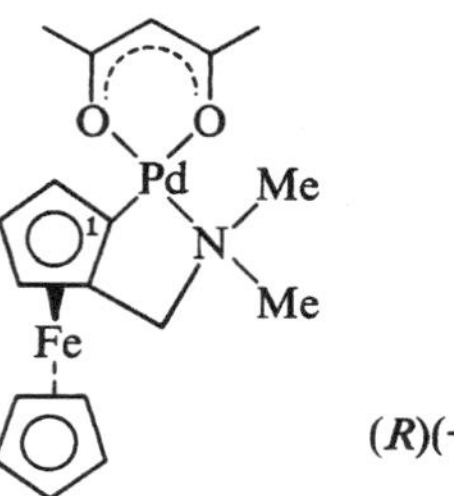

M 447.652
Yellow cryst.

(*1R*)-*form* [73609-66-2]
R_{planar}-*form*
Yellow cryst. $[\alpha]_D^{20}$ +494° (c, 0.04 in MeOH), +370° (c, 0.5 in CH_2Cl_2).

(1S)-form
S_{planar}-*form*
Yellow cryst. $[\alpha]^{20}_{D}$ −300° (c, 4.15 in CH_2Cl_2).
(±)-form
Yellow cryst. (pentane). Mp 123-4°.

Gaunt, J.C. *et al*, *J. Organomet. Chem.*, 1975, **102**, 511 (*synth*)
Sokolov, V.I. *et al*, *Chimia*, 1978, **32**, 122.
Sokolov, V.I. *et al*, *J. Organomet. Chem.*, 1979, **182**, 537 (*abs config*)
Komatsu, T. *et al*, *Bull. Chem. Soc. Jpn.*, 1981, **54**, 186 (*resoln*)

$C_{18}H_{24}Cl_2N_2Pd_2$ Pd-00148

Di-μ-chlorobis[2-[(dimethylamino)methyl]phenyl-*C,N*]dipalladium, 9CI
Di-μ-chlorobis[α-(dimethylamino)-o-tolyl]dipalladium, 8CI. Di-μ-chlorobis(N,N-dimethylbenzylamine-2-C,N)dipalladium
[18987-59-2]

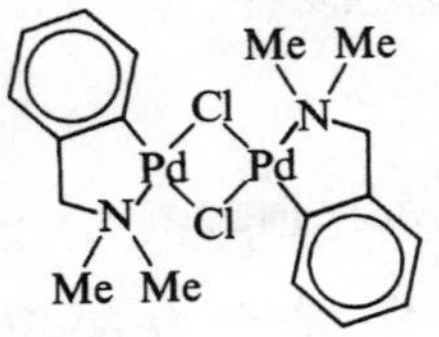

M 552.147
Yellow cryst. (C_6H_6/hexane). Mp 185-7° dec.
Monomer: Chloro[2-[(dimethylamino)methyl]phenyl-C,N]palladium.
$C_9H_{12}ClNPd$ M 276.074
Unknown.

Cope, A.C. *et al*, *J. Am. Chem. Soc.*, 1968, **90**, 909 (*synth, cmr*)
Crociani, B. *et al*, *J. Chem. Soc. (A)*, 1970, 531 (*ir*)
Cockburn, B.N. *et al*, *J. Chem. Soc., Dalton Trans.*, 1973, 404 (*synth*)
Dehand, J. *et al*, *Spectrochim. Acta, Part A*, 1977, **33**, 1101 (*ir, raman*)

$C_{18}H_{24}N_2Pd$ Pd-00149

Bis[2-[(dimethylamino)methyl]phenyl-*C,N*]palladium, 9CI
Bis[α-(dimethylamino)-o-tolyl]palladium, 8CI

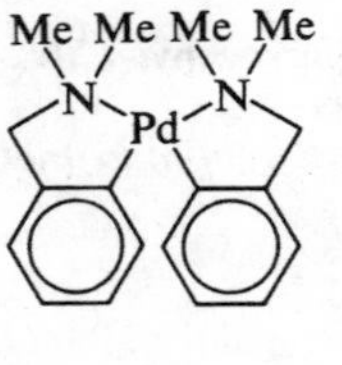

cis-form

M 374.821
cis-form [38437-97-7]
Cryst. (THF). Mp 221° (141°) dec.
trans-form [23626-48-4]
Yellow cryst. (C_6H_6). Mp 209-10° dec.

Kasahara, A. *et al*, *Bull. Chem. Soc. Jpn.*, 1969, **42**, 1765 (*synth, ir, pmr*)
Longoni, G. *et al*, *J. Organomet. Chem.*, 1972, **39**, 413 (*synth, pmr*)
Garbo, A.R. *et al*, *J. Organomet. Chem.*, 1975, **86**, 219 (*cmr*)
Murahashi, S. *et al*, *J. Org. Chem.*, 1978, **43**, 4099 (*synth*)

$C_{18}H_{26}O_4Pd$ Pd-00150

[8-(1-Acetylacetonyl)-π-4-cycloocten-1-yl](2,4-pentanedionato)palladium, 8CI

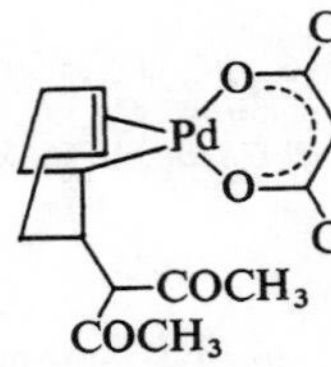

M 412.821
Cryst. ($CHCl_3/Et_2O$). Mp 123° dec.

Johnson, B.F.G. *et al*, *J. Chem. Soc. (A)*, 1968, 1993 (*synth, pmr, ir*)

$C_{18}H_{28}Cl_2N_2O_2Pd_2$ Pd-00151

Bis(η^3-1-acetyl-4-ethylidenepiperidinyl)di-μ-chlorodipalladium, 10CI
[67450-36-6]

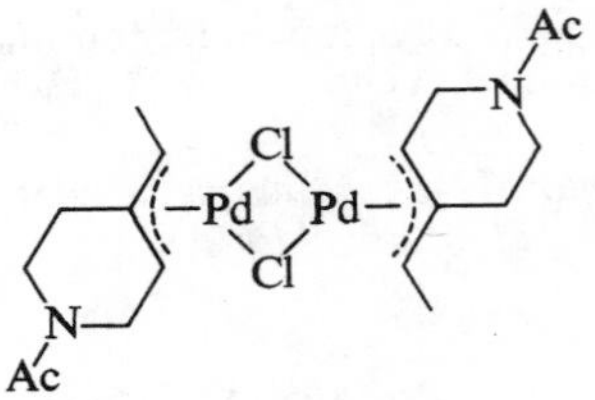

M 588.177
Bridged dimer. Solid. Mp 142-52° dec.
Monomer: (1-Acetyl-4-ethylidenepiperidinyl)-chloropalladium.
$C_9H_{14}ClNOPd$ M 294.089
Unknown.

Trost, B.M. *et al*, *J. Am. Chem. Soc.*, 1978, **100**, 3407.

$C_{18}H_{30}BrF_5P_2Pd$ Pd-00152

Bromo(pentafluorophenyl)bis(triethylphosphine)palladium, 9CI
Bis(triethylphosphine)pentafluorophenylpalladium bromide. Pentafluorophenylbromobis(triethylphosphine)-palladium. Perfluorophenylbromobis(triethylphosphine)-palladium

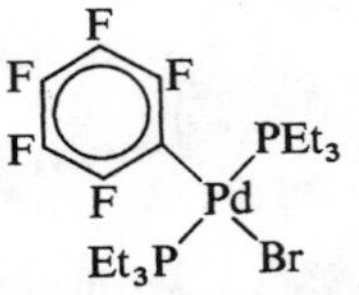

M 589.699
trans-form [63700-80-1]
Cryst. (hexane or MeOH). Mp 125-6°.

Klabunde, K.J. *et al*, *J. Am. Chem. Soc.*, 1974, **96**, 7674 (*synth, ir, pmr, ms*)
Fahey, D.R. *et al*, *J. Am. Chem. Soc.*, 1976, **98**, 4499 (*synth*)
Rieke, R.D. *et al*, *J. Org. Chem.*, 1979, **44**, 3069 (*synth*)

$C_{18}H_{30}Cl_2O_2Pd_2$ Pd-00153

Di-μ-chlorobis[(1,4,5-η)-8-methoxy-4-cycloocten-1-yl]dipalladium, 9CI

Di-μ-chlorobis(2-methoxy-5-cyclooctenyl)dipalladium. Di-(8-methoxy-4-cyclooctenyl)-μ,μ'-dichorodipalladium

[35502-73-9]

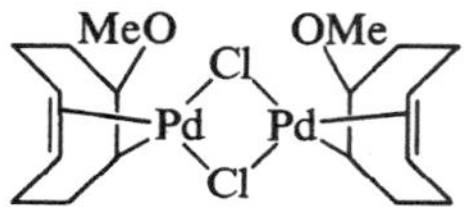

M 562.180

Pale-yellow cryst. (MeOH). Mp 150-5° (136-40°) dec.

Monomer: Chloro[(1,4,5-η)-8-methoxy-4-cycloocten-1-yl]palladium.
$C_9H_{15}ClOPd$ M 281.090
Unknown.

Chatt, J. *et al*, *J. Chem. Soc.*, 1957, 3413 (*synth*)
Schultz, R.G., *J. Organomet. Chem.*, 1966, **6**, 435 (*synth*)
Tsuji, J. *et al*, *Bull. Chem. Soc. Jpn.*, 1966, **39**, 141 (*struct*)
Anderson, C.B. *et al*, *J. Organomet. Chem.*, 1967, **7**, 181 (*pmr*)

$C_{18}H_{30}Cl_6P_2Pd$ Pd-00154

Chloro(pentachlorophenyl)bis(triethylphosphine)palladium, 9CI

Pentachlorophenylbis(triethylphosphine)palladium chloride. (Perchlorophenyl)bis(triethylphosphine)palladium chloride. Bis(triethylphosphine)-chloro(pentachlorophenyl)palladium

[63700-76-5]

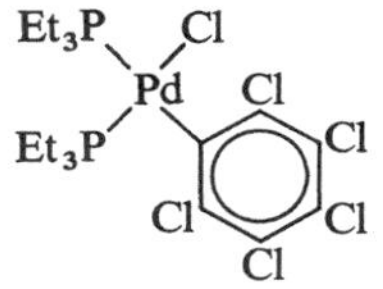

cis-form

M 627.521

cis-form [71536-70-4]
Cryst. ($EtOH/CH_2Cl_2$). Mp 129-31° dec. Isom. slowly to *trans*-form in $CHCl_3$ soln.

trans-form [60337-04-4]
Cryst. (EtOH). Mp 181-2°.

Corones, J.M. *et al*, *Synth. React. Inorg. Metal-Org. Chem.*, 1976, **6**, 217 (*synth, ir, pmr*)
Ceder, R. *et al*, *J. Organomet. Chem.*, 1979, **174**, 115 (*synth*)

$C_{18}H_{30}F_6P_2Pd$ Pd-00155

Bis(triethylphosphine)bis(3,3,3-trifluoro-1-propynyl)palladium, 8CI

Bis(triethylphosphine)bis(trifluoromethylethynyl)palladium

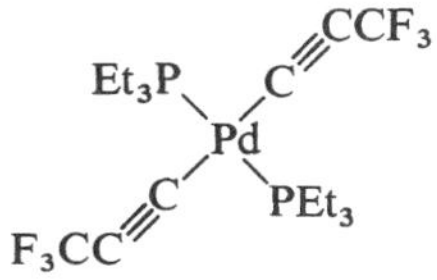

M 528.793

trans-form [18194-43-9]
Cryst. (pet. ether). Mp 95-7°.

Bruce, M.I. *et al*, *J. Chem. Soc. (A)*, 1968, 356 (*synth, ir, pmr, nmr*)

$C_{18}H_{33}PPd$ Pd-00156

(π-Cyclopentadienyl)(2-methyl-2-propenyl)(triisopropylphosphine)palladium

(η^5-2,4-Cyclopentadien-1-yl)(2-methyl-2-propenyl)[tris(1-methylethyl)phosphine]palladium, 9CI

[63511-32-0]

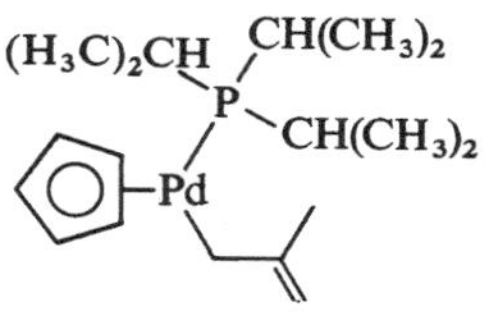

M 386.852

Isomeric with (η^1-2,4-Cyclopentadien-1-yl)[(1,2,3-η)-2-methyl-2-propenyl][tris(1-methylethyl)phosphine]palladium, Pd-00157 equilibrium mixt. of both in soln. Pale-yellow solid. Mp 55° dec.

Werner, H. *et al*, *Chem. Ber.*, 1977, **110**, 1763 (*synth, pmr*)
Werner, H. *et al*, *Angew. Chem., Int. Ed. Engl.*, 1979, **18**, 416 (*pmr*)
Werner, H. *et al*, *Chem. Ber.*, 1980, **113**, 2291 (*synth, pmr, cmr, ms, config*)

$C_{18}H_{33}PPd$ Pd-00157

(η^1-2,4-Cyclopentadien-1-yl)[(1,2,3-η)-2-methyl-2-propenyl][tris(1-methylethyl)phosphine]palladium, 9CI

(σ-Cyclopentadienyl)(π-2-methylallyl)(triisopropylphosphine)palladium

[70072-33-2]

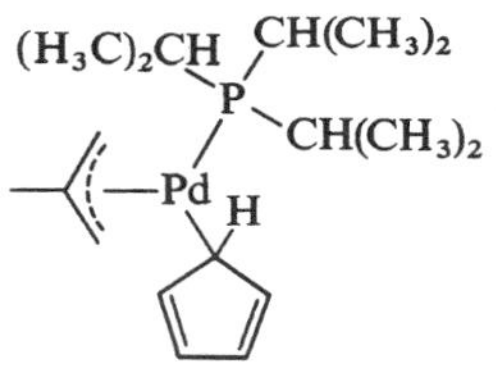

M 386.852

Isomeric with (π-Cyclopentadienyl)(2-methyl-2-propenyl)(triisopropylphosphine)palladium, Pd-00156 equilibrium mixt. of both in soln. Pale-yellow solid. Mp 55° dec.

Werner, H. *et al*, *Angew. Chem., Int. Ed. Engl.*, 1979, **18**, 416 (*pmr*)
Werner, H. *et al*, *Chem. Ber.*, 1980, **113**, 2291 (*synth, pmr, cmr, ms, config*)

$C_{18}H_{35}BrP_2Pd$ Pd-00158

Bromo(phenyl)bis(triethylphosphine)palladium, 9CI

Phenylbis(triethylphosphine)palladium bromide. Bis-(triethylphosphine)bromo(phenyl)palladium

[57029-73-9]

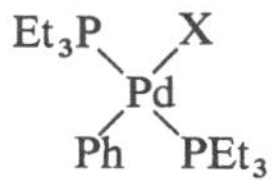

X = Br

M 499.746

trans-form [52230-30-5]
Cryst. (Et_2O, hexane or pentane). Mp 105-7° (88-91° dec., 96-8°).

Calvin, G. *et al*, *J. Chem. Soc.*, 1960, 2008 (*synth*)
Fahey, D.R. *et al*, *J. Am. Chem. Soc.*, 1976, **98**, 4499 (*synth*)
Garrou, P.E. *et al*, *J. Am. Chem. Soc.*, 1976, **98**, 4115 (*synth, nmr*)

Schunn, R.A., *Inorg. Chem.*, 1976, **15**, 208 (*synth, pmr*)
Rieke, R.D. *et al*, *J. Org. Chem.*, 1979, **44**, 3069 (*synth*)

$C_{18}H_{35}ClP_2Pd$ Pd-00159

Chloro(phenyl)bis(triethylphosphine)palladium, 9CI
Phenylbis(triethylphosphine)palladium chloride. Bis-(triethylphosphine)chloro(phenyl)palladium
[63701-76-8]
As Bromo(phenyl)bis(triethylphosphine)palladium, Pd-00158 with

X = Cl

M 455.295
trans-form [15697-59-3]
Cryst. (hexane or EtOH/hexane). Mp 101-2° (98.5-99°).

Cross, R.J. *et al*, *J. Chem. Soc. (A)*, 1970, 840 (*synth, pmr, ir*)
Rieke, R.D. *et al*, *J. Org. Chem.*, 1979, **44**, 3069 (*synth*)

$C_{18}H_{43}ClP_2Pd$ Pd-00160

Chlorohydrobis(triisopropylphosphine)palladium, 8CI
Chlorohydrobis[tris(1-methylethyl)phosphine]palladium, 9CI. Bis(triisopropylphosphine)palladium hydridochloride. Hydridochlorobis(triisopropylphosphine)-palladium
[27900-91-0]

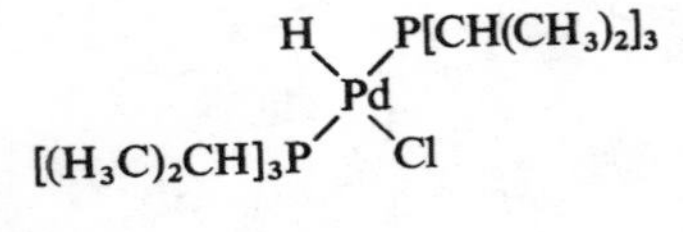

H, P[CH(CH₃)₂]₃, Pd, [(H₃C)₂CH]₃P, Cl

M 463.358
trans-form
Catalyses oligomerisation of butadiene. Cryst. (pet. ether); thermally stable. Mp 108-10°.

Green, M.L.H. *et al*, *J. Chem. Soc. (A)*, 1971, 469 (*synth, ir, pmr*)
Green, M.L.H. *et al*, *J. Chem. Soc., Dalton Trans.*, 1974, 269 (*use*)
Goel, A.B. *et al*, *Inorg. Chim. Acta*, 1980, **45**, 85 (*synth, ir, pmr, nmr*)

$C_{19}F_{15}NPd^{\ominus\ominus}$ Pd-00161

(Cyano-*C*)tris(pentafluorophenyl)palladate(2−)
Tris(pentafluorophenyl)cyanopalladate(2−)

$[PdCN(C_6F_5)_3]^{\ominus\ominus}$

M 633.612 (ion)
Bis(tetrabutylammonium) salt: [76083-06-2].
$C_{51}H_{72}F_{15}N_3Pd$ M 1118.546
White solid (hexane).

Uson, R. *et al*, *J. Organomet. Chem.*, 1980, **199**, 111 (*synth, ir*)

$C_{19}H_{25}FeNO_2Pd$ Pd-00162

[2-[1-(Dimethylamino)ethyl]ferrocenyl-*C,N*](2,4-pentanedionato-*O,O'*)palladium, 10CI
Cyclo-1-(1'-dimethylaminoethyl)ferrocene-2-(acetylacetonato)palladium
[64913-26-4]

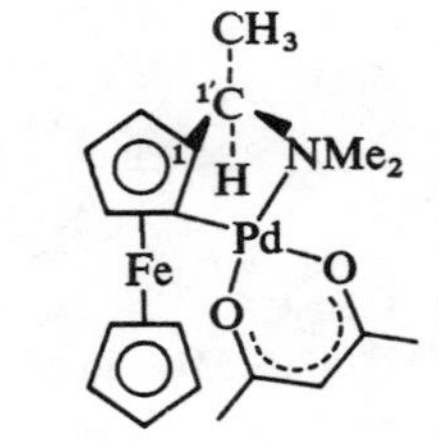

CH₃, 1'C, 1, H, NMe₂, Pd, Fe, O, O

M 461.679
(*1S,1'R*)-*form*
R,S$_{planar}$-*form*
Cryst. (hexane). Mp 124°. $[\alpha]_D$ −450° (c, 0.5 in CH_2Cl_2).

Troitskaya, L.L. *et al*, *Dokl. Akad. Nauk SSSR, Ser. Sci. Khim.*, 1977, **236**, 371; *Dokl. Chem. (Engl. Transl.)*, 1977, **236**, 527; *CA*, **88**, 7023k (*synth*)
Kuz'min, L.G. *et al*, *Izv. Akad. Nauk SSSR, Ser. Khim.*, 1979, 1528; *Bull. Acad. Sci. USSR, Div. Chem. Sci. (Engl. Transl.)*, 1979, **28**, 1417; *CA*, **92**, 42096r (*struct, abs config*)

$C_{19}H_{27}PPd$ Pd-00163

[2-(*tert*-Butylphenylphosphino)-2-methylpropyl]cyclopentadienylpalladium
(η^5-2,4-Cyclopentadien-1-yl)[2-[(1,1-dimethylethyl)-phenylphosphino]-2-methylpropyl]palladium, 10CI
[77933-00-7]

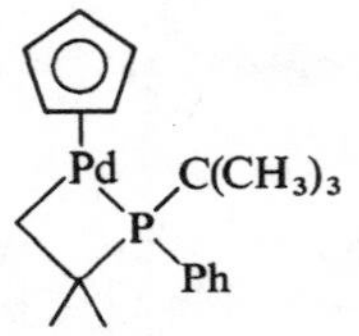

Pd, C(CH₃)₃, P, Ph

M 392.816
Orange-brown cryst. (pentane). Mp 66-8° dec.

Werner, H. *et al*, *J. Organomet. Chem.*, 1981, **204**, 415 (*synth, struct, pmr, cmr, nmr*)

$C_{19}H_{27}P_2Pd^{\oplus}$ Pd-00164

Bis(dimethylphenylphosphine)(η^3-2-propenyl)palladium(1+), 9CI
π-Allylbis(dimethylphenylphosphine)palladium(1+). π-Enylbis(dimethylphenylphosphine)palladium(1+)

PMe₂Ph, Pd, PMe₂Ph, ⊕

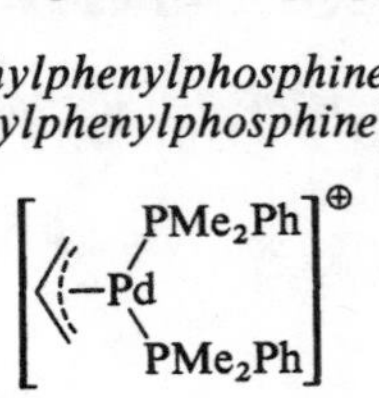

M 423.790 (ion)
2-Pyridinecarboxylate: [36540-79-1].
$C_{25}H_{31}NO_2P_2Pd$ M 545.893
No physical data available, observed only in soln.
2,4-Pentanedionate: [36569-64-9].
$C_{24}H_{34}O_2P_2Pd$ M 522.899
No physical data available, observed only in soln.

Powell, J. *et al*, *J. Organomet. Chem.*, 1972, **35**, 203 (*pmr*)

$C_{19}H_{28}PPd^{\oplus}$ Pd-00165

Cyclopentadienyl(styrene)(triethylphosphine)palladium(1+)
(η^5-2,4-Cyclopentadien-1-yl)[(η^2-ethenyl)benzene](triethylphosphine)palladium(1+), 9CI. *(η^5-2,4-Cyclopentadien-1-yl)(phenylethene)(triethylphosphine)palladium(1+)*

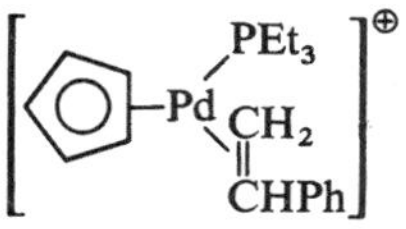

M 393.824 (ion)
Perchlorate: [75345-58-3].
$C_{19}H_{28}ClO_4PPd$ M 493.275
Violet cryst. (hexane/EtOH). Mp 120° dec.

Kurosawa, H. *et al*, *J. Am. Chem. Soc.*, 1980, **102**, 6996 (*synth, pmr*)
Miki, K. *et al*, *J. Organomet. Chem.*, 1982, **239**, 417.

$C_{19}H_{31}PPd$ Pd-00166

2,4-Cyclopentadien-1-yl(η^5-2,4-cyclopentadien-1-yl)[tris(1-methylethyl)phosphine]palladium, 9CI
Bis(cyclopentadienyl)(triisopropylphosphine)palladium. Dicyclopentadienyltriisopropylphosphinepalladium
[72244-78-1]

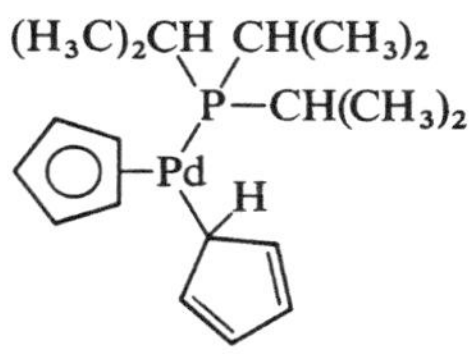

M 396.848
Green cryst. (pentane), slightly air-sensitive.

Werner, H. *et al*, *Angew. Chem., Int. Ed. Engl.*, 1979, **18**, 948 (*synth, ms, pmr, cmr*)

$C_{19}H_{35}NP_2Pd$ Pd-00167

Cyano(phenyl)bis(triethylphosphine)palladium, 9CI
Bis(triethylphosphine)phenyl(cyano)palladium. Phenylbis(triethylphosphine)palladium cyanide
[56960-34-0]

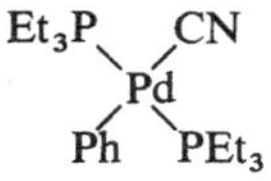

M 445.860

***trans*-form**
Cryst. (hexane or hexane/THF). Mp 85°, 112-6° dec.

Schunn, R.A., *Inorg. Chem.*, 1976, **15**, 208 (*synth, ir, pmr*)
Rieke, R.D. *et al*, *J. Org. Chem.*, 1979, **44**, 3069 (*synth, ir*)

$C_{19}H_{37}P_2Pd^{\oplus}$ Pd-00168

(η^3-6-Methylene-2,4-cyclohexadien-1-yl)bis(triethylphosphine)palladium(1+), 9CI
π-Benzylbis(triethylphosphine)palladium(1+)

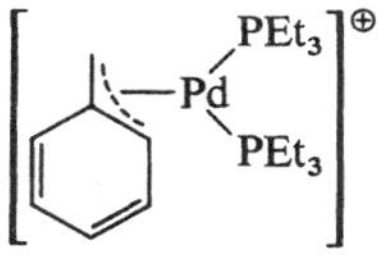

M 433.869 (ion)
Tetrafluoroborate: [32965-48-3].
$C_{19}H_{37}BF_4P_2Pd$ M 520.672
Yellow cryst. (Et_2O).

Stevens, R.R. *et al*, *J. Organomet. Chem.*, 1970, **21**, 495 (*synth, ir, pmr*)

$C_{20}H_{16}Cl_2N_2Pd_2$ Pd-00169

Di-μ-chlorobis(8-quinolinylmethyl-*C,N*)dipalladium, 9CI
*μ-Dichlorobis(8-methylquinoline-*C,N*)dipalladium*
[28377-73-3]

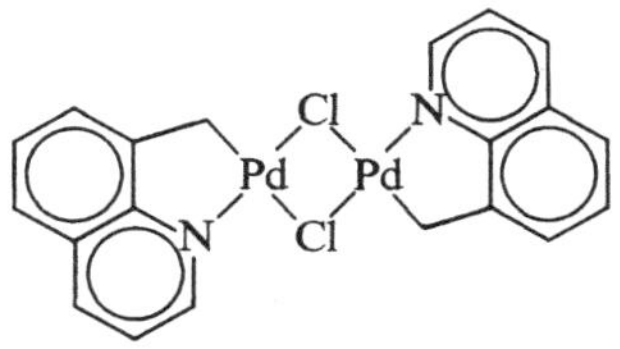

M 568.106
Yellow solid.

Hartwell, G.E. *et al*, *J. Chem. Soc., Chem. Commun.*, 1970, 912 (*synth, pmr*)
Dehand, J. *et al*, *Spectrochim. Acta, Part A*, 1977, **33**, 1101 (*ir, raman*)
Deeming, A.J. *et al*, *J. Chem. Soc., Dalton Trans.*, 1978, 1490.

$C_{20}H_{20}ClPPdS$ Pd-00170

Chloro[(methylthio)methyl-*C,S*](triphenylphosphine)palladium, 9CI
Chlorothiomethoxymethyltriphenylphosphinepalladium
[57300-11-5]

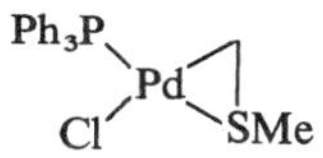

M 465.285
Yellow cryst. (CH_2Cl_2/Et_2O). Mp 210° dec.

Yoshida, G. *et al*, *J. Organomet. Chem.*, 1976, **113**, 85 (*synth, ir, pmr*)
Chivers, T. *et al*, *J. Organomet. Chem.*, 1976, **118**, C37 (*synth*)
Miki, K. *et al*, *J. Organomet. Chem.*, 1977, **135**, 53 (*struct*)

$C_{20}H_{20}Cl_2N_2O_2Pd_2$ Pd-00171

Di-μ-chlorobis[5,6,7,8-tetrahydro-8-(hydroxyimino)-1-naphthalenyl-*C,N*]dipalladium, 9CI
*Di-μ-chlorobis(1-tetralone oxime-*C,N*)dipalladium*
[77674-65-8]

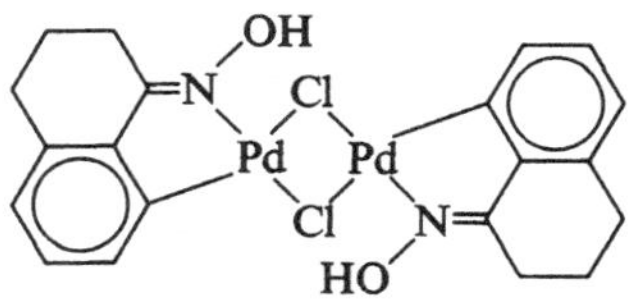

M 604.136

Solid ($MeOH/Et_2O$). Mp 302° dec.

Nielson, A.J., *J. Chem. Soc., Dalton Trans.*, 1981, 205 (*synth, ir, pmr*)

$C_{20}H_{22}F_6P_2Pd$ **Pd-00172**

[(2,3-η)-Hexafluoro-2-butyne]bis(dimethylphenylphosphine)palladium

[Bis(trifluoromethyl)vinylene]bis(dimethylphenylphosphine)palladium, 8CI. *[Bis(trifluoromethyl)acetylene]-bis(dimethylphenylphosphine)palladium*

[23715-25-5]

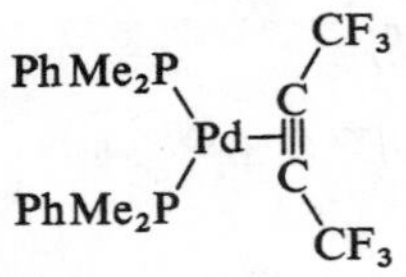

M 544.752

Cryst. (MeOH aq.). Mp 118-9° dec.

Greaves, E.O. *et al*, *Can. J. Chem.*, 1968, **46**, 3879 (*synth, ir*)

$C_{20}H_{26}Cl_2O_2Pd_2$ **Pd-00173**

Di-μ-chlorobis[μ-[(1,2,3-η)-2-(4-methyl-5-oxo-3-cyclohexen-1-yl)-2-propenyl]]dipalladium, 10CI

Bis[chloro(η³-2-(4-methyl-5-oxo-3-cyclohexen-1-yl)-2-propenyl)palladium]

[67719-68-0]

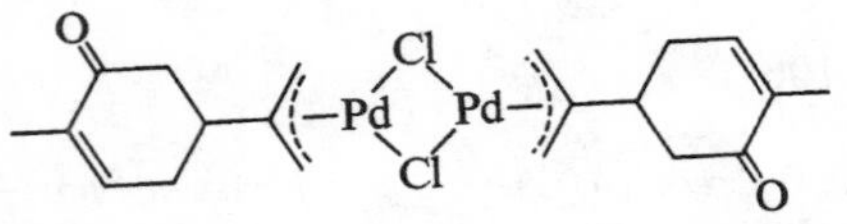

M 582.170

Chloride bridged dimer. Yellow cryst. (hexane). Mp 152-6° dec.

Monomer: Chloro[2-(4-methyl-5-oxo-3-cyclohexen-1-yl)-2-propenyl]palladium.
$C_{10}H_{13}ClOPd$ M 291.085
Unknown.

Trost, B.M. *et al*, *J. Am. Chem. Soc.*, 1978, **100**, 3407.
Muzart, J. *et al*, *J. Chem. Soc., Chem. Commun.*, 1980, 257; 1981, 668.

$C_{20}H_{30}Cl_2Pd_2$ **Pd-00174**

Di-μ-chlorobis(η³-6,6-dimethyl-4-methylenebicyclo-[3.1.1]hept-3-yl)dipalladium, 10CI

Bis[chloro-(7,1,2-η³-pinene)palladium]

[34829-33-9]

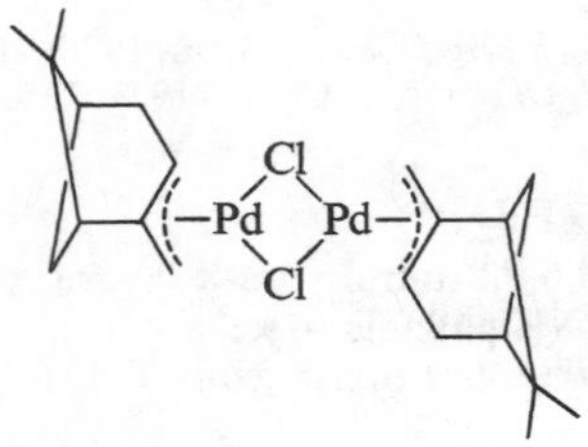

M 554.203

Chloride bridged dimer. Catalyses polymerisation of olefins. Yellow cryst. (hexane). Mp 169-71° dec. $[\alpha]_D$ +32.8°.

Monomer: Chloro(η³-6,6-dimethyl-4-methylenebicyclo[3.1.1]hept-3-yl)palladium. Chloro(7,1,2-η³-pinene)palladium.
$C_{10}H_{15}ClPd$ M 277.102
Unknown.

Dunne, K. *et al*, *J. Chem. Soc. (C)*, 1970, 2200 (*stereochem*)
Scott, A.I. *et al*, *Tetrahedron*, 1971, **27**, 2339 (*stereochem*)
Hoajbri, F., *J. Appl. Chem. Biotechnol.*, 1973, **23**, 601 (*use*)
Hojabri, F., *Polymer*, 1976, **17**, 58 (*use*)
Trost, B.M. *et al*, *J. Am. Chem. Soc.*, 1978, **100**, 3407 (*synth*)
Muzart, J. *et al*, *J. Chem. Soc., Chem. Commun.*, 1980, 257.

$C_{20}H_{32}Cl_4Pd_2$ **Pd-00175**

Di-μ-chlorobis[(1,4,5-η)-8-(1-chloroethyl)-4-cycloocten-1-yl]dipalladium, 9CI

Bis(μ-chloro)bis[(1,4,5-η)-8-(α-chloroethyl)cyclooctenyl]dipalladium

[79188-47-9]

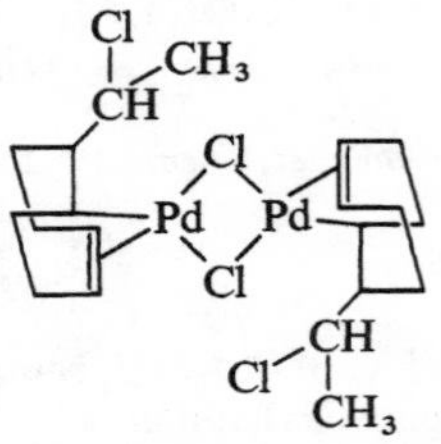

M 627.125

Bridged dimer. Yellow cryst. (CH_2Cl_2).

Monomer: Chloro[(1,4,5-η)-8-(1-chloroethyl)-4-cycloocten-1-yl]palladium.
$C_{10}H_{16}Cl_2Pd$ M 313.562
Unknown.

Rettig, M.F. *et al*, *J. Organomet. Chem.*, 1981, **214**, 261 (*synth, ir, pmr*)
Parra-Hake, M. *et al*, *Organometallics*, 1982, **1**, 1478 (*struct*)

$C_{20}H_{33}ClPPdSi^{\oplus}$ **Pd-00176**

Chloro[(1,2,5,6-η)-1,5-cyclooctadiene][dimethylphenylphosphonium(1-η)-(trimethylsilyl)methylide]palladium(1+), 9CI

Chloro[dimethylphenylphosphonium(trimethylsilyl)-methylide](1,5-cyclooctadiene)palladium(1+)

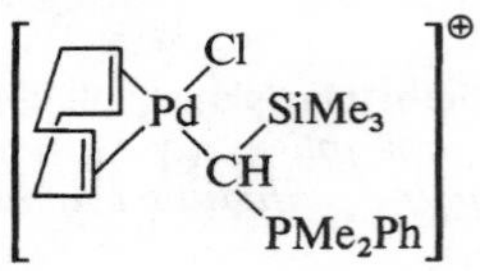

M 474.413 (ion)

Hexafluorophosphate: [63133-32-4].
$C_{20}H_{33}ClF_6P_2PdSi$ M 619.377
Yellow cryst. (CH_2Cl_2/Et_2O). Mp 124-6° dec.

Itoh, K. *et al*, *J. Organomet. Chem.*, 1977, **129**, 259 (*synth, pmr, nmr*)
Buchanan, R.M. *et al*, *Inorg. Chem.*, 1979, **18**, 3608 (*struct*)

$C_{20}H_{35}ClP_2Pd$ **Pd-00177**

Chloro(phenylethynyl)bis(triethylphosphine)palladium

(Phenylacetylenyl)chlorobis(triethylphosphine)palladium

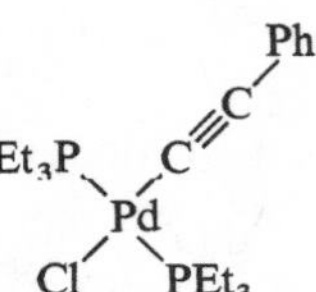

M 479.317

No physical data available.

Tohda, Y. *et al*, *J. Chem. Soc., Chem. Commun.*, 1975, 54.

$C_{20}H_{36}Cl_2N_4Pd_2$ Pd-00178

Di-μ-chlorotetrakis[2-isocyano-2-methylpropane]dipalladium, 9CI

Dichlorotetrakis(tert-*butylisonitrile*)*dipalladium. Dichlorotetrakis*(tert-*butylisocyanide*)*dipalladium. Tetrakis*(tert-*butylisocyanide*)*di-μ-chlorodipalladium*

[34742-93-3]

$[[(H_3C)_3CNC]_2PdCl]_2$

M 616.277

Though originally formulated with bridging chlorides, a Pd-Pd linked dimer with terminal Cl's cannot be ruled out. Yellow solid (CH_2Cl_2/Et_2O or chlorobenzene); fairly air-stable. Sol. common org. solvs. Mp 155-210° dec. Diamagnetic.

Monomer: Chlorobis(2-isocyano-2-methylpropane)-palladium.
$C_{10}H_{18}ClN_2Pd$ M 308.139
Unknown.

Otsuka, S. *et al*, *J. Am. Chem. Soc.*, 1971, **93**, 6705 (*synth*)
Rettig, M.F. *et al*, *J. Organomet. Chem.*, 1976, **111**, 113 (*synth, pmr, ir*)
Inorg. Synth., 1977, **17**, 134 (*synth, ir, pmr*)

$C_{20}H_{36}Cl_4Pd_2$ Pd-00179

Di-μ-chlorodichlorobis[(3,4-η)-2,2,5,5-tetramethyl-3-hexyne]dipalladium

Di-μ-chlorodichlorobis(*di*-tert-*butylacetylene*)*dipalladium*

M 631.156

Red needles (C_6H_6/pet. ether). Mp 164-5° dec.

Hosokawa, T. *et al*, *Tetrahedron Lett.*, 1969, 3833 (*synth, ir, pmr*)

$C_{21}H_{15}F_5N_3Pd^{\oplus}$ Pd-00180

(Pentafluorophenyl)tris(pyridine)palladium(1+)

$[Pd(C_6F_5)(C_5H_5N)_3]^{\oplus}$

M 510.782 (ion)

Perchlorate: [59053-34-8].
$C_{21}H_{15}ClF_5N_3O_4Pd$ M 610.232
White solid. Mp 159° dec.

Uson, R. *et al*, *J. Organomet. Chem.*, 1976, **104**, 253 (*synth, ir*)

$C_{21}H_{20}Cl_3PPdSn$ Pd-00181

(η^3-2-Propenyl)(trichlorostannyl)(triphenylphosphine)palladium, 9CI

π-Allyl(trichlorostannyl)(triphenylphosphine)palladium, 8CI. *π-Allyl(triphenylphosphine)palladium trichlorotin*

[32679-68-8]

M 634.832

Yellow cryst. (Me_2CO or toluene). Mp 138-40° dec.

Mason, R. *et al*, *J. Chem. Soc. (A)*, 1969, 2709 (*synth, struct*)
Crosby, J.N. *et al*, *J. Organomet. Chem.*, 1971, **26**, 277 (*synth, ir, nmr*)
Sakakibara, M. *et al*, *J. Organomet. Chem.*, 1971, **27**, 139 (*pmr*)

$C_{22}H_8Cl_2F_{10}N_2Pd$ Pd-00182

Dichloro(2,2′-bipyridine)bis(pentafluorophenyl)palladium

*Dichlorobis(pentafluorophenyl)(2,2-bipyridine)palladium. (2,2′-Bipyridine-*N,N′*)-dichlorobis(pentafluorophenyl)palladium*

[57209-02-6]

$PdCl_2(C_6F_5)_2(bipy)$

M 667.629

Yellow cryst. Mp 303° dec.

Uson, R. *et al*, *J. Organomet. Chem.*, 1975, **96**, 307 (*synth, ir*)

$C_{22}H_8F_{10}N_2Pd$ Pd-00183

(2,2′-Bipyridine)bis(pentafluorophenyl)palladium, 8CI

Bis(pentafluorophenyl)(2,2′-bipyridine)palladium

[25916-94-3]

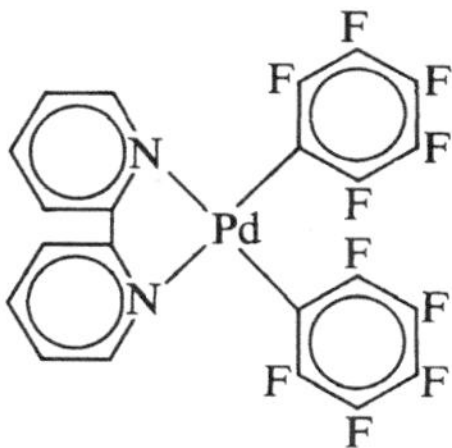

M 596.723

White needles (Me_2CO/MeOH). Mp 334-5°.

Rausch, M.D. *et al*, *J. Organomet. Chem.*, 1970, **21**, 487 (*synth, ir*)
Uson, R. *et al*, *J. Organomet. Chem.*, 1975, **96**, 307.

$C_{22}H_{16}Cl_2N_2Pd_2$ Pd-00184

Di-μ-chlorobis[2-(2-pyridinyl)phenyl-*C,N*]dipalladium, 9CI

[20832-86-4]

M 592.128

Pale-yellow. Mp 327° (270°) dec.

Kasahara, A., *Bull. Chem. Soc. Jpn.*, 1968, **41**, 1272 (*synth, ir*)
Cockburn, B.N. *et al*, *J. Chem. Soc., Dalton Trans.*, 1973, 404 (*synth*)
Gutierrez, M.A. *et al*, *J. Organomet. Chem.*, 1980, **202**, 341 (*synth*)

$C_{22}H_{22}AsClPd$ — Pd-00185

Chloro[(1,2,3-η)-2-methyl-2-propenyl](triphenylarsine)palladium, 9CI

Chloro(2-methyl-π-allyl)(triphenylarsine)palladium, 8CI. (2-Methylallyl)chloro(triphenylarsine)palladium

[12113-96-1]

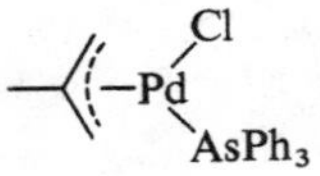

M 503.210

Yellow cryst. (EtOH). Mp 205-8° dec.

Hegarty, B.F. *et al*, *J. Organomet. Chem.*, 1966, **6**, 578 (*uv*)
Ramey, K.C. *et al*, *J. Am. Chem. Soc.*, 1966, **88**, 4387 (*pmr*)
Powell, J. *et al*, *J. Chem. Soc. (A)*, 1967, 1839 (*synth, pmr, ir*)

$C_{22}H_{22}ClPPd$ — Pd-00186

Chloro[(1,2,3-η)-2-methyl-2-propenyl)](triphenylphosphine)palladium, 9CI

Chloro(2-methyl-π-allyl)(triphenylphosphine)palladium, 8CI. (2-Methylallyl)chloro(triphenylphosphine)-palladium

[12098-21-4]

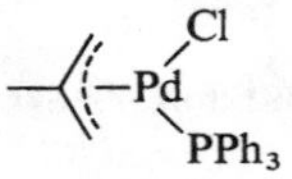

M 459.263

Catalyses hydrogenation of allene to propene. Yellow cryst. (EtOH). Mp 210-6° dec.

Hegarty, B.F. *et al*, *J. Organomet. Chem.*, 1966, **6**, 578 (*uv*)
Powell, J. *et al*, *J. Chem. Soc. (A)*, 1967, 1839 (*synth, ir, pmr*)
Vrieze, K. *et al*, *J. Organomet. Chem.*, 1968, **12**, 533 (*pmr*)
Sakakibara, M. *et al*, *J. Organomet. Chem.*, 1971, **27**, 139 (*pmr*)
Shaw, B.L. *et al*, *J. Chem. Soc., Chem. Commun.*, 1971, 790 (*cmr*)
Van Leeuwen, P.W.N.M. *et al*, *J. Organomet. Chem.*, 1971, **29**, 433 (*pmr*)
Carturan, G. *et al*, *J. Organomet. Chem.*, 1978, **157**, 475 (*use*)

The first digit of the Entry number defines the Supplement in which the Entry is found. 0 indicates the Main Work

$C_{22}H_{30}Cl_2O_2Pd_2$ — Pd-00187

Di-μ-chlorobis[(2,3,5-η)-3a,4,5,6,7,7a-hexahydro-6-methoxy-4,7-methano-1*H*-inden-5-yl]dipalladium, 9CI

Di-μ-chlorobis(2-methoxydicyclopentadien-1-yl)dipalladium. Bis(dicyclopentadienemethoxide)-μ,μ′-dichlorodipalladium

[33218-61-0]

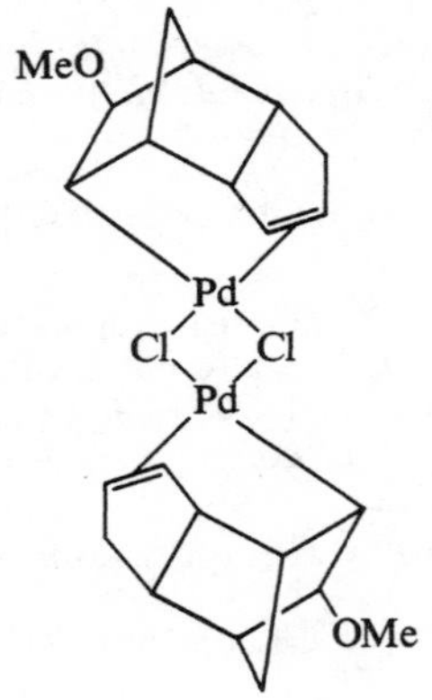

M 610.224

Bridged dimer. Yellow cryst. ($CHCl_3/Et_2O$). Mp 166-70° dec.

*Monomer: Chloro[(2,3,5-η)-3*a*,4,5,6,7,7*a*-hexahydro-6-methoxy-4,7-methano-1*H*-inden-5-yl]palladium. Chloro(2-methoxydicyclopentadienyl)palladium.*
$C_{11}H_{15}ClOPd$ M 305.112
Unknown.

Chatt, J. *et al*, *J. Chem. Soc.*, 1957, 3413 (*synth*)
Stille, J.K. *et al*, *J. Am. Chem. Soc.*, 1966, **88**, 5135 (*synth, cmr*)

$C_{22}H_{34}Cl_2O_4Pd_2$ — Pd-00188

Di-μ-chlorobis[(1,2,3-η)-8-methoxy-2,6-dimethyl-8-oxo-2,6-octadienyl]dipalladium, 10CI

[57731-30-3]

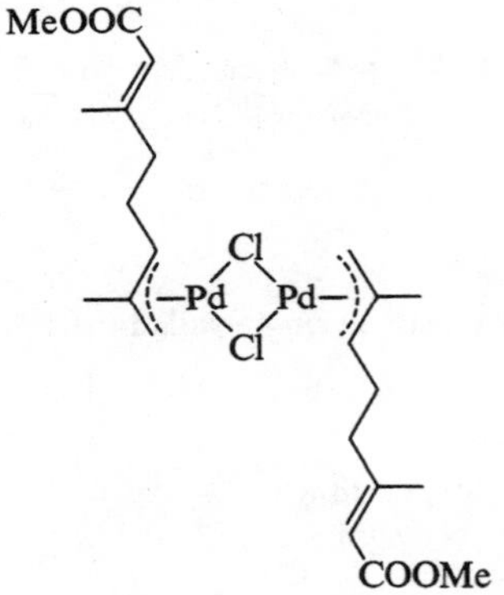

M 646.254

Chloride bridged dimer. Yellow cryst. (hexane). Mp 117-8° dec.

Monomer: Chloro[(1,2,3-η)-8-methoxy-2,6-dimethyl-8-oxo-2,6-octadienyl]palladium.
$C_{11}H_{17}ClO_2Pd$ M 323.127
Unknown.

Trost, B.M. *et al*, *J. Org. Chem.*, 1975, **40**, 3617 (*pmr*)
Trost, B.M. *et al*, *J. Am. Chem. Soc.*, 1978, **100**, 3407 (*synth*)

$C_{22}H_{34}Cl_2Pd_2$ Pd-00189

Di-μ-chlorobis(η³-2-ethylidene-6,6-dimethylbicyclo-[3.1.1]hept-3-yl)dipalladium, 10CI

[55684-63-4]

M 582.257

Bridged dimer. Solid. Mp 155-65° dec.

Monomer: Chloro(2-ethylidene-6,6-dimethylbicyclo[3.1.1]hept-3-yl)palladium.

$C_{11}H_{17}ClPd$ M 291.128

Unknown.

Trost, B.M. *et al*, *J. Am. Chem. Soc.*, 1978, **100**, 3407 (*synth*)

$C_{22}H_{38}Cl_2Pd_2$ Pd-00190

Di-μ-chlorobis(η³-5-*tert*-butyl-2-methylenecyclohexyl)dipalladium

Di-μ-chlorobis[η³-5-(1,1-dimethylethyl)2-methylenecyclohexyl]dipalladium, 10CI. *Bis[chloro(η³-5-tert-butyl-2-methylenecyclohexyl)palladium]*

[55940-14-2]

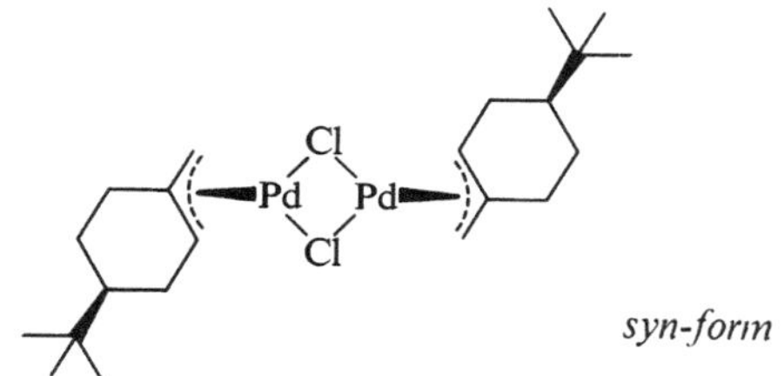

syn-form

M 586.288

Obt. as a 3:2 mixt. of *syn-* and *anti*-isomers. Yellow cryst. (hexane). Mp 165-70° dec.

Monomer:

$C_{11}H_{19}ClPd$ M 293.144

Unknown.

Trost, B.M. *et al*, *J. Am. Chem. Soc.*, 1978, **100**, 3407, 3416 (*synth*, *pmr*)

Muzart, J. *et al*, *J. Chem. Soc., Chem. Commun.*, 1981, 668 (*synth*)

$C_{22}H_{42}Cl_2Pd_2$ Pd-00191

Di-μ-chlorobis[(1,2,3-η)-1,1,5-trimethyl-2-octenyl]dipalladium, 10CI

Di-μ-chlorobis[(2,3,4-η)-2,6-dimethyl-3-nonen-2-yl]dipalladium

[67719-73-7]

M 590.320

Bridged dimer. Solid. Mp 108-15° dec.

Monomer: Chloro(1,1,5-trimethyl-2-octenyl)palladium.

$C_{11}H_{21}ClPd$ M 295.160

Unknown.

Trost, B.M. *et al*, *J. Am. Chem. Soc.*, 1978, **100**, 3407.

$C_{23}H_{20}BrPPd$ Pd-00192

Bromo(η⁵-2,4-cyclopentadien-1-yl)(triphenylphosphine)palladium, 9CI

Cyclopentadienyl(bromo)(triphenylphosphine)palladium

[31741-89-6]

M 513.709

Green solid. Mp 129-30° dec.

Cross, R.J. *et al*, *J. Chem. Soc. (A)*, 1971, 2000 (*ir*, *pmr*, *synth*)

$C_{24}Br_2F_{20}Pd_2^{\ominus\ominus}$ Pd-00193

Di-μ-bromotetrakis(pentafluorophenyl)dipalladate(2−), 9CI

Tetrakis(pentafluorophenyl)di-μ-bromodipalladate-(2−)

M 1040.880 (ion)

Bis(tetrabutylammonium) salt: [74436-10-5].

$C_{56}H_{72}Br_2F_{20}N_2Pd_2$ M 1525.814

Cryst. (butanol). Mp 147°.

Usón, R. *et al*, *J. Chem. Soc., Dalton Trans.*, 1980, 888 (*synth*)

$C_{24}Cl_2F_{20}Pd_2^{\ominus\ominus}$ Pd-00194

Di-μ-chlorotetrakis(pentafluorophenyl)dipalladate(2−)

Di-μ-chlorobis[bis(pentafluorophenyl)palladate](2−). Tetrabis(pentafluorophenyl)di-μ-chlorodipalladate-(2−)

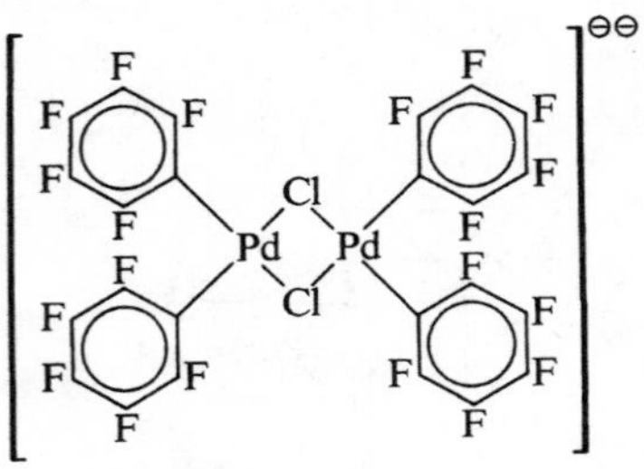

M 951.978 (ion)

Bis(tetrabutylammonium) salt: [74436-08-1].
$C_{56}H_{72}Cl_2F_{20}N_2Pd_2$ M 1436.912
Cryst. (2-propanol). Mp 159° dec.

Monomer: Chlorobis(pentafluorophenyl)palladate(1−).
$C_{12}ClF_{10}Pd^{\ominus}$ M 475.989 (ion)
Unknown.

Uson, R. *et al*, *J. Chem. Soc., Dalton Trans.*, 1980, 888 (*synth*)
Uson, R. *et al*, *J. Chem. Soc., Dalton Trans.*, 1981, 463 (*use*)

$C_{24}F_{20}Pd^{\ominus\ominus}$ Pd-00195

Tetrakis(pentafluorophenyl)palladate(2−), 9CI

Tetrakis(perfluorophenyl)palladate(2−)

$[Pd(C_6F_5)_4]^{\ominus\ominus}$ (D_{4h})

M 774.652 (ion)

Bistetrabutylammonium salt: [66302-88-3].
$C_{56}H_{72}F_{20}N_2Pd$ M 1259.586
Cryst. (2-propanol). Mp 158°.

Usón, R. *et al*, *J. Chem. Soc., Dalton Trans.*, 1980, 888 (*synth*)

$C_{24}H_{18}Cl_2N_4Pd_2$ Pd-00196

Di-μ-chlorobis[2-(phenylazo)phenyl]dipalladium, 9CI

Bis(azobenzeneyl)di-μ-chlorodipalladium. Di-μ-chlorodi(phenylazophenyl-C²,N′)dipalladium

[54865-84-8]

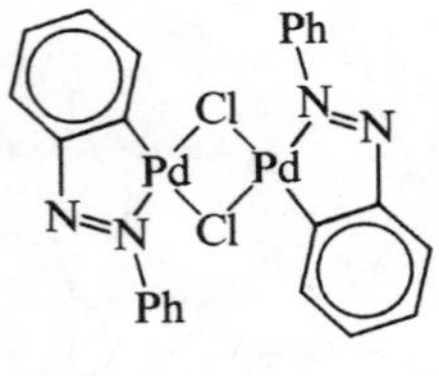

M 646.179
Maroon cryst. (C_6H_6). Mp 279-81° dec.

Monomer: Chloro[2-(phenylazo)phenyl]palladium.
$C_{12}H_9ClN_2Pd$ M 323.090
Unknown.

Cope, A.C. *et al*, *J. Am. Chem. Soc.*, 1965, **87**, 3272 (*synth*)
Crociani, B. *et al*, *J. Chem. Soc. (A)*, 1970, 531 (*ir*)
Cross, R.J. *et al*, *J. Organomet. Chem.*, 1974, **72**, 21 (*synth*)
Dehand, J. *et al*, *Spectrochim. Acta, Part A*, 1977, **33**, 1101 (*ir, raman*)

$C_{24}H_{18}N_4Pd$ Pd-00197

Bis[2-phenylazo(phenyl)-*C,N*]palladium, 9CI

Bis-o-C,N-(azobenzene)palladium

[57286-37-0]

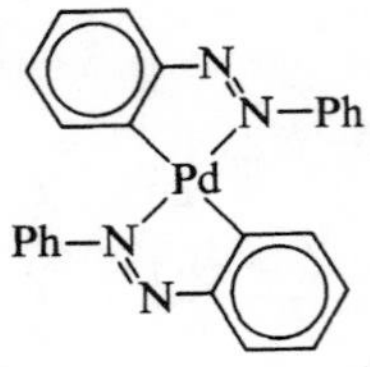

M 468.853
Red cryst. (C_6H_6/pet. ether). Mp 163-164.5° dec.

Sokolov, V.I. *et al*, *J. Organomet. Chem.*, 1975, **93**, C11 (*synth*)

$C_{24}H_{20}OPPd^{\oplus}$ Pd-00198

Carbonyl(η⁵-2,4-cyclopentadien-1-yl)(triphenylphosphine)palladium(1+), 9CI

(π-Cyclopentadienyl)carbonyl(triphenylphosphine)palladium(1+)

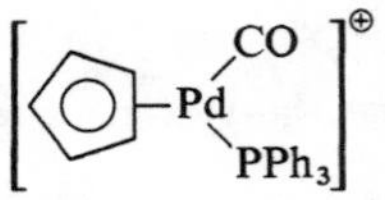

M 461.815 (ion)

Perchlorate: [64040-88-6].
$C_{24}H_{20}ClO_5PPd$ M 561.266
Violet powder. Mp 167° dec.

Majima, T. *et al*, *J. Organomet. Chem.*, 1977, **134**, C45 (*ir, pmr*)
Kurosawa, H. *et al*, *J. Am. Chem. Soc.*, 1980, **102**, 6996 (*synth*)

$C_{24}H_{22}O_2Pd$ Pd-00199

[η³-6-(Diphenylmethylene)-2,4-cyclohexadien-1-yl](2,4-pentanedionato-*O,O′*)palladium

(2,4-Pentanedionato-O,O′)(η³-triphenylmethyl)palladium. Acetylacetonato(triphenylmethyl)palladium

[56050-88-5]

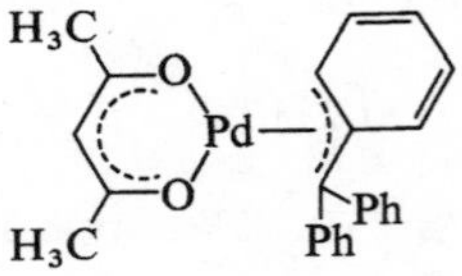

M 448.857
Orange-yellow cryst. (C_6H_6/pet. ether). Mp 176-8° dec.

Mann, B.E. *et al*, *J. Chem. Soc., Dalton Trans.*, 1979, 338 (*synth, cmr, pmr*)

$C_{24}H_{23}PPd$ Pd-00200

(η⁵-2,4-Cyclopentadien-1-yl)methyl(triphenylphosphine)palladium, 9CI

Cyclopentadienylmethyl(triphenylphosphine)palladium

[62483-32-3]

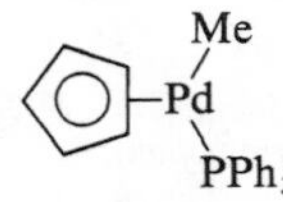

M 448.839
Red-orange cryst. (pentane/toluene). Mp 130-2° dec.

Turner, G.K. *et al*, *J. Organomet. Chem.*, 1976, **121**, C29 (*synth, pmr*)

$C_{24}H_{30}Cl_5F_5P_2Pd$ Pd-00201

(Pentachlorophenyl)(pentafluorophenyl)bis(triethylphosphine)palladium

Bis(triethylphosphine)(pentachlorophenyl)(pentafluorophenyl)palladium. (Perchlorophenyl)(perfluorophenyl)bis(triethylphosphine)palladium

[63643-19-6]

$Pd(C_6Cl_5)(C_6F_5)(PEt_3)_2$

M 759.126

Cryst. (EtOH). Mp 249°.

Usón, R. *et al*, *J. Organomet. Chem.*, 1976, **132**, 429 (*synth, ir*)

$C_{24}H_{30}F_6O_4Pd_2$ Pd-00202

Bis(η^3-6,6-dimethyl-4-methylenebicyclo[3.1.1]hept-3-yl)di-μ-(trifluoroacetato)dipalladium

Bis[trifluoroacetato(7,1,2-η^3-pinene)palladium]

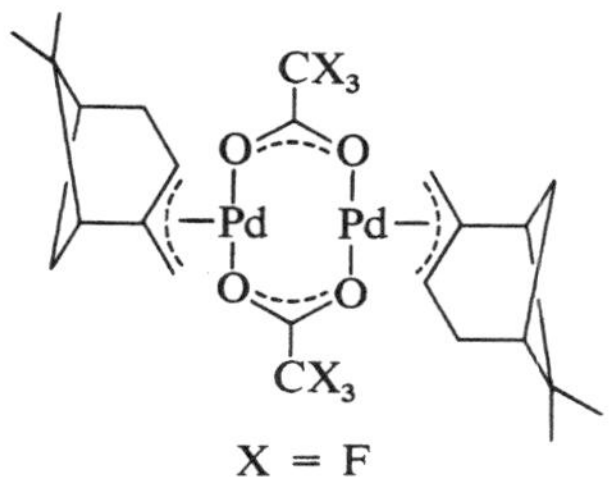

CX_3 Pd Pd O O CX_3

X = F

M 709.329

Trifluoroacetate bridged dimer. Yellow-green cryst. (hexane). Mp 116-8° dec.

Monomer: (η^3-6,6-Dimethyl-4-methylenebicyclo[3.3.1]hept-3-yl)palladium trifluoroacetate. Trifluoroacetato(η^3-pinene)palladium.

$C_{12}H_{15}F_3O_2Pd$ M 354.665

Unknown.

Trost, B.M. *et al*, *J. Am. Chem. Soc.*, 1980, **102**, 3572 (*synth, ir, pmr, cmr*)

$C_{24}H_{32}O_2Pd$ Pd-00203

[η^3-2-(4-Methylphenyl)-2-(1,2,3,4,5-pentamethyl-2,4-cyclopentadien-1-yl)ethyl](2,4-pentanedionato-*O,O'*)palladium, 9CI

[38959-94-3]

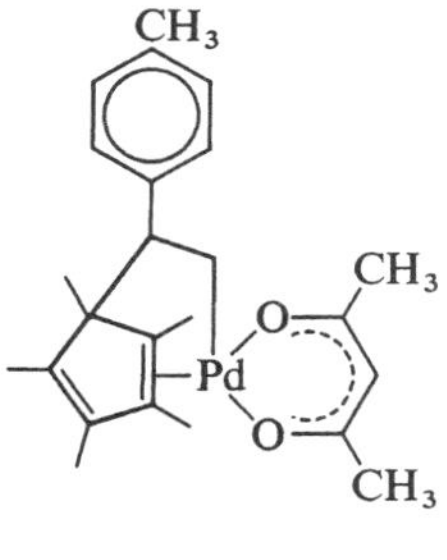

CH_3 Pd O O CH_3 CH_3

M 458.936

Calvo, C. *et al*, *J. Am. Chem. Soc.*, 1972, **94**, 3237.
Hosokawa, T. *et al*, *J. Am. Chem. Soc.*, 1972, **94**, 3238.
Hosokawa, T. *et al*, *J. Am. Chem. Soc.*, 1973, **95**, 4914 (*struct*)

$C_{24}H_{34}Cl_2Pd_2$ Pd-00204

Di-μ-chlorobis(η^3-1,2,4,5,6-pentamethyl-3-methylenebicyclo[2.2.0]hex-5-en-2-yl)dipalladium, 9CI

[33111-51-2]

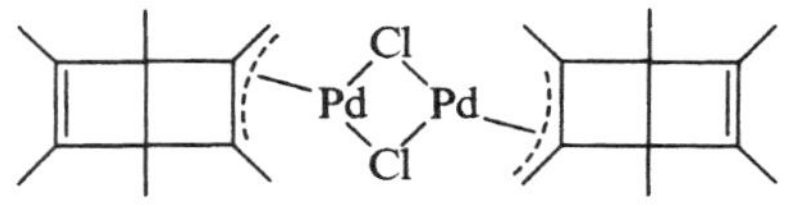

Cl Pd Pd Cl

M 606.279

Yellow cryst. (C_6H_6/pet. ether). Mp 159-60° (170-4°).

Monomer: Chloro(1,2,4,5,6-pentamethyl-3-methylenebicyclo[2.2.0]hex-5-en-2-yl)palladium.

$C_{12}H_{17}ClPd$ M 303.139

Unknown.

Shaw, B.L. *et al*, *J. Chem. Soc. (A)*, 1969, 602 (*pmr, synth, ir*)
Koser, G.F. *et al*, *J. Org. Chem.*, 1973, **38**, 4452 (*synth, ir, pmr*)

$C_{24}H_{36}O_4Pd_2$ Pd-00205

Bis[μ-(acetato-*O:O*)](η^3-6,6-dimethyl-2-methylenebicyclo[3.1.1]hept-3-yl)dipalladium, 10CI

Bis[acetoxy(3,2,10-η-pinene)palladium]. Bis-μ-acetatobis[(7,1,2-η)-pinene]dipalladium

[77481-48-2]

As Bis(η^3-6,6-dimethyl-4-methylenebicyclo[3.1.1]hept-3-yl)di-μ-(trifluoroacetato)dipalladium, Pd-00202 with

X = H

M 601.386

Acetate bridged dimer. Catalyses asymmetric oxidative cyclisation of 2-allylphenols. Yellow cryst. (hexane). Mp 125-7° dec. $[\alpha]_D^{25}$ +48.35°.

Monomer: (Acetato)(6,6-dimethyl-2-methylenebicyclo[3.3.1]hept-3-yl)palladium. Acetoxy(3,2,10-η-pinene)palladium.

$C_{12}H_{18}O_2Pd$ M 300.693

Unknown.

Hosokawa, T. *et al*, *J. Am. Chem. Soc.*, 1981, **103**, 2318 (*synth, pmr, use*)

$C_{24}H_{38}Cl_2O_4Pd_2$ Pd-00206

Bis[η^3-2-[2-(acetyloxy)ethylidene]-6-methyl-5-heptenyl]-di-μ-chlorodipalladium, 10CI

[70003-08-6]

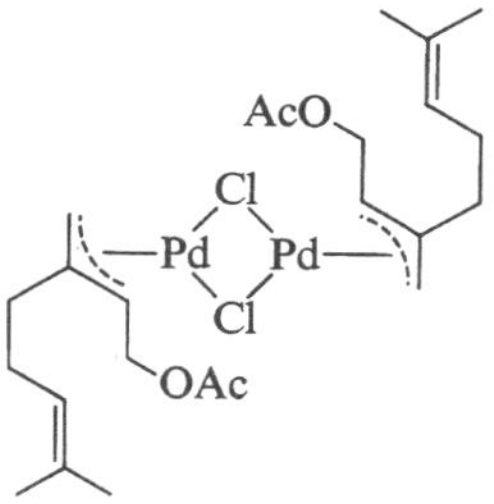

AcO Cl Pd Pd Cl OAc

M 674.308

Chloride bridged dimer. Yellow cryst. (CH_2Cl_2). Mp 121-122.5°.

Monomer: [η^3-2-[2-(Acetyloxy)ethylidene]-6-methyl-5-heptenyl]chloropalladium.

$C_{12}H_{19}ClO_2Pd$ M 337.154

Unknown.

Takahashi, M. *et al*, *Chem. Lett.*, 1979, 53.

$C_{24}H_{39}ClN_2P_2Pd$ Pd-00207

Chloro[2-(phenylazo)phenyl]bis(triethylphosphine)palladium, 9CI

Azobenzenyl(chloro)bis(triethylphosphine)palladium

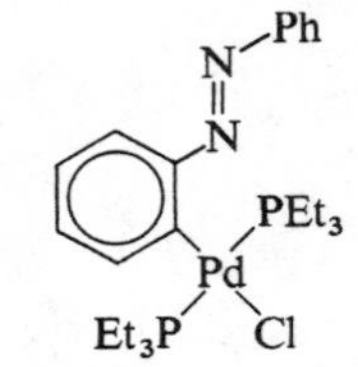

M 559.406

trans-form [29259-31-2]

Orange cryst. (hexane). Mp 116-8°.

Weaver, D.L., *Inorg. Chem.*, 1970, **9**, 2250 (*struct*)
Cross, R.J. *et al*, *J. Organomet. Chem.*, 1974, **72**, 21 (*synth*)

$C_{24}H_{42}Cl_2O_2Pd_2$ Pd-00208

Bis[chloro(9,10,11-η)methyl-10-undecenoate)palladium]

Di-μ-chlorobis[(1,2,3-η)-11-oxo-11-methoxy-2-undecenyl]dipalladium

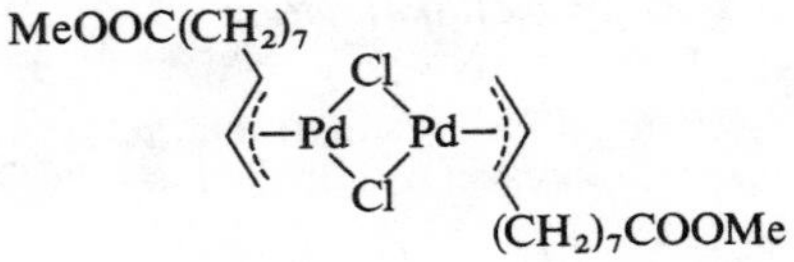

$MeOOC(CH_2)_7$ … $(CH_2)_7COOMe$

M 646.341

Chloride bridged dimer. Yellow cryst. (hexane/$CHCl_3$). Mp 86-7° dec.

Monomer: Chloro(methyl 10-undecenoate)palladium.
$C_{12}H_{21}ClOPd$ M 323.170
Unknown.

Trost, B.M. *et al*, *J. Am. Chem. Soc.*, 1980, **102**, 3572 (*synth, ir, pmr*)

$C_{24}H_{45}F_5P_3Pd^{\oplus}$ Pd-00209

(Pentafluorophenyl)tris(triethylphosphine)palladium(1+)

$[Pd(C_6F_5)(PEt_3)_3]^{\oplus}$

M 627.953 (ion)

Perchlorate: [59053-38-2].
$C_{24}H_{45}ClF_5O_4P_3Pd$ M 727.403
White solid. Mp 95° dec.

Uson, R. *et al*, *J. Organomet. Chem.*, 1976, **104**, 253 (*synth, ir*)

$C_{24}H_{54}As_2Pd_2$ Pd-00210

Bis[(2,2-di-*tert*-butylarsino)-2-methylpropyl]di-μ-hydridodipalladium

Bis[2-[bis(1,1-dimethylethyl)arsino]-2-methylpropyl-As,C]di-μ-hydrodipalladium, 9CI

[74281-64-4]

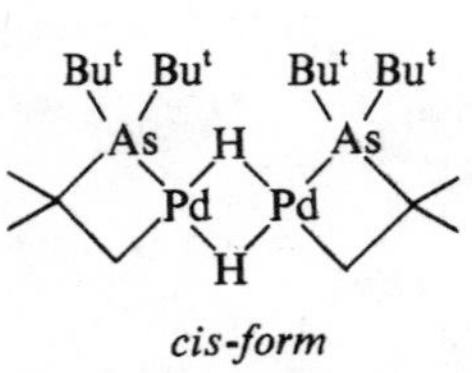

cis-form

M 705.374

Observed only in soln. as mixt. of both isomers.

Monomer:
$C_{12}H_{27}AsPd$ M 352.687
Unknown.

Goel, R.G. *et al*, *Inorg. Chim. Acta*, 1980, **44**, L165 (*pmr, struct*)

$C_{24}H_{54}P_2Pd$ Pd-00211

Bis(tri-*tert*-butylphosphine)palladium

Bis[tris-(1,1-dimethylethyl)phosphine]palladium, 9CI

[53199-31-8]

$[(H_3C)_3C]_3PPdP[C(CH_3)_3]_3$

M 511.058

Cryst. (hexane); air-stable. Mp 160-63° dec. (150-3° dec.).

Matsumoto, M. *et al*, *J. Am. Chem. Soc.*, 1974, **96**, 3322 (*synth, struct, pmr*)
Otsuka, S. *et al*, *J. Am. Chem. Soc.*, 1976, **98**, 5850 (*synth, pmr, struct*)
Werner, H. *et al*, *Angew. Chem., Int. Ed. Engl.*, 1977, **16**, 412 (*use*)
Inorg. Synth., 1979, **19**, 101 (*synth, pmr*)
Clark, H.C. *et al*, *Inorg. Chem.*, 1979, **18**, 2803.

$C_{24}H_{55}ClP_2Pd$ Pd-00212

Chlorohydrobis(tri-*tert*-butylphosphine)palladium

*Chlorohydrobis[tris(2-methyl-2-propyl)phosphine]palladium. Hydridochloridebis[tri-*tert*-butylphosphine]-palladium*

[63166-71-2]

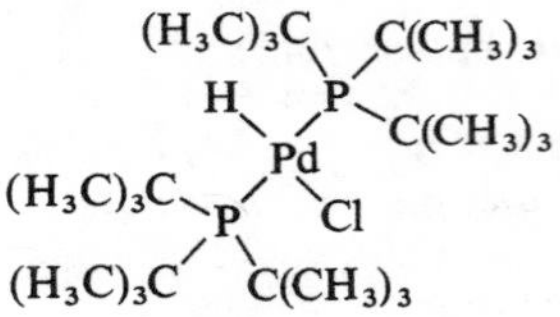

M 547.519

trans-form

Cryst. (C_6H_6/hexane), air-stable in solid state. Mp 144-7° dec.

Clark, H.C. *et al*, *Inorg. Chem.*, 1979, **18**, 2803 (*synth, ir, pmr, nmr*)

$C_{24}H_{60}O_{12}P_4Pd$ Pd-00213

Tetrakis(triethylphosphite-*P*)palladium, 9CI

Tetrakis(phosphorous acid)palladium dodecaethyl ester, 8CI

[23066-14-0]

$Pd[P(OEt)_3]_4$ (T_d)

M 771.046

White solid (H_2O or MeOH aq.); air-sensitive. Mp 65° dec., 112° dec. (under N_2).

Meier, M. *et al*, *Inorg. Chem.*, 1969, **8**, 795 (*synth*)
Myers, V.G. *et al*, *Inorg. Chem.*, 1969, **8**, 1204 (*ir*)
Inorg. Synth., 1971, **13**, 112 (*synth*)

$C_{25}H_{20}AsCl_2NPd$ Pd-00214

Dichloro(isocyanobenzene)(triphenylarsine)palladium, 9CI

Dichloro(phenylisocyanide)(triphenylarsine)palladium, 8CI. Dichloro(phenylisonitrile)(triphenylarsine)palladium. Isocyanobenzene(triphenylarsine)palladium dichloride

[29827-43-8]

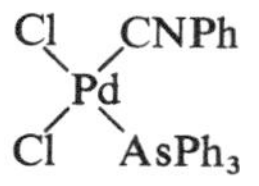

M 586.687

cis-form

Yellow cryst. Mp 192°.

Crociani, B. *et al*, Inorg. Chem., 1970, **9**, 2021 (*synth, ir*)

$C_{25}H_{20}Cl_2NPPd$ Pd-00215

Dichloro(isocyanobenzene)(triphenylphosphine)palladium, 9CI

Dichloro(phenyl isocyanide)(triphenylphosphine)palladium, 8CI. Dichloro(phenylisonitrile)-(triphenylphosphine)palladium

[29827-42-7]

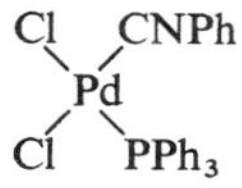

M 542.739

cis-form

Cream solid. Mp 248°.

Crociani, B. *et al*, Inorg. Chem., 1970, **9**, 2021 (*synth, ir*)

$C_{25}H_{22}Cl_2N_2OPPd$ Pd-00216

Chloro[2-(methylnitrosoamino)phenyl](triphenylphosphine)-palladium, 9CI

[76137-81-0]

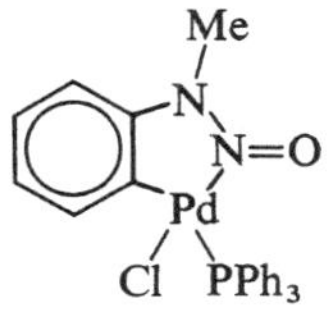

M 574.761

Orange cryst. Mp 185-90° dec.

Constable, A.G. *et al*, J. Chem. Soc., Dalton Trans., 1980, 2282 (*synth, struct, ir, pmr, nmr*)

$C_{25}H_{24}PPd^{\oplus}$ Pd-00217

(π-Cyclopentadienyl)ethylene(triphenylphosphine)palladium(1+)

(η^5-2,4-Cyclopentadien-1-yl)(η^2-ethene)(triphenylphosphine)palladium(1+), 9CI

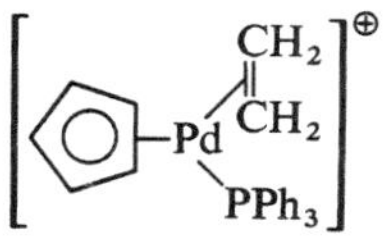

M 461.858 (ion)

Perchlorate: [64040-90-0].

$C_{25}H_{24}ClO_4PPd$ M 561.309

Violet cryst. (hexane). Mp 156° dec.

▷Potentially explosive

Majima, T. *et al*, J. Organomet. Chem., 1977, **134**, C45 (*synth, pmr*)

Kurosawa, H. *et al*, J. Am. Chem. Soc., 1980, **102**, 6996 (*synth, pmr*)

$C_{25}H_{25}PPdS$ Pd-00218

(η^5-2,4-Cyclopentadien-1-yl)[(methylthio)methyl](triphenylphosphine)palladium, 9CI

(Methylthiomethyl)(π-cyclopentadienyl)(triphenylphosphine)palladium

[61824-12-2]

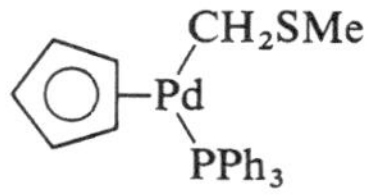

M 494.926

Red cryst. (Et_2O/pet. ether).

Suzuki, K. *et al*, Inorg. Chim. Acta, 1976, **20**, L15 (*synth, pmr*)

$C_{25}H_{50}O_2P_2Pd_2$ Pd-00219

(μ-π-Cyclopentadienyl)(μ-acetato)bis(triisopropylphosphine)dipalladium

[μ-(Acetato-O:O′)][μ-[1-η:2,3-η)-2,4-cyclopentadien-1-yl]]bis[tris(1-methylethyl)phosphine]dipalladium, 9CI

[72981-39-6]

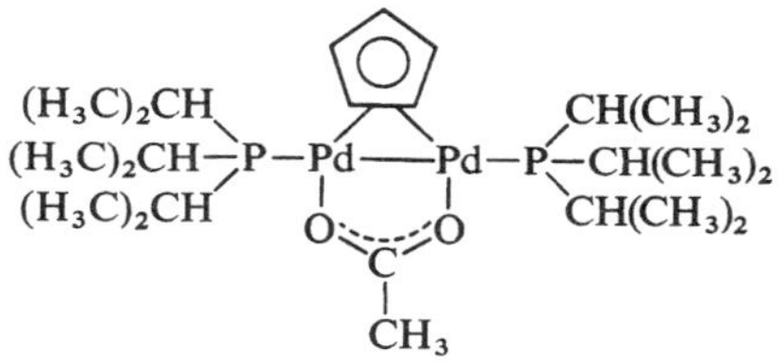

M 657.456

Orange solid. Mp 80° dec.

Werner, H. *et al*, Chem. Ber., 1980, **113**, 1072 (*synth, ms*)

$C_{26}H_{32}Cl_2Fe_2N_2Pd_2$ Pd-00220

Di-μ-chlorobis[2-[(dimethylamino)methyl]ferrocenyl-*C,N*]dipalladium, 10CI, 9CI

[58616-62-9]

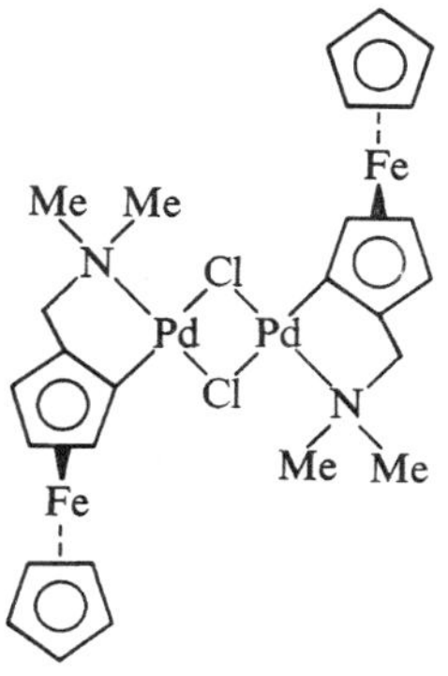

(*S*)-form

M 767.992

Orange cryst. (MeOH). Mp 172-5° dec.

(*R*)-form [71214-61-4]

Red cryst. (C_6H_6/heptane). Mp 172°. $[\alpha]_D^{20}$ +511° (c, 0.35 in CH_2Cl_2), $[\alpha]_D$ +664° (c, 0.15 in CH_2Cl_2).

(*S*)-form

$[\alpha]_D^{20}$ −470° (c, 0.4 in CH_2Cl_2).

Gaunt, J.C. *et al*, J. Organomet. Chem., 1975, **102**, 511 (*synth*)

Sokolov, V.I. *et al*, *Chimia*, 1978, **32**, 122.
Sokolov, V.I. *et al*, *J. Organomet. Chem.*, 1979, **182**, 537 (*synth, pmr*)
Komatsu, T. *et al*, *Bull. Chem. Soc. Jpn.*, 1981, **54**, 186 (*resoln, uv, pmr, cd*)

$C_{26}H_{46}Cl_2Pd_2$ Pd-00221

Di-μ-chlorobis[(1,2,3-η)-2,8-dimethyl-2,10-undecadienyl]dipalladium, 10CI
[67719-72-6]

M 642.395
Bridged dimer. Solid. Mp 95-8° dec.
Monomer: Chloro(2,8-dimethyl-2,10-undecadienyl)-palladium.
$C_{13}H_{23}ClPd$ M 321.198
Unknown.

Trost, B.M. *et al*, *J. Am. Chem. Soc.*, 1978, **100**, 3407.

$C_{26}H_{56}P_2Pd_2$ Pd-00222

Bis[μ-[(1-η:2,3-η)-2-methyl-2-propenyl]]bis[tris(1-methylethyl)phosphine]dipalladium, 9CI
Bis(μ-2-methyl-π-allyl)bis(triisopropylphosphine)dipalladium
[62586-39-4]

M 643.516
Yellow cryst. (pentane). Mp 99° dec.

Werner, H. *et al*, *J. Organomet. Chem.*, 1979, **179**, 439 (*synth, struct, pmr, cmr, nmr, ms*)

$C_{27}H_{24}F_3IP_2Pd$ Pd-00223

[Ethylenebis[diphenylphosphine]]iodo(trifluoromethyl)palladium, 8CI
[1,2-Ethanediylbis[diphenylphosphine]-P,P′]iodo(trifluoromethyl)palladium. 1,2-Bis(diphenylphosphino)-ethaneperfluoromethyliodopalladium. (Trifluoromethyl)iodo[1,2-bis(diphenylphosphino)ethane]palladium
[19469-53-5]

M 700.754
Yellow cryst. (Me_2CO/pet. ether). Mp 273° dec.

Rosevear, D.T. *et al*, *J. Chem. Soc. (A)*, 1968, 164 (*synth, ir*)

$C_{27}H_{29}IP_2Pd$ Pd-00224

Iodo(methyl)bis(methyldiphenylphosphine)palladium
Bis(methyldiphenylphosphine)methyliodopalladium. Methylbis(methyldiphenylphosphine)palladium iodide

M 648.798
trans-form [42582-53-6]
Cryst. Mp 140-2° dec.

Yamamoto, Y. *et al*, *Inorg. Chem.*, 1974, **13**, 438 (*synth, pmr*)

$C_{27}H_{29}PPd$ Pd-00225

Butyl(η⁵-2,4-cyclopentadien-1-yl)(triphenylphosphine)palladium, 9CI
(η⁵-2,4-Cyclopentadien-1-yl)butyl(triphenylphosphine)-palladium
[62483-34-5]

M 490.920
Orange cryst. Mp 59-62° dec. Dec. at 35° in $CDCl_3$ or C_6D_6.

Turner, G.K. *et al*, *J. Organomet. Chem.*, 1976, **121**, C29 (*synth, pmr*)

$C_{28}H_{27}P_2Pd^{\oplus}$ Pd-00226

[Methylenebis[diphenylphosphine]-*P,P′*](η³-2-propenyl)palladium(1+), 9CI
π-Allyl[methylenebis[diphenylphosphine]-P,P′]palladium(1+).
π-Enyl[methylenebis(diphenylphosphine)-P,P′]palladium(1+)

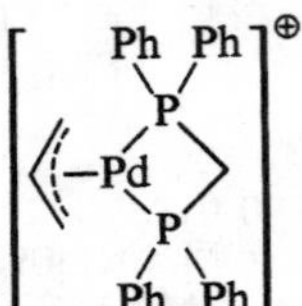

M 531.889 (ion)

Chloride: [35915-74-3]. *Chloro[methylenebis[diphenylphosphine]-P,P′](η³-2-propenyl)palladium, 9CI.*
$C_{28}H_{27}ClP_2Pd$ M 567.342
Orange-yellow cryst. Mp 238-40°.

Issleib, K. *et al*, *Z. Anorg. Allg. Chem.*, 1972, **388**, 89 (*synth, ir, uv*)

$C_{28}H_{29}O_4PPd$ Pd-00227

(1-Acetyl-2-oxopropyl)(2,4-pentanedionato-*O,O′*)(triphenylphosphine)palladium, 9CI

Acetylacetonatoacetylacetonyltriphenylphosphinepalladium. Bis(acetylacetonato)(triphenylphosphine)-palladium

[34710-54-8]

H_3C, O, PPh_3, Pd, O, $CH(COCH_3)_2$, H_3C

M 566.928
Yellow cryst. (C_6H_6/pet. ether). Mp 142° dec.

Baba, S. *et al*, *Inorg. Nucl. Chem. Lett.*, 1971, **7**, 1195 (*synth*)
Baba, S. *et al*, *Bull. Chem. Soc. Jpn.*, 1974, **47**, 665 (*ir, pmr*)
Horike, M. *et al*, *J. Organomet. Chem.*, 1974, **72**, 441 (*struct*)

$C_{28}H_{30}P_2Pd$ Pd-00228

[Ethylenebis[diphenylphosphine]]dimethylpalladium

[1,2-Ethanediylbis[diphenylphosphine]-P,P′]dimethylpalladium, 9CI. 1,2-Bis(diphenylphosphino)ethane(dimethyl)palladium. Dimethyl[1,2-bis(diphenylphosphino)-ethane]palladium

[63455-39-0]

Ph Ph P Me Pd P Me Ph Ph

M 534.913
Cryst. (Me_2CO). Mp 166-8° (105°) dec.

Calvin, G. *et al*, *J. Chem. Soc.*, 1960, 2008 (*synth, ir*)
Ito, T. *et al*, *Bull. Chem. Soc. Jpn.*, 1977, **50**, 1319 (*synth, ir, pmr*)
Gillie, A. *et al*, *J. Am. Chem. Soc.*, 1980, **102**, 4933 (*ir, pmr, cmr, nmr*)

$C_{28}H_{32}P_2Pd$ Pd-00229

Dimethylbis(methyldiphenylphosphine)palladium, 9CI

Dimethylbis(diphenylmethylphosphine)palladium

[70354-76-6]

Me PPh_2Me Pd Me PPh_2Me *cis-form*

M 536.928

cis-form [60885-30-5]
White cryst. (Me_2CO). Mp 110-5° dec.

trans-form [74345-90-7]
White solid (C_6H_6/pentane). Mp 112-6° dec.

Ito, T. *et al*, *Bull. Chem. Soc. Jpn.*, 1977, **50**, 1319 (*synth, ir, pmr*)
Gillie, A. *et al*, *J. Am. Chem. Soc.*, 1980, **102**, 4933 (*synth, ir, pmr, cmr, nmr*)
Ozawa, F. *et al*, *Bull. Chem. Soc. Jpn.*, 1981, **54**, 1868 (*synth, ir, pmr*)

$C_{28}H_{40}P_2Pd$ Pd-00230

Bis(phenylethynyl)bis(triethylphosphine)palladium, 8CI

Bis(triethylphosphine)bis(phenylethynyl)palladium. Bis(phenylacetylide)bis(triethylphosphine)palladium

[31386-97-7]

$[Pd(C{\equiv}CPh)_2(PEt_3)_2]$ (D_{2h})

M 544.992
Cryst. (toluene). Mp 162-4° dec., 170° dec.

Calvin, G. *et al*, *J. Chem. Soc.*, 1960, 2008 (*synth*)
Masai, H. *et al*, *Bull. Chem. Soc. Jpn.*, 1971, **44**, 2226 (*uv*)
Masai, H. *et al*, *J. Organomet. Chem.*, 1971, **26**, 271 (*ir*)

$C_{28}H_{46}P_2Pd$ Pd-00231

Bis(di-*tert*-butylphenylphosphine)palladium

Bis[bis-(1,1-dimethylethyl)phenylphosphine]palladium, 9CI

[52359-17-8]

$[(H_3C)_3C]_2PPhPdPPh[C(CH_3)_3]_2$

M 551.039
Catalyses co-oligomerization of butadiene and CO. Air-stable, yellow cryst. (hexane or toluene/MeOH). Mp 122-6° dec. (161-2° dec. under N_2).

Immirzi, A. *et al*, *J. Chem. Soc., Chem. Commun.*, 1974, 400 (*struct*)
Matsumoto, M. *et al*, *J. Am. Chem. Soc.*, 1974, **96**, 3322 (*synth, pmr, struct, stereochem*)
Kuran, W. *et al*, *Inorg. Chim. Acta*, 1975, **12**, 187 (*synth, cmr, pmr*)
Mann, B.E. *et al*, *J. Chem. Soc., Dalton Trans.*, 1975, 1673 (*nmr*)
Otsuka, S. *et al*, *J. Am. Chem. Soc.*, 1976, **98**, 5850 (*synth, struct, pmr*)
Inorg. Synth., 1979, **19**, 101 (*synth, pmr*)
Musco, A., *J. Chem. Soc., Perkin Trans. 1*, 1980, 693 (*use*)

$C_{28}H_{48}P_4Pd$ Pd-00232

Bis[1,2-bis(diethylphosphino)benzene]palladium

Bis[o-phenylenebis(diethylphosphine)]palladium, 8CI. Di-o-phenylenebisdiethylphosphinepalladium

[31989-53-4]

Et Et Et Et P P Pd P P Et Et Et Et

M 615.002
Yellow/orange cryst. (C_6H_6/MeOH); less air-sensitive than Ni(O) analogue. Mp 229-30°.

Chatt, J. *et al*, *J. Chem. Soc.*, 1961, 5504 (*synth*)

$C_{28}H_{52}P_2Pd_2$ Pd-00233

Di-μ-cyclopentadienylbis(triisopropylphosphine)dipalladium

Bis(η⁵-2,4-cyclopentadien-1-yl)bis[tris(1-methylethyl)-phosphine]dipalladium, 9CI

[72317-94-3]

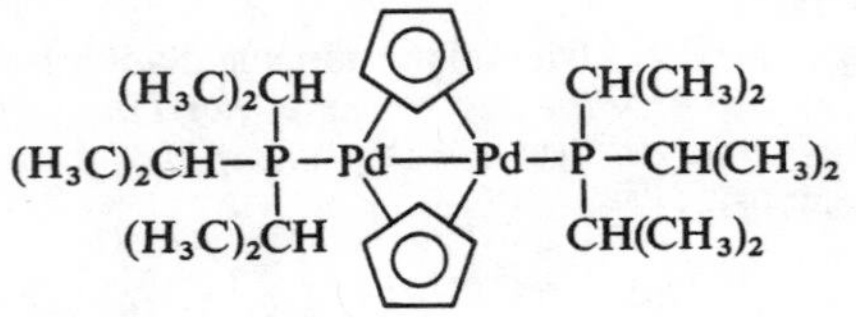

M 663.506

No physical data available.

Werner, H. *et al*, *J. Chem. Soc., Chem. Commun.*, 1979, 814 (*synth, pmr, struct*)

$C_{29}H_{25}BrNPPd$ Pd-00234

Bromo[1-(8-quinolinyl)ethyl-*C,N*](triphenylphosphine)palladium, 9CI

*(8-Ethylquinoline)bromo(triphenylphosphine)palladium. Triphenylphosphine(8-ethylquinoline-*C,N*)palladium bromide*

[81894-23-7]

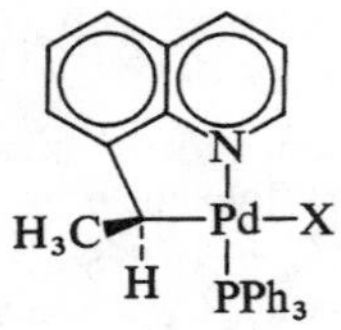

X = Br

M 604.821

(S)-form

Solid (hexane). Mp 125-30° dec. $[\alpha]_D^{20}$ +6.9° (c, 1 in CH_2Cl_2).

Sokolov, V.I. *et al*, *J. Organomet. Chem.*, 1982, **225**, 57.

$C_{29}H_{25}ClNPPd$ Pd-00235

Chloro[1-(8-quinolinyl)ethyl-*C,N*](triphenylphosphine)palladium, 9CI

*(8-Ethylquinoline)chloro(triphenylphosphine)palladium. Triphenylphosphine(8-ethylquinoline-*C,N*)palladium chloride*

[36571-82-1]

As Bromo[1-(8-quinolinyl)ethyl-*C,N*]-(triphenylphosphine)palladium, Pd-00234 with

X = Cl

M 560.370

(S)-form

$[\alpha]_D^{20}$ +41.5° (c, 4.5 in CH_2Cl_2).

Sokolov, V.I. *et al*, *J. Organomet. Chem.*, 1972, **36**, 389.

$C_{29}H_{25}PPd$ Pd-00236

(η⁵-2,4-Cyclopentadien-1-yl)phenyl(triphenylphosphine)palladium, 9CI

Phenyl(cyclopentadienyl)(triphenylphosphine)palladium

[62483-33-4]

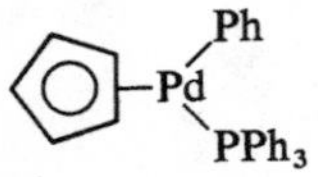

M 510.910

Orange cryst. (toluene/pentane). Mp 110-5° dec.

Turner, G.K. *et al*, *J. Organomet. Chem.*, 1976, **121**, C29 (*synth, pmr*)

$C_{30}H_{26}O_3P_2Pd$ Pd-00237

[1,2-Ethanediylbis(diphenylphosphine)-*P,P'*][(3,4-η)-2,5-furandione]palladium, 9CI

[Ethylenebis(diphenylphosphine)](maleic anhydride)-palladium, 8CI

[33292-27-2]

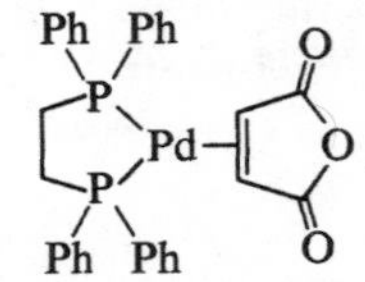

M 602.901

Solid. Mp 207-10° dec.

Takahashi, S. *et al*, *Nippon Kagaku Zasshi*, 1967, **88**, 1306; *CA*, **69**, 27514g (*ir, nmr*)

$C_{30}H_{26}P_2Pd$ Pd-00238

[1,2-Ethanediylbis(diphenylphosphine)-*P,P'*]diethynylpalladium, 9CI

[Ethylenebis[diphenylphosphine]]diethynylpalladium. [1,2-Bis(diphenylphosphino)ethane]diethynylpalladium. Diethynyl[1,2-bis(diphenylphosphino)ethane]-palladium

[66986-71-8]

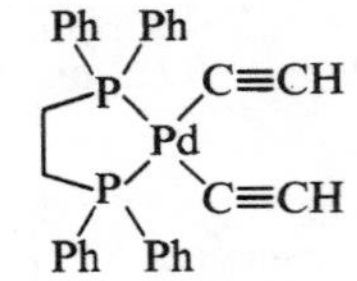

M 554.903

Brown-yellow powder.

Nast, R. *et al*, *Chem. Ber.*, 1978, **111**, 1627 (*synth, ir*)

$C_{30}H_{28}N_2P_2Pd$ Pd-00239

Bis(cyanomethyl)[1,2-ethanediylbis[diphenylphosphine]-*P,P'*]palladium, 9CI

Di(cyanomethyl)[ethylenebis[diphenylphosphine]]palladium

[55257-10-8]

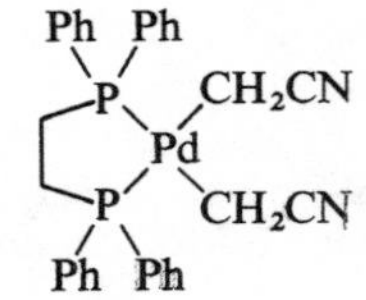

M 584.932

No physical data available.

Oehme, G. *et al*, *Z. Anorg. Allg. Chem.*, 1979, **449**, 157 (*ir*)

$C_{30}H_{34}P_2Pd$ Pd-00240

Diethyl[ethylenebis[diphenylphosphine]]palladium

[1,2-Ethanediylbis[diphenylphosphine]-P,P′]diethylpalladium, 9CI. Diethyl[1,2-ethanediylbis[diphenylphosphine]-P,P′]palladium. Diethyl[1,2-bis(diphenylphosphino)ethane]palladium

[63455-40-3]

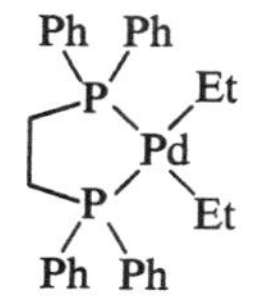

M 562.966

Non-cryst. solid. Poorly sol. Mp 144-8° dec.

Ito, T. *et al*, *Bull. Chem. Soc. Jpn.*, 1977, **50**, 1319 (*synth, ir, pmr*)

Ozawa, F. *et al*, *Bull. Chem. Soc. Jpn.*, 1981, **59**, 1868.

$C_{30}H_{36}P_2Pd$ Pd-00241

Diethylbis(methyldiphenylphosphine)palladium, 9CI

[60876-08-6]

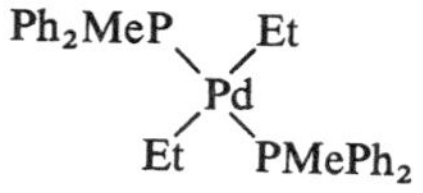

M 564.982

trans-form

Solid. Poorly sol. Mp 73-6° dec. Difficult to crystallise.

Ito, T. *et al*, *Bull. Chem. Soc. Jpn.*, 1977, **50**, 1319 (*synth, ir, pmr*)

Ozawa, F. *et al*, *J. Am. Chem. Soc.*, 1980, **102**, 6457 (*ir, pmr*)

$C_{30}H_{54}N_6Pd_2^{\oplus\oplus}$ Pd-00242

Hexakis(2-isocyano-2-methylpropane)dipalladium(2+), 9CI

Hexakis(tert-butylisonitrile)dipalladium(2+)

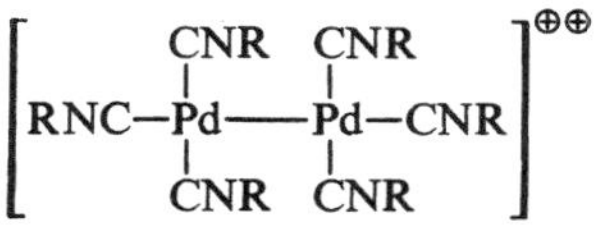

R = $(H_3C)_3C-$

M 711.637 (ion)

Bis(hexafluorophosphate): [59561-00-1].

$C_{30}H_{54}F_{12}N_6P_2Pd_2$ M 1001.565

White cryst. (2-propanol).

Boehm, J.R. *et al*, *Inorg. Chem.*, 1977, **16**, 778 (*synth, ir, pmr*)

$C_{31}H_{35}P_3Pd$ Pd-00243

[(Diethylphosphinidenio)bis(methylene)][[methylenebis(diphenylphosphinato)](1−)-*P,P′*]palladium, 9CI

Palladium[bis(diphenylphosphino)methanide][diethylphosphoniumbis(methylide)]

[63528-03-0]

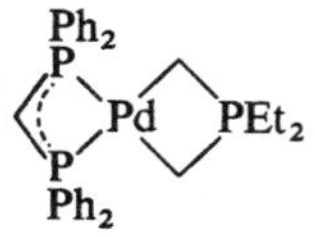

M 606.959

Yellow cryst. (pentane); high thermal stability. Mp 150°.

Schmidbaur, H. *et al*, *Angew. Chem., Int. Ed. Engl.*, 1977, **16**, 640 (*synth, ms, pmr, nmr*)

Bassett, J.M. *et al*, *Chem. Ber.*, 1980, **113**, 1145 (*synth, pmr, cmr, nmr*)

$C_{32}H_{20}Pd^{\ominus\ominus}$ Pd-00244

Tetrakis(phenylethynyl)palladate(2−)

Tetrakis(phenylacetylide)palladate(2−)

$Pd(C{\equiv}CPh)_4^{\ominus\ominus}$ (D_{4h})

M 510.930 (ion)

Di-K salt:

$C_{32}H_{20}K_2Pd$ M 589.127

Yellow powder.

Nast, R. *et al*, *Chem. Ber.*, 1978, **111**, 1627 (*synth, ir*)

$C_{32}H_{24}N_4P_2Pd$ Pd-00245

[Ethylenebis[diphenylphosphine]](tetracyanoethylene)palladium

[1,2-Ethanediylbis[diphenylphosphine]-P,P′](tetracyanoethene)palladium, 10CI. (Ethenetetracarbonitrile)-[ethylenebis[diphenylphosphine]]palladium, 8CI. [1,2-Bis(diphenylphosphino)ethane](tetracyanoethylene)palladium

[34742-01-3]

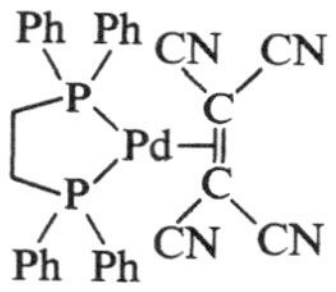

M 632.936

Yellow cryst. (Et_2O/pet. ether).

Boschi, T. *et al*, *J. Organomet. Chem.*, 1971, **30**, 283 (*ir, synth*)

$C_{32}H_{26}ClF_5P_2Pd$ Pd-00246

Chlorobis(methyldiphenylphosphine)(pentafluorophenyl)palladium, 9CI

Bis(diphenylmethylphosphine)(σ-pentafluorophenyl)-chloropalladium. (Pentafluorophenyl)chlorobis(methyldiphenylphosphine)palladium

[56298-20-5]

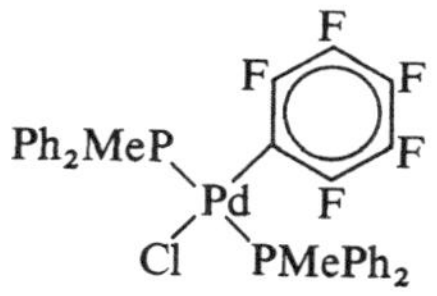

M 709.370

trans-form

Yellow cryst. (EtOH/CH_2Cl_2 or C_6H_6/hexane). Mp 203-4° (195-7°).

Mukhedkar, A.J. *et al*, *J. Chem. Soc. (A)*, 1969, 3023 (*synth, ir, pmr*)

Rausch, M.D. *et al*, *J. Organomet. Chem.*, 1970, **21**, 487 (*synth, ir, pmr*)

Uson, R. *et al*, *J. Organomet. Chem.*, 1975, **90**, 367 (*synth*)

$C_{32}H_{30}P_2Pd$ Pd-00247

[Ethylenebis[diphenylphosphine]]bis(propynyl)palladium

[1,2-Ethanediylbis(diphenylphosphine)-P,P′]bis(propynyl)palladium. (1,2-Bis(diphenylphosphino)ethane)bis(methylethynyl)palladium. Dipropynyl[1,2-bis(diphenylphosphino)ethane]palladium

M 582.957

Orange-yellow powder.

Nast, R. *et al*, *Chem. Ber.*, 1978, **111**, 1627 (*synth*, *ir*)

$C_{32}H_{35}B_9Pd$ Pd-00248

(1,2,3,4-Tetraphenyl-1,3-cyclobutadiene)[nonahydro-1,2-dimethyl-1,2-dicarbaundecaborato(2−)]palladium, 8CI

[12118-93-3]

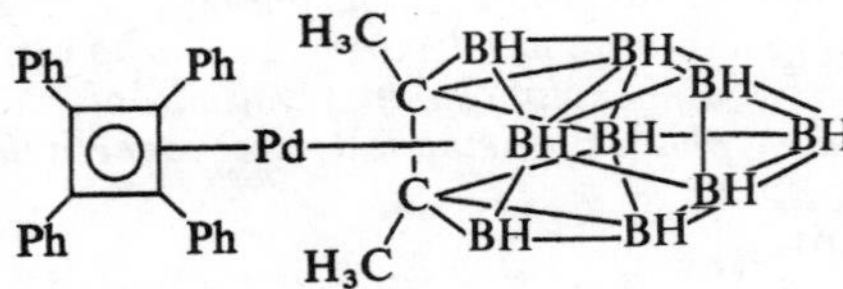

M 623.339

Cryst. (CH_2Cl_2/hexane). Mp >325° dec.

Wegner, P.A. *et al*, *J. Chem. Soc., Chem. Commun.*, 1966, 861 (*synth*, *ir*, *pmr*, *nmr*)

$C_{32}H_{50}Cl_2O_4Pd_2$ Pd-00249

Di-μ-chlorobis[(1,2,3-η)-12-methoxy-2,6,10-trimethyl-12-oxo-2,6,10-dodecatrienyl]dipalladium, 10CI

Bis[chloro(η³-12-methoxy-2,6,10-trimethyl-12-oxo-2,6,10-dodecatrienyl)palladium]

[57731-28-9]

M 782.491

Chloride bridged dimer. Yellow cryst. (hexane). Mp 114-21° dec.

Monomer: Chloro(12-methoxy-2,6,10-trimethyl-12-oxo-2,6,10-dodecatrienyl)palladium.

$C_{16}H_{25}ClO_2Pd$ M 391.245

Unknown.

Trost, B.M. *et al*, *J. Org. Chem.*, 1975, **40**, 3617 (*pmr*)
Trost, B.M. *et al*, *J. Am. Chem. Soc.*, 1978, **100**, 3407 (*synth*)

$C_{33}H_{25}Pd^{\oplus}$ Pd-00250

(η⁵-2,4-Cyclopentadien-1-yl)(tetraphenyl-1,3-cyclobutadiene)palladium(1+)

(Tetraphenyl-1,3-cyclobutadiene)(cyclopentadienyl)palladium

M 527.981 (ion)

Bromide:

$C_{33}H_{25}BrPd$ M 607.885

Air-stable orange cryst. (CH_2Cl_2/pet. ether). Mp 193° dec.

Tetrabromoferrate:

$C_{33}H_{25}Br_4FePd$ M 903.444

Cryst. (pet. ether); air-stable.

Maitlis, P.M. *et al*, *J. Am. Chem. Soc.*, 1965, **87**, 719 (*synth*, *struct*, *pmr*)

$C_{33}H_{35}P_2Pd^{\oplus}$ Pd-00251

[1,2-Ethanediylbis[diphenylphosphine]-*P*,*P′*](η³-2-methylenecyclohexyl)palladium(1+), 10CI

(η³-2-Methylenecyclohexyl)[1,2-bis(diphenylphosphino)ethane]palladium(1+)

M 600.007 (ion)

Tetrafluoroborate: [67423-87-4].

$C_{33}H_{35}BF_4P_2Pd$ M 686.811

Yellow powder.

Trost, B.M. *et al*, *J. Am. Chem. Soc.*, 1978, **100**, 3416 (*synth*, *pmr*)

$C_{34}H_{28}Cl_2FeP_2Pd$ Pd-00252

[1,1′-Bis(diphenylphosphino)ferrocene-*P*,*P′*]dichloropalladium, 9CI

Dichloro[1,1′-bis(diphenylphosphino)ferrocene]palladium

[72287-26-4]

M 731.716

Catalyses cross-coupling reactions and regioselective allylation of Grignard reagents and synth. of acetylenic ketones. Cryst. ($CHCl_3$/C_6H_6). Mp 265-8° dec.

Hayashi, T. *et al*, *Tetrahedron Lett.*, 1979, 1871 (*synth*, *use*)
Hayashi, T. *et al*, *Chem. Lett.*, 1980, 767 (*use*)

Hayashi, T. *et al*, *J. Organomet. Chem.*, 1980, **186**, C1 (*use*)
Hayashi, T. *et al*, *J. Chem. Soc., Chem. Commun.*, 1981, 313 (*use*)
Kobayashi, T. *et al*, *J. Chem. Soc., Chem. Commun.*, 1981, 333 (*use*)

$C_{34}H_{28}O_2Pd$ Pd-00253

Bis[η^2-1,5-diphenyl-1,4-pentadien-3-one]palladium, 9CI
Bis(dibenzylideneacetone)palladium
[32005-36-0]

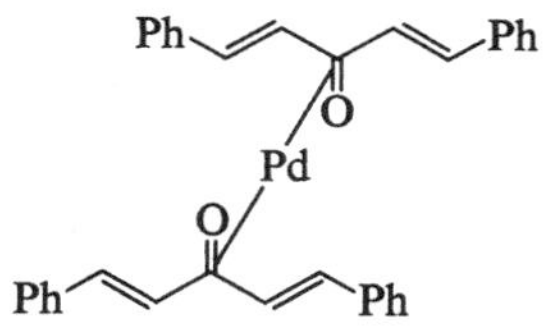

M 575.014
Structure may be ketonic bonded as shown, but olefinic bonding has also been postulated. Catalyses allylic alkylation of olefins, cyclopropene oligomerisations, reactions of nitro-aromatics with CO, arylation of ethylene, and cycloadditions of olefins and methylene cyclopropane. Brownish solid. Mp 135° dec.

Takahashi, Y. *et al*, *J. Chem. Soc., Chem. Commun.*, 1970, 1065 (*synth, ir*)
Moseley, K. *et al*, *J. Chem. Soc., Chem. Commun.*, 1971, 982.

$C_{34}H_{34}P_2Pd$ Pd-00254

Bis(methyldiphenylphosphine)(styrene)palladium
Bis(methyldiphenylphosphine)(phenylethene)palladium. [(η^2-*Ethenyl*)*benzene*]*bis*(*methyldiphenylphosphine*)*palladium*, 9CI
[70316-76-6]

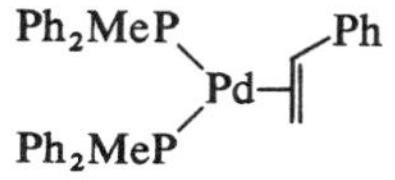

M 611.010
Yellow cryst. (hexane).

Ito, T. *et al*, *J. Organomet. Chem.*, 1979, **168**, 375 (*synth, ir, pmr*)

$C_{34}H_{36}P_2Pd^{\oplus\oplus}$ Pd-00255

[(1,2,5,6-η)-1,5-Cyclooctadiene][1,2-ethanediylbis[diphenylphosphine]-*P,P'*]palladium(2+), 9CI
(*1,5-Cyclooctadiene*)[*ethylenebis*[*diphenylphosphine*]]-*palladium*(*2+*). (*1,5-Cyclooctadiene*)[*1,2-bis*(*diphenylphosphino*)*ethane*]*palladium*(*2+*)

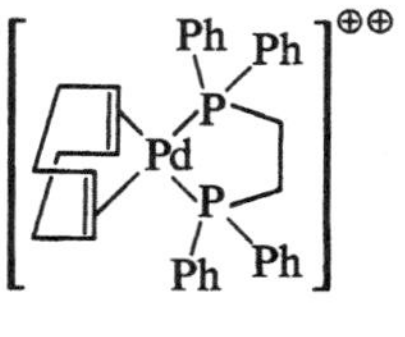

M 613.026 (ion)
Bis(hexafluorophosphate): [55046-52-1].
$C_{34}H_{36}F_{12}P_4Pd$ M 902.954
Not fully descr. Olefin readily attacked by nucleophiles.

Roulet, R. *et al*, *Helv. Chim. Acta*, 1974, **57**, 2139 (*synth*)

$C_{34}H_{64}Cl_2P_4Pd_2$ Pd-00256

Dichloro[μ-(1,4-phenylenedi-1,2-ethynediyl)]tetrakis(triethylphosphine)dipalladium, 9CI
[75345-86-7]

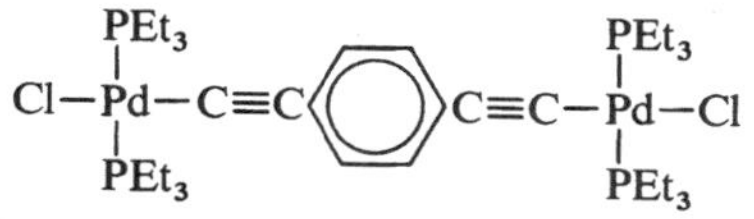

M 880.521
Brown cryst. (EtOH).

Nast, R. *et al*, *J. Organomet. Chem.*, 1980, **194**, 125 (*synth, ir, nmr*)

$C_{35}H_{25}NOPd$ Pd-00257

Nitrosyl[(1,2,3,4,5-η)-1,2,3,4,5-pentaphenyl-2,4-cyclopentadien-1-yl]palladium, 9CI
η^5-*Pentaphenylcyclopentadienylnitrosylpalladium*
[63946-61-2]

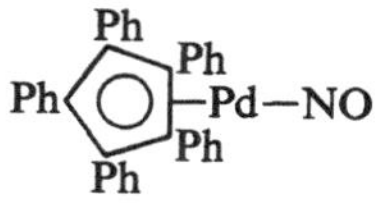

M 582.009
Purple cryst. Mp 151-4°.

Jack, T.R. *et al*, *J. Am. Chem. Soc.*, 1977, **99**, 4707 (*synth, ir, uv, ms*)

$C_{35}H_{30}OPd$ Pd-00258

(η^5-2,4-Cyclopentadien-1-yl)[(1,2,3-η)-4-ethoxy-1,2,3,4-tetraphenyl-2-cyclobuten-1-yl]palladium
Cyclopentadienyl(1-ethoxy-1,2,3,4-tetraphenylcyclobutenyl)palladium

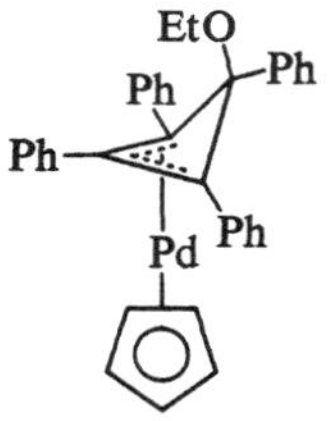

M 573.041
Dark-red cryst. (C_6H_6/MeOH). Mp 149-52° dec.

Maitlis, P.M. *et al*, *J. Am. Chem. Soc.*, 1965, **87**, 719 (*synth, pmr, struct*)

$C_{36}H_{28}Cl_2N_2O_2P_2Pd_2$ Pd-00259

Dicarbonyldichlorobis[2-(diphenylphosphino)pyridine-*P*]dipalladium, 9CI
[78055-59-1]

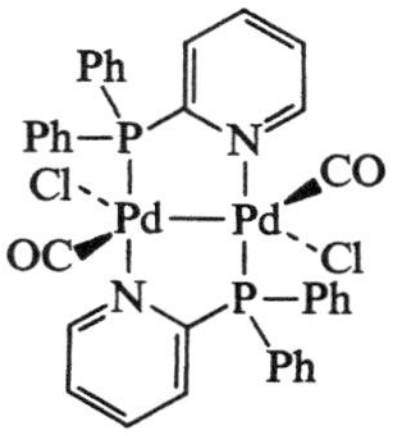

M 866.323
Loses CO on attempted purifn.

Maisonnat, A. *et al*, *Inorg. Chim. Acta*, 1981, **53**, L217 (*synth, ir, struct*)

$C_{36}H_{30}Cl_2P_2Pd$ Pd-00260

Dichlorobis(triphenylphosphine)palladium, 10CI, 9CI, 8CI

Bis(triphenylphosphine)palladium dichloride

[13965-03-2]

$Pd(PPh_3)_2Cl_2$

M 701.907

Catalyst for carboalkylation of halides to carboxylic acid and amides. Bright-yellow cryst. (toluene). Mp 297-8° dec.

▷ATP-ase inhibitor

***cis*-form** [15604-37-2]

Not separately characterised.

***trans*-form** [28966-81-6]

Not separately characterised.

Chatt, J. *et al*, *J. Chem. Soc.*, 1939, 1631 (*synth*)
Coates, G.E. *et al*, *J. Chem. Soc.*, 1963, 421 (*ir*)
Cookson, R.C. *et al*, *J. Chem. Soc.*, 1965, 1881 (*synth*)
Druding, L.F. *et al*, *J. Chromatogr.*, 1966, **24**, 491.
Goodall, D.C., *J. Chem. Soc. (A)*, 1968, 887 (*synth, ir*)
Grim, S.O., *Inorg. Chim. Acta*, 1970, **4**, 56 (*nmr*)
Shobatke, K. *et al*, *J. Am. Chem. Soc.*, 1970, **92**, 3332 (*ir*)
Tayim, H.A. *et al*, *J. Inorg. Nucl. Chem.*, 1970, 3799 (*synth*)
Fieser, M. *et al*, *Reagents for Organic Synthesis*, Wiley, 1967-83, **3**, 81; **6**, 59; **8**, 151.

$C_{36}H_{30}NOP_2Pd$ Pd-00261

Nitrosylbis(triphenylphosphine)palladium

$(NO)(PPh_3)_2Pd—Pd(PPh_3)_2(NO)$

M 661.007

Dimeric.

Dimer: [23064-67-7]. *Dinitrosyltetrakis(triphenylphosphine)dipalladium*, 8CI. *Tetrakis(triphenylphosphine)-dinitrosyldipalladium.*

$C_{72}H_{60}N_2O_2P_4Pd_2$ M 1322.013

Solid. Mp 208° dec.

Pneumaticakis, G.A., *J. Chem. Soc., Chem. Commun.*, 1968, 275 (*synth, ir*)

$C_{36}H_{31}ClP_2Pd$ Pd-00262

Chlorohydrobis(triphenylphosphine)palladium, 9CI, 8CI

Bis(triphenylphosphine)palladium hydridochloride. Chlorohydridobis(triphenylphosphine)palladium. Hydridochlorobis(triphenylphosphine)palladium

[29893-78-5]

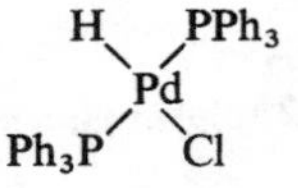

H PPh₃ / Pd / Ph₃P Cl

M 667.461

***trans*-form**

Pale-yellow solid.

Kudo, K. *et al*, *J. Chem. Soc., Chem. Commun.*, 1970, 1701 (*synth, ir*)

$C_{36}H_{46}Cl_2Pd_2$ Pd-00263

Di-μ-chlorobis[2-[(2,3-η)-1,2,3,4,5-pentamethyl-2,4-cyclopentadien-1-yl]-2-phenylethyl]dipalladium, 9CI

[38960-16-6]

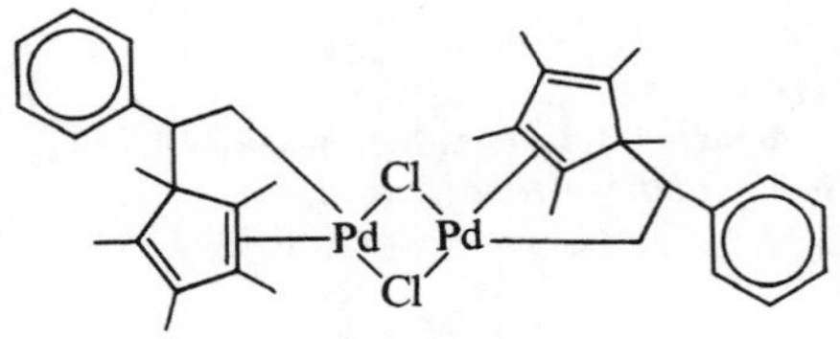

M 762.505

Yellow cryst. (pet. ether). Mp 125-6° dec.

Hosokawa, T. *et al*, *J. Am. Chem. Soc.*, 1973, **95**, 4914 (*synth, struct, ir, pmr*)
Mabbott, D.J. *et al*, *J. Chem. Soc., Dalton Trans.*, 1976, 2156.
Mabbott, D.J. *et al*, *J. Chem. Soc., Dalton Trans.*, 1977, 254 (*synth, cmr*)

$C_{36}H_{67}ClP_2Pd$ Pd-00264

Chlorohydrobis(tricyclohexylphosphine)palladium, 9CI, 8CI

Chlorohydridobis(tricyclohexylphosphine)palladium. Hydridobis(tricyclohexylphosphine)palladium chloride

[28016-71-9]

$[(C_6H_{11})_3P]_2PdClH$

M 703.746

Slightly air-sensitive cryst. (pentane or toluene/MeOH). Mp 218-20° dec.

Green, M.L.H., *J. Chem. Soc., Chem. Commun.*, 1970, 881 (*synth, ir, pmr*)
Kudo, K. *et al*, *J. Chem. Soc., Chem. Commun.*, 1970, 1701 (*synth, ir*)
Inorg. Synth., 1977, **17**, 83 (*synth, ir, pmr*)
Goel, A.B. *et al*, *Inorg. Chim. Acta*, 1980, **45**, L85 (*synth, ir, pmr, nmr*)

$C_{36}H_{68}P_2Pd$ Pd-00265

Dihydrobis(tricyclohexylphosphine)palladium, 9CI

Bis(tricyclohexylphosphine)palladium dihydride

[54083-05-5]

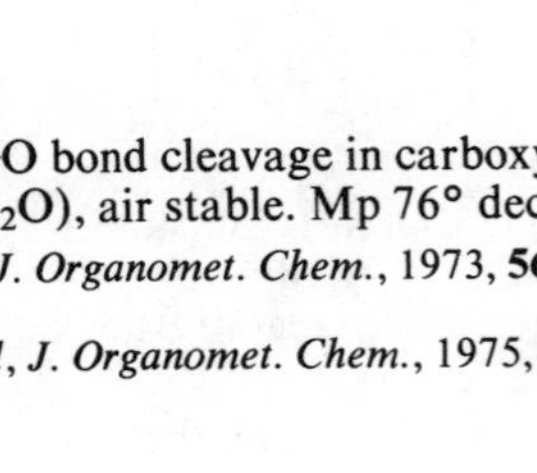

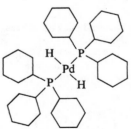

M 669.301

***trans*-form**

Promotes C—O bond cleavage in carboxylates. Cryst. (hexane/Et_2O), air stable. Mp 76° dec.

Kudo, K. *et al*, *J. Organomet. Chem.*, 1973, **56**, 413 (*synth, ir, pmr*)
Komiya, S. *et al*, *J. Organomet. Chem.*, 1975, **87**, 333 (*use*)

$C_{36}H_{71}BP_2Pd$ Pd-00266

Hydro[tetrahydroborato(1−)-*H,H'*]bis(tricyclohexylphosphine)palladium, 9CI

Bis(tricyclohexylphosphine)hydridopalladium tetrahydroborate.
Hydridoborohydridobis(tricyclohexylphosphine)palladium
[30916-06-4]

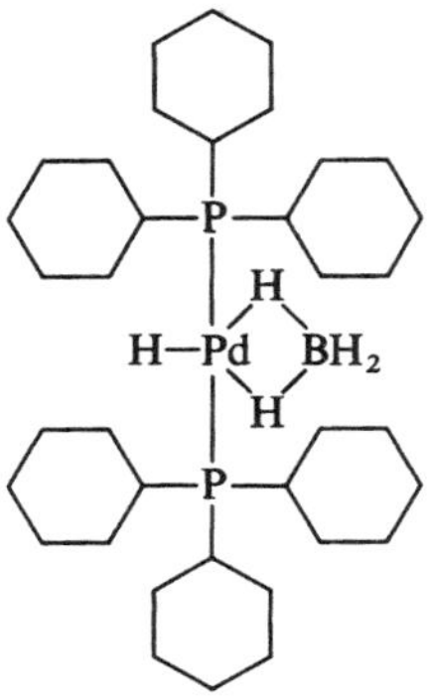

M 683.134
Precursor of catalyst for oligomerization of butadiene. Cryst. (EtOH aq.). Mp 135-8° dec.

Green, M.L.H. *et al*, *J. Chem. Soc. (A)*, 1971, 469 (*synth, ir, pmr*)
Green, M.L.H. *et al*, *J. Chem. Soc., Dalton Trans.*, 1974, 269 (*use*)
Inorg. Synth., 1977, **17**, 88 (*synth, ir, pmr*)

$C_{37}H_{30}F_3IP_2Pd$ Pd-00267

Iodotrifluoromethylbis(triphenylphosphine)palladium, 8CI

Trifluoromethylbis(triphenylphosphine)palladium iodide. Bis(triphenylphosphine)-perfluoromethyliodopalladium
[23868-37-3]

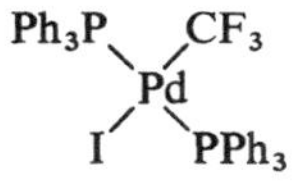

M 826.911

***trans*-form** [19469-52-4]
Orange cryst. (C_6H_6/MeOH). Mp 255° dec.

Rosevear, D.T. *et al*, *J. Chem. Soc. (A)*, 1968, 164 (*synth, ir*)
Johnson, M.P., *Inorg. Chim. Acta*, 1969, **3**, 232 (*ir*)

$C_{37}H_{30}P_2PdS_2$ Pd-00268

[(*C,S*-η)-Carbon disulfide]bis(triphenylphosphine)palladium, 9CI

Bis(triphenylphosphine)(carbon disulfide)palladium
[74593-76-3]

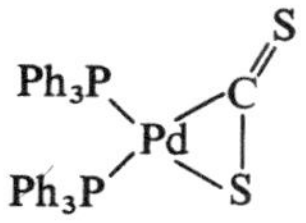

M 707.132
Orange cryst. (CH_2Cl_2/Et_2O or CS_2). Mp 112-22° dec.

Baird, M.C. *et al*, *J. Chem. Soc. (A)*, 1967, 865 (*synth, ir, struct*)

$C_{37}H_{33}IP_2Pd$ Pd-00269

Iodomethylbis(triphenylphosphine)palladium, 9CI, 8CI

Methylbis(triphenylphosphine)palladium iodide.
Methyliodobis(triphenylphosphine)palladium
[53228-65-2]

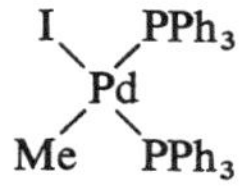

cis-form

M 772.940
Kudo *et al* detected two isomers: pink, Mp 168° dec., and yellow, Mp 130° dec., without determining structure.

***cis*-form** [35655-02-8]
Not unequivocally descr.

***trans*-form** [18115-58-7]
Mp 150-5° dec. (151-4°).

Fitton, P. *et al*, *J. Chem. Soc., Chem. Commun.*, 1968, 6 (*synth, pmr*)
Kudo, K. *et al*, *J. Organomet. Chem.*, 1971, **33**, 393.
Garrou, P.E. *et al*, *J. Am. Chem. Soc.*, 1976, **98**, 4115 (*synth, pmr*)

$C_{38}H_{24}Cl_{10}P_2Pd$ Pd-00270

[Ethylenebis[diphenylphosphine]]bis(pentachlorophenyl)palladium

[1,2-Ethanediylbis[diphenylphosphine]-P,P']bis(pentachlorophenyl)palladium. [1,2-Bis(diphenylphosphino)-ethane]bis(pentachlorophenyl)palladium
[71480-03-0]

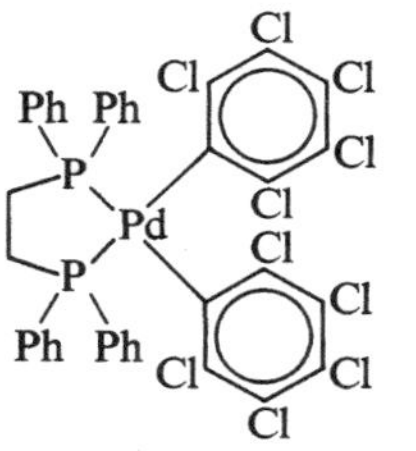

M 1003.505
Cryst. (MeOH/Me_2CO). Mp 275-6° dec.

Ceder, R. *et al*, *J. Organomet. Chem.*, 1979, **174**, 115 (*synth*)

$C_{38}H_{30}Cl_4P_2Pd$ Pd-00271

Chloro(trichlorovinyl)bis(triphenylphosphine)palladium, 8CI

Chloro(trichloroethenyl)bis(triphenylphosphine)palladium, 9CI. *(Trichlorovinyl)bis(triphenylphosphine)palladium chloride. Bis(triphenylphosphine)chloro(trichlorovinyl)palladium. Bis(triphenylphosphine)-(trichlorovinyl)chloropalladium*
[17764-61-3]

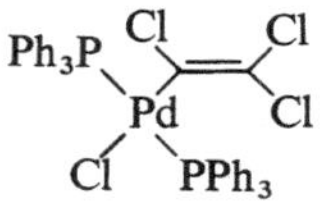

M 796.835

***trans*-form**
Mp 259-62° dec.

Fitton, P. *et al*, *J. Chem. Soc., Chem. Commun.*, 1968, 4 (*synth, ir*)

$C_{38}H_{31}Cl_3P_2Pd$ Pd-00272

Chloro(2,2-dichlorovinyl)bis(triphenylphosphine)palladium, 8CI

Chloro(2,2-dichloroethenyl)bis(triphenylphosphine)-palladium. (2,2-Dichlorovinyl)-chlorobis(triphenylphosphine)palladium

[31871-49-5]

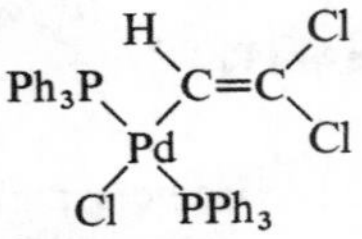

M 762.389

Stable solid. Mp 310-2° dec.

Fitton, P. *et al*, *J. Chem. Soc., Chem. Commun.*, 1968, 4 (*synth*, *ir*, *pmr*)

$C_{38}H_{32}ClNP_2Pd$ Pd-00273

Chloro(cyanomethyl)bis(triphenylphosphine)palladium, 9CI

(Cyanomethyl)chlorobis(triphenylphosphine)palladium

[55298-20-9]

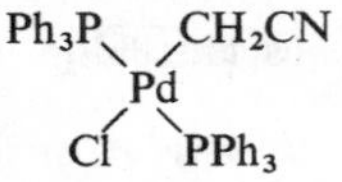

M 706.498

Yellow cryst. (Me_2CO). Mp 190-2° dec.

Suzuki, K. *et al*, *J. Organomet. Chem.*, 1973, **54**, 385 (*synth*, *ir*, *pmr*)
Suzuki, K. *et al*, *Inorg. Chim. Acta*, 1979, **32**, L3.

$C_{38}H_{32}Cl_2P_2Pd$ Pd-00274

Chloro(2-chlorovinyl)bis(triphenylphosphine)palladium, 8CI

Chloro(2-chloroethenyl)bis(triphenylphosphine)palladium. (β-Chlorovinyl)chlorobis(triphenylphosphine)-palladium

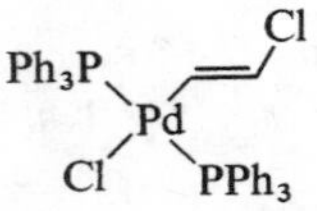

(E)-trans-form

M 727.944

(E)-trans-form [17764-63-5]

Mp 272-7° dec.

(Z)-trans-form [17830-49-8]

Mp 279-83° dec.

Fitton, P. *et al*, *J. Chem. Soc., Chem. Commun.*, 1968, 4 (*synth*, *pmr*, *ir*)

$C_{38}H_{33}ClOP_2Pd$ Pd-00275

Acetylchlorobis(triphenylphosphine)palladium, 9CI

Chloro(acetyl)bis(triphenylphosphine)palladium

[41910-22-9]

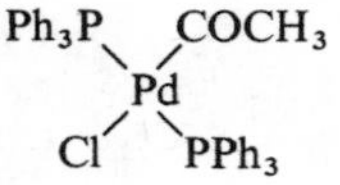

M 709.499

Catalyses carboxylation or alkoxycarbonylation of unsaturated hydrocarbons. Cryst. Mp 166-72° dec.

Otsuka, S. *et al*, *J. Am. Chem. Soc.*, 1973, **95**, 3180 (*synth*, *ir*, *pmr*)

$C_{38}H_{34}P_2Pd$ Pd-00276

Ethylenebis(triphenylphosphine)palladium, 8CI

η^2-Ethenebis(triphenylphosphine)palladium, 9CI

[33395-22-1]

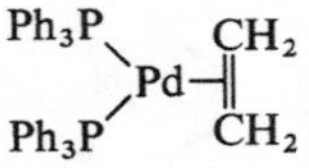

M 659.054

Catalyses synth. of silyl-substituted alkenes and allylic alkylations. Air-sensitive, white cryst. (Et_2O).

Van der Linde, R. *et al*, *J. Chem. Soc., Chem. Commun.*, 1971, 563 (*synth*)
Inorg. Synth., 1976, **16**, 127 (*synth*, *ir*)
Czech. Pat., 174 583, (*1978*); *CA*, **90**, 87657z (*use*)
Trost, B.M. *et al*, *J. Am. Chem. Soc.*, 1980, **102**, 4730 (*use*)

$C_{38}H_{35}ClP_2PdS$ Pd-00277

Chloro[(methylthio)methyl]bis(triphenylphosphine)palladium, 9CI

Chlorothiomethoxymethylbis(triphenylphosphine)palladium

[60619-21-8]

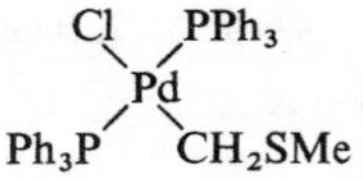

M 727.575

trans-form

Yellow cryst. + $1CH_2Cl_2$(CH_2Cl_2/hexane). Mp 144° dec.

Yoshida, G. *et al*, *J. Organomet. Chem.*, 1976, **113**, 85 (*synth*, *ir*, *pmr*)
Miki, K. *et al*, *J. Organomet. Chem.*, 1979, **165**, 79 (*struct*)

$C_{38}H_{36}P_2Pd$ Pd-00278

Dimethylbis(triphenylphosphine)palladium, 9CI

Bis(triphenylphosphine)dimethylpalladium

[36485-69-5]

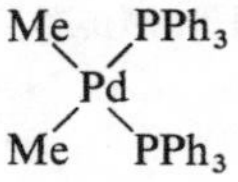

cis-form

M 661.070

cis-form [71830-11-0]

Cryst. (THF or butanone). Mp 197-8° (128°) dec.

trans-form [74345-39-4]

No physical data available.

Calvin, G. *et al*, *J. Chem. Soc.*, 1960, 2008 (*synth*, *ir*)
Garty, N. *et al*, *J. Organomet. Chem.*, 1972, **36**, 391 (*synth*, *ir*, *pmr*)
Gillie, A. *et al*, *J. Am. Chem. Soc.*, 1980, **102**, 4933 (*synth*, *ir*, *pmr*, *cmr*, *nmr*)

$C_{38}H_{70}P_2Pd$ Pd-00279

Ethylenebis(tricyclohexylphosphine)palladium, 8CI
η^2-Ethenebis(tricyclohexylphosphine)palladium, 9CI
[33395-48-1]

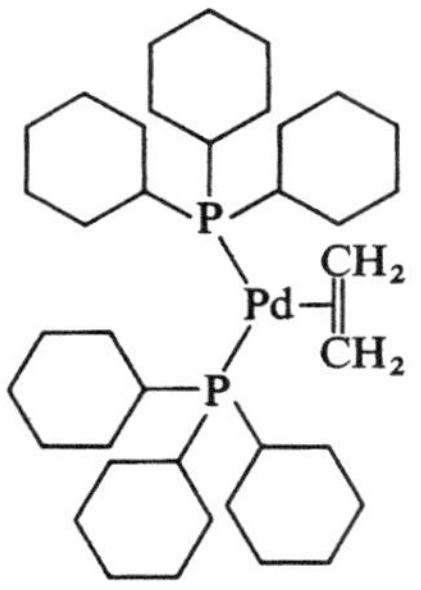

M 695.339
Cryst. (Et_2O/ethylene at 0°). Air-sensitive.
Inorg. Synth., 1976, **16**, 127 (*synth, ir*)

$C_{39}H_{30}F_6OP_2Pd$ Pd-00280

(1,1,1,3,3,3-Hexafluoro-2-propanone)bis(triphenylphosphine)palladium, 9CI
[Oxy[trifluoro-1-(trifluoromethyl)ethylidene]]bis(triphenylphosphine)palladium, 8CI. *η^2-Perfluoroacetonebis(triphenylphosphine)palladium*
[19554-17-7]

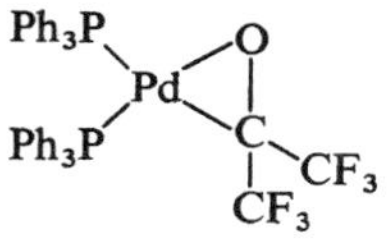

M 797.023
Cryst. (C_6H_6/pet. ether or CH_2Cl_2/hexane). Mp 187-9° (*in vacuo*).
Clarke, B. *et al*, *J. Chem. Soc.* (*A*), 1968, 167 (*synth, ir, nmr*)

$C_{39}H_{35}IP_2Pd_2$ Pd-00281

μ-Iodo[μ-(1-η:2,3-η)-2-propenyl]bis(triphenylphosphine)dipalladium, 9CI
(μ-π-Allyl)μ-iodobis(triphenylphosphine)dipalladium
[36548-51-3]

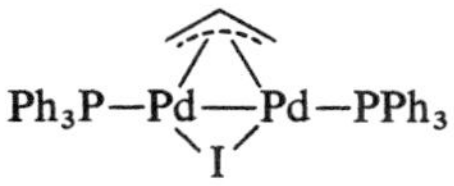

M 905.398
Yellow cryst. (CH_2Cl_2/hexane). Mp 150°.
Kobayashi, Y. *et al*, *Acta Crystallogr., Sect. B*, 1972, **28**, 899 (*synth, pmr, struct*)

$C_{39}H_{35}P_2Pd^{\oplus}$ Pd-00282

(η^3-2-Propenyl)bis(triphenylphosphine)palladium(1+), 9CI
(π-Allyl)bis(triphenylphosphine)palladium(1+). Bis(triphenylphosphine)allylpalladium(1+). π-Enylbis(triphenylphosphine)palladium(1+)

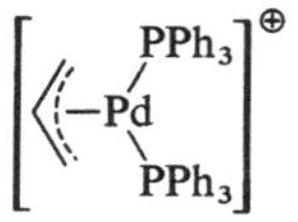

M 672.073 (ion)
Perchlorate: [38497-96-0].
$C_{39}H_{35}ClO_4P_2Pd$ M 771.524
Cryst.
Tetrafluoroborate: [36540-72-4].
$C_{39}H_{35}BF_4P_2Pd$ M 758.877
Solid.
Johnson, B.F.G. *et al*, *Synth. React. Inorg. Metal-Org. Chem.*, 1971, **1**, 235 (*synth, pmr*)
Takahashi, Y. *et al*, *Inorg. Chem.*, 1972, **11**, 1516 (*synth*)

$C_{40}H_{30}F_6P_2Pd$ Pd-00283

[(2,3-η)-1,1,1,4,4,4-Hexafluoro-2-butyne]bis(triphenylphosphine)palladium, 9CI
Bis(triphenylphosphine)hexafluoro-2-butynepalladium
[15629-87-5]

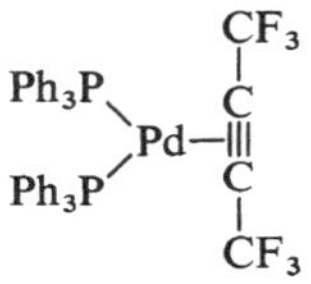

M 793.035
Cryst. Mp 194-5°.
Burgess, J. *et al*, *J. Organomet. Chem.*, 1973, **56**, 405 (*synth*)

$C_{40}H_{32}O_3P_2Pd$ Pd-00284

[(3,4-η)-2,5-Furandione]bis(triphenylphosphine)palladium, 9CI
(Maleic anhydride)bis(triphenylphosphine)palladium, 8CI. *Bis(triphenylphosphine)(maleic anhydride)palladium*
[17830-50-1]

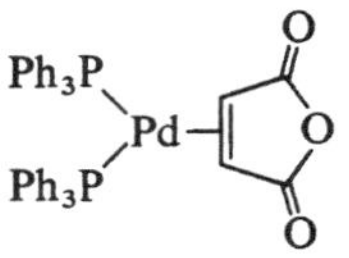

M 729.059
Catalyses dimerisation, oligomerisation, codimerisation, cyclization, cocyclization and hydrosilylation of dienes, and disilane metathesis. Air stable cryst. Mp 147-51° dec.

Takahashi, S. *et al*, *J. Chem. Soc. Jpn.* (*Pure Chem. Sect.*), 1967, **88**, 1306 (*synth*)
Fitton, P. *et al*, *J. Chem. Soc., Chem. Commun.*, 1968, 4 (*synth, ir, pmr*)
Takahashi, S. *et al*, *Bull. Chem. Soc. Jpn.*, 1968, **41**, 254; 1972, **45**, 230 (*use*)
Coulson, R.D., *J. Org. Chem.*, 1972, **37**, 1253; 1973, **38**, 1483.
Minematsu, H. *et al*, *J. Organomet. Chem.*, 1973, **59**, 395 (*struct*)
Kiji, J. *et al*, *Bull. Chem. Soc. Jpn.*, 1974, **47**, 2523 (*use*)
Sakurai, H. *et al*, *J. Organomet. Chem.*, 1977, **131**, 147 (*use*)
Tamaru, Y. *et al*, *Tetrahedron Lett.*, 1980, **21**, 3787 (*use*)

$C_{40}H_{35}ClN_2O_2P_2Pd$ Pd-00285

Chloro(1-diazo-2-ethoxy-2-oxoethyl)bis(triphenylphosphine)-palladium, 9CI

Chloro[diazo(ethoxycarbonyl)methyl]bistriphenylphosphinepalladium

[72034-34-5]

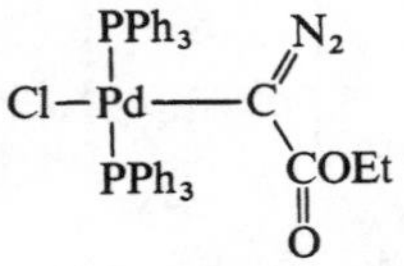

M 779.549

Red cryst. (CH_2Cl_2/hexane). Mp 146-8° dec.

Murahashi, S.-I. *et al*, *J. Chem. Soc., Chem. Commun.*, 1979, 450 (*synth, ir, pmr, cmr, struct*)

$C_{40}H_{36}O_4P_2Pd$ Pd-00286

Bis(acetato-*O*)bis(triphenylphosphine)palladium, 9CI

Diethanoatobis(triphenylphosphine)palladium. Bis(triphenylphosphine)palladium acetate. Diacetoxybis(triphenylphosphine)palladium

[14588-08-0]

$Pd(OAc)_2(PPh_3)_2$

M 749.090

Config. uncertain. Catalyses oligomerisation and carbonylation of conjugated dienes; hydrogenation; aryl coupling; dehalogenation of aryl halides and arylation of allylic alcohols. Yellow cryst. (Et_2O). Mp 118-20°, 135-6°.

Stephenson, T.A. *et al*, *J. Chem. Soc.*, 1965, 3632 (*synth, ir*)
Yoshimoto, H. *et al*, *Bull. Chem. Soc. Jpn.*, 1973, **46**, 2490 (*synth, use*)
Goodfellow, J.A. *et al*, *J. Chem. Soc., Dalton Trans.*, 1978, 1195 (*pmr, nmr*)

$C_{40}H_{36}P_2Pd$ Pd-00287

(2-Methylene-1,3-propanediyl)bis(triphenylphosphine)palladium, 9CI

Trimethylenemethanebis(triphenylphosphine)palladium

[74977-22-3]

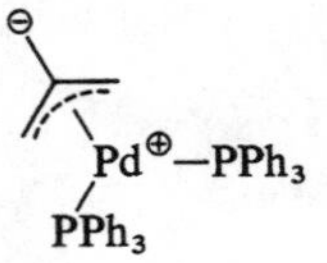

M 685.092

No physical data available.

Trost, B.M. *et al*, *J. Am. Chem. Soc.*, 1980, **102**, 6359 (*struct*)

$C_{40}H_{37}P_2Pd^{\oplus}$ Pd-00288

[(1,2,3-η)-2-Methyl-2-propenyl]bis(triphenylphosphine)palladium(1+), 9CI

(2-Methyl-π-allyl)bis(triphenylphosphine)palladium(1+), 8CI

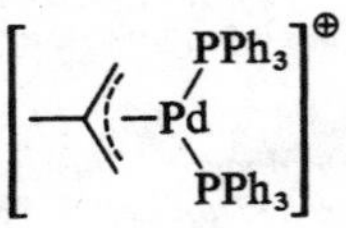

M 686.100 (ion)

Chloride: [12309-85-2].
$C_{40}H_{37}ClP_2Pd$ M 721.553
White cryst. $+2H_2O$ (C_6H_6). Mp 90-100°.

Tetraphenylborate: [12309-86-3].
$C_{64}H_{57}BP_2Pd$ M 1005.332
White cryst. (CH_2Cl_2/EtOH). Mp 114-16° dec.

Hexafluorophosphate: [74397-58-3].
$C_{40}H_{37}F_6P_3Pd$ M 831.064
White cryst. (MeCN). Mp 230° dec.

Tetrafluoroborate: [36543-50-7].
$C_{40}H_{37}BF_4P_2Pd$ M 772.903
No physical data available.

Powell, J. *et al*, *J. Chem. Soc. (A)*, 1968, 774 (*synth*)
Johnson, B.F.G. *et al*, *Synth. Inorg. Metal-Org. Chem.*, 1971, **1**, 235 (*synth, pmr*)
Grenouillet, P. *et al*, *Inorg. Chem.*, 1980, **19**, 3189 (*synth, pmr*)

$C_{40}H_{73}ClP_2Pd_2$ Pd-00289

μ-Chloro[μ-[(1-η:2,3-η)-2-methyl-2-propenyl]]bis(tricyclohexylphosphine)dipalladium, 9CI

μ-Chloro-μ-(2-methylallyl)bis(tricyclohexylphosphine)dipalladium

[72533-19-8]

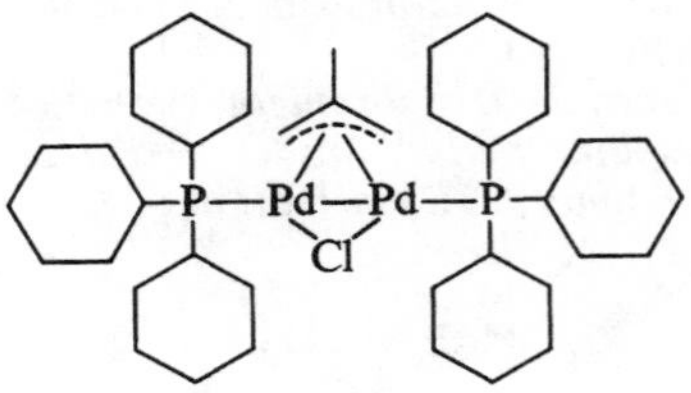

M 864.257

Yellow cryst. (pentane). Mp 115° dec.

Werner, H. *et al*, *J. Organomet. Chem.*, 1979, **179**, 439 (*synth, struct, pmr*)

$C_{41}H_{35}As_2Pd^{\oplus}$ Pd-00290

(η^5-2,4-Cyclopentadien-1-yl)bis(triphenylarsine)palladium(1+)

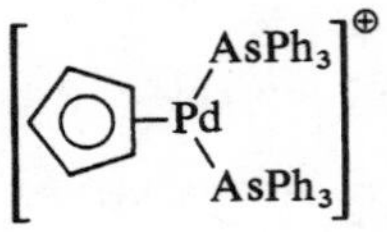

M 783.991 (ion)

Hexafluorophosphate:
$C_{41}H_{35}As_2F_6PPd$ M 928.955
Blue cryst. (CH_2Cl_2/Et_2O); air-stable. Mp 191-2°.

Roberts, N.K. *et al*, *J. Chem. Soc., Dalton Trans.*, 1982, 2093 (*synth, pmr, uv*)

$C_{41}H_{35}BrP_2Pd_2$ Pd-00291

μ-Bromo-μ-(2,4-cyclopentadien-1-yl)bis(triphenylphosphine)palladium, 9CI

μ-(η^3-Cyclopentadienyl)-μ-bromobis[triphenylphosphinepalladium]

[57363-43-6]

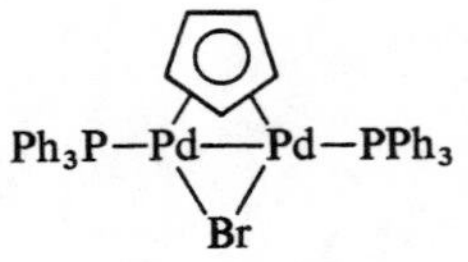

M 882.419

Cryst. (toluene/hexane or CH_2Cl_2). Mp 180-92° dec.

Ducruiz, A. *et al*, *J. Chem. Soc., Chem. Commun.*, 1975, 615 (*synth*)
Felkin, H. *et al*, *J. Organomet. Chem.*, 1977, **129**, 429 (*synth, pmr, struct*)

$C_{41}H_{35}P_2Pd^{\oplus}$ Pd-00292

η5-2,4-Cyclopentadien-1-yl)bis(triphenylphosphine)palladium(1+)

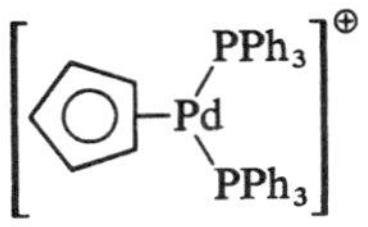

M 696.095 (ion)

Hexafluorophosphate:

$C_{41}H_{35}F_6P_3Pd$ M 841.059

Air-stable purple cryst. (bromodichloroethane/Et_2O). Mp 194-6°.

Roberts, N.K. *et al*, *J. Chem. Soc., Dalton Trans.*, 1982, 2093 (*synth, pmr, uv*)

$C_{41}H_{35}PdSb_2^{\oplus}$ Pd-00293

η5-2,4-Cyclopentadien-1-yl)bis(triphenylantimony)palladium(1+)

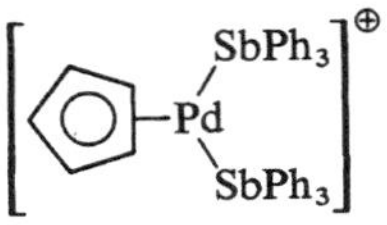

M 877.648 (ion)

Hexafluorophosphate:

$C_{41}H_{35}F_6PPdSb_2$ M 1022.612

Blue cryst. (CH_2Cl_2/Et_2O); air-stable. Mp 145-8°.

Roberts, N.K. *et al*, *J. Chem. Soc., Dalton Trans.*, 1982, 2093 (*synth, pmr, uv, struct*)

$C_{42}H_{30}As_2BrF_5Pd$ Pd-00294

Bromo(pentafluorophenyl)bis(triphenylarsine)palladium, 9CI

(*Pentafluorophenyl*)*bromobis*(*triphenylarsine*)*palladium*

[59091-10-0]

$[PdBr(C_6F_5)(AsPh_3)_2]$

M 965.858

Pale-yellow or yellow-brown solid. Mp 235° dec., 160-70° dec. Mps may refer to different isomers.

Uson, R. *et al*, *J. Organomet. Chem.*, 1976, **104**, 253 (*synth, ir*)
Klabunde, K.J. *et al*, *Inorg. Chem.*, 1980, **19**, 3719 (*synth, ir, pmr, nmr*)

$C_{42}H_{30}BrF_5P_2Pd$ Pd-00295

Bromo(pentafluorophenyl)bis(triphenylphosphine)palladium

Bis(*triphenylphosphine*)*pentafluorophenylpalladium bromide.*

Pentafluorophenylbromobis(*triphenylphosphine*)*palladium*

[53022-32-5]

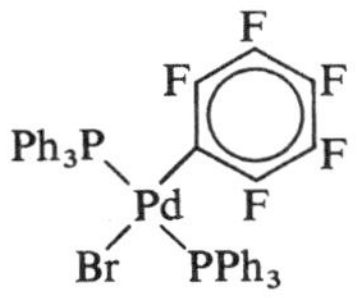

trans-form

M 877.963

cis-form [74465-03-5]

Cryst. (Me_2CO/EtOH). Mp 257° dec.

trans-form [41588-04-9]

Cryst. (Me_2CO/EtOH). Mp 284°.

Klabunde, K.J. *et al*, *J. Am. Chem. Soc.*, 1974, **96**, 7674 (*synth, ir, pmr*)
Uson, R. *et al*, *J. Chem. Soc., Dalton Trans.*, 1980, 888 (*synth*)

$C_{42}H_{30}ClF_5P_2Pd$ Pd-00296

Chloro(pentafluorophenyl)bis(triphenylphosphine)palladium, 9CI

Pentafluorophenylbis(*triphenylphosphine*)*palladium chloride. Chlorobis*(*triphenylphosphine*)-*pentafluorophenylpalladium*

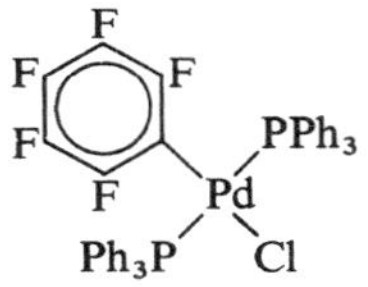

M 833.512

trans-form [56272-19-6]

Cryst. (EtOH). Mp 230° dec.

Usón, R. *et al*, *J. Organomet. Chem.*, 1975, **90**, 367 (*synth*)

$C_{42}H_{30}Cl_4Pd_3$ Pd-00297

Tetra-μ-chlorobis(1,2,3-triphenylcyclopropenyl)tripalladium

Bis(*triphenylcyclopropenyl*)*tetrachlorotripalladium*

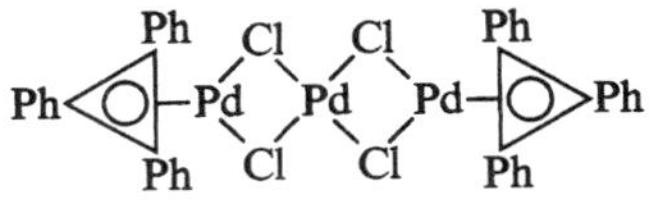

M 995.771

Orange-red solid. Mp 253-4° dec.

Moiseev, I.I. *et al*, *Izv. Akad. Nauk SSSR, Ser. Khim.*, 1964, 775; *CA*, **61**, 3146g (*synth, struct*)

$C_{42}H_{31}F_5OP_2Pd$ Pd-00298

Hydroxy(pentafluorophenyl)bis(triphenylphosphine)palladium

(Pentafluorophenyl)hydroxobis(triphenylphosphine)-palladium

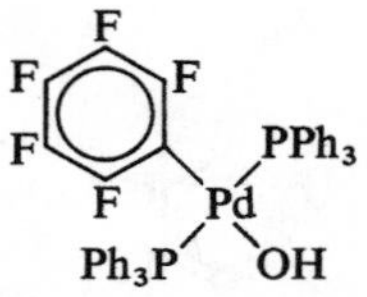

M 815.066

trans-form

Cryst. (hexane). Mp 180° dec.

Yoshida, T. *et al*, *J. Chem. Soc., Dalton Trans.*, 1976, 993 (*synth*)

$C_{42}H_{34}O_2P_2Pd$ Pd-00299

(*p*-Benzoquinone)bis(triphenylphosphine)palladium, 8CI

[(2,3,5,6-η)-2,5-Cyclohexadiene-1,4-dione]bis(triphenylphosphine)palladium, 9CI. *Bis(triphenylphosphine)-(p-benzoquinone)palladium*

[52462-73-4]

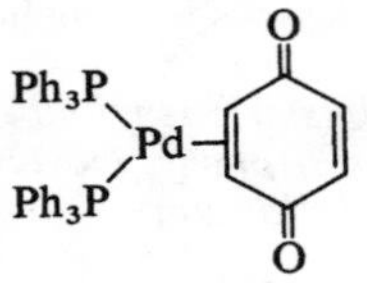

M 739.097

Catalyses hydrosilylation of butadiene. Dark-red solid. Mp 155-7° dec.

Takahashi, S. *et al*, *Organomet. Chem. Synth.*, 1971, **1**, 193 (*use*)
Ukai, T. *et al*, *J. Organomet. Chem.*, 1974, **65**, 253 (*synth, ir*)
Minematsu, H. *et al*, *J. Organomet. Chem.*, 1975, **91**, 389 (*ir, pmr*)
Roffia, P. *et al*, *J. Mol. Catal.*, 1977, **2**, 191; *CA*, **87**, 44675z (*synth*)

$C_{42}H_{34}P_2Pd$ Pd-00300

[1,2-Ethanediylbis(diphenylphosphine)-*P,P'*]bis(phenylethynyl)palladium

[Ethylenebis(diphenylphosphine)]bis(phenylethynyl)-palladium. [1,2-Bis(diphenylphosphino)ethane]bis-(phenylethynyl)palladium. Bis(phenylethynyl)[1,2-bis-(diphenylphosphino)ethane]palladium

[66986-72-9]

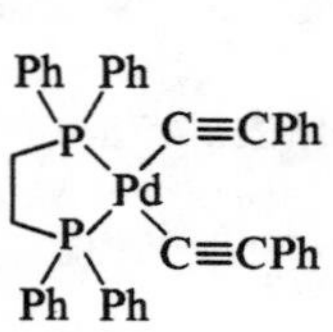

M 707.098

Brown-yellow powder.

Nast, R. *et al*, *Chem. Ber.*, 1978, **111**, 1627 (*synth, ir, pmr*)

$C_{42}H_{35}ClP_2Pd$ Pd-003

Chlorophenylbis(triphenylphosphine)palladium, 9CI

Phenylbis(triphenylphosphine)palladium chloride

[22605-84-1]

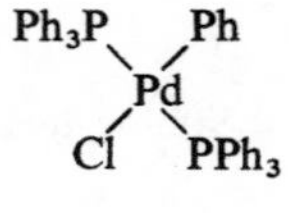

M 743.559

trans-form

Catalyses diakylurea synth. and carboxylation and alkoxycarbonylation of unsatd. hydrocarbons. Cryst. (CH_2Cl_2/MeOH). Mp 240-3° dec.

Coulson, D.R. *et al*, *J. Chem. Soc., Chem. Commun.*, 1968, 1530 (*synth*)
Dieck, H.T. *et al*, *J. Org. Chem.*, 1975, **40**, 2819 (*use*)
Garrou, P.E. *et al*, *J. Am. Chem. Soc.*, 1976, **98**, 4115 (*synth, nmr*)

$C_{42}H_{35}IP_2Pd$ Pd-003

Iodophenylbis(triphenylphosphine)palladium, 9CI

Phenylbis(triphenylphosphine)palladium iodide

[18115-61-2]

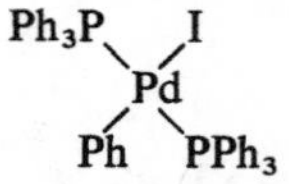

M 835.011

trans-form [55123-60-9]

Catalyses ethylene/styrene codimerisation, asymm. ketone and arylacetylene synth. and coupling of organotin compds. with aryl halides. Mp 171-86° dec.

Fitton, P. *et al*, *J. Chem. Soc., Chem. Commun.*, 1968, 6 (*synth, ir*)
Nozima, H. *et al*, *Chem. Lett.*, 1973, 1163 (*use*)
Cassar, L., *J. Organomet. Chem.*, 1975, **93**, 253 (*use*)
Sekiya, A. *et al*, *J. Organomet. Chem.*, 1976, **118**, 349 (*use*)
Tanaka, M., *Tetrahedron Lett.*, 1979, 2601 (*use*)
Kashin, A.N. *et al*, *Izv. Akad. Nauk SSSR, Ser. Khim.*, 1980, 479; *CA*, **93**, 26019h (*use*)
Tanaka, M., *Bull. Chem. Soc. Jpn.*, 1981, **54**, 637 (*use*)

$C_{42}H_{36}O_4P_2Pd$ Pd-0030

[(2,3-η)-Dimethyl-2-butynedioate]bis(triphenylphosphine)palladium, 9CI

(Dicarboxyvinylene)bis(triphenylphosphine)palladium dimethyl ester, 8CI. *[1,2-Bis(carbomethoxy)ethyne]bis-(triphenylphosphine)palladium. (Dimethyl acetylenedicarboxylate)bis(triphenylphosphine)palladium*

[15629-88-6]

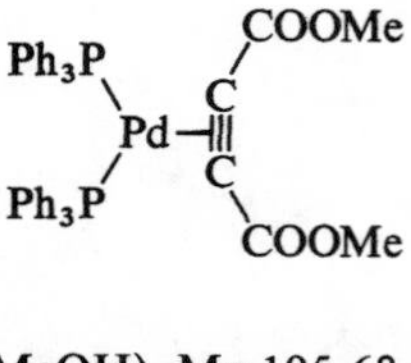

M 773.112

Cryst. (CH_2Cl_2/MeOH). Mp 195-6° dec. Slowly yellow on exp. to air.

Greaves, E.O. *et al*, *Can. J. Chem.*, 1968, **46**, 3879 (*synth, ir*)
McGinnety, J.A., *J. Chem. Soc., Dalton Trans.*, 1974, 1038 (*struct*)
Ito, T., *et al*, *J. Organomet. Chem.*, 1974, **73**, 401 (*synth*)

$C_{42}H_{37}ClOP_2Pd$ Pd-00304

Chloro(3-oxo-1-cyclohexen-1-yl)bis(triphenylphosphine)palladium, 9CI

[67721-17-9]

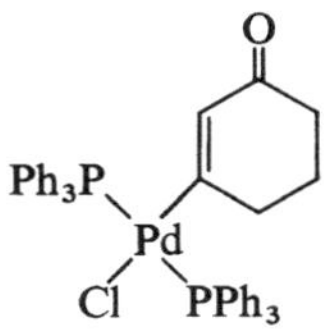

M 761.574

Pale-yellow powder (C_6H_6). Mp >191° dec.

Onishi, M. *et al, Bull. Chem. Soc. Jpn.*, 1978, **51**, 1856 (*synth, ir, pmr*)
Onishi, M. *et al, Bull. Chem. Soc. Jpn.*, 1980, **53**, 2540.

$C_{42}H_{54}Cl_2O_2Pd_2$ Pd-00305

Di-μ-chlorobis[(16,17,20-η)-3-methoxy-19-nor-1,3,5(10),17(20)-pregnatetraene]dipalladium, 10CI

Bis[chloro-(16,17,20-η)-3-methoxy-19-nor-1,3,5(10),17(20)-pregnatetraene)palladium]

[58527-00-7]

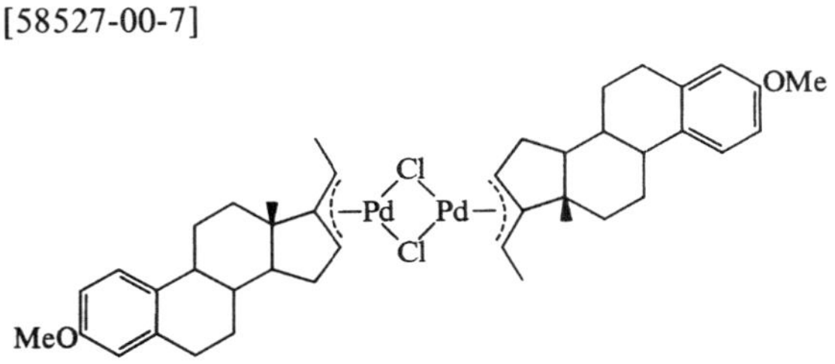

M 874.633

Chloride bridged dimer. Yellow solid. Mp 161-82° dec.

Monomer: Chloro(16,17,20-η)-3-methoxy-19-nor-1,3,5(10),17(20)-pregnatetraenepalladium.
$C_{21}H_{27}ClOPd$ M 437.317
Unknown.

Trost, B.M. *et al, J. Am. Chem. Soc.*, 1976, **98**, 630; 1978, **100**, 3435 (*synth, pmr*)

$C_{42}H_{65}ClP_5Pd_3^{\oplus}$ Pd-00306

μ-Chlorobis[μ-(diphenylphosphino)]tris(triethylphosphine)tripalladium(1+), 9CI

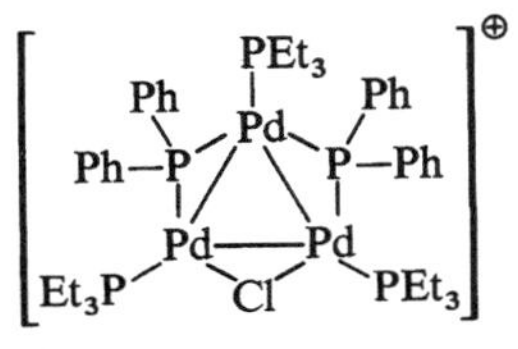

M 1079.557 (ion)

Tetrafluoroborate: [65916-06-5].
$C_{42}H_{65}BClF_4P_5Pd_3$ M 1166.361
Orange-red solid.

Bushnell, G.W. *et al, J. Chem. Soc., Chem. Commun.*, 1977, 709.
Dixon, K.R. *et al, Inorg. Chem.*, 1978, **17**, 1099 (*synth, struct, pmr*)

$C_{43}H_{30}F_5OP_2Pd^{\oplus}$ Pd-00307

Carbonylbis(triphenylphosphine)(pentafluorophenyl)palladium(1+), 9CI

Carbonyl(pentafluorophenyl)bis(triphenylphosphine)palladium(1+). Pentafluorophenyl(carbonyl)bis(triphenylphosphine)palladium(1+)

$[Pd(CO)(C_6F_5)(PPh_3)_2]^{\oplus}$

M 826.069 (ion)

Perchlorate: [60102-01-4].
$C_{43}H_{30}ClF_5O_5P_2Pd$ M 925.520
White, air-sensitive solid.

Uson, R. *et al, J. Organomet. Chem.*, 1976, **112**, 105 (*synth, ir*)

$C_{43}H_{35}ClOP_2Pd$ Pd-00308

Benzoylchlorobis(triphenylphosphine)palladium, 9CI, 8CI

Chloro(benzoyl)bis(triphenylphosphine)palladium

[50417-59-9]

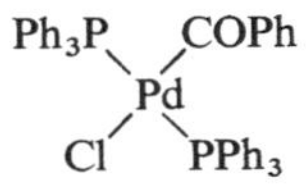

M 771.569

trans-form

Catalyses synth. of long-chain nitro and amino compds., benzoylation and phenylation of methyl methoxylate and aldehyde synth. from acyl chlorides and tributyltin hydride. Pale-yellow cryst. (Et_2O).

Ger. Pat., 1 960 929, (*1970*); *CA*, **73**, 120066e (*use*)
Suzuki, K. *et al, Bull. Chem. Soc. Jpn.*, 1973, **46**, 2887 (*synth, ir*)
Biavati, A. *et al, Transition Met. Chem.*, 1979, **4**, 398 (*use*)
Four, P. *et al, J. Org. Chem.*, 1981, **46**, 4439 (*use*)

$C_{43}H_{37}ClP_2Pd$ Pd-00309

Benzylchlorobis(triphenylphosphine)palladium, 8CI

Chloro(phenylmethyl)bis(triphenylphosphine)palladium, 9CI. Benzylbis(triphenylphosphine)palladium chloride

[22784-59-4]

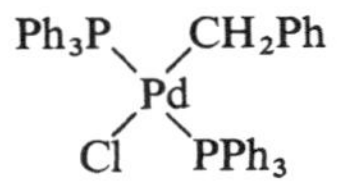

M 757.586

trans-form

Catalyses ketone synth. from acid chlorides and organotin compds. Cryst. (CH_2Cl_2/Et_2O contg. PPh_3). Mp 147-51° dec. Dimerises to Dibenzyldi-μ-chlorobis(triphenylphosphine)dipalladium, Pd-00320 by loss of PPh_3.

Fitton, P. *et al, J. Chem. Soc., Chem. Commun.*, 1969, 370 (*synth, pmr*)
Ros, R. *et al, Inorg. Chim. Acta*, 1977, **25**, 61 (*synth, ir, pmr*)
Milstein, D. *et al, J. Am. Chem. Soc.*, 1979, **101**, 4992 (*use*)
Milstein, D. *et al, J. Org. Chem.*, 1979, **44**, 1613 (*use*)
Four, P. *et al, J. Org. Chem.*, 1981, **46**, 4439 (*use*)

$C_{44}H_{35}ClP_2Pd$ Pd-00310

Chloro(phenylethynyl)bis(triphenylphosphine)palladium, 9CI

Bis(triphenylphosphine)chloro(phenylethynyl)palladium. (Phenylacetylide)bis(triphenylphosphine)palladium chloride

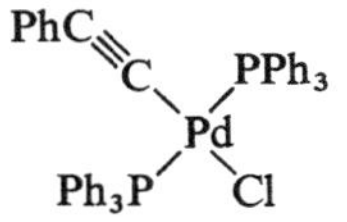

M 767.581

***trans*-form** [69291-32-3]
Yellow solid. Mp 149-57° dec.

Burgess, J. *et al*, *J. Chem. Soc., Dalton Trans.*, 1978, 1577 (*synth, ir*)

$C_{44}H_{36}P_2Pd$ Pd-00311

Hydrido(phenylethynyl)bis(triphenylphosphine)palladium
Hydro(phenylethynyl)bis(triphenylphosphine)palladium, 9CI
[56550-78-8]

$(Ph_3P)_2PdH(C{\equiv}CPh)$

M 733.136
Yellowish-brown solid. Mp 100°.

Chakhadzhyan, G.A. *et al*, *Zh. Obshch. Khim.*, 1975, **45**, 1114; *J. Gen. Chem. USSR (Engl. Transl.)*, **45**, 1096 (*synth, struct*)

$C_{44}H_{40}P_2Pd_2$ Pd-00312

[μ-[(1-η:2,3-η)-2,4-Cyclopentadien-1-yl-]][μ-[(1-η:2,3-η)-2-propenyl]]bis(triphenylphosphine)dipalladium, 9CI
(μ-π-Allyl)(μ-π-cyclopentadienyl)bis(triphenylphosphine)dipalladium
[63600-82-8]

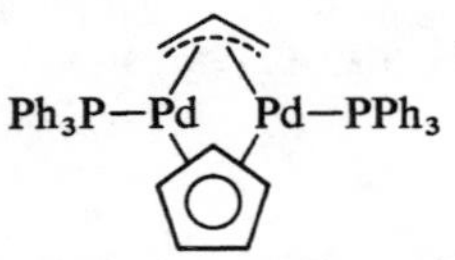

Ph3P—Pd Pd—PPh3

M 843.588
Orange-yellow cryst. (C_6H_6/pentane). Mp 130° dec.

Werner, H. *et al*, *Chem. Ber.*, 1977, **110**, 1763 (*synth, pmr, struct*)

$C_{44}H_{46}O_6P_2Pd$ Pd-00313

(η^2-Ethene)bis[tris(2-methylphenyl)phosphite-*P*]palladium, 9CI
*Ethylenebis(tri-*o*-tolylphosphite)palladium. (Ethylene)bis(phosphorous acid)palladium hexa-*o*-tolyl ester*, 8CI
[33395-49-2]

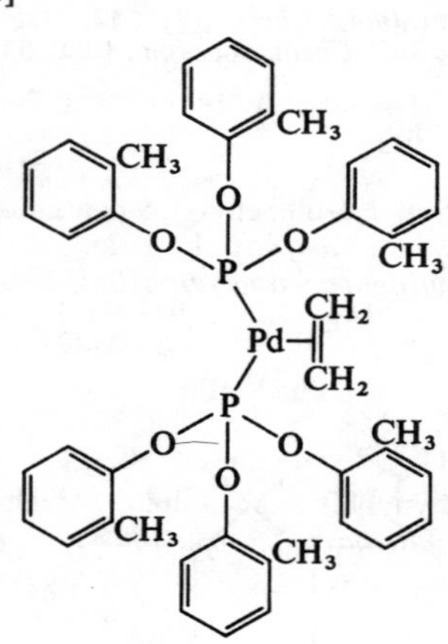

M 839.211
Cryst. (Et_2O saturated with ethylene, −30°). Air-sensitive.

Van der Linde, R. *et al*, *J. Chem. Soc., Chem. Commun.*, 1971, 563 (*synth*)
Inorg. Synth., 1976, **16**, 127 (*synth, ir*)

$C_{44}H_{58}P_3Pd^{\oplus}$ Pd-00314

[Ethylenebis[diphenylphosphine]]hydro(tricyclohexylphosphine)palladium(1+), 8CI
[1,2-Ethanediylbis[diphenylphosphine]-P,P′]hydro(tricyclohexylphosphine)palladium(1+), 9CI. *Hydridotricyclohexylphosphine[1,2-bis(diphenylphosphino)ethane]-palladium*

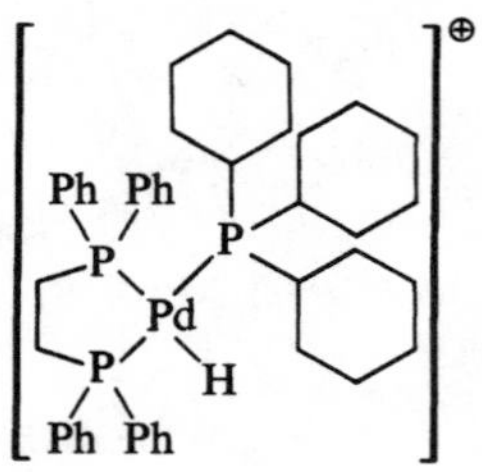

M 786.283 (ion)
Hexafluorophosphate: [31901-96-9].
$C_{44}H_{58}F_6P_4Pd$ M 931.248
Cryst. Mp 190-2° dec.

Green, M.L.H. *et al*, *J. Chem. Soc., Dalton Trans.*, 1974, 269 (*synth, ir, pmr*)

$C_{44}H_{80}P_2Pd_2$ Pd-00315

Bis[μ-[(1-η:2,3-η)-2-methyl-2-propenyl]]bis(tricyclohexylphosphine)dipalladium, 10CI
Bis(μ-2-methylallyl)bis(tricyclohexylphosphine)dipalladium
[72533-18-7]

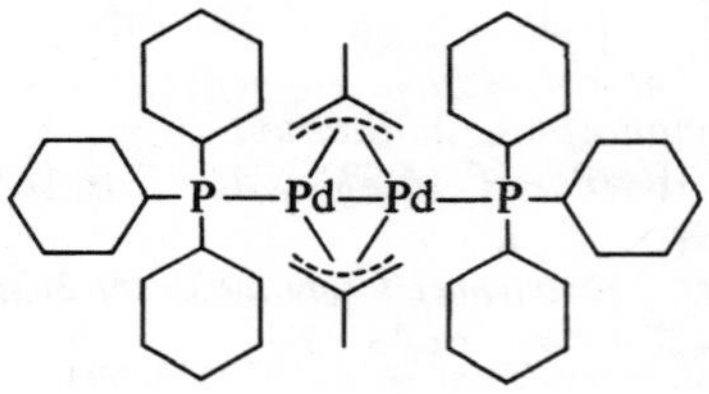

M 883.904
Yellow solid.

Werner, H. *et al*, *J. Organomet. Chem.*, 1979, **179**, 439 (*synth, struct, pmr*)

$C_{46}H_{66}Cl_2O_4Pd_2$ Pd-00316

Bis[(16,17-20-η)-(3β)-3-(acetyloxy)-pregna-5,16-dien-20-yl-]di-μ-chlorodipalladium, 10CI
Bis[chloro(16,17,20-η)-3β-acetoxy-17-ethylidene-5-androstene)palladium]
[74494-13-6]

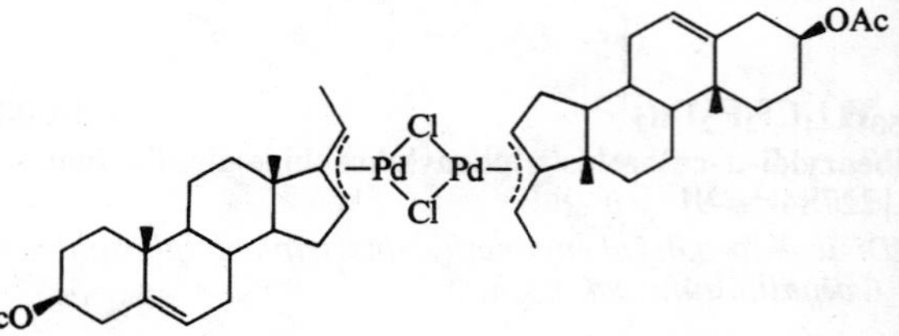

M 966.771
Chloride bridged dimer. Cryst. (hexane). Mp 189-94° dec.

Monomer: Chloro(16,17,20-η)-3β-acetoxy-17-ethylidene-5-androstenepalladium.
$C_{23}H_{33}ClO_2Pd$ M 483.386
Unknown.

Trost, B.M. *et al*, *J. Am. Chem. Soc.*, 1980, **102**, 3572 (*synth, ir pmr*)

$_{47}H_{35}Cl_5NP_2Pd^{\oplus}$ **Pd-00317**
entachlorophenyl(pyridine)bis(triphenylphosphine)palladium(1+)

$[Pd(C_6Cl_5)(C_5H_5N)(PPh_3)_2]^{\oplus}$

M 959.433 (ion)
Perchlorate: [73821-19-9].
$C_{47}H_{35}Cl_6NO_4P_2Pd$ M 1058.883
Cryst. (Me_2CO or $CHCl_3$). Mp 248-9° dec.

Coronas, J.M. *et al*, *Synth. React. Inorg. Metal-Org. Chem.*, 1980, **10**, 53 (*synth, ir*)

$_{48}H_{30}Cl_2F_{10}P_2Pd_2$ **Pd-00318**
i-μ-chlorobis(pentafluorophenyl)bis(triphenylphosphine)dipalladium, 9CI
Bis(pentafluorophenyl)di-μ-chlorobis(triphenylphosphine)dipalladium. Bis(triphenylphosphine)bis(pentafluorophenyl)dichlorodipalladium
[70681-67-3]

M 1142.443
Bridged dimer. Yellow cryst. (Et_2O). Mp 250° dec.
Monomer: Chloro(pentafluorophenyl)-(triphenylphosphine)palladium.
$C_{24}H_{15}ClF_5PPd$ M 571.221
Unknown.

Uson, R. *et al*, *J. Organomet. Chem.*, 1975, **90**, 367 (*synth, ir, struct*)
Uson, R. *et al*, *Inorg. Chim. Acta*, 1979, **33**, 69 (*synth, ir, struct*)

$_{48}H_{60}Ge_2P_2Pd$ **Pd-00319**
is(triethylphosphine)bis(triphenylgermyl)palladium
Bis(triphenylgermyl)bis(triethylphosphine)palladium

$Pd(GePh_3)_2(PEt_3)_2$

M 950.550
Geometry not assigned. Yellow solid (toluene/pet. ether). Dec. at 97-107°.

Brooks, E.H. *et al*, *J. Chem. Soc. (A)*, 1966, 1241 (*synth*)

$_{50}H_{44}Cl_2P_2Pd_2$ **Pd-00320**
ibenzyldi-μ-chlorobis(triphenylphosphine)dipalladium, 8CI
[22784-54-9].
Di-μ-chlorobis(phenylmethyl)bis(triphenylphosphine)-dipalladium, 9CI.

M 990.591
Yellow cryst. ($CHCl_3$/hexane). Mp 205-7° dec. Formed from Benzylchlorobis(triphenylphosphine)palladium, Pd-00309 by loss of $2PPh_3$.

Monomer: Benzylchloro(triphenylphosphine)palladium.
$C_{25}H_{22}ClPPd$ M 495.296
Unknown.

Ros, R. *et al*, *Inorg. Chim. Acta*, 1977, **25**, 61 (*synth, ir, pmr*)
Zanello, P. *et al*, *J. Inorg. Nucl. Chem.*, 1981, **43**, 1095.

$C_{50}H_{46}O_2P_2Pd$ **Pd-00321**
[(5,6-η-1-Ethenyl-1,2,3,3a,3b,7a,8,8a-octahydrocyclopent[a]indene-4,7-dione]bis(triphenylphosphine)palladium, 9CI
[57127-90-9]

M 847.280
Yellow cryst. Mp 128-32° dec.

Minematsu, H. *et al*, *J. Chem. Soc., Chem. Commun.*, 1975, 466 (*synth, struct*)

$C_{51}H_{42}O_3Pd$ **Pd-00322**
Tris[(1,2-η)-1,5-diphenyl-1,4-pentadien-2-one]palladium, 10CI
Tris(dibenzylideneacetone)palladium
[48243-18-1]

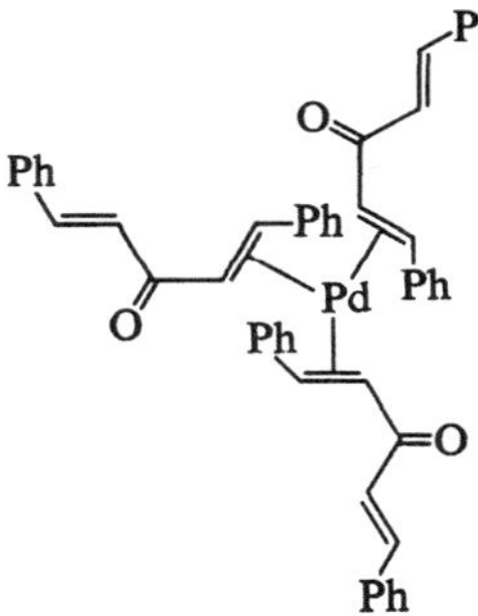

M 809.311
Orange-brown cryst. + $1C_6H_6$ (C_6H_6).

Mazza, M.C. *et al*, *Inorg. Chem.*, 1973, **12**, 2955 (*synth, struct*)
Tanaka, H. *et al*, *Bull. Chem. Soc. Jpn.*, 1980, **53**, 1743 (*pmr*)

$C_{51}H_{42}O_3Pd_2$ **Pd-00323**
Tris[μ-[(1,2-η:4,5-η)-1,5-diphenyl-1,4-pentadien-3-one]]dipalladium, 9CI
Tris(μ-dibenzylideneacetone)dipalladium
[51364-51-3]

M 915.731
Catalyses dimerization of butadiene.
Mono-C_6H_6 solvate: Deep purple cryst. Mp 142-4° dec.

Mono-toluene solvate: Deep purple cryst. Mp 140-1° dec.
Mono-$CHCl_3$ solvate: Deep purple cryst. Mp 122-4° dec.

Ukai, T. *et al*, *J. Organomet. Chem.*, 1974, **65**, 253 (*synth*, *ir*, *pmr*, *ms*, *struct*)
Kawazura, H. *et al*, *Bull. Chem. Soc. Jpn.*, 1978, **51**, 3466 (*pmr*)

$C_{52}H_{40}P_2Pd$ Pd-00324

Bis(phenylethynyl)bis(triphenylphosphine)palladium, 9CI
Bis(triphenylphosphine)bis(phenylethynyl)palladium

$Pd(C{\equiv}CPh)_2(PPh_3)_2$

M 833.256

***trans*-form** [31387-03-8]
Cryst. (Et_2O). Mp 118-20° dec., 145-7° dec.

Masai, H. *et al*, *J. Organomet. Chem.*, 1971, **26**, 271 (*synth*, *ir*, *struct*)
Nelson, J.H. *et al*, *Inorg. Chem.*, 1974, **13**, 27 (*synth*, *ir*, *pmr*)

$C_{52}H_{44}O_4Pd_3$ Pd-00325

Bis(2,4-pentanedionato-*O,O′*)bis[*μ*-[(1,2,3-*η*:1,3-*η*)-1,2,3-triphenyl-1-propen-1-yl-3-ylidene]]tripalladium, 9CI
Bis(acetylacetonato)bis(triphenylcyclopropenyl)tripalladium
[69645-86-9]

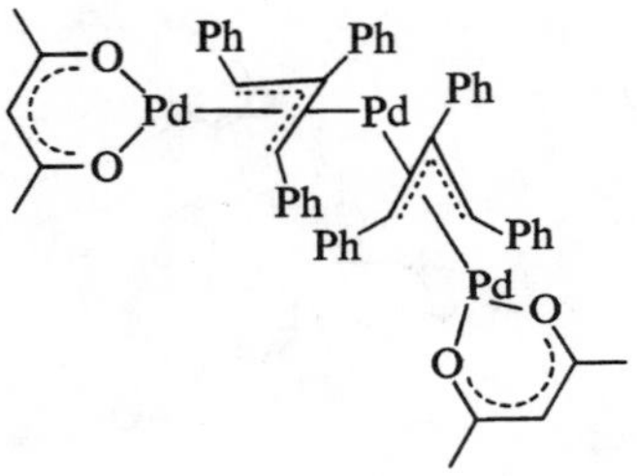

Ph Ph Ph Pd Pd O O Ph Ph Ph Pd O O

M 1052.177
Red cryst. (CH_2Cl_2). Mp 220° dec. C—C bond of cyclopropenyl ligand broken during formation of complex.

Keasey, A. *et al*, *J. Chem. Soc., Dalton Trans.*, 1978, 1830 (*pmr*, *struct*, *synth*)

$C_{53}H_{108}O_5P_4Pd_4$ Pd-00326

Pentacarbonyltetrakis(tributylphosphine)tetrapalladium
Tetrakis(tributylphosphine)pentacarbonyltetrapalladium

$Pd_4(CO)_5[P(CH_2CH_2CH_2CH_3)_3]_4$

M 1375.008
Solid. Prep. and operations should be conducted under CO atm.

Mednikov, E.G. *et al*, *J. Organomet. Chem.*, 1982, **239**, 401 (*synth*, *ir*)

$C_{54}H_{86}Cl_2O_2Pd_2$ Pd-0032

Di-*μ*-chlorobis[(4,5,6-*η*)-3-oxo-5-cholesten-4-yl]dipalladiu 10CI
[59487-94-4]

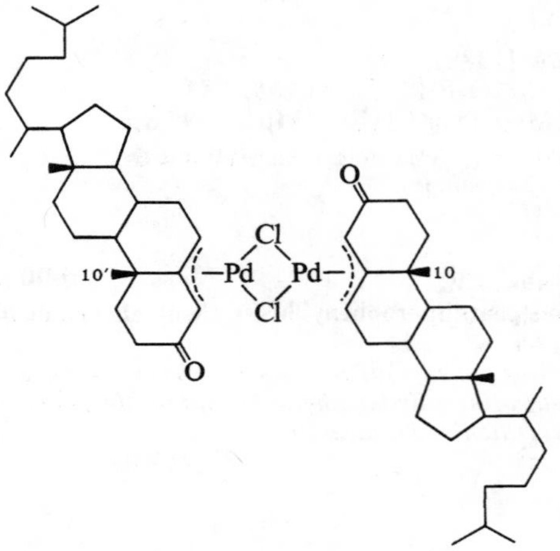

O Cl 10′ Pd Pd 10 Cl O *α-form*

M 1051.018
Chloride bridged dimer. Intermed. in conversion of enon to dienone.

***α*-form**
Yellow cryst. (pet. ether). Mp 167-9°. $[\alpha]_D$ +259°.

***β*-form**
Yellow cryst. (pet. ether). Mp 164-7°. This form has the Pd atoms *cis* to the 10-methyl groups.
Monomer: Chloro[(4,5,6-η)-3-oxo-5-cholesten-4-yl]palladium.
$C_{27}H_{43}ClOPd$ M 525.509
Unknown.

Howsam, R.W. *et al*, *Tetrahedron Lett.*, 1968, 3667 (*ir*, *uv*)
Jones, D.N. *et al*, *J. Chem. Soc., Chem. Commun.*, 1975, 165 (*stereochem*)
Collins, D.J. *et al*, *Aust. J. Chem.*, 1977, **30**, 2167 (*synth*, *pmr*, *cmr*, *ir*)
Henderson, K. *et al*, *J. Chem. Soc., Chem. Commun.*, 1978, 15 (*pmr*)
Collins, D.J. *et al*, *Aust. J. Chem.*, 1980, **33**, 2663 (*stereochem*, *ms*, *pmr*)
Haynes, R.K. *et al*, *Aust. J. Chem.*, 1980, **33**, 1537 (*use*)

$C_{54}H_{108}O_6P_4Pd_4$ Pd-0032

Hexa-*μ*-carbonyltetrakis(tributylphosphine)tetrapalladium
Tetrakis(tributylphosphine)hexa-μ-carbonyltetrapalladium

$(CH_2)_3CH_3$ $H_3C(CH_2)_3$ P $(CH_2)_3CH_3$ Pd OC CO CO O C $H_3C(CH_2)_3$ $(CH_2)_3CH_3$ $H_3C(CH_2)_3$–P–Pd Pd–P–$(CH_2)_3CH_3$ $H_3C(CH_2)_3$ OC–Pd–CO $(CH_2)_3CH_3$ $H_3C(CH_2)_3$ P $(CH_2)_3CH_3$ $(CH_2)_3CH_3$

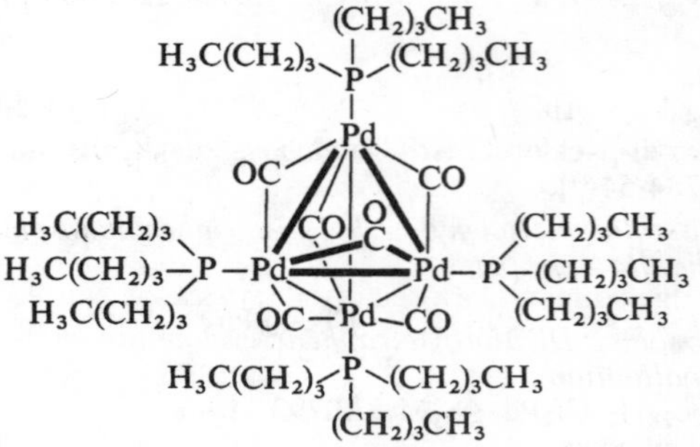

M 1403.019
Red cryst. Prep. and operations should by conducted under CO atm.

Mednikov, E.G. *et al*, *J. Organomet. Chem.*, 1982, **239**, 401 (*synth*, *ir*, *struct*)

$C_{55}H_{45}OP_3Pd$ Pd-00329

Carbonyltris(triphenylphosphine)palladium, 9CI

Tris(triphenylphosphine)carbonylpalladium

[24670-32-4]

$PdCO(PPh_3)_3$ (C_{3v})

M 921.301

Catalyses carboxymethylation of organic halides; cocatalyst in preparation of oxalic acid esters. Yellow cryst. (hexane or C_6H_6/heptane); dec. slowly in air. Mp 110° dec. (190-200° dec.).

Kudo, K. *et al*, *J. Organomet. Chem.*, 1971, **33**, 393 (*synth*, *ir*)
Hidai, M. *et al*, *Bull. Chem. Soc. Jpn.*, 1975, **48**, 2075 (*use*)
Morandini, F. *et al*, *Helv. Chim. Acta*, 1979, **62**, 59 (*synth*, *ir*, *pmr*, *cmr*)

$C_{56}H_{40}Br_4Pd_2$ Pd-00330

Dibromodi-μ-bromobis(tetraphenylcyclobutadiene)dipalladium

Tetrabromobis(tetraphenyl-1,3-cyclobutadiene)dipalladium. Di-μ-bromodibromobis[1,1′,1″,1‴-(η⁴-1,3-cyclobutadiene-1,2,3,4-tetrayl)tetrakis[benzene]]dipalladium

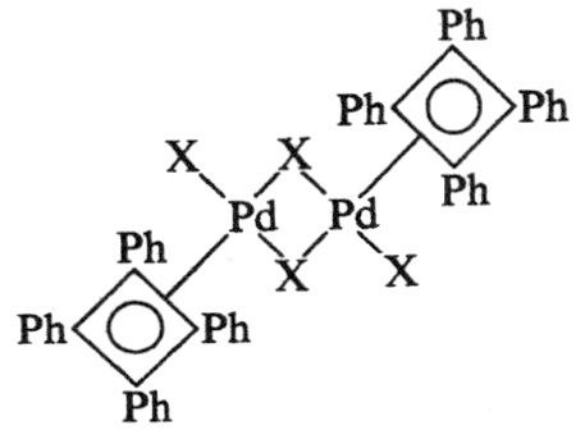

X = Br

M 1245.388

Bridged dimer. Cryst. (colour not reported). Mp 347-8° dec.

Monomer: Dibromo(tetraphenylcyclobutadiene)-palladium.
$C_{28}H_{20}Br_2Pd$ M 622.694
Unknown.

Maitlis, P.M. *et al*, *Can. J. Chem.*, 1964, **42**, 183 (*synth*)

$C_{56}H_{40}Cl_4Pd_2$ Pd-00331

Di-μ-chlorodichlorobis(tetraphenylcyclobutadiene)dipalladium

Di-μ-chlorodichlorobis[1,1′,1″,1‴-(η⁴-1,3-cyclobutadiene-1,2,3,4-tetrayl)-tetrakis[benzene]]dipalladium, 9CI. *Tetrachlorobis(tetraphenylcyclobutadiene)-dipalladium*

[12124-57-1]

As Dibromodi-μ-bromobis(tetraphenylcyclobutadiene)dipalladium, Pd-00330 with

X = Cl

M 1067.584

Bridged dimer. Dark-red cryst.; air-stable. Mp >330°.

Monomer: Dichloro(tetraphenylcyclobutadiene)-palladium.
$C_{28}H_{20}Cl_2Pd$ M 533.792
Unknown.

Blomquist, A.T. *et al*, *J. Am. Chem. Soc.*, 1962, **84**, 2329 (*synth*, *pmr*, *ir*, *struct*)

$C_{56}H_{40}Cl_6Pd_3$ Pd-00332

Tetra-μ-chlorodichlorobis(tetraphenyl-1,3-cyclobutadiene-)tripalladium

Hexachlorobis(tetraphenyl-1,3-cyclobutadiene)tripalladium

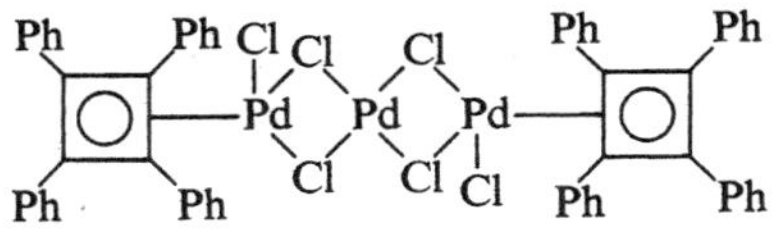

M 1244.910

Red-brown solid. Mp 305-7° dec.

Huettel, R. *et al*, *Tetrahedron Lett.*, 1964, 3541 (*synth*, *ir*, *uv*)

$C_{56}H_{40}Pd$ Pd-00333

Bis(tetraphenylcyclobutadiene)palladium

Bis(1,1′,1″,1‴-(η⁴-1,3-cyclobutadiene-1,2,3,4-tetrayl)-tetrakis[benzene]]palladium, 9CI

[75811-07-3]

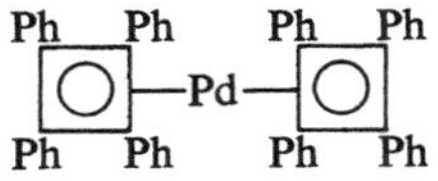

M 819.352

Blue cryst.

Hoberg, H. *et al*, *J. Organomet. Chem.*, 1980, **197**, 105 (*synth*, *cmr*, *struct*)

$C_{57}H_{45}O_3P_3Pd_3$ Pd-00334

Tri-μ-carbonyltris(triphenylphosphine)tripalladium, 9CI

[36642-60-1]

$Pd_3(CO)_3(PPh_3)_3$

M 1190.162

Catalyses carboxymethylation of organic halides. Red cryst. (hexane), dec. slowly in air. Mp 73° dec., 75°.

Kudo, K. *et al*, *J. Organomet. Chem.*, 1971, **33**, 393 (*synth*, *ir*)
Von Werner, K. *et al*, *Chem. Ber.*, 1972, **105**, 3947 (*synth*)
Hidai, M. *et al*, *Bull. Chem. Soc. Jpn.*, 1975, **48**, 2075 (*use*)

$C_{60}H_{45}As_3F_5Pd^{\oplus}$ Pd-00335

(Pentafluorophenyl)tris(triphenylarsine)palladium(1+), 9CI

$[Pd(C_6F_5)(AsPh_3)_3]^{\oplus}$

M 1192.192 (ion)

Perchlorate: [59053-42-8].
$C_{60}H_{45}As_3ClF_5O_4Pd$ M 1291.643
White solid. Mp 170-90° dec.

Uson, R. *et al*, *J. Organomet. Chem.*, 1976, **104**, 253 (*synth*, *ir*)

$C_{60}H_{50}Cl_2O_2Pd_2$ Pd-00336

Di-μ-chlorobis[(1,2,3-η)-4-ethoxy-1,2,3,4-tetraphenyl-2-cyclobuten-1-yl]dipalladium, 9CI

[57194-51-1]

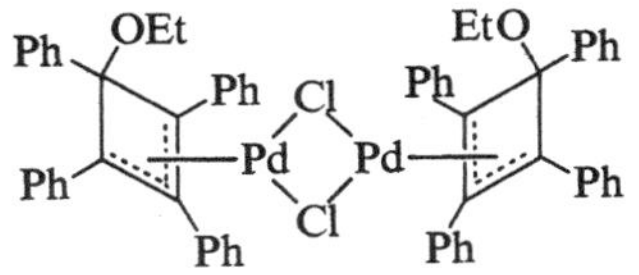

M 1086.800

Bridged dimer. Orange-red cryst. (CH_2Cl_2); air-stable. Mp >190° dec.

Monomer: Chloro[(1,2,3-η)-4-ethoxy-1,2,3,4-tetraphenyl-2-cyclobuten-1-yl]palladium. 4-Ethoxy-π-1,2,3,4-tetraphenylcyclobutenylpalladium chloride.

$C_{30}H_{25}ClOPd$ M 543.400

Unknown.

Blomquist, A.T. *et al*, *J. Am. Chem. Soc.*, 1962, **84**, 2329 (*synth*)

Cheng, P.K. *et al*, *J. Chem. Soc., Chem. Commun.*, 1975, 369 (*struct*)

$C_{62}H_{108}O_{14}P_4Pd_{10}$ Pd-00337

Tetradecacarbonyltetrakis(tributylphosphine)decapalladium

Octa-μ-carbonyltetra-μ₃-carbonyldicarbonyltetrakis(tributylphosphine)decapalladium, 10CI

[79305-04-7]

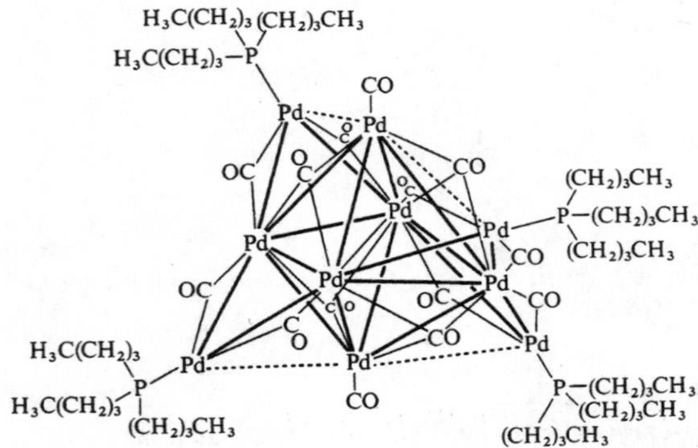

M 2265.622

Cryst. (dioxan/Me_2CO). Prep. and operations should be conducted under CO atm.

Mednikov, E.G. *et al*, *J. Chem. Soc., Chem. Commun.*, 1981, 989 (*ir, nmr*)

Mednikov, E.G. *et al*, *J. Organomet. Chem.*, 1982, **239**, 401.

Suggestions for new Entries are welcomed. Please write to the Editor, Dictionary of Organometallic Compounds, Chapman and Hall Ltd, 11 New Fetter Lane, London EC4P 4EE

$C_{64}H_{56}Cl_4Pd_2$ Pd-00338

Di-μ-chlorodichlorobis[tetrakis(4-methylphenyl)cyclobutadiene]dipalladium

Di-μ-chlorodichlorobis[1,1′,1″,1‴-(η⁴-1,3-cyclobutadiene-1,2,3,4-tetrayl)tetrakis[4-methylbenzene]]dipalladium, 9CI. Di-μ-chlorodichlorobis(1,2,3,4-tetra-p-tolyl-1,3-cyclobutadiene)dipalladium, 8CI. Tetrachlorobis-[tetrakis(4-methylphenyl)cyclobutadiene]dipalladium

[32761-47-0]

M 1179.798

Bridged dimer. Red cryst. (CH_2Cl_2/pet. ether).

Monomer: Dichloro[tetrakis(4-methylphenyl)-cyclobutadiene]palladium.

$C_{32}H_{28}Cl_2Pd$ M 589.899

Unknown.

Maitlis, P.M. *et al*, *J. Organomet. Chem.*, 1971, **26**, 407 (*synth, nmr*)

Taylor, S.H. *et al*, *J. Am. Chem. Soc.*, 1978, **100**, 4700.

$C_{72}H_{60}As_4Pd$ Pd-00339

Tetrakis(triphenylarsine)palladium, 9CI

[23732-79-8]

$Pd(AsPh_3)_4$ (T_d)

M 1331.372

Catalyses alkenylation of amines and ketones. Cryst. (pet. ether). Mp 80-100° dec.

Malatesta, L. *et al*, *J. Chem. Soc.*, 1957, 1186 (*synth*)

$C_{72}H_{60}P_2Pb_2Pd$ Pd-00340

Bis(triphenylphosphine)bis(triphenylplumbyl)palladium, 9CI

Bis(triphenylplumbyl)bis(triphenylphosphine)palladium. Bis(triphenyllead)bis(triphenylphosphine)-palladium

[41705-71-9]

$Pd(PbPh_3)_2(PPh_3)_2$

M 1508.034

Configuration not determined. Yellow-greenish solid (pet. ether). Mp 90-5° dec.

Crociani, B. *et al*, *J. Organomet. Chem.*, 1973, **49**, 249 (*synth, ir*)

$C_{72}H_{60}P_4Pd$ Pd-00341

Tetrakis(triphenylphosphine)palladium

[14221-01-3]

$Pd(PPh_3)_4$ (T_d)

M 1155.581

Extremely versatile catalyst for alkene reactions, additions and oligomerisations; condensation reactions, coupling of organic halides and organometallics; hydrosilylations; carbonylations and cleavage reactions of organosilanes and organostannanes. Yellow solid. Mp 100-5°. Unstable in air, dec. at 115°.

Malatesta, L. *et al*, *J. Chem. Soc.*, 1957, 1118 (*synth*)
Inorg. Synth., 1972, **13**, 121 (*synth*)
Townsend, J.M. *et al*, *J. Org. Chem.*, 1975, **40**, 2976 (*synth*, *ir*)
Fieser, M. *et al*, *Reagents for Organic Synthesis*, Wiley, 1967-83, **8**, 472 (*use*)

$C_{72}H_{60}PdSb_4$ Pd-00342

Tetrakis(triphenylstibine)palladium, 10CI, 9CI
Tetrakis(triphenylantimony)palladium
[23854-68-4]

$Pd(SbPh_3)_4$ (T_d)

M 1518.686

Catalyses polymerisation of haloanilines and diamines with CO. Solid.

Garrou, P.E. *et al*, *Inorg. Chem.*, 1976, **15**, 730 (*synth*, *pmr*)
Koketsu, J. *et al*, *CA*, 1981, **95**, 149437s (*synth*)

$C_{75}H_{60}O_3P_4Pd_3$ Pd-00343

Tri-μ-carbonyltetrakis(triphenylphosphine)tripalladium, 9CI
[36733-08-1]

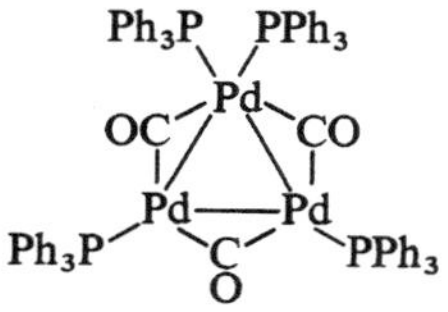

Ph₃P PPh₃ / OC Pd CO / Pd—Pd / Ph₃P C PPh₃ / O

M 1452.452

Catalyses carboxymethylation of organic halides. Orange-yellow cryst.; dec. slowly in air. Mp 70° dec.

Kudo, K. *et al*, *J. Organomet. Chem.*, 1971, **33**, 393 (*synth*, *ir*)
Hidai, M. *et al*, *J. Organomet. Chem.*, 1973, **52**, 431 (*synth*)
Hidai, M. *et al*, *Bull. Chem. Soc. Jpn.*, 1975, **48**, 2075 (*use*)

$C_{84}H_{60}Pd_2$ Pd-00344

μ-Diphenylacetylenebis(η^5-pentaphenylcyclopentadienyl)dipalladium
[*μ*-[*1,1'*-[(η^2:η^2)-*1,2-Ethynediyl*]*bis*[*benzene*-]]*bis*[(*1,2,3,4,5*-*η*)-*1,2,3,4,5-pentaphenyl-2,4-cyclopentadien-1-yl*]*dipalladium*, 9CI. (*μ-Diphenylethyne*)*bis*-(*pentaphenylcyclopentadienyl*)*dipalladium*
[39459-32-0]

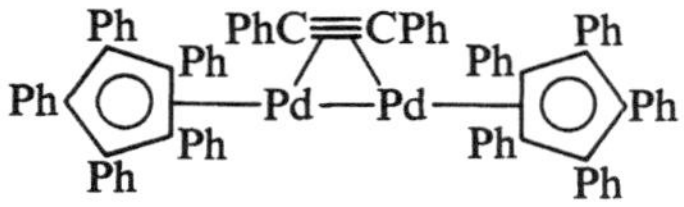

M 1282.238

Green cryst. ($CHCl_3$ or C_6H_6). Mp 240° dec.

Ban, E. *et al*, *J. Chem. Soc., Chem. Commun.*, 1973, 368 (*struct*)
Jack, T.R. *et al*, *J. Am. Chem. Soc.*, 1977, **99**, 4707 (*synth*, *uv*, *ms*, *struct*)

$C_{84}H_{162}O_{12}P_6Pd_{10}$ Pd-00345

Octa-μ-carbonyltetra-μ_3-carbonylhexakis(tributylphosphine)decapalladium, 9CI
Hexakis(tributylphosphine)dodecacarbonyldecapalladium. Dodecacarbonylhexakis(tributylphosphine)-decapalladium
[79305-05-8]

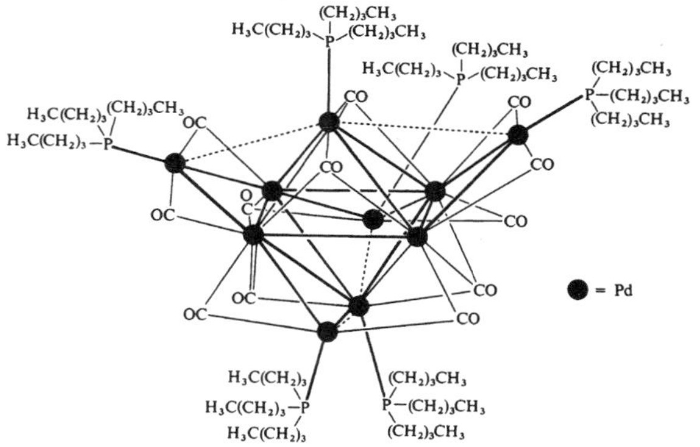

M 2614.239

Cryst. (Me_2CO). Prep. and operations should be conducted under CO atmosphere.

Mednikov, E.G. *et al*, *J. Organomet. Chem.*, 1982, **239**, 401 (*synth*, *struct*)

$F_{12}P_4Pd$ Pd-00346

Tetrakis(trifluorophosphine)palladium
Tetrakis(phosphorus trifluoride)palladium, 9CI
[13815-33-3]

$Pd(PF_3)_4$ (T_d)

M 458.296

Unstable, volatile liquid at r.t., cryst. <−41°. Mp −41°. Dec. at 100°.

Kruck, T. *et al*, *Z. Anorg. Allg. Chem.*, 1969, **364**, 192 (*synth*, *ir*, *nmr*)
Edwards, H.G.M. *et al*, *Spectrochim. Acta, Part A*, 1970, **26**, 897 (*synth*, *ir*, *raman*)
Timms, P.L., *J. Chem. Soc. (A)*, 1970, 2526 (*synth*)

Pt Platinum

R. J. Cross

Platine (Fr.), Platin (Ger.), Platino (Sp., Ital.), Платина (Platina) (Russ.), 白金 (Japan.)

Atomic Number. 78

Atomic Weight. 195.09. An uncertainty of ±0.03 limits the accuracy of the quoted molecular weights for entries in this section.

Electronic Configuration. [Xe] $5d^9\,6s^1$

Oxidation States. The most common oxidation levels are 0 (d^{10}), +2 (d^8), and +4 (d^6). Pt(IV) compounds are usually 18-electron molecules, but both 16- and 18-electron molecules are common for Pt(0) and Pt(II). A growing number of platinum—platinum bonded compounds is establishing Pt(I) as an important oxidation level also.

Coordination Number. Conventional (η^1) ligands usually form four-coordinate tetrahedral complexes with Pt(0), square-planar complexes with Pt(II), and six-coordinate octahedral with Pt(IV).

Colour. Variable.

Availability. The price of platinum exceeds that of gold, and like that of gold, it fluctuates on the world market. Common starting materials are K_2PtCl_4 and $PtCl_2$.

Handling. Most platinum complexes are air- and moisture-stable, and can be handled conventionally at ordinary temperatures. Their price makes small-scale operations attractive, however.

Toxicity. Whilst platinum compounds are not normally regarded as being very toxic, some molecules have a high biological activity (including a few with carcinostatic properties) and so caution should be exercised.

Isotopic Abundance. ^{192}Pt, 0.79%; ^{194}Pt, 32.9%; ^{195}Pt, 33.8%; ^{196}Pt, 25.3%; ^{198}Pt, 7.2%.

Spectroscopy. ^{195}Pt, $I = \frac{1}{2}$, has a relative sensitivity of 9.94×10^{-3} (^{1}H = 1.000), and is becoming a useful nmr probe. See Pregosin, P. S., *Coord. Chem. Rev.*, 1982, **44,** 247. Most platinum complexes are diamagnetic, and other nuclei (^{1}H, ^{13}C, ^{31}P) make valuable nmr spectroscopic handles.

Analysis. Analysis for platinum is gravimetrically as Pt metal, after digestion of the compound by nitric acid and reduction with formic acid at pH 6. Atomic absorption spectroscopy can also be used. Response is linear to 75 ppm, and the sensitivity is 2 μg cm^{-3}.

References. Compounds of platinum are the least reactive of the Ni, Pd, Pt triad, and consequently many more have been isolated and examined. The corollary is, of course, that platinum complexes are less useful catalytically.

In addition to reviews listed in the introduction to the *Sourcebook* the reader is referred to:

Belluco, U., *The Organometallic and Coordination Chemistry of Platinum*, Academic Press, New York, 1974.

Hartley, F. R., *The Chemistry of Platinum and Palladium*, Applied Science, 1973.

$PtBr_3(CO)^{\ominus}$

Pt-00001

$[PtCl_3(CO)]^{\ominus}$ (C_{2v})

Pt-00002

$[Pt(CO)Cl_5]^{\ominus}$

Pt-00003

$[PtCl_5Me]^{\ominus\ominus}$

Pt-00004

$PtI_3(CO)^{\ominus}$

Pt-00005

Pt-00006

cis-form

Pt-00007

Pt-00008

$PtBr_3(C_2H_4)^{\ominus}$ (C_{2v})

Pt-00009

Pt-00010

$[PtMe_2Br_2]_n$

Pt-00011

$Pt(OH)_2Me_2$

Pt-00012

Pt-00013

Tetramer

Pt-00014

Pt-00015

As Pt-00017 with
X = OH

Pt-00016

X = H

Pt-00017

X = Cl

Pt-00018

Pt-00019

As Pt-00018 with
X = OH

Pt-00020

Pt-00021

$[PtMe_3(OH_2)_3]^{\oplus}$

Pt-00022

cis-form

Pt-00023

Pt-00024

$PtMe_2(CO)_2$

Pt-00025

$PtCl_2(C_2H_4)_2$

Pt-00026

Pt-00027

Pt-00028

Pt-00029

$PtMe_4^{\ominus\ominus}$ (D_{4h})

Pt-00030

R = Me

Pt-00031

$Pt(CO)_4$ (T_d)

Pt-00032

Pt-00033

Pt-00034

Pt-00035

$[PtBr(CNMe)_3]^{\oplus}$ (C_{2v})

Pt-00036

$[PtMe_3(CN)_3]^{\ominus\ominus}$

Pt-00037

Pt-00038

Pt-00039

Pt-00040

Pt-00041

Pt-00042

Pt-00043

Pt-00044

R = Me

Pt-00045

$PtMe_6^{\ominus\ominus}$ (O_h)

Pt-00046

Pt-00047

$[Pt_3(CO)_3(\mu\text{-}CO)_3]^{\ominus\ominus}$

Pt-00048

X = Br

Pt-00049

As Pt-00049 with
X = Cl

Pt-00050

As Pt-00049 with
X = I

Pt-00051

cis-form

Pt-00052

Pt-00053

cis-form

$R^1 = R^2 = Et$

Pt-00054

Pt-00055

$PtClMe(AsMe_3)_2$

Pt-00056

X = Br

Pt-00057

As Pt-00057 with
X = Cl

Pt-00058

Pt-00059

As Pt-00057 with
X = I

Pt-00060

Pt-00061

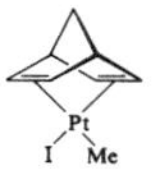

Pt-00062

Pt-00063

Pt-00064

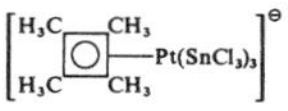

Pt-00065

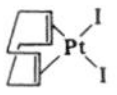

Pt-00066

$[Pt(MeCN)_4]^{\oplus\oplus}$ (D_{4h})

Pt-00067

$[Pt(CNMe)_4]^{\oplus\oplus}$ (D_{4h})

Pt-00068

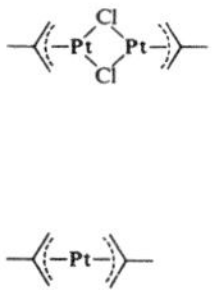

Pt-00069

Pt-00070

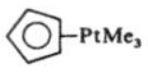

Pt-00071

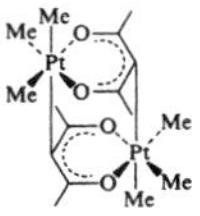

Pt-00072

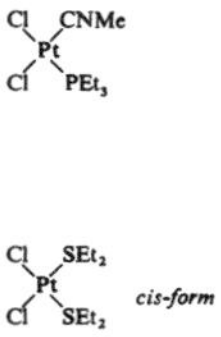

Pt-00073

cis-form

Pt-00074

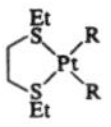

R = Me

Pt-00075

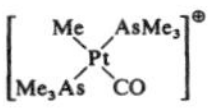

trans-form

Pt-00076

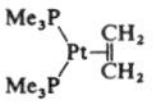

Pt-00077

$PtMe_2(AsMe_3)_2$

Pt-00078

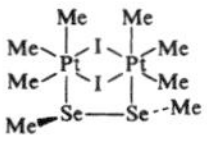

Pt-00079

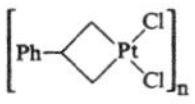

Pt-00080

As Pt-00054 with
R^1 = Me, R^2 = Ph

Pt-00081

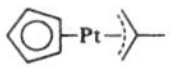

Pt-00082

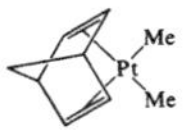

Pt-00083

As Pt-00031 with
R = Ph

Pt-00084

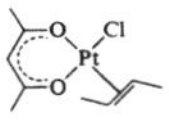

(E)-form

Pt-00085

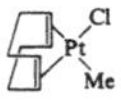

Pt-00086

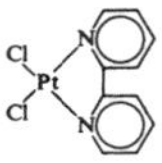

Pt-00087

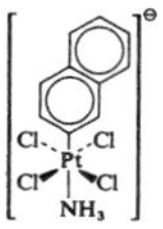

Pt-00088

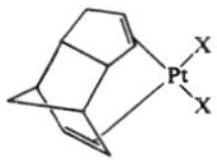

X = Br

Pt-00089

As Pt-00089 with
X = Cl

Pt-00090

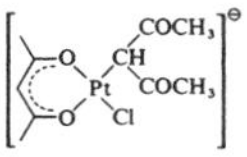

Pt-00091

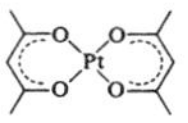

Pt-00092

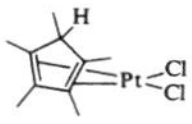

Pt-00093

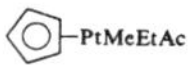

Pt-00094

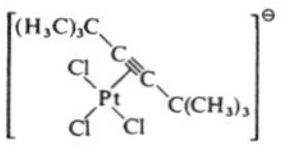

Pt-00095

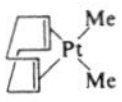

Pt-00096

$(Me_3PCH_2)_2PtMe_2$

Pt-00097

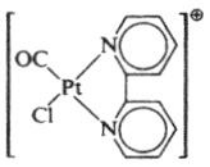

Pt-00098

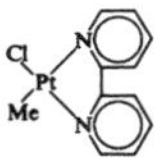

Pt-00099

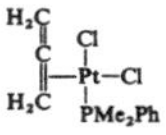

Pt-00100

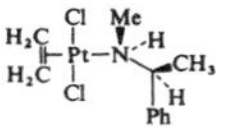

(S,S)-trans-form

Pt-00101

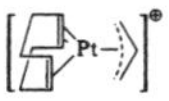

Pt-00102

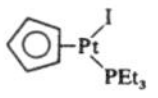

Pt-00103

$Pt(C_2F_4)(Bipy)$

Pt-00104

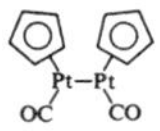

Pt-00105

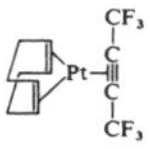

Pt-00106

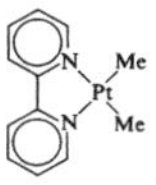

Pt-00107

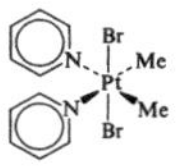

Pt-00108

$PtMe_2Py_2$

Pt-00109

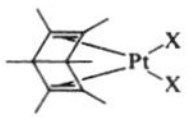

X = Br

Pt-00110

As Pt-00110 with
X = Cl

Pt-00111

As Pt-00110 with
X = I

Pt-00112

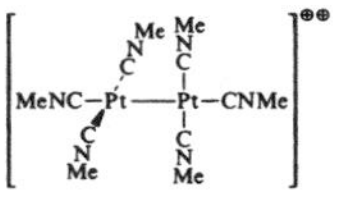

Pt-00113

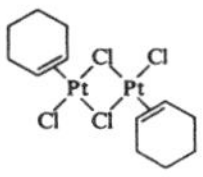

Pt-00114

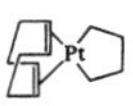

Pt-00115

Pt-00116

$(Bu^tC{\equiv}CBu^t)PtCl(SnCl_3)(NCCH_3)$

Pt-00117

$Pt(C{\equiv}CCH_3)_2(AsMe_3)_2$

Pt-00118

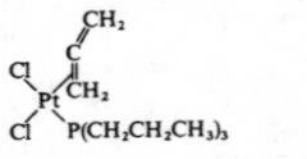

Pt-00119

$[PtCl(SnCl_3)(PEt_3)_2]$

Pt-00120

$[Pt(SnCl_3)_2(PEt_3)_2]$

Pt-00121

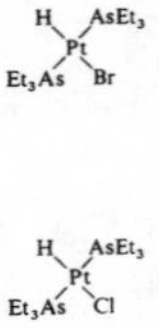

Pt-00122

Pt-00123

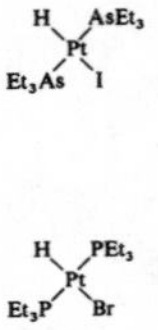

Pt-00124

Pt-00125

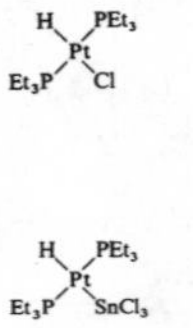

Pt-00126

Pt-00127

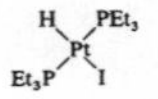

Pt-00128

$[PtH(NO_2)(PEt_3)_2]$ (C_{2v})

Pt-00129

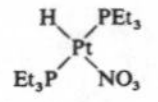

Pt-00130

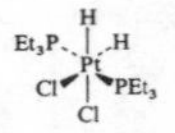

Pt-00131

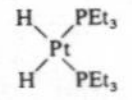

cis-form

Pt-00132

$[Pt(B_8H_{12})(PEt_3)_2]$

Pt-00133

$[Pt(B_{10}H_{12})(PEt_3)_2]$

Pt-00134

$[Ni_3Pt_3(CO)_{12}]^{\ominus\ominus}$

Pt-00135

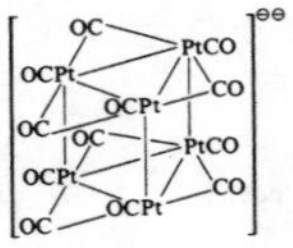

Pt-00136

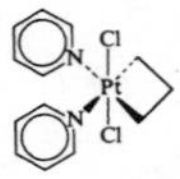

Pt-00137

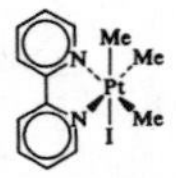

Pt-00138

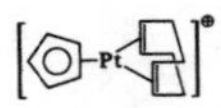

Pt-00139

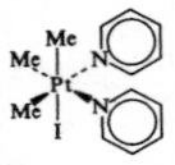

Pt-00140

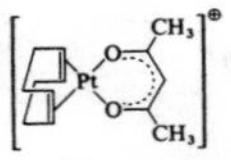

Pt-00141

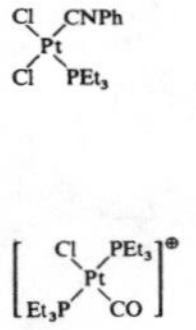

Pt-00142

Pt-00143

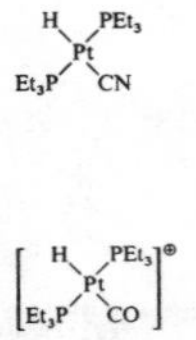

Pt-00144

Pt-00145

cis-form

Pt-00146

cis-form

Pt-00147

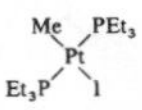

Pt-00148

cis-form

Pt-00149

Pt-00150

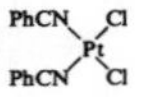

cis-form

Pt-00151

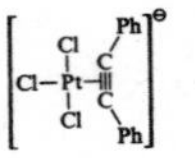

Pt-00152

$PtPh_2(CO)_2$

Pt-00153

As Pt-00054 with
R^1 = Ph, R^2 = Me

Pt-00154

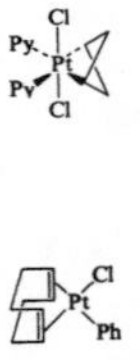

Pt-00155

Pt-00156

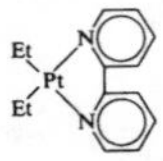

Pt-00157

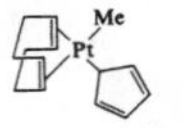

Pt-00158

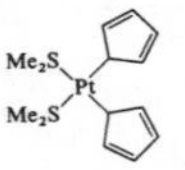

cis-form

Pt-00159

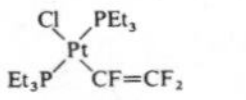

Pt-00160

$[Pt(CO)_2(PEt_3)_2]$ (C_{2v})

Pt-00161

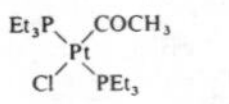

Pt-00162

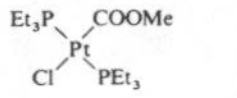

Pt-00163

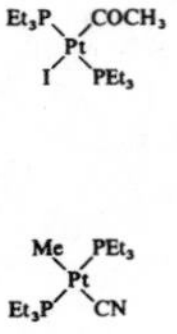

Pt-00164

Pt-00165

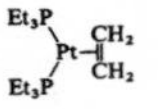

Pt-00166

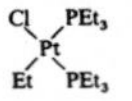

cis-form

Pt-00167

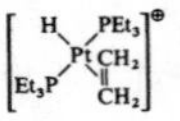

Pt-00168

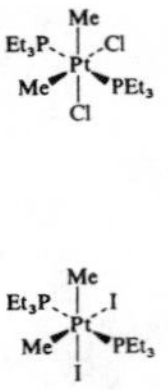

Pt-00169

Pt-00170

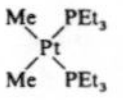

cis-form

Pt-00171

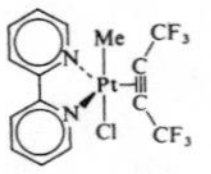

Pt-00172

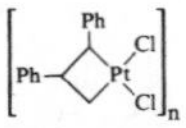

Pt-00173

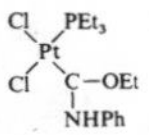

Pt-00174

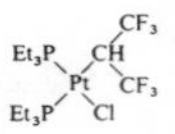

cis-form

Pt-00175

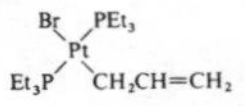

Pt-00176

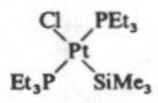

Pt-00177

Pt-00178

As Pt-00045 with
R = Ph

Pt-00179

Pt-00180

R = CH_3

Pt-00181

Pt-00182

Pt-00183

Pt-00184

(E)-cis-form

Pt-00185

cis-form

Pt-00186

Pt-00187

Pt-00188

$Me_4Pt(PEt_3)_2$

Pt-00189

$R^1 = Me, R^2 = Ph$

Pt-00190

Pt-00191

cis-form

Pt-00192

Pt-00193

$(C_5H_5)PtPh(PEt_3)_2$

Pt-00194

Pt-00195

Pt-00196

Pt-00197

Pt-00198

Pt-00199

$Pt(C_2F_4)(PMe_2Ph)_2$

Pt-00200

As Pt-00075 with
R = Ph

Pt-00201

Pt-00202

Pt-00203

ab-dibromo-*ce*-diphosphine-*df*-dimethyl-*form*

Pt-00204

ab-dichloro-*ce*-diphosphine-*df*-dimethyl-*form*

Pt-00205

af-diphosphine-*bc*-diiodo-*de*-dimethyl-*form*

Pt-00206

$[PtMe_5(PMePh_2)]^{\ominus}$

Pt-00207

Pt-00208

cis-form

Pt-00209

mer-trans-form *mer-cis-form*

Pt-00210

Pt-00211

cis-form

Pt-00212

Pt-00213

Pt-00214

cis-form

Pt-00215

Pt-00216

Pt-00217

Pt-00218

$[Pt(PEt_3)_3]$

Pt-00219

$[PtH(PEt_3)_3]^{\oplus}$ (C_{2v})

Pt-00220

Pt-00221

cis-form

Pt-00222

As Pt-00054 with
$R^1 = R^2 = Ph$

Pt-00223

Pt-00224

Pt-00225

Pt-00226

Pt-00227

Pt-00228

Pt-00229

Pt-00230

(±)-form *meso-form*

Pt-00231

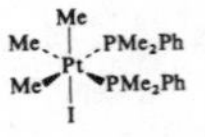

Pt-00232

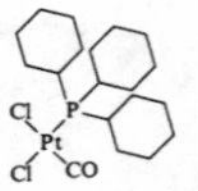

cis-form

Pt-00233

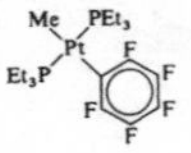

Pt-00234

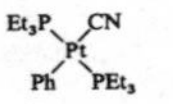

Pt-00235

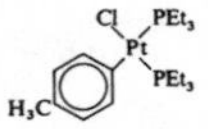

Pt-00236

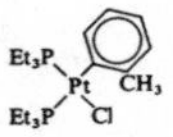

cis-form

Pt-00237

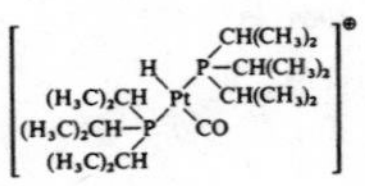

trans-form

Pt-00239

$Pt(CO)(PEt_3)_3$ (C_{3v})

Pt-00240

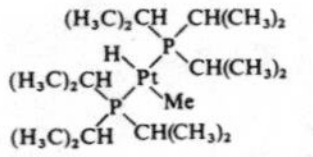

Pt-00241

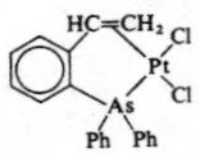

Pt-00242

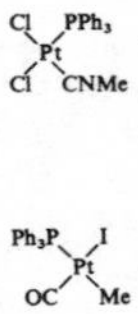

Pt-00243

Pt-00244

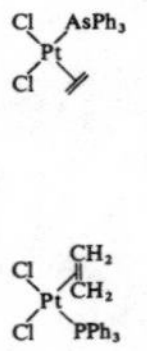

Pt-00245

Pt-00246

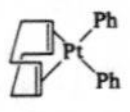

Pt-00247

$(H_2C{=}CCl)_2Pt(PMe_2Ph)_2$

Pt-00248

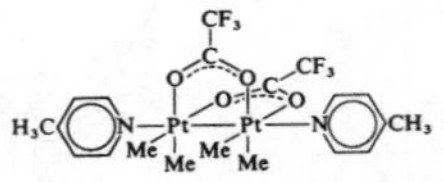

Pt-00249

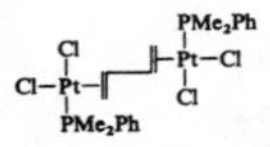

Pt-00250

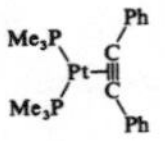

Pt-00251

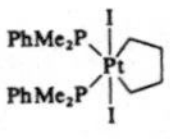

Pt-00252

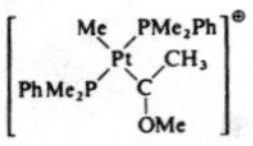

Pt-00253

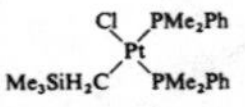

cis-form

Pt-00254

$Me_4Pt(AsMe_2Ph)_2$

Pt-00255

$Me_4Pt(PMe_2Ph)_2$

Pt-00256

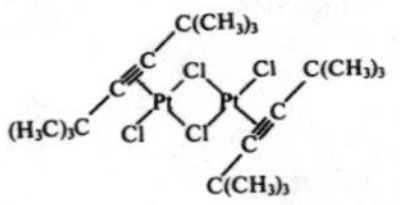

Pt = 00257

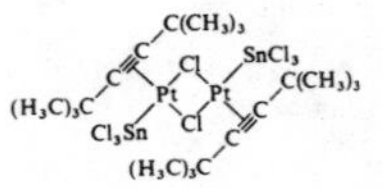

Pt-00258

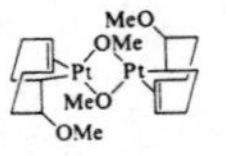

Pt-00259

$Pt(CO)_3(PPh_3)$ (C_{3v})

Pt-00260

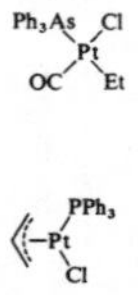

Pt-00261

Pt-00262

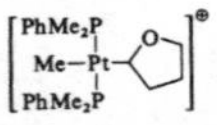

Pt-00263

$[PtMe(CH_3C{\equiv}CCH_3)(PMe_2Ph)_2]^{\oplus}$

Pt-00264

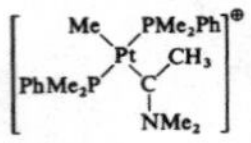

Pt-00265

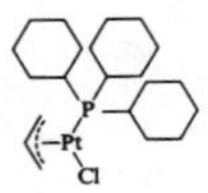

Pt-00266

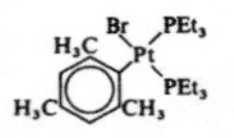

cis-form

Pt-00267

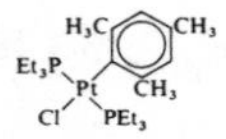

Pt-00268

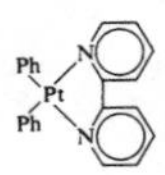

Pt-00269

$PtPh_2Py_2$

Pt-00270

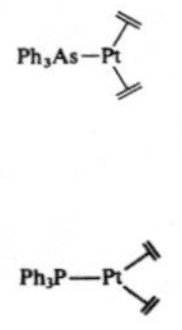

Pt-00271

Pt-00272

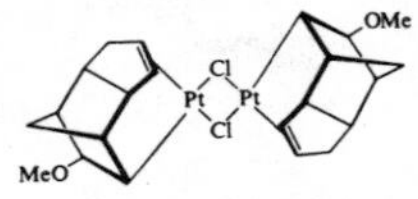

Pt-00273

$PtCl(CH{=}CH_2)(PEt_2Ph)_2$

Pt-00274

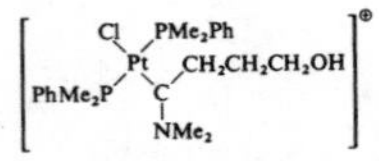

Pt-00275

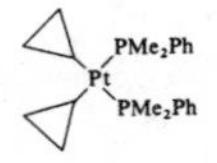

Pt-00276

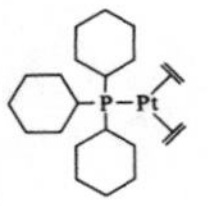

Pt-00277

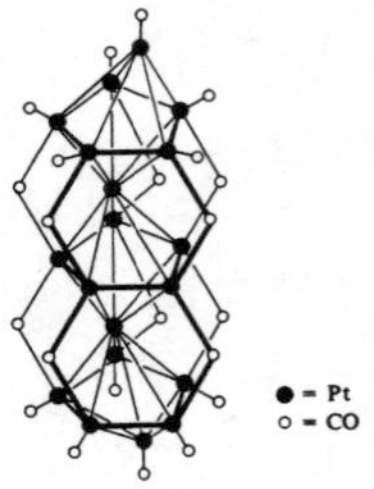

● = Pt
○ = CO

Pt-00278

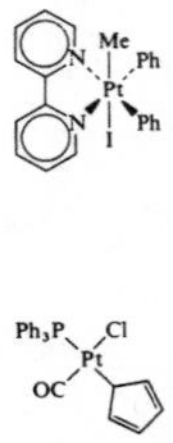

Pt-00279

Pt-00280

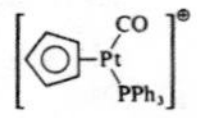

Pt-00281

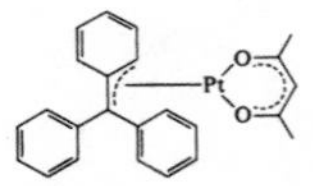

Pt-00282

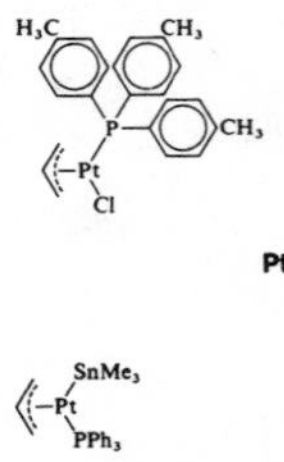

Pt-00283

Pt-00284

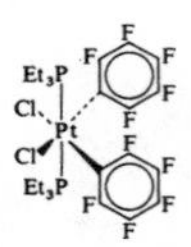

Pt-00285

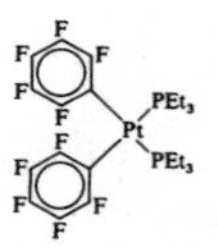

cis-form

Pt-00286

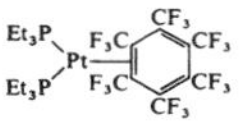

Pt-00287

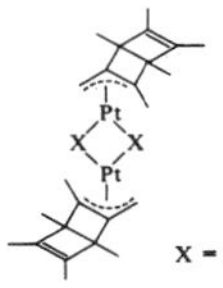

X = Br

Pt-00288

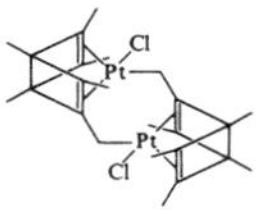

Pt-00289

As Pt-00288 with
X = Cl

Pt-00290

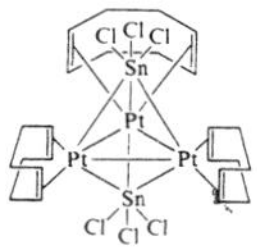

Pt-00291

$(MeOCH_2CH{=}CH)_2Pt(PMe_2Ph)_2$

Pt-00292

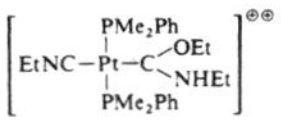

Pt-00293

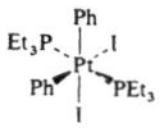

Pt-00294

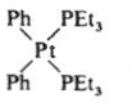

cis-form

Pt-00295

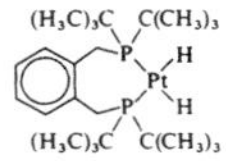

Pt-00296

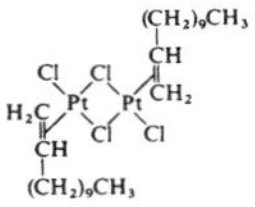

Pt-00297

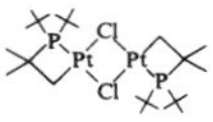

Pt-00298

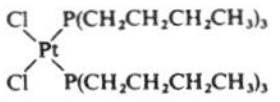

cis-form

Pt-00299

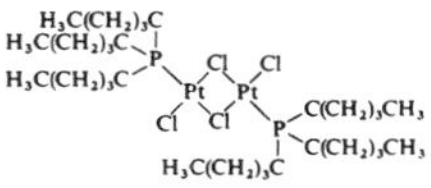

Pt-00300

$[(H_3C)_3C]_3PPtP[C(CH_3)_3]_3$

Pt-00301

$[(H_3C)_3C]_3PPtHP[C(CH_3)_3]_3{}^{\oplus}$

Pt-00302

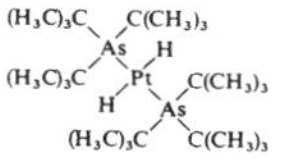

Pt-00303

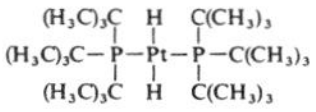

Pt-00304

$Pt[P(OEt)_3]_4$ (T_d)

Pt-00305

$[Pt(PEt_3)_4]$ (T_d)

Pt-00306

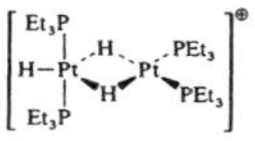

Pt-00307

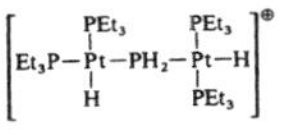

cis,trans-form

Pt-00308

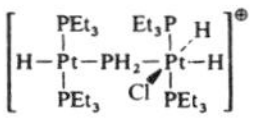

Pt-00309

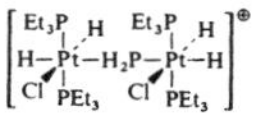

Pt-00310

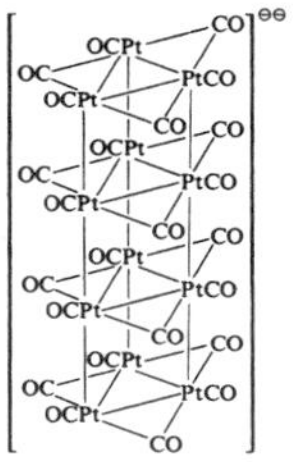

Pt-00311

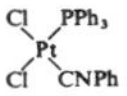

Pt-00312

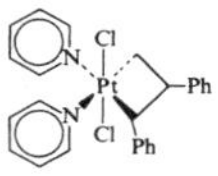

Pt-00313

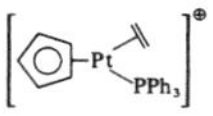

Pt-00314

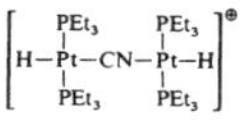

Pt-00315

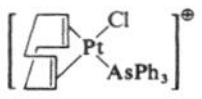

Pt-00316

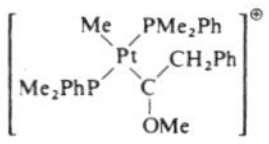

Pt-00317

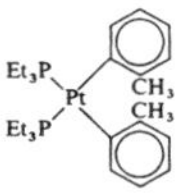

cis-form

Pt-00318

Pt-00319

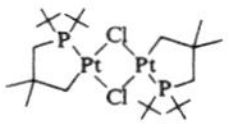

Pt-00320

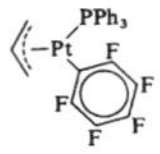

Pt-00321

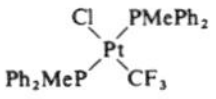

Pt-00322

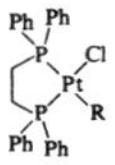

R = Me

Pt-00323

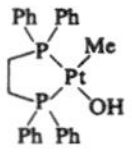

Pt-00324

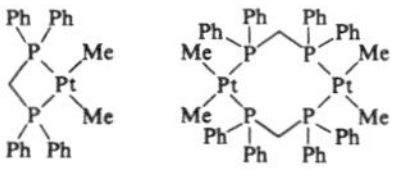

monomer dimer

Pt-00325

cis-form

Pt-00326

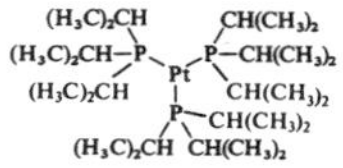

Pt-00327

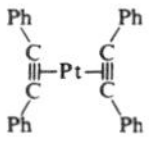

Pt-00328

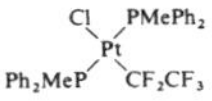

Pt-00329

As Pt-00323 with
R = Et

Pt-00330

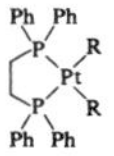

R = Me

Pt-00331

Pt-00332

cis-form

Pt-00333

$PtCl(C{\equiv}CPh)(PEt_2Ph)_2$

Pt-00334

$Pt(C{\equiv}CPh)_2(AsEt_3)_2$

Pt-00335

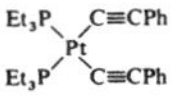

cis-form

Pt-00336

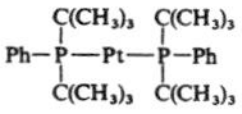

Pt-00337

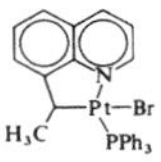

Pt-00338

$Pt(CO)_2(PPh_2Et)_2$ (C_{2v})

Pt-00339

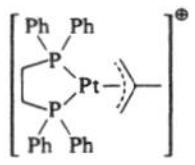

Pt-00340

As Pt-00331 with
R = Et

Pt-00341

$Me_4Pt(PMePh_2)_2$

Pt-00342

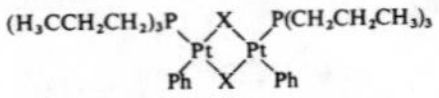

X = Br

Pt-00343

As Pt-00343 with
X = I

Pt-00344

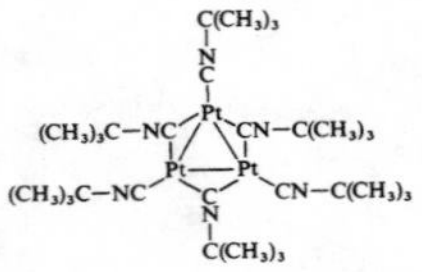

Pt-00345

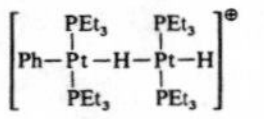

Pt-00346

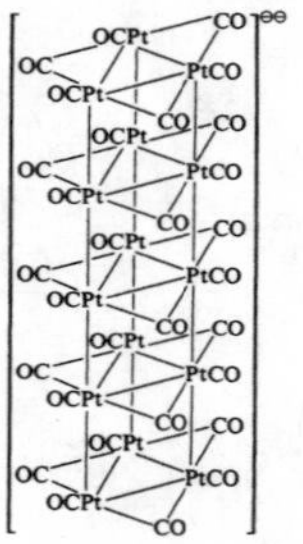

Pt-00347

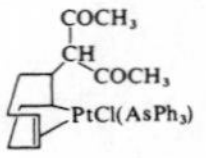

Pt-00348

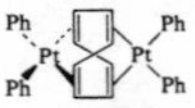

Pt-00349

As Pt-00323 with
R = Ph

Pt-00350

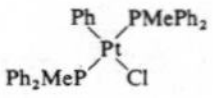

Pt-00351

$[Pt(C{\equiv}CPh)_2(PMe_2Ph)_2](D_{2h})$

Pt-00352

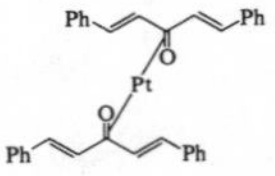

Pt-00353

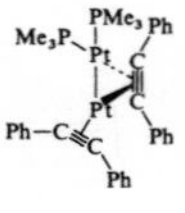

Pt-00354

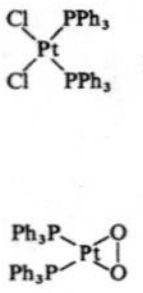

cis-form

Pt-00355

Pt-00356

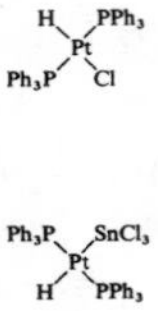

Pt-00357

Pt-00358

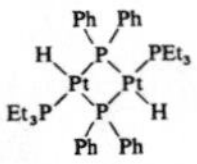

Pt-00359

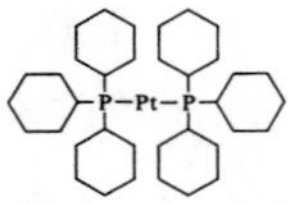

Pt-00360

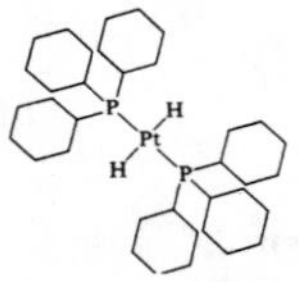

Pt-00361

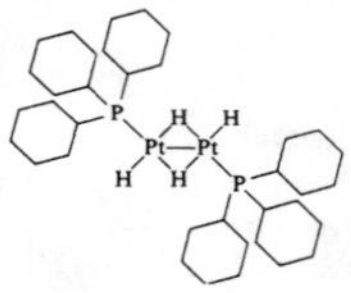

Pt-00362

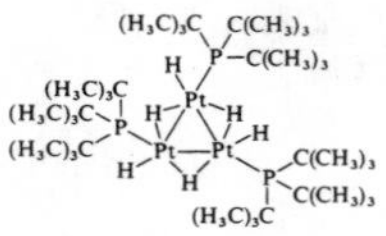

Pt-00363

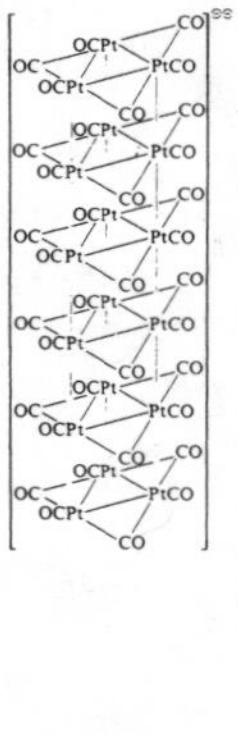

Pt-00364

As Pt-00190 with
$R^1 = R^2 = Ph$

Pt-00365

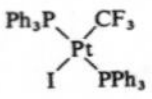

Pt-00366

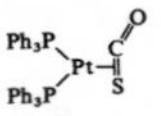

Pt-00367

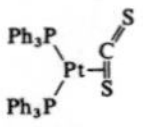

Pt-00368

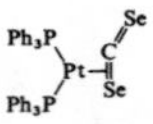

Pt-00369

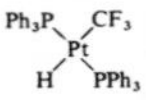

Pt-00370

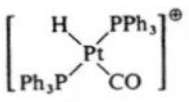

Pt-00371

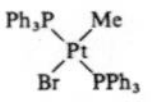

trans-form

Pt-00372

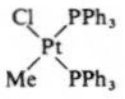

cis-form

Pt-00373

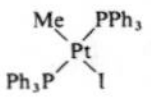

Pt-00374

$PtI_3Me(PPh_3)_2$

Pt-00375

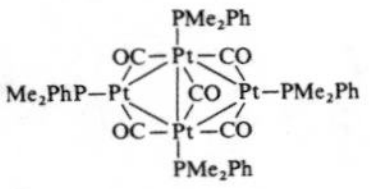

Pt-00376

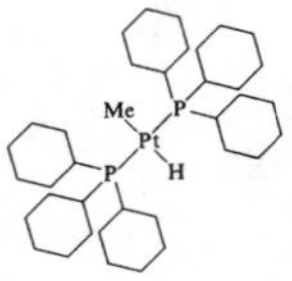

Pt-00377

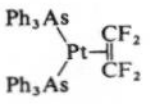

Pt-00378

As Pt-00381 with
X = Cl

Pt-00379

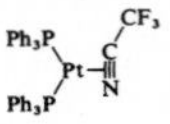

Pt-00380

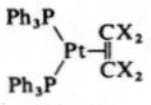

X = F

Pt-00381

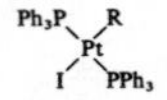

$R = -CF_2CF_3$

Pt-00382

$Pt(CO)_2(PPh_3)_2\ (C_{2v})$

Pt-00383

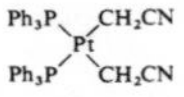

cis-form

Pt-00384

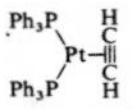

Pt-00385

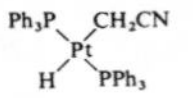

Pt-00386

As Pt-00331 with
R = Ph

Pt-00387

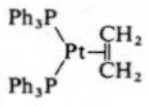

Pt-00388

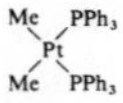

cis-form

Pt-00389

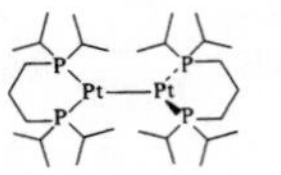

Pt-00390

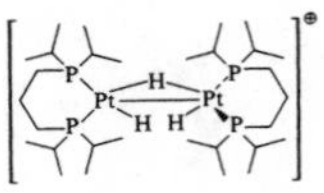

Pt-00391

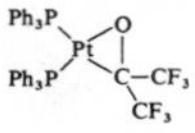

Pt-00392

As Pt-00382 with
R = —$CF_2CF_2CF_3$

Pt-00393

Pt-00394

Pt-00395

Pt-00396

Pt-00397

Pt-00398

Pt-00399

Pt-00400

Pt-00401

Pt-00402

Pt-00403

Pt-00404

Pt-00405

Pt-00406

Pt-00407

Pt-00408

$Et_2Pt(PPh_3)_2$

Pt-00409

$Me_3PbPtMe(PPh_3)_2$

Pt-00410

Pt-00411

Pt-00412

Pt-00413

Pt-00414

As Pt-00416 with
X = Br

Pt-00415

Pt-00416

Pt-00417

Pt-00418

Pt-00419

Pt-00420

Pt-00421

Pt-00422

Pt-00423

Pt-00424

Pt-00425

Pt-00426

Pt-00427

Pt-00428

Pt-00429

Pt-00430

$(Ph_3P)_2Pt(C_6F_6)_2$

Pt-00431

Pt-00432

$Pt(GePh_3)_2(PEt_3)_2$

Pt-00433

Pt-00434

Pt-00435

Pt-00436

Pt-00437

Pt-00438

Pt-00439

Pt-00440

Pt-00441

Pt-00442

Pt-00443

Pt-00444

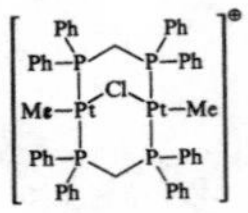

Pt-00445

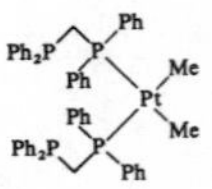

Pt-00446

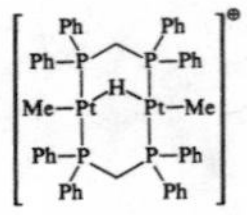

Pt-00447

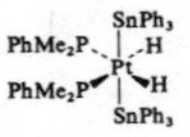

Pt-00448

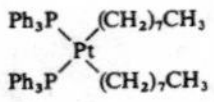

Pt-00449

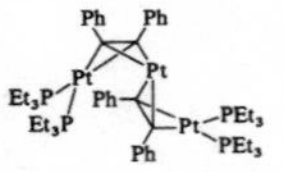

Pt-00450

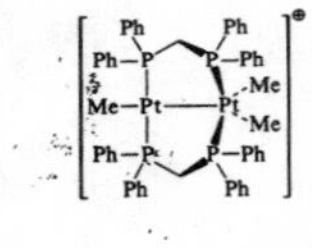

Pt-00451

$Pt(PPh_3)_3$

Pt-00452

$[PtH(PPh_3)_3]^{\oplus}$ (C_{2v})

Pt-00453

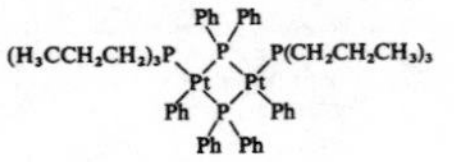

Pt-00454

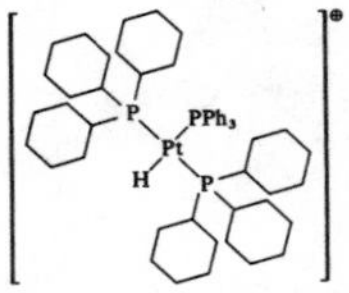

Pt-00455

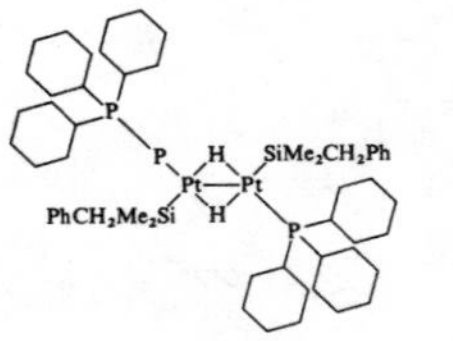

Pt-00456

$Pt(CO)(PPh_3)_3$ (C_{3v})

Pt-00457

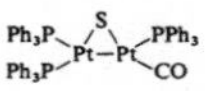

Pt-00458

$(Ph_3P)_3PtMe^{\oplus}$ (C_{2v})

Pt-00459

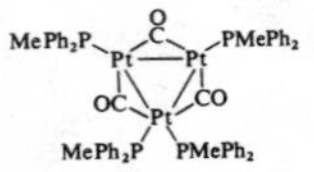

Pt-00460

As Pt-00181 with
R = Ph

Pt-00461

$(Ph_3P)_3PtEt^{\oplus}$ (C_{2v})

Pt-00462

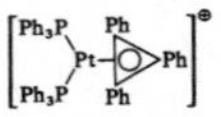

Pt-00463

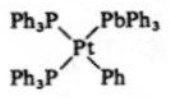

Pt-00464

$(Ph_3P)_3PtCH_2Ph^{\oplus}$ (C_{2v})

Pt-00465

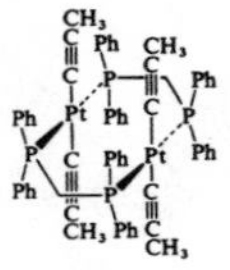

Pt-00466

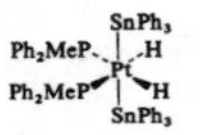

Pt-00467

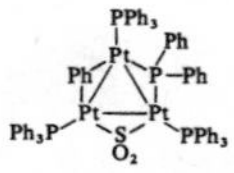

Pt-00468

$Pt[P(OPh)_3]_4$ (T_d)

Pt-00469

$(Ph_3Pb)_2Pt(PPh_3)_2$

Pt-00470

$Pt(PPh_3)_4$ (T_d)

Pt-00471

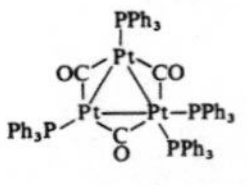

Pt-00472

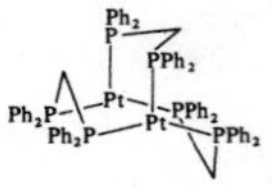

Pt-00473

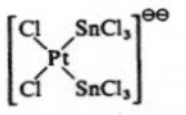

Pt-00474

$[PtH(SnCl_3)_4]^{\ominus\ominus\ominus}$

Pt-00475

$Pt(SnCl_3)_5^{\ominus\ominus\ominus}$

Pt-00476

$Pt(PF_3)_4$ (T_d)

Pt-00477

$CBr_3OPt^{\ominus}$ Pt-00001

Tribromocarbonylplatinate(1−)

[66197-25-9]

$PtBr_3(CO)^{\ominus}$

M 462.802 (ion)

K salt:

CBr_3KOPt M 501.901

Yellow-orange cryst. Mp 100° dec.

Tetrapropylammonium salt:

$C_{13}H_{28}Br_3NOPt$ M 649.162

Yellow cryst. (Me_2CO/Et_2O). Mp 121°.

Malatesta, L. *et al*, *Gazz. Chim. Ital.*, 1960, **90**, 1505 (*synth*)
Browning, J. *et al*, *J. Chem. Soc., Dalton Trans.*, 1977, 2061 (*synth, ir, nmr, raman*)

$CCl_3OPt^{\ominus}$ Pt-00002

Carbonyltrichloroplatinate(1−)

[21710-57-6]

$[PtCl_3(CO)]^{\ominus}$ (C_{2v})

M 329.449 (ion)

Tetrabutylammonium salt: [34964-16-4].

$C_{17}H_{36}Cl_3NOPt$ M 571.917

Pale-yellow cryst.

*(2,2′-Bipyridine-*N,N′*)carbonylchloroplatinum(1+) salt:* [33679-79-7].

$C_{12}H_8Cl_4N_2O_2Pt_2$ M 744.179

Yellow, moisture-sensitive solid.

Spaulding, L. *et al*, *Inorg. Chem.*, 1972, **11**, 2092 (*synth, ir*)
Cherwinski, W.J. *et al*, *J. Chem. Soc., Dalton Trans.*, 1975, 1156 (*ir*)
Russell, D.R. *et al*, *J. Organomet. Chem.*, 1976, **104**, 387 (*struct*)
Calderazzo, F. *et al*, *Inorg. Chem.*, 1981, **20**, 1310 (*ir*)

$CCl_5OPt^{\ominus}$ Pt-00003

Carbonylpentachloroplatinate(1−)

$[Pt(CO)Cl_5]^{\ominus}$

M 400.355 (ion)

Possible chlorination catalyst.

Diisopropylammonium salt:

$C_7H_{14}ClNOPt$ M 358.727

Yellow-orange solid. Loses Cl_2 in soln. Dec. by H_2O. ir ν(CO)2191cm^{-1}.

Crocker, C. *et al*, *J. Chem. Soc., Chem. Commun.*, 1978, 1056.
Dell'Amico, D.B. *et al*, *J. Chem. Soc., Dalton Trans.*, 1982, 2257.

$CH_3Cl_5Pt^{\ominus\ominus}$ Pt-00004

Pentachloro(methyl)platinate(2−)

Methylpentachloroplatinate(2−)

$[PtCl_5Me]^{\ominus\ominus}$

M 387.380 (ion)

Obt. only in soln. as K salt.

Fanchiang, Y.-T. *et al*, *J. Am. Chem. Soc.*, 1979, **101**, 1442.

$CI_3OPt^{\ominus}$ Pt-00005

Carbonyltriiodoplatinate(1−)

[66213-26-1]

$PtI_3(CO)^{\ominus}$

M 603.804 (ion)

K salt:

CI_3KOPt M 642.902

Red cryst. Mp 100° dec.

Tetrabutylammonium salt: [66213-27-2].

$C_{17}H_{36}I_3NOPt$ M 846.271

Orange cryst. (Me_2CO/Et_2O). Mp 128°.

Malatesta, L. *et al*, *Gazz. Chim. Ital.*, 1960, **90**, 1505 (*synth*)
Browning, J. *et al*, *J. Chem. Soc., Dalton Trans.*, 1977, 2061 (*synth, ir, raman, nmr*)

$C_2Br_2O_2Pt$ Pt-00006

Dibromodicarbonylplatinum, 10CI

Dibromoplatinum dicarbonyl. Dicarbonylplatinum dibromide

Br CO
Pt
Br CO

M 410.909

***cis*-form** [20963-52-4]

Cryst. Bp 220° subl. (under CO).

Browning, J. *et al*, *J. Chem. Soc., Dalton Trans.*, 1977, 2061 (*synth, ir, raman, nmr*)

$C_2Cl_2O_2Pt$ Pt-00007

Dicarbonyldichloroplatinum

Dichloroplatinum dicarbonyl. Dicarbonylplatinum chloride

[25478-60-8]

Cl CO
Pt *cis-form*
Cl CO

M 322.007

Hydroformylation catalyst.

***cis*-form** [15020-32-3]

Cryst., stored in sealed tube under refrigeration. Subl. at 220°.

***trans*-form** [62841-60-5]

Not fully descr.

Saito, Y. *et al*, *Seisan Kenkyu*, 1976, **28**, 440; *CA*, **86**, 170267k (*synth, ir, nmr*)
Browning, J. *et al*, *J. Chem. Soc., Dalton Trans.*, 1977, 2061 (*synth, ir, raman, nmr*)
Dell'Amico, D.B. *et al*, *Gazz. Chim. Ital.*, 1977, **107**, 101 (*synth*)

$C_2Cl_4O_2Pt_2^{\ominus\ominus}$ Pt-00008

Dicarbonyltetrachlorodiplatinate(2−), 9CI

Tetrachlorodicarbonyldiplatinate(2−)

[OC CO; Cl−Pt−Pt−Cl; Cl Cl]$^{\ominus\ominus}$

M 587.993 (ion)

Bistetrapropylammonium salt: [52538-93-9].

$C_{26}H_{56}Cl_4N_2O_2Pt_2$ M 960.713

Yellow solid (Et_2O). Mp 188° dec.

Goggin, P.L. *et al*, *J. Chem. Soc., Dalton Trans.*, 1973, 2355 (*synth, ir*)
Modinos, A. *et al*, *J. Chem. Soc., Dalton Trans.*, 1975, 1516 (*struct*)

$C_2H_4Br_3Pt^{\ominus}$ Pt-00009

Tribromo(ethylene)platinate(1−)

Tribromo(ethene)platinate(1−), 9CI

[56191-55-0]

$PtBr_3(C_2H_4)^{\ominus}$ (C_{2v})

M 462.846 (ion)

K salt: [12175-83-6].
$C_2H_4Br_3KPt$ M 501.944
Orange-yellow cryst. (H_2O).

Bokii, G.B. *et al*, *Kristallografiya*, 1957, **2**, 400 (*struct*)
Pesa, F. *et al*, *J. Coord. Chem.*, 1975, **4**, 225 (*synth*)

$C_2H_4Cl_3Pt^{\ominus}$ Pt-00010

Trichloro(η^2-ethene)platinate(1−), 10CI, 9CI
Trichloro(ethylene)platinate(1−)

$$\left[\begin{matrix} CH_2 \\ \| \!\!—PtCl_3 \\ CH_2 \end{matrix}\right]^{\ominus}$$

M 329.493 (ion)

K salt: Zeise's salt.
$C_2H_4Cl_3KPt$ M 368.591
Golden-orange cryst. Mp 180° dec.

Hiraishi, J.N. *et al*, *Spectrochim. Acta, Part A*, 1969, **25**, 744 (*ir, raman*)
Jarvis, J.A. *et al*, *Acta Crystallogr., Sect. B*, 1971, **27**, 366 (*cryst struct*)
Inorg. Synth., 1973, **14**, 90 (*synth*)
Hall, P.W. *et al*, *J. Organomet. Chem.*, 1974, **71**, 145 (*pmr, cmr*)

$C_2H_6Br_2Pt$ Pt-00011

Dibromodimethylplatinum, 9CI
Dimethylplatinum dibromide
[31926-36-0]

$[PtMe_2Br_2]_n$

M 384.957
Polymeric. Probably octahedral platinum with bridging bromides. Yellow cryst. ($CHCl_3$/EtOH), dec. at 180-90°. Sol. MeOH, insol. H_2O, spar. sol. most org. solvs.

Hall, J.R. *et al*, *J. Organomet. Chem.*, 1973, **56**, 419 (*ir*)
Inorg. Synth., 1980, **20**, 185 (*synth, ir*)

$C_2H_8O_2Pt$ Pt-00012

Dihydroxydimethylplatinum, 9CI
Dimethylplatinum dihydroxide
[68565-21-9]

$Pt(OH)_2Me_2$

M 259.164
Polymeric sesquihydrate. Cryst. + $1\frac{1}{2}H_2O$ (H_2O). Sol. H_2O, insol. org. solvs. Dec. ~125°.
▷Explodes at about 170°

Inorg. Synth., 1980, **20**, 185 (*synth*)

$C_2I_2O_2Pt$ Pt-00013

Dicarbonyldiiodoplatinum
Diiodoplatinum dicarbonyl. Dicarbonylplatinum diiodide

M 504.910

cis-form
Red cryst. Subl. from 40°, dec. at 150°. Dec. in C_6H_6 to give $Pt_2I_4(CO)_2$.

Malatesta, L. *et al*, *Gazz. Chim. Ital.*, 1960, **90**, 1505 (*synth*)

C_3H_5ClPt Pt-00014

Chloro(η^3-2-propenyl)platinum
Allylchloroplatinum. Allylplatinum chloride
[12145-01-6]

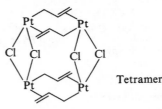

Tetramer

M 271.606
Tetrameric; in one paper descr. as dimeric, but this appears to be identical with the tetramer.
Tetramer: [32216-28-7]. *Tetra-μ-chlorotetrakis[(1-η:2,3-η)-2-propenyl]tetraplatinum*, 9CI. *Tetra-μ-allyltetra-μ-chlorotetraplatinum.*
$C_{12}H_{20}Cl_4Pt_4$ M 1086.422
Catalyses butadiene oligomerisation. Orange-yellow cryst. (CH_2Cl_2). Dec. without melting at 173-84°.

Lukas, J.H. *et al*, *J. Organomet. Chem.*, 1971, **26**, C25 (*synth*)
Mann, B.E. *et al*, *J. Chem. Soc. (A)*, 1971, 3536 (*synth, ir, pmr*)
Raper, G. *et al*, *J. Chem. Soc., Dalton Trans.*, 1972, 265 (*struct*)

$C_3H_6Cl_2Pt$ Pt-00015

Dichloro-1,3-propanediylplatinum, 9CI
[60409-64-5]

M 308.066
Polymeric, thought to be tetrameric. Pale-yellow solid. Highly insol. Mp 148° dec. Once thought to be a cyclopropane deriv.

Tipper, C.F.H., *J. Chem. Soc.*, 1955, 2045.
Gillard, R.D. *et al*, *J. Organomet. Chem.*, 1971, **32**, 247 (*props*)
Inorg. Synth., 1976, **16**, 113 (*synth*)

$C_3H_6Cl_3OPt^{\ominus}$ Pt-00016

Trichloro[(2,3-η)-2-propen-1-ol]platinate(1−), 9CI
Trichloro(3-hydroxypropene)platinate(1−). (Allyl alcohol)trichloroplatinate(1−), 8CI
[12275-05-7]
As Trichloro[(1,2-η)-1-propene]platinate(1−), Pt-00017 with

X = OH

M 359.519 (ion)
K salt: [12075-58-0].
$C_3H_6Cl_3KOPt$ M 398.617
Yellow cryst. (Me_2CO/Et_2O).
Tetrabutylammonium salt: [73413-50-0].
$C_{19}H_{42}Cl_3NOPt$ M 601.986

Yellow cryst. (2-propen-1-ol). Mp 87-93°.

Hartley, F.R. *et al*, *J. Chem. Soc. (A)*, 1967, 330.
Hartley, F.R. *et al*, *J. Chem. Soc. (A)*, 1967, 1322 (*uv*)
Hubert, J. *et al*, *J. Organomet. Chem.*, 1975, 265 (*synth, pmr*)
Briggs, J.R. *et al*, *J. Chem. Soc., Dalton Trans.*, 1980, 64 (*synth, ir*)

$C_3H_6Cl_3Pt^{\ominus}$ Pt-00017

Trichloro[(1,2-η)-1-propene]platinate(1−), 9CI
Trichloro(propylene)platinate(1−)

X = H

M 343.519 (ion)
K salt: [12075-59-1].
$C_3H_6Cl_3KPt$ M 382.618
No phys. props. reported.
Tetrabutylammonium salt: [34808-06-5].
$C_{19}H_{42}Cl_3NPt$ M 585.987
Yellow cryst. (propanol). Mp 97-8°.

Hartley, F.R., *Inorg. Chim. Acta*, 1971, **5**, 197 (*synth*)
Meester, M.A.M. *et al*, *Inorg. Chim. Acta*, 1977, **21**, 251 (*synth, ir, raman, uv, nmr*)

C_3H_9ClPt Pt-00018

Chlorotrimethylplatinum, 9CI, 8CI
Trimethylplatinum chloride
[4250-72-0]

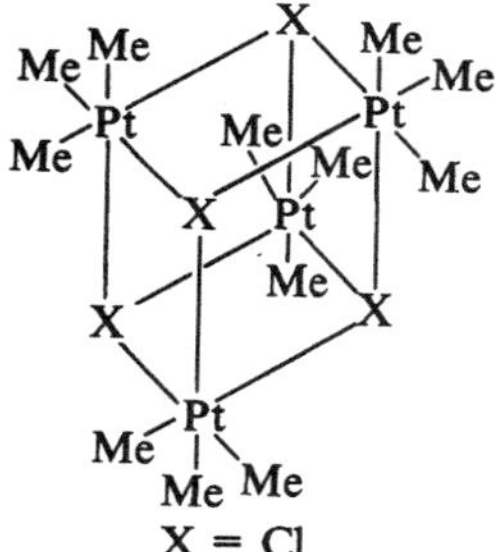

X = Cl

M 275.637
Tetrameric.
Tetramer: Tetra-μ₃-chlorododecamethyltetraplatinum, 9CI, 8CI. *Tetrakis[chlorotrimethylplatinum]*.
$C_{12}H_{36}Cl_4Pt_4$ M 1102.548
Cryst. ($CHCl_3$). Insol. H_2O, sol. C_6H_6, $CHCl_3$.

Pope, W.J. *et al*, *J. Chem. Soc.*, 1909, 571 (*synth*)
Bulliner, P.A. *et al*, *Inorg. Chem.*, 1970, **9**, 1887 (*ir, raman*)
Appleton, T.G. *et al*, *Aust. J. Chem.*, 1980, **33**, 2387 (*nmr*)

C_3H_9IPt Pt-00019

Iodotrimethylplatinum, 9CI
Trimethylplatinum iodide
[14364-93-3]

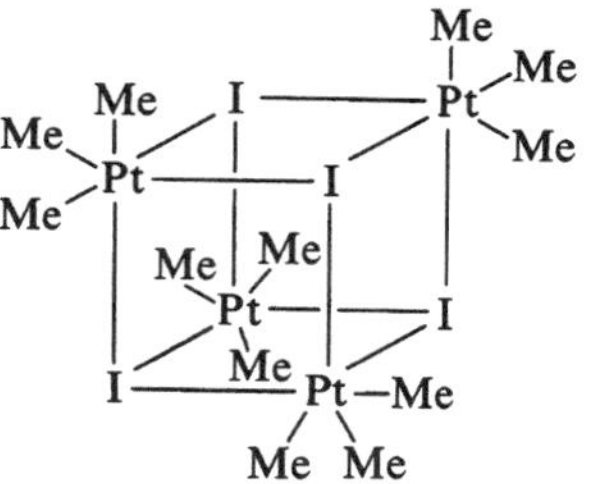

M 367.089
Tetrameric.
Tetramer: [18253-26-4]. *Tetra-μ₃-iodododecamethyltetraplatinum*, 10CI, 9CI.
$C_{12}H_{36}I_4Pt_4$ M 1468.354
Commonly yellow cryst., white when pure. Sol. nonpolar solvs. insol. Me_2CO, H_2O. Mp 190-5°, 195° dec.

Kile, K. *et al*, *J. Chem. Soc.*, 1966, 1744 (*nmr*)
Inorg. Synth., 1967, **10**, 71 (*synth*)
Clegg, D.E. *et al*, *J. Organomet. Chem.*, 1970, **22**, 491 (*ir, raman*)
Baldwin, J.C. *et al*, *Inorg. Chem.*, 1975, **14**, 2020 (*synth*)

$C_3H_{10}OPt$ Pt-00020

Trimethylplatinum hydroxide
Hydroxytrimethylplatinum, 9CI, 8CI.
Hydroxotrimethylplatinum
As Chlorotrimethylplatinum, Pt-00018 with

X = OH

M 257.191
Tetrameric.
Tetramer: [18785-97-2]. *Tetra-μ₃-hydroxydodecamethyltetraplatinum*, 9CI, 8CI. *Tetrakis[hydroxotrimethylplatinum]*.
$C_{12}H_{40}O_4Pt_4$ M 1028.766
Cryst. (C_6H_6). Sol. Et_2O, Me_2CO, $CHCl_3$, C_6H_6, EtOH, insol. H_2O, pet. ether. The compound previously characterised as $[PtMe_4]_4$ is in fact this material.

Pope, W.J. *et al*, *J. Chem. Soc.*, 1909, 571 (*synth*)
Cowan, D.O. *et al*, *Acta Crystallogr., Sect. B*, 1968, **24**, 287 (*struct*)
Bulliner, P.A. *et al*, *Inorg. Chem.*, 1970, **9**, 1887 (*ir, raman*)
Appleton, T.G. *et al*, *Aust. J. Chem.*, 1980, **33**, 2387 (*nmr*)

$C_3H_{15}IN_2Pt$ Pt-00021

Diammineiodotrimethylplatinum, 9CI, 8CI
Trimethyliodoplatinumbis(ammine). Bis(ammine)iodotrimethylplatinum
[17362-76-4]

M 401.149
Cryst. Sol. EtOH, Me_2CO, C_6H_6, insol. H_2O, $CHCl_3$, pet. ether.

Pope, W.J. *et al*, *J. Chem. Soc.*, 1909, 571 (*synth*)
Hall, J.R. *et al*, *J. Organomet. Chem.*, 1972, **42**, 479 (*synth, nmr*)

$C_3H_{15}O_3Pt^{\oplus}$ Pt-00022

Tri(aqua)trimethylplatinum(1+), 9CI, 8CI

[24418-93-7]

$[PtMe_3(OH_2)_3]^{\oplus}$

M 294.230 (ion)

fac-config. Can be obt. in water from $(PtMe_3)_2SO_4$.

Fluoride: [65153-42-6].
$C_3H_{15}FO_3Pt$ M 313.228
Characterised spectroscopically.

Hexafluoroplatinate(2–): [65153-45-9].
$C_6H_{30}F_6O_6Pt_3$ M 897.530
Characterised spectroscopically.

Hexafluorosilicate(2–): [65153-46-0].
$C_6H_{30}F_6O_6Pt_2Si$ M 730.535
Characterised spectroscopically.

Clegg, D.E. *et al, Aust. J. Chem.*, 1967, **20**, 2025 (*pmr*)
Glass, G.E. *et al, J. Am. Chem. Soc.*, 1967, **89**, 6372 (*nmr*)
Zharkova, G.I. *et al, Izv. Sib. Otd. Akad. Nauk. SSSR, Ser. Khim. Nauk.*, 1977, **5**, 105; *CA*, **88**, 23124z (*synth*)

$C_4H_6Cl_2N_2Pt$ Pt-00023

Bis(acetonitrile)dichloroplatinum, 9CI, 8CI

Dichlorobis(methyl cyanide)platinum

[13869-38-0]

cis-form

M 348.091

Useful starting complex as acetonitrile ligands are easily displaced.

cis-form [21264-32-4]
Yellow cryst. (MeCN).
▷TP2180000.

Walton, R.A., *Can. J. Chem.*, 1968, **46**, 2347 (*ir, raman*)
Hartley, F.R. *et al, Inorg. Chem.*, 1979, **18**, 1394 (*synth*)

$C_4H_6Cl_6Pt_2^{\ominus\ominus}$ Pt-00024

μ-[(1,2:3,4-η)-Butadiene]hexachlorodiplatinate(2–)

Hexachloro(μ-butadiene)diplatinate(2–)

M 656.969 (ion)

Dipotassium salt:
$C_4H_6Cl_6K_2Pt_2$ M 735.166
Orange-red cryst. Mp 240-5°.

Slade, P.E. *et al, J. Am. Chem. Soc.*, 1957, **79**, 1277 (*synth, ir*)
Grogan, M.J. *et al, Inorg. Chim. Acta*, 1967, **1**, 228 (*ir, struct*)
Lodewijk, E. *et al, J. Chem. Soc. (A)*, 1968, 119 (*synth*)

$C_4H_6O_2Pt$ Pt-00025

Dicarbonyldimethylplatinum, 10CI

Dimethyldicarbonylplatinum

[76705-05-0]

$PtMe_2(CO)_2$

M 281.170

Observed in soln. and characterised spectroscopically.

Anderson, G.K. *et al, Inorg. Chem.*, 1981, **20**, 1636 (*synth, ir, nmr*)

$C_4H_8Cl_2Pt$ Pt-00026

Dichlorobis(ethylene)platinum, 8CI

Dichlorobis(η²-ethene)platinum, 9CI

[31781-68-7]

$PtCl_2(C_2H_4)_2$

M 322.093

Solid materials described as white, yellow or red-brown have been assigned this composition. *cis-* and *trans-*forms should be possible.

Inorg. Synth., 1957, **5**, 210.
Hall, P.W. *et al, J. Organomet. Chem.*, 1975, **84**, 407.

$C_4H_8Cl_4Pt_2$ Pt-00027

Di-μ-chlorodichlorobis(η²-ethene)diplatinum, 10CI, 9CI

Bis(ethylenedichloroplatinum). Zeise's dimer

[12073-36-8]

M 588.079

Dimeric. Pale-orange needles or granular cryst. (toluene or C_6H_6). Mp 160-5°, 180-5°, 190° dec.

Monomer: Dichloro(η²-ethene)platinum. Dichloroethyleneplatinum. Ethylenedichloroplatinum.
$C_2H_4Cl_2Pt$ M 294.040
Unknown.

Inorg. Synth., 1950, **5**, 210 (*synth*)
Grogan, M.J. *et al, J. Am. Chem. Soc.*, 1968, **90**, 918 (*ir*)
Busse, P. *et al, J. Organomet. Chem.*, 1977, **128**, 85 (*synth*)

$C_4H_9Cl_2OPPt$ Pt-00028

Carbonyldichloro(trimethylphosphine)platinum, 10CI

Dichloro(trimethylphosphine)platinum carbonyl

CO

M 370.074

cis-form [66219-24-7]
Cryst. (CH_2Cl_2/Et_2O). Mp 196-8°.

Browning, J. *et al, J. Chem. Soc., Dalton Trans.*, 1977, 2061 (*synth, ir, raman, nmr*)

$C_4H_{11}Cl_2NPt$ Pt-00029

Dichloro(ethylene)(dimethylamine)platinum

Dichloro(η²-ethene)(N-methylmethanamine)platinum, 9CI. Dichloro(dimethylamino)(ethene)platinum, 8CI

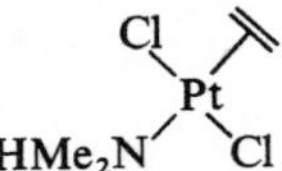

M 339.124

trans-form [33409-87-9]
Yellow cryst. (pet. ether).

Alderman, P.R.H. *et al*, *Acta Crystallogr.*, 1960, **13**, 149 (*struct*)
Fritz, H.P. *et al*, *Z. Naturforsch.*, *B*, 1967, **22**, 610 (*pmr*)
Meester, M.A.M. *et al*, *Inorg. Chim. Acta*, 1976, **16**, 191 (*synth, ir, nmr, raman, nqr*)
Green, M. *et al*, *Transition Met. Chem.*, 1979, **4**, 308 (*nmr*)
Green, M. *et al*, *Inorg. Chim. Acta*, 1981, **54**, L67 (*cmr*)

$C_4H_{12}Pt^{\ominus\ominus}$ Pt-00030

Tetramethylplatinate(2−), 9CI

$PtMe_4^{\ominus\ominus}$ (D_{4h})

M 255.219 (ion)
Reacts with MeI to form Hexamethylplatinate(2−), Pt-00046 in the presence of MeLi.
Di-Li salt: [62685-89-6].
$C_4H_{12}Li_2Pt$ M 269.101
Air-sensitive soln. in Et_2O.

Rice, G.W. *et al*, *J. Am. Chem. Soc.*, 1977, **99**, 2141 (*synth, ir, pmr*)
Pearson, R.G. *et al*, *J. Am. Chem. Soc.*, 1980, **102**, 1541.

$C_4H_{12}PtS$ Pt-00031

Trimethyl(methylthio)platinum

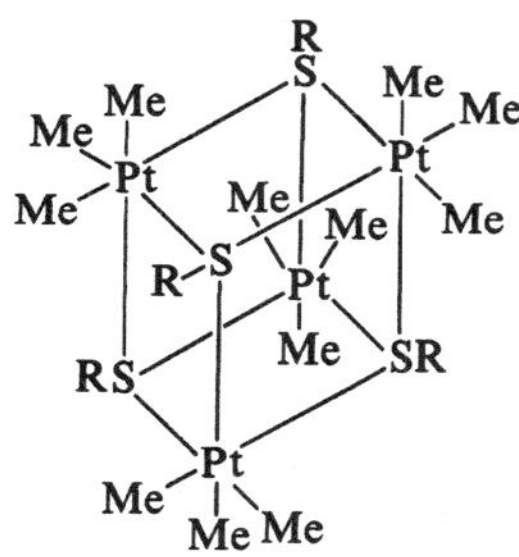

R = Me

M 287.279
Tetrameric.
Tetramer: [71743-38-9]. *Tetrakis*[μ_3-(*methanethiolato*)-]*dodecamethyltetraplatinum*, 9CI.
$C_{16}H_{48}Pt_4S_4$ M 1149.115
Lemon-yellow cryst. ($CHCl_3$/EtOH). Mp 225-50° dec.

Appleton, T.G. *et al*, *Aust. J. Chem.*, 1980, **33**, 2387 (*nmr*)
Abel, E.W. *et al*, *J. Organomet. Chem.*, 1982, **231**, 271 (*synth, nmr, ir, raman*)

C_4O_4Pt Pt-00032

Tetracarbonylplatinum
Platinum tetracarbonyl

$Pt(CO)_4$ (T_d)

M 307.122
Obt. only by matrix isolation techniques. Dec. below r.t.

Kündig, E.P. *et al*, *J. Am. Chem. Soc.*, 1973, **95**, 7234 (*ir, raman*)

C_5H_5NOPt Pt-00033

(η^5-2,4-Cyclopentadien-1-yl)nitrosylplatinum

M 290.181
Orange volatile cryst. Mp 64° (sealed tube). Subl. at 5°.

Fischer, E.O. *et al*, *Z. Naturforsch.*, *B*, 1964, **19**, 766 (*synth, pmr*)

$C_5H_8Cl_2N_2Pt$ Pt-00034

Dichloro(ethylene)(pyrazole)platinum
Dichloro(η^2-*ethene*)(*1*H-*pyrazole*-N[2])*platinum*, 10CI
[74065-29-5]

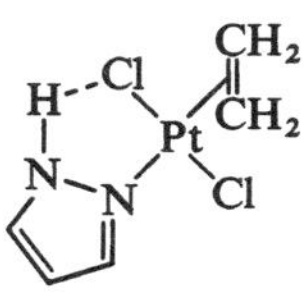

M 362.118
Yellow cryst. (CCl_4).

Johnson, D.A. *et al*, *Acta Crystallogr., Sect. B*, 1981, **37**, 2220 (*struct*)

C_6H_5IOPt Pt-00035

Carbonyl(η^5-2,4-cyclopentadien-1-yl)iodoplatinum
Cyclopentadienyl(*carbonyl*)*iodoplatinum*

M 415.089
Black cryst. (pentane). Mp 55° dec. (under N_2).

Fischer, E.O. *et al*, *Z. Naturforsch.*, *B*, 1963, **18**, 429 (*synth, ir, pmr*)
Fritz, H.P. *et al*, *Chem. Ber.*, 1963, **96**, 2008 (*pmr*)

$C_6H_9BrN_3Pt^{\oplus}$ Pt-00036

Bromotris(isocyanomethane)platinum(1+), 9CI
Bromotris(*methylisonitrile*)*platinum*(*1*+)

$[PtBr(CNMe)_3]^{\oplus}$ (C_{2v})

M 398.141 (ion)
Hexafluorophosphate: [38317-64-5].
$C_6H_9BrF_6N_3PPt$ M 543.105
Cryst. ($MeCN/Et_2O$). ir υ (C≡N) 2286 cm^{-1}.

Miller, J.S. *et al*, *Inorg. Chem.*, 1972, **11**, 2069 (*synth, ir, pmr*)
Boehm, J.R. *et al*, *J. Am. Chem. Soc.*, 1976, **98**, 4845 (*synth, ir, pmr*)

$C_6H_9N_3Pt^{\ominus\ominus}$ Pt-00037

Tricyanotrimethylplatinate(2−), 8CI
Trimethylplatinumtricyanide(*2*−)
[19401-20-8]

$[PtMe_3(CN)_3]^{\ominus\ominus}$

M 318.237 (ion)

fac-form
Ion can be obtained in soln. by treatment of $[Me_3PtX]_n$ compds. with $CN^{\ominus}$.

Clegg, D.E. *et al*, *Aust. J. Chem.*, 1967, **20**, 2025 (*pmr*)

$C_6H_{10}Cl_2Pt$ Pt-00038

Dichloro[(1,2,5,6-η)-1,5-hexadiene]platinum, 9CI
(1,5-Hexadiene)dichloroplatinum
[12266-61-4]

M 348.131
Pale-yellow cryst. ($CHCl_3$). Mp 172-3° dec.

Jensen, K.A., *Acta Chem. Scand.*, 1953, **7**, 866 (*synth*)
Zakharova, I.A. *et al*, *J. Organomet. Chem.*, 1974, **72**, 283 (*ir, raman*)

$C_6H_{10}I_2Pt_2$ Pt-00039

Di-μ-iodobis(η^3-2-propenyl)diplatinum, 9CI
Bis(π-allyl)di-μ-iododiplatinum
[52176-24-6]

M 726.114
Bridged dimer. Catalyses butadiene oligomerisation.
Monomer: Iodo(η^3-2-propenyl)platinum. Allyliodoplatinum.
C_3H_5IPt M 363.057
Unknown.

Yurchenko, Ê.N. *et al*, *J. Struct. Chem.*, 1975, **16**, 639 (*ir*)

$C_6H_{10}Pt$ Pt-00040

Bis(η^3-2-propenyl)platinum
Bis(allyl)platinum. Diallylplatinum
[12240-88-9]

M 277.225
Catalyses oligomerisation of butadiene. Volatile cryst. Mp 40-2°. Subl. at r.t./10^{-4} torr.

Wilke, G. *et al*, *Angew. Chem., Int. Ed. Engl.*, 1966, **5**, 151 (*synth*)
Becconsall, J.K. *et al*, *J. Chem. Soc. (A)*, 1967, 423 (*synth, pmr*)
Mann, B.E. *et al*, *J. Chem. Soc. (A)*, 1971, 3536 (*pmr*)
Andrews, D.C. *et al*, *J. Organomet. Chem.*, 1973, **55**, 383 (*ir, raman*)

$C_6H_{12}Pt$ Pt-00041

Tris(ethylene)platinum
Tris(η^2-ethene)platinum, 9CI
[56009-87-1]

M 279.241
Evil-smelling cryst. (pentane or pet. ether). Can be kept for weeks under C_2H_4 at −20°. Dec. to Pt in min. at r.t. in absence of ethylene. Volatile.

Inorg. Synth., 1979, **19**, 213 (*synth, pmr*)

$C_6H_{14}ClPPt$ Pt-00042

Chloro(η^3-2-propenyl)(trimethylphosphine)platinum, 10CI
Allylchloro(trimethylphosphine)platinum
[71035-53-5]

M 347.683
Cryst. (hexane). Mp 102-5°.

Carturan, G. *et al*, *J. Organomet. Chem.*, 1979, **172**, 91 (*synth, nmr*)

$C_6H_{15}ClPt$ Pt-00043

Chlorotriethylplatinum, 8CI
Triethylplatinum chloride
[4250-73-1]

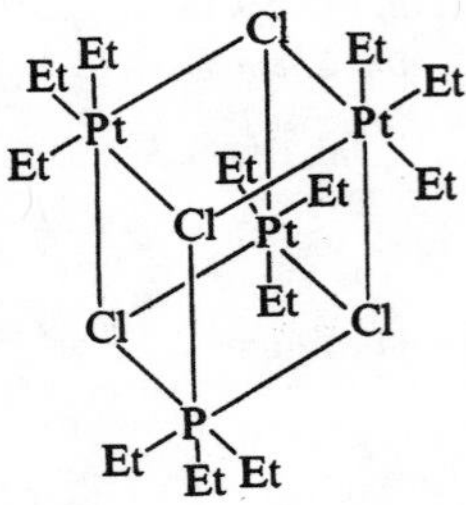

M 317.718
Tetrameric.
Tetramer: Tetra-μ_3-chlorododecaethyltetraplatinum, 8CI.
$C_{24}H_{60}Cl_4Pt_4$ M 1270.870
Cryst. (C_6H_6).

Kettle, F.S.A., *J. Chem. Soc.*, 1965, 5737 (*synth*)
Hargreaves, R.N. *et al*, *J. Chem. Soc. (A)*, 1971, 90 (*struct*)

$C_6H_{18}As_2Cl_9PtSn_3^{\ominus}$ Pt-00044

Tris(trichlorostannyl)bis(trimethylarsine)platinate(1−)
Tris(trichlorotin)bis(trimethylarsine)platinate(1−)

M 1110.278 (ion)
Bis(triphenylphosphine)iminium salt:
$C_{42}H_{48}As_2Cl_9NP_2PtSn_3$ M 1648.866
Cryst. (Me_2CO).

Albinati, A. *et al*, *Angew. Chem., Int. Ed. Engl.*, 1982, **21**, 284 (*synth, nmr, struct*)

$C_6H_{18}O_2PtS_2$ Pt-00045

Dimethylbis(dimethylsulfoxide)platinum
Dimethylbis[sulfinylbis[methane]-S]platinum, 10CI

R = Me

M 381.407

cis-form [70423-98-2]
Cryst. (CH_2Cl_2/Et_2O). Sol. C_6H_6, polar org. solvs., insol. H_2O. Dec. at 122°.

Eaborn, C. *et al*, *J. Chem. Soc., Dalton Trans.*, 1981, 933 (*synth, pmr, ir*)

$C_6H_{18}Pt^{\ominus\ominus}$ — Pt-00046

Hexamethylplatinate(2−), 9CI

$PtMe_6^{\ominus\ominus}$ (O_h)

M 285.288 (ion)

Di-Li salt: [58659-23-7].
$C_6H_{18}Li_2Pt$ M 299.170
Unstable air-sensitive soln. in Et_2O, more stable in presence of LiMe.

Bis(tetrabutylammonium) salt: [68220-42-8].
$C_{38}H_{90}N_2Pt$ M 770.222
Air-sensitive solid.

Rice, G.W. *et al*, *J. Am. Chem. Soc.*, 1977, **99**, 2141 (*synth, ir, pmr*)
Creaser, C.S. *et al*, *J. Chem. Soc., Chem. Commun.*, 1978, **157**, 243 (*synth*)

$C_6H_{19}ClP_2Pt$ — Pt-00047

Chlorohydrobis(trimethylphosphine)platinum

Bis(trimethylphosphine)platinum hydridochloride. Hydridochlorobis(trimethylphosphine)platinum

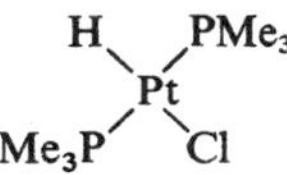

M 383.697

trans-form
Cryst.; reported as unstable. Mp 132-7° dec.

Chatt, J. *et al*, *J. Chem. Soc.*, 1962, 5075 (*synth, ir*)

$C_6O_6Pt_3^{\ominus\ominus}$ — Pt-00048

Tri-μ-carbonyltricarbonyltriplatinate(2−)

Hexacarbonyltriplatinate(2−)

[63993-21-5]

$[Pt_3(CO)_3(\mu\text{-}CO)_3]^{\ominus\ominus}$

M 753.302 (ion)

Di-K salt:
$C_6K_2O_6Pt_3$ M 831.499
Pink-red soln., dec. on attempt to precipitate.

Longoni, G. *et al*, *J. Am. Chem. Soc.*, 1976, **98**, 7225 (*synth, ir*)
Brown, C. *et al*, *J. Organomet. Chem.*, 1979, **181**, 233 (*nmr*)

$C_7H_8Br_2Pt$ — Pt-00049

[(2,3,5,6-η)-Bicyclo[2.2.1]hepta-2,5-diene]dibromoplatinum, 9CI

Dibromo(2,5-norbornadiene)platinum, 8CI. Dibromo(bicyclo[2.2.1]hepta-2,5-diene)platinum

[58356-22-2]

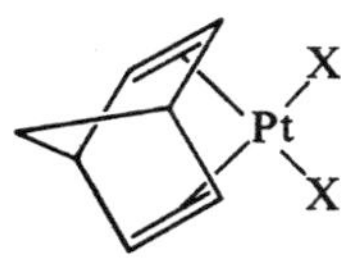

X = Br

M 447.028

Pale-yellow cryst. (CH_2Cl_2).

Alexander, R.A. *et al*, *J. Am. Chem. Soc.*, 1960, **82**, 535 (*synth, ir*)
Zakharova, I.A. *et al*, *J. Organomet. Chem.*, 1975, **102**, 227 (*ir, raman*)

$C_7H_8Cl_2Pt$ — Pt-00050

[(2,3,5,6-η)-Bicyclo[2.2.1]hepta-2,5-diene]dichloroplatinum, 9CI

Dichloro(2,5-norbornadiene)platinum, 8CI. Dichloro(bicyclo[2.2.1]hepta-2,5-diene]platinum

[12152-26-0]

As [(2,3,5,6-η)-Bicyclo[2.2.1]hepta-2,5-diene]dibromoplatinum, Pt-00049 with

X = Cl

M 358.126

Fuel additive. Used to platinum-coat alumina or resins for catalysts. Precursor of catalysts for carboalkoxylations. Catalyst for hydrosilylation of olefins. Cryst. (CH_2Cl_2). Mp 230-80° dec.

Abel, E.W. *et al*, *J. Chem. Soc.*, 1959, 3179 (*synth, ir*)
Alexander, R.A. *et al*, *J. Am. Chem. Soc.*, 1960, **82**, 535 (*synth, ir*)
Brown, T.L. *et al*, *Inorg. Chem.*, 1971, **10**, 1097 (*nqr*)
Zakharova, I.A. *et al*, *J. Organomet. Chem.*, 1975, **102**, 227 (*ir, raman*)
Wertz, D.A. *et al*, *Spectrochim. Acta, Part A*, 1980, **36**, 467.

$C_7H_8I_2Pt$ — Pt-00051

[(2,3,5,6-η)-Bicyclo[2.2.1]hepta-2,5-diene]diiodoplatinum, 9CI

Diiodo(2,5-norbornadiene)platinum, 8CI. 2,5-Norbornadienediiodoplatinum

[53789-85-8]

As [(2,3,5,6-η)-Bicyclo[2.2.1]hepta-2,5-diene]dibromoplatinum, Pt-00049 with

X = I

M 541.029

Orange cryst. (CH_2Cl_2).

Alexander, R.A. *et al*, *J. Am. Chem. Soc.*, 1960, **82**, 535 (*synth, ir*)
Zakharova, I.A. *et al*, *J. Organomet. Chem.*, 1975, **102**, 227 (*ir, raman*)

$C_7H_9Cl_2NPt$ — Pt-00052

Dichloro(ethylene)(pyridine)platinum

Dichloro(η²-ethene)(pyridine)platinum, 9CI, 8CI

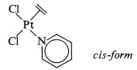

cis-form

M 373.141

Catalyses cleavage of Si—C bonds in organosilanes and alkoxide exchange of vinyl ethers.

cis-form [57918-48-6]
Characterised spectroscopically.

trans-form [12078-66-9]
Yellow solid. Sol. org. solvs. except hydrocarbons. Mp 125-7°.

Lazzaroni, R. *et al*, *J. Organomet. Chem.*, 1971, **33**, 131 (*nmr*)
Meester, M.A.M. *et al*, *Inorg. Chim. Acta*, 1975, **14**, 25, 33; 1977, **21**, 251 (*ir, nmr, raman, uv*)

Courtot, P. *et al*, *J. Organomet. Chem.*, 1978, **14**, 337.
Inorg. Synth., 1980, **20**, 181 (*synth*, *nmr*)

$C_7H_9Cl_4N_2O_2Pt^\ominus$ Pt-00053

Amminetetrachloro(4-methyl-3-nitrophenyl)platinate(1−), 9CI
(4-Methyl-3-nitrophenyl)(ammine)tetrachloroplatinate(1−)

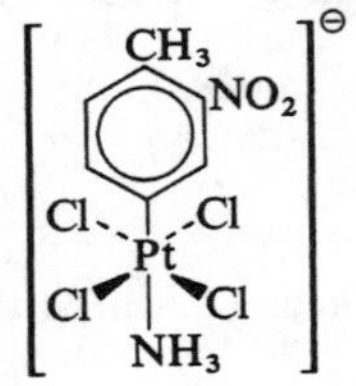

M 490.052 (ion)
NH_4 salt: [80183-93-3].
$C_7H_{13}Cl_4N_3O_2Pt$ M 508.091
Yellow cryst. (Me_2CO). Mp 250°.

Shibaeva, R.P. *et al*, *J. Organomet. Chem.*, 1981, **220**, 271 (*struct*)
Shul'pin, G.B., *Zh. Obshch. Khim.*, 1981, **59**, 2100 (*synth*)

$C_7H_{15}Cl_2OPPt$ Pt-00054

Carbonyldichloro(triethylphosphine)platinum, 10CI
Dichlorocarbonyl(triethylphosphine)platinum

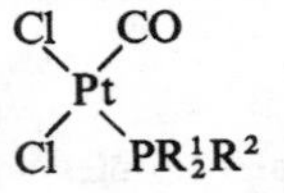

cis-form

$R^1 = R^2 = Et$

M 412.155
cis-form [65466-58-2]
Cryst. (EtOH). Mp 134-6°. Dipole moment 10.0 D.
trans-form [73347-27-0]
Obt. in soln. only. Readily isom. to *cis*-form, isom. catalysed by CO.

Chatt, J. *et al*, *J. Chem. Soc.*, 1964, 1662 (*synth*, *ir*)
Manojlović-Muir, L. *et al*, *J. Organomet. Chem.*, 1977, **142**, 265 (*struct*)
Anderson, G.K. *et al*, *J. Chem. Res. (S)*, 1979, **5**, 120 (*nmr*)
Anderson, G.K. *et al*, *J. Chem. Soc., Dalton Trans.*, 1980, 1988 (*synth*, *ir*, *nmr*)

$C_7H_{17}PPt$ Pt-00055

Bis(ethylene)(trimethylphosphine)platinum
Bis(ethene)(trimethylphosphine)platinum, 9CI
[57158-82-4]

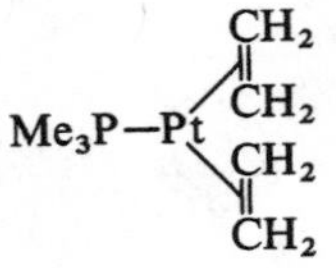

M 327.265
Cryst. (pet. ether). Mp 30-5° dec. Dec. at r.t. after a few hours. Best stored under C_2H_4.

Harrison, N.C. *et al*, *J. Chem. Soc., Dalton Trans.*, 1978, 1337 (*synth*, *ir*, *nmr*)

$C_7H_{21}As_2ClPt$ Pt-00056

Chloro(methyl)bis(trimethylarsine)platinum, 9CI, 8CI
Methylbis(trimethylarsine)platinum chloride

$PtClMe(AsMe_3)_2$

M 485.619
trans-form [30179-97-6]
Cryst. (pet. ether). Mp 159-60°.

Clark, H.C. *et al*, *Inorg. Chem.*, 1970, **9**, 2670 (*synth*, *nmr*)
Chisholm, M.H. *et al*, *J. Chem. Soc., Chem. Commun.*, 1971, 1627 (*nmr*)
Appleton, T.G. *et al*, *J. Organomet. Chem.*, 1974, **65**, 275 (*synth*)
Clark, H.C. *et al*, *Can. J. Chem.*, 1974, **52**, 1165 (*nmr*)

$C_8H_8Br_2Pt$ Pt-00057

Dibromo[(1,2,5,6-η)-1,3,5,7-cyclooctatetraene)platinum, 9CI
[12266-68-1]

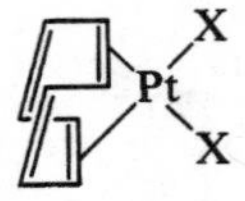

X = Br

M 459.039
Orange cryst.

Fritz, H.P. *et al*, *Spectrochim. Acta, Part A*, 1967, **23**, 1991 (*pmr*)
Fritz, H.P. *et al*, *Z. Naturforsch., B*, 1967, **22**, 20 (*ir*, *pmr*)
Inorg. Synth., 1972, **13**, 47 (*synth*)

$C_8H_8Cl_2Pt$ Pt-00058

Dichloro[(1,2,5,6-η)-1,3,5,7-cyclooctatetraene]platinum, 9CI
[12266-69-2]
As Dibromo[(1,2,5,6-η)-1,3,5,7-cyclooctatetraene)platinum, Pt-00057 with

X = Cl

M 370.137
Orange solid.

Jensen, K.A., *Acta Chem. Scand.*, 1953, **7**, 868 (*synth*)
Fritz, H.P. *et al*, *Spectrochim. Acta, Part A*, 1967, **23**, 1991 (*pmr*)
Fritz, H.P. *et al*, *Z. Naturforsch., B*, 1967, **22**, 20 (*ir*, *pmr*)
Inorg. Synth., 1972, **13**, 47 (*synth*)

$C_8H_8Cl_3Pt^\ominus$ Pt-00059

Trichloro(styrene)platinate(1−), 8CI
Trichloro[(η^2-ethenyl)benzene]platinate(1−), 9CI. Trichloro(phenylethene)platinate(1−)

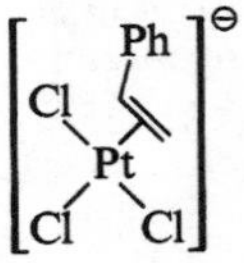

M 405.590 (ion)
K salt: [12080-15-8].
$C_8H_8Cl_3KPt$ M 444.689
Deep-yellow cryst. (EtOH aq.).
Tetraammineplatinum(2+) salt:
$C_{16}H_{28}Cl_6N_4Pt_3$ M 1074.382
Golden-yellow cryst. (EtOH aq.).

Anderson, J.S., *J. Chem. Soc.*, 1936, 1042 (*synth*)
Brown, T.L. *et al*, *Inorg. Chem.*, 1971, **10**, 1097 (*nqr*)
Cooper, D.G. *et al*, *Inorg. Chem.*, 1976, **15**, 1959 (*ir*, *nmr*)

$C_8H_8I_2Pt$ Pt-00060

[(1,2,5,6-η)-1,3,5,7-Cyclooctatetraene]diiodoplatinum, 9CI
[12266-70-5]

As Dibromo[(1,2,5,6-η)-1,3,5,7-cyclooctatetraene)platinum, Pt-00057 with

X = I

M 553.040

Orange-red cryst. ($CHCl_3$).

Jensen, K.A., *Acta Chem. Scand.*, 1953, **7**, 868 (*synth*)
Kistner, C.R. *et al*, *Inorg. Chem.*, 1963, **2**, 1255 (*synth*)
Fritz, H.P. *et al*, *Spectrochim. Acta, Part A*, 1967, **23**, 1991 (*pmr*)
Fritz, H.P. *et al*, *Z. Naturforsch.*, *B*, 1967, **22**, 20 (*ir*)
Inorg. Synth., 1972, **13**, 47 (*synth*)

$C_8H_{10}Pt$ **Pt-00061**

(η^5-2,4-Cyclopentadien-1-yl)(η^3-2-propenyl)platinum, 9CI

Allylcyclopentadienylplatinum. Cyclopentadienyl(allyl)-platinum

[35770-29-7]

M 301.247

Yellow volatile cryst. Mp 63-4°. $Bp_{0.01}$ 25° subl.

Mann, B.E. *et al*, *J. Chem. Soc. (A)*, 1971, 3537 (*synth, ir, pmr*)

$C_8H_{11}IPt$ **Pt-00062**

[(2,3,5,6-η)-Bicyclo[2.2.1]hepta-2,5-diene]iodomethylplatinum, 9CI

Iodomethyl(2,5-norbornadiene)platinum, 8CI. *Methyliodo(2,5-norbornadiene)platinum*

[53789-86-9]

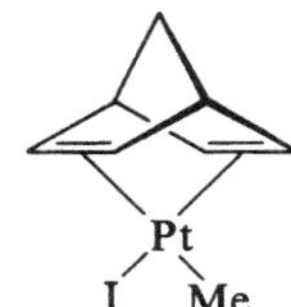

M 429.159

Orange cryst. (CH_2Cl_2). Mp 122-4°.

Kistner, C. *et al*, *Inorg. Chem.*, 1963, **2**, 1255 (*synth, pmr*)

$C_8H_{12}Br_2Pt$ **Pt-00063**

Dibromo[(1,2,5,6-η)-1,5-cyclooctadiene]platinum, 9CI

1,5-Cyclooctadienedibromoplatinum

[12145-48-1]

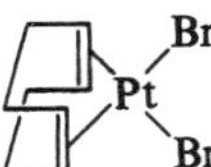

M 463.071

Pale-yellow cryst. (AcOH). Mp 200-70° dec.

Chatt, J. *et al*, *J. Chem. Soc.*, 1957, 2496.
Fritz, H.P. *et al*, *Spectrochim. Acta, Part A*, 1967, **23**, 1991 (*pmr*)
Inorg. Synth., 1972, **13**, 50 (*synth*)

$C_8H_{12}Cl_2Pt$ **Pt-00064**

Dichloro[(1,2,5,6-η)-1,5-cyclooctadiene]platinum, 9CI

1,5-Cyclooctadienedichloroplatinum

[12080-32-9]

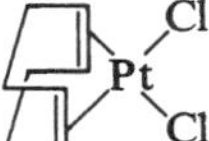

M 374.169

Catalyst for hydroformylation or hydrosilylation of alkenes. Used to deposit platinum on Al_2O_3 or SiO_2 for hydrogenation catalysts. Versatile starting material for synthesis of platinum and organoplatinum compds. Cryst. (CH_2Cl_2/pet. ether). Mp 220-78° dec.

Chatt, J. *et al*, *J. Chem. Soc.*, 1957, 2496.
Brown, T.L. *et al*, *Inorg. Chem.*, 1971, **10**, 1097 (*nqr*)
Inorg. Synth., 1972, **13**, 48 (*synth*)
Riggs, W.M., *Anal. Chem.*, 1972, **44**, 830 (*pe*)
Kennedy, J.D. *et al*, *J. Chem. Soc., Dalton Trans.*, 1976, 874 (*nmr*)
Wertz, D.W. *et al*, *Inorg. Chem.*, 1980, **19**, 705 (*ir, raman*)

$C_8H_{12}Cl_9PtSn_3^{\ominus}$ **Pt-00065**

[(1,2,3,4-η)-1,2,3,4-Tetramethyl-1,3-cyclobutadiene]tris(trichlorostannyl)platinate(1–), 10CI

Tris(trichlorostannyl)[tetramethylcyclobutadiene]platinate(1–)

M 978.410 (ion)

Bis(triphenylphosphine)iminium salt: [75517-62-3]. $C_{44}H_{42}Cl_9NP_2PtSn_3$ M 1516.997
Cryst. (Me_2CO).

Trichlorobis(tetramethylcyclobutadiene)diplatinum salt: [75517-56-5]. $C_{24}H_{36}Cl_{12}Pt_3Sn_3$ M 1691.294
Yellow cryst. (CH_2Cl_2).

Moreto, J. *et al*, *J. Chem. Soc., Dalton Trans.*, 1980, 1368 (*synth, ir, nmr*)

$C_8H_{12}I_2Pt$ **Pt-00066**

[(1,2,5,6-η)-1,5-Cyclooctadiene]diiodoplatinum, 9CI

Diiodo(1,5-cyclooctadiene)platinum

[12266-72-7]

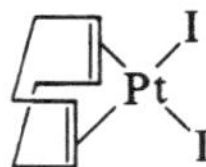

M 557.072

Yellow cryst. (CH_2Cl_2/pet. ether). Mp 250° dec.

Chatt, J. *et al*, *J. Chem. Soc.*, 1957, 2496.
Fritz, H.P. *et al*, *Spectrochim. Acta, Part A*, 1967, **23**, 1991 (*pmr*)
Inorg. Synth., 1972, **13**, 50 (*synth*)
Chisholm, M.H. *et al*, *J. Am. Chem. Soc.*, 1975, **97**, 721 (*cmr*)

$C_8H_{12}N_4Pt^{\oplus\oplus}$ **Pt-00067**

Tetrakis(acetonitrile)platinum(2+)

Tetrakis(methyl cyanide)platinum(2+)

$[Pt(MeCN)_4]^{\oplus\oplus}$ (D_{4h})

M 359.290 (ion)

Bis(tetrafluoroborate): [59218-69-8].
$C_8H_{12}B_2F_8N_4Pt$ M 532.897
Used for catalytic dimerisation of olefins. Cryst. (MeONO).

de Renzi, A. *et al*, *J. Chem. Soc., Chem. Commun.*, 1976, 47 (*synth, use*)

$C_8H_{12}N_4Pt^{\oplus\oplus}$ Pt-00068

Tetrakis(isocyanomethane)platinum(2+), 9CI
Tetrakis(methylisonitrile)platinum(2+)
[45073-89-0]

$[Pt(CNMe)_4]^{\oplus\oplus}$ (D_{4h})

M 359.290 (ion)
Bis(hexafluorophosphate): [38317-61-2].
$C_8H_{12}F_{12}N_4P_2Pt$ M 649.218
Cryst. (MeCN). ir ν_{CN} 2308 cm^{-1}.
Bis(tetrafluoroborate): [33989-89-8].
$C_8H_{12}B_2F_8N_4Pt$ M 532.897
Cryst. (MeCN/EtOAc). Mp 224-7°. ir ν_{CN} 2300 cm^{-1}.
Tetrakis(cyano-C)platinate(2−): [50600-86-7].
$C_{12}H_{12}N_8Pt_2$ M 658.440
Bright-yellow fluorescent cryst. (CH_2Cl_2).

Treichel, P.M. *et al*, *J. Am. Chem. Soc.*, 1971, **93**, 5424 (*synth, ir, pmr*)
Miller, J.S. *et al*, *Inorg. Chem.*, 1972, **11**, 2069 (*synth, ir, pmr*)
Isci, H. *et al*, *Inorg. Chem.*, 1974, **13**, 1175; 1975, **14**, 913 (*synth, ir, pmr, uv*)

$C_8H_{14}Cl_2Pt_2$ Pt-00069

Di-μ-chlorobis[(1,2,3,-η)-2-methyl-2-propenyl]diplatinum, 9CI
Di-μ-chlorobis(2-methylallyl)diplatinum
[35770-44-6]

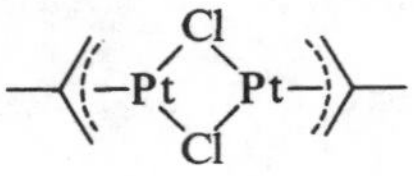

M 571.265
Bridged dimer. Pale-yellow cryst. Mp 150-4° dec.
Monomer: Chloro[(1,2,3-η)-2-methyl-2-propenyl]platinum.
C_4H_7ClPt M 285.632
Unknown.

Mann, B.E. *et al*, *J. Chem. Soc. (A)*, 1971, 3536 (*synth, pmr*)

$C_8H_{14}Pt$ Pt-00070

Bis[(1,2,3-η)-2-methyl-2-propenyl]platinum, 9CI
Bis(2-methylallyl)platinum
[33010-07-0]

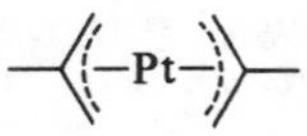

M 305.279
Colourless, volatile cryst. (pentane at −80°). Mp 68-70°. Subl. at r.t., 10^{-4} mm.

O'Brien, S., *J. Chem. Soc. (A)*, 1970, 9 (*synth, pmr*)
Mann, B.E. *et al*, *J. Chem. Soc. (A)*, 1971, 3536 (*synth, pmr*)
Boehm, M.C. *et al*, *Helv. Chim. Acta*, 1980, **63**, 990 (*pe*)

$C_8H_{14}Pt$ Pt-00071

(η^5-2,4-Cyclopentadien-1-yl)trimethylplatinum, 9CI
Trimethyl(cyclopentadienyl)platinum
[1271-07-4]

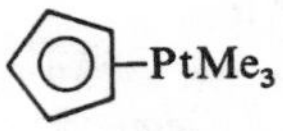

M 305.279
Volatile cryst. (MeOH). Mp 65°. $Bp_{0.01}$ 20° subl.

Robinson, S.D. *et al*, *J. Chem. Soc.*, 1965, 1529 (*synth, ir, pmr*)
Egger, K.W. *et al*, *J. Organomet. Chem.*, 1970, **24**, 501 (*ms*)
Daly, F.J.J. *et al*, *J. Chem. Soc. (A)*, 1971, 2616 (*struct*)
Hall, J.R. *et al*, *Aust. J. Chem.*, 1971, **24**, 911 (*ir, raman*)
Hamer, G. *et al*, *Can. J. Chem.*, 1980, **58**, 2011 (*nmr*)

$C_8H_{16}O_2Pt$ Pt-00072

(Acetylacetonato)trimethylplatinum
Trimethyl(2,4-pentanedionato)platinum

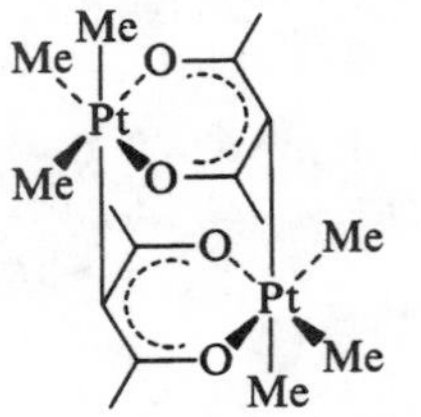

M 339.293
Dimeric.
Dimer: [17362-49-1]. *Hexamethylbis(μ-(2,4-pentanedionato-C^3:O^2,O^4))diplatinum, 9CI. Bis[μ-(1-acetylacetonyl)]hexamethyldiplatinum, 8CI. Bis[trimethyl(2,4-pentanedionato)platinum].*
$C_{16}H_{32}O_4Pt_2$ M 678.586
Cryst. (Et_2O or hexane). Dec. without melting ~ 200°.

Menzies, R.C. *et al*, *J. Chem. Soc.*, 1933, 21 (*synth*)
Kite, K. *et al*, *J. Chem. Soc. (A)*, 1966, 1744 (*pmr*)
Kite, K. *et al*, *J. Chem. Soc. (A)*, 1968, 934 (*ir, uv*)
Zharkova, G.L. *et al*, *Koord. Khim.*, 1979, **5**, 743, 1376; *Soviet J. Coord. Chem.*, 586, 1073 (*synth, ir, uv*)

$C_8H_{18}Cl_2NPPt$ Pt-00073

Dichloro(isocyanomethane)(triethylphosphine)platinuum, 9CI
Dichloro(methyl isocyanide)(triethylphosphine)platinum, 8CI. Dichloro(methylisonitrile)(triethylphosphine)-platinum

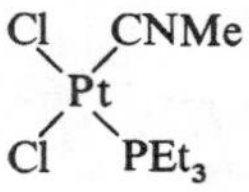

M 425.197
cis-form [32492-31-2]
Cryst. (EtOH). Mp 174-6°.

Richards, R.L. *et al*, *J. Chem. Soc. (A)*, 1971, 21 (*synth, ir, pmr*)
Crociani, B. *et al*, *J. Organomet. Chem.*, 1978, **144**, 85 (*cmr*)

$C_8H_{20}Cl_2PtS_2$ Pt-00074

Dichlorobis(diethyl sulfide)platinum

Dichlorobis[1,1'-thiobis[ethane]]platinum, 9CI. *Dichlorobis(ethyl sulfide)platinum*, 8CI. *Bis(diethyl sulfide)-dichloroplatinum*

[14873-92-8]

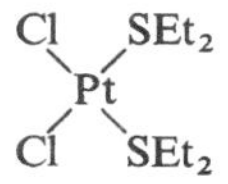

cis-form

M 446.352

Catalyses cross-linking of polysiloxanes.

cis-form [15442-57-6]

Pale-yellow cryst. (Me_2CO/pet. ether). Mp 107-8°.

trans-form [15337-84-5]

Yellow cryst. (EtOH aq.). Mp 107-8° (93-100°).

Inorg. Synth., 1960, **6**, 211 (*synth*)

Cross, R.J. *et al*, *J. Chem. Soc., Dalton Trans.*, 1976, 1150 (*nmr*)

$C_8H_{20}PtS_2$ Pt-00075

[1,2-Bis(ethylthio)ethane-*S,S'*]dimethylplatinum

[Ethylenebis(ethylsulfide)]dimethylplatinum. (3,6-Dithiaoctane)dimethylplatinum

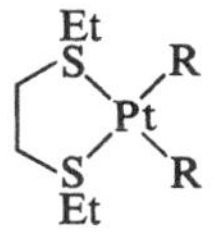

R = Me

M 375.446

Cryst. (pet. ether). Mp 74.5-75.5°. Dipole moment 6.7 D.

Chatt, J. *et al*, *J. Chem. Soc.*, 1959, 705 (*synth*)

Chatt, J. *et al*, *J. Chem. Soc.*, 1960, 2047 (*ir*)

$C_8H_{21}As_2OPt^{\oplus}$ Pt-00076

Carbonylmethylbis(trimethylarsine)platinum(1+), 9CI

Methylbis(trimethylarsine)carbonylplatinum(1+)

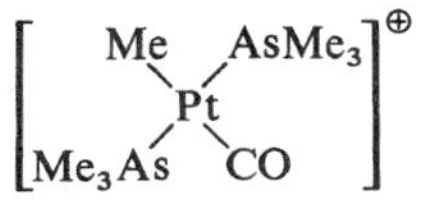

trans-form

M 478.177 (ion)

trans-form

Hexafluorophosphate: [36604-68-9].

$C_8H_{21}As_2F_6OPPt$ M 623.141

Cryst. (Me_2CO/Et_2O). Mp 131-2°.

Chisholm, M.H. *et al*, *J. Am. Chem. Soc.*, 1973, **95**, 8574 (*synth, ir, nmr*)

$C_8H_{22}P_2Pt$ Pt-00077

Ethylenebis(trimethylphosphine)platinum

Ethenebis(trimethylphosphine)platinum, 9CI

[69547-16-6]

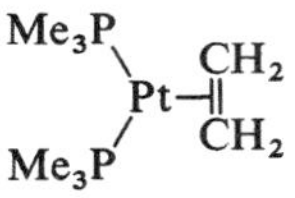

M 375.289

Nuzzo, R.G. *et al*, *Inorg. Chem.*, 1981, **20**, 1312 (*synth, nmr*)

$C_8H_{24}As_2Pt$ Pt-00078

Dimethylbis(trimethylarsine)platinum, 9CI, 8CI

Bis(trimethylarsine)dimethylplatinum

$PtMe_2(AsMe_3)_2$

M 465.201

cis-form [15413-98-6]

Cryst. (pet. ether). Mp 127-9°.

Clark, H.C. *et al*, *Inorg. Chem.*, 1970, **9**, 2670 (*synth, ir, nmr*)

Chisholm, M.H. *et al*, *J. Chem. Soc., Chem. Commun.*, 1971, 1627 (*nmr*)

Clark, H.C. *et al*, *Can. J. Chem.*, 1974, **52**, 1165.

$C_8H_{24}I_2Pt_2Se_2$ Pt-00079

Di-μ-iodohexamethyl[μ-(dimethyldiselenide)-*Se,Se*]diplatinum

[μ-[Dimethyl diselenide-Se:Se')]di-μ-iodohexamethyldiplatinum, 10CI

[75592-28-8]

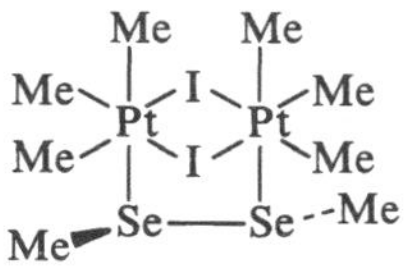

M 922.167

Cryst.

Abel, E.W. *et al*, *J. Organomet. Chem.*, 1982, **235**, 121 (*struct*)

$C_9H_{10}Cl_2Pt$ Pt-00080

Dichloro(2-phenyl-1,3-propanediyl)platinum

(2-Phenyl-1,3-propanediyl)dichloroplatinum

[60379-96-6]

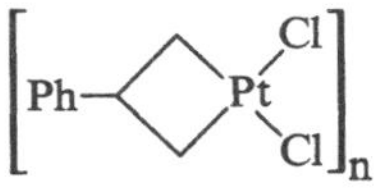

M 384.164

Chloride-bridged polymer. Pale-yellow solid. Insol. Mp 135° dec.

Inorg. Synth., 1976, **16**, 113 (*synth*)

$C_9H_{11}Cl_2OPPt$ Pt-00081

Carbonyldichloro(dimethylphenylphosphine)platinum

As Carbonyldichloro(triethylphosphine)platinum, Pt-00054 with

R^1 = Me, R^2 = Ph

M 432.145

cis-form [19618-86-1]

Cryst. ($CHCl_3$/hexane). Mp 184-91°, 181-91° dec.

trans-form [73347-18-9]

Yellow. Obt. in soln. only; readily isom. to *cis*-form.

Jenkins, J.M., *J. Chem. Soc. (A)*, 1966, 770 (*synth, pmr*)

Smithies, A.L. *et al*, *J. Organomet. Chem.*, 1968, **12**, 199 (*synth, ir*)

Anderson, G.K. *et al*, *J. Chem. Res. (S)*, 1979, 120 (*cmr*)

Anderson, G.K. *et al*, *J. Chem. Soc., Dalton Trans.*, 1980, 1988 (*synth, nmr, ir*)

$C_9H_{12}Pt$ **Pt-00082**

(η^5-2,4-Cyclopentadien-1-yl)[(1,2,3-η)-2-methyl-2-propenyl-]platinum, 9CI

2-Methylallyl(cyclopentadienyl)platinum

[35770-30-0]

M 315.274

Yellow cryst. by subl. Mp 54-5°.

Mann, B.E. *et al*, *J. Chem. Soc.* (*A*), 1971, 3536 (*synth, pmr*)

$C_9H_{14}Pt$ **Pt-00083**

[(2,3,5,6-η)-Bicyclo[2.2.1]hepta-2,5-diene]dimethylplatinum, 9CI

Dimethyl(norbornadiene)platinum

[53199-36-3]

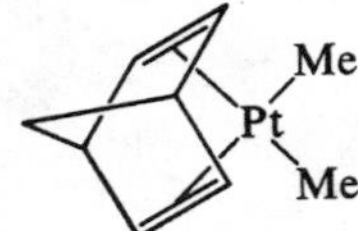

M 317.290

No details available.

Clark, H.C. *et al*, *Can. J. Chem.*, 1974, **52**, 1165 (*cmr*)

$C_9H_{14}PtS$ **Pt-00084**

Trimethyl(phenylthio)platinum

As Trimethyl(methylthio)platinum, Pt-00031 with

R = Ph

M 349.350

Tetrameric.

Tetramer: [76830-24-5]. *Tetrakis[μ_3-(benzenethiolato)-]dodecamethyltetraplatinum, 9CI.*

$C_{36}H_{56}Pt_4S_4$ M 1397.398

Orange cryst. (C_6H_6/hexane). Mp 175-240° dec.

Appleton, T.G. *et al*, *Aust. J. Chem.*, 1980, **33**, 2387 (*nmr*)
Abel, E.W. *et al*, *J. Organomet. Chem.*, 1982, **231**, 271 (*synth, nmr, ir, raman*)

$C_9H_{15}ClO_2Pt$ **Pt-00085**

[(2,3-η)-2-Butene]chloro(2,4-pentanedionato-*O,O'*)platinum, 9CI

(Acetylacetonato)(2-butene)chloroplatinum

[31989-13-6]

(*E*)-*form*

M 385.749

(*E*)-*form* [31941-76-1]

Yellow cryst. (C_6H_6/Et_2O).

(*Z*)-*form* [31941-79-4]

Yellow cryst. (C_6H_6/Et_2O).

Holloway, C.E. *et al*, *J. Chem. Soc.* (*A*), 1970, 1653 (*synth, pmr*)
Hulley, G. *et al*, *J. Chem. Soc.* (*A*), 1970, 1732 (*ir*)
Ashley-Smith, J. *et al*, *J. Chem. Soc., Dalton Trans.*, 1974, 128 (*pmr*)

$C_9H_{15}ClPt$ **Pt-00086**

Chloro[(1,2,5,6-η)-1,5-cyclooctadiene]methylplatinum, 9CI

Methylchloro(1,5-cyclooctadiene)platinum

[50978-00-2]

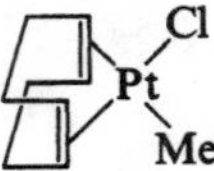

M 353.751

Cryst. (MeOH). Mp 166-7°.

Clark, H.C. *et al*, *J. Organomet. Chem.*, 1973, **59**, 411 (*synth*)
Chisholm, M.H. *et al*, *J. Am. Chem. Soc.*, 1975, **97**, 721 (*cmr*)

$C_{10}H_8Cl_2N_2Pt$ **Pt-00087**

(2,2'-Bipyridine-*N,N'*)dichloroplatinum, 9CI

Dichloro(2,2'-bipyridine)platinum

[13965-31-6]

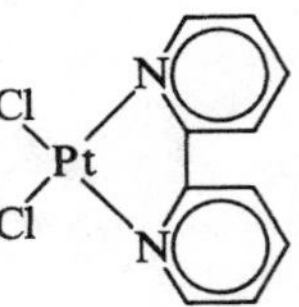

M 422.173

Exists as two cryst. modifications, red and yellow. Yellow form more common. Yellow cryst. (H_2O); red cryst. (HCl aq.). Spar. sol. $CHCl_3$, CH_2Cl_2.

Morgan, G.T. *et al*, *J. Chem. Soc.*, 1934, 965 (*synth*)
Clark, D.T. *et al*, *J. Chem. Soc., Dalton Trans.*, 1973, 169 (*nqr, pe*)
Norbury, A.H. *et al*, *J. Inorg. Nucl. Chem.*, 1973, **35**, 1211 (*ir*)
Osborn, R.S. *et al*, *J. Chem. Soc., Dalton Trans.*, 1974, 1002 (*struct*)
Bielli, E. *et al*, *J. Chem. Soc., Dalton Trans.*, 1974, 2133 (*synth, ir, pmr, uv*)

$C_{10}H_{10}Cl_4NPt^{\ominus}$ **Pt-00088**

Amminetetrachloro-2-naphthalenylplatinate(1–)

Amminetetrachloro(2-naphthyl)platinate(1–). Naphthyl(ammine)tetrachloroplatinate(1–)

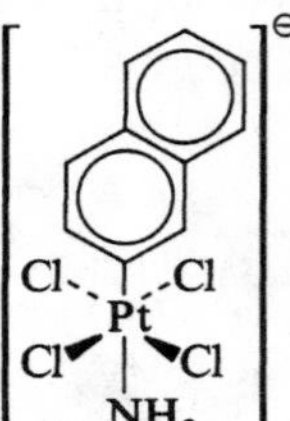

M 481.088 (ion)

NH_4 salt: [80123-62-2].

$C_{10}H_{14}Cl_4N_2Pt$ M 499.126

Yellow cryst. (Me_2CO). Mp 178°.

Shibaeva, R.P. *et al*, *J. Organomet. Chem.*, 1981, **220**, 271 (*struct*)
Shul'pin, G.B., *Zh. Obshch. Khim.*, 1981, **59**, 2100 (*synth*)

$C_{10}H_{12}Br_2Pt$ Pt-00089

Dibromo(dicyclopentadiene)platinum

Dibromo[(*2,3,5,6-η*)-*3*a,*4,7,7*a-*tetrahydro-4,7-methano-1*H-*indene*]*platinum*

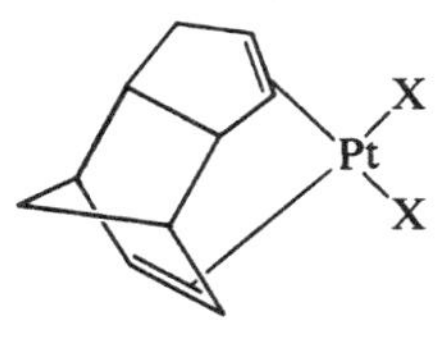

X = Br

M 487.093

Canary-yellow cryst. (Me_2CO). Mp 200-25° dec.

Chatt, J. *et al*, *J. Chem. Soc.*, 1957, 2496 (*synth*)

$C_{10}H_{12}Cl_2Pt$ Pt-00090

Dichloro(dicyclopentadiene)platinum

Dichloro[(*2,3,5,6-η*)-*3*a,*4,7,7*a-*tetrahydro-4,7-methano-1*H-*indene*]*platinum*, *9CI*

[12083-92-0]

As Dibromo(dicyclopentadiene)platinum, Pt-00089 with

X = Cl

M 398.191

Cryst. ($CHCl_3/Et_2O$). Mp 200-20° dec.

Chatt, J. *et al*, *J. Chem. Soc.*, 1957, 2496 (*synth*)
Avitabile, G. *et al*, *Inorg. Chim. Acta*, 1973, **7**, 329 (*struct*)

$C_{10}H_{14}ClO_4Pt^{\ominus}$ Pt-00091

(1-Acetyl-2-oxopropyl)chloro(2,4-pentanedionato-*O,O'*)platinate(1−), 9CI

(*1-Acetylacetonyl*)*chloro*(*2,4-pentanedionato*)-*platinate*(*1*−), *8CI*. *Bis*(*acetylacetonato*)-*chloroplatinate*(*1*−)

M 428.751 (ion)

H deriv.: [12129-03-2].
$C_{10}H_{15}ClO_4Pt$ M 429.759
Yellow solid (H_2O). The $H^{\oplus}$ ion is attached to the oxygens of the carbon-bonded acac$^{\ominus}$.

K salt: [15258-91-0].
$C_{10}H_{14}ClKO_4Pt$ M 467.850
Yellow cryst. (H_2O).

Figgis, B.N. *et al*, *Nature (London)*, 1962, **195**, 1278 (*synth*)
Gibson, D. *et al*, *J. Chem. Soc.* (*A*), 1967, 72 (*synth*, *ir*, *pmr*)
Behnke, G.T. *et al*, *Inorg. Chem.*, 1968, **7**, 330 (*ir*, *synth*)
Nakamura, Y. *et al*, *Inorg. Chem.*, 1975, **14**, 63 (*ir*)
Christian, D.F. *et al*, *Can. J. Chem.*, 1978, **56**, 2516 (*synth*)

> *The symbol ▷ in Entries highlights hazard or toxicity information*

$C_{10}H_{14}O_4Pt$ Pt-00092

Bis(2,4-pentanedionato-*O,O'*)platinum, 9CI

Bis(*acetylacetonato*)*platinum*

[15170-57-7]

M 393.298

Catalyses selective autooxidn. of cyclohexene, butadiene dimerisation, silicone rubber vulcanisation and olefin oxidn. Yellow cryst. (C_6H_6).

Lewis, J. *et al*, *J. Chem. Soc.*, 1965, 6740 (*ir*, *pmr*)
Inorg. Synth., 1980, **20**, 65 (*synth*, *uv*)

$C_{10}H_{16}Cl_2Pt$ Pt-00093

Dichloro[(1,2,3,4-η)-1,2,3,4,5-pentamethyl-1,3-cyclopentadiene]platinum, 9CI

(*Pentamethylcyclopentadiene*)*dichloroplatinum*

[33677-86-0]

M 402.222

Yellow cryst. (CH_2Cl_2/Et_2O). Mp 218-20° dec.

Balakrishnan, P.V. *et al*, *J. Chem. Soc.* (*A*), 1971, 1715 (*synth*, *ir*, *pmr*)
Shaw, B.L. *et al*, *J. Chem. Soc.*, *Dalton Trans.*, 1973, 264 (*synth*, *ir*, *pmr*)

$C_{10}H_{16}OPt$ Pt-00094

Acetyl(η⁵-2,4-cyclopentadien-1-yl)ethylmethylplatinum, 9CI

π-Cyclopentadienylethylmethylacetylplatinum

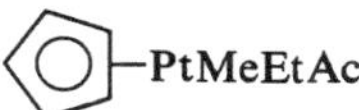

M 347.316

Clear liq., turns yellow when distilled. Mushroom odour.

Shaver, A., *Can. J. Chem.*, 1978, **56**, 2281 (*synth*)
Eisenberg, A. *et al*, *J. Am. Chem. Soc.*, 1980, **102**, 1416.
Hamer, G. *et al*, *Can. J. Chem.*, 1980, **58**, 2011 (*pmr*, *cmr*)

$C_{10}H_{18}Cl_3Pt^{\ominus}$ Pt-00095

Trichloro(2,2,5,5-tetramethyl-3-hexyne)platinate(1−)

Trichloro(*di*-tert-*butylacetylene*)*platinate*(*1*−)

M 439.691 (ion)

Na salt:
$C_{10}H_{18}Cl_3NaPt$ M 462.681
Yellow cryst. (Me_2CO). Mp 200-10° dec.

K salt:
$C_{10}H_{18}Cl_3KPt$ M 478.790
Yellow cryst. (Me_2CO). Mp 210-20° dec.

Chatt, J. *et al*, *J. Chem. Soc.*, 1961, 827 (*synth*, *ir*)

$C_{10}H_{18}Pt$ Pt-00096

[(1,2,5,6-η)-1,5-Cyclooctadiene]dimethylplatinum, 9CI

Dimethyl(1,5-cyclooctadiene)platinum

[12266-92-1]

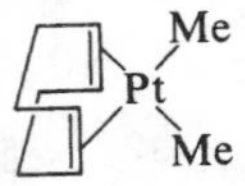

M 333.332

Cryst. (CH_2Cl_2). Mp 94-5°.

Kistner, C.R. *et al*, *Inorg. Chem.*, 1963, **2**, 1255.
Fritz, H.P. *et al*, *Spectrochim. Acta, Part A*, 1967, **23**, 1991 (*pmr*)
Clark, H.C. *et al*, *J. Organomet. Chem.*, 1973, **59**, 411 (*synth*)
Chisholm, M.H. *et al*, *J. Am. Chem. Soc.*, 1975, **97**, 721 (*cmr*)
Kennedy, J.D. *et al*, *J. Chem. Soc., Dalton Trans.*, 1976, 874 (*nmr*)

$C_{10}H_{28}P_2Pt$ Pt-00097

Dimethylbis(trimethylphosphonium-η-methylide)platinum, 9CI

Dimethylplatinumbis(trimethylphosphinemethylene ylide)

[72707-32-5]

$(Me_3PCH_2)_2PtMe_2$

M 405.359

cis-form

Solid. Mp 154°.

Blaschke, G. *et al*, *J. Organomet. Chem.*, 1979, **182**, 251 (*synth, pmr*)

$C_{11}H_8ClN_2OPt^{\oplus}$ Pt-00098

(2,2′-Bipyridine-*N,N′*)carbonylchloroplatinum(1+)

Carbonylchloro(bipyridine)platinum(1+)

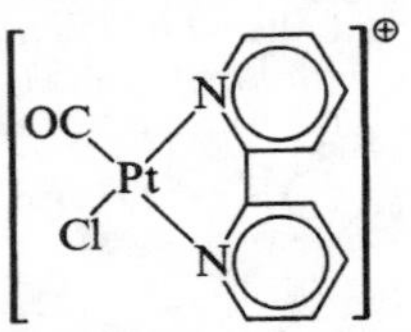

M 414.730 (ion)

Carbonyltrichloroplatinate(1−): see Carbonyltrichloroplatinate(1−), Pt-00002

Irving, R.J. *et al*, *J. Chem. Soc.*, 1956, 1860 (*synth, ir*)
Varshavsky, Ju.S. *et al*, *J. Organomet. Chem.*, 1971, **31**, 119 (*synth*)

$C_{11}H_{11}ClN_2Pt$ Pt-00099

(2,2′-Bipyridine-*N,N′*)chloromethylplatinum, 9CI

Methylchloro(bipyridine)platinum

[50726-77-7]

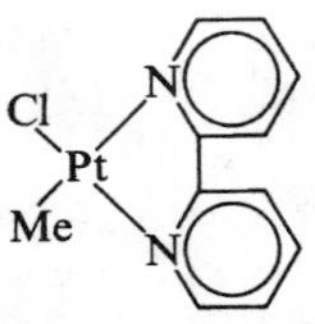

M 401.754

Yellow-orange cryst. (CH_2Cl_2/Et_2O). Mp 248-52°.

Clark, H.C. *et al*, *J. Organomet. Chem.*, 1973, **59**, 411 (*synth, pmr*)
Kuyper, J., *Inorg. Chem.*, 1978, **17**, 77 (*pmr*)

$C_{11}H_{15}Cl_2PPt$ Pt-00100

Dichloro(dimethylphenylphosphine)[(1,2-η)-1,2-propadiene-]platinum, 9CI

(Allene)dichloro(dimethylphenylphosphine)platinum

[77681-85-7]

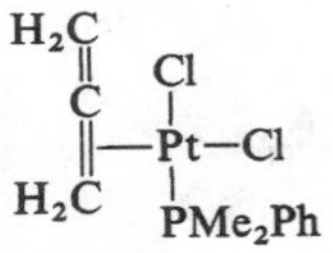

M 444.199

Cryst. (pet. ether), dec. >140°.

Briggs, J.R. *et al*, *J. Chem. Soc., Dalton Trans.*, 1981, 121 (*synth, pmr, struct*)

$C_{11}H_{17}Cl_2NPt$ Pt-00101

Dichloro(ethylene)(*N*-methyl-α-methylbenzylamine)platinum

Dichloro(N,α-dimethylbenzenemethanamine)(η²-ethene)platinum, 9CI. Dichloro(ethene)[methyl(1-phenylethyl)amine]platinum

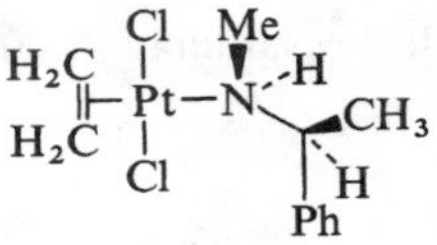

(S,S)-trans-form

M 429.248

Cryst. Sol. $CHCl_3$. Cryst. as a single (*S,S*) diastereomer. In soln. the two diastereomers interconvert rapidly.

Salvadori, P. *et al*, *J. Chem. Soc., Chem. Commun.*, 1974, 635 (*struct, pmr*)
Pregosin, P.S. *et al*, *Helv. Chim. Acta*, 1977, **60**, 2514 (*nmr*)

$C_{11}H_{17}Pt^{\oplus}$ Pt-00102

[(1,2,5,6-η)-1,5-Cyclooctadiene](η³-2-propenyl)platinum(1+), 9CI

(π-Allyl)(1,5-cyclooctadiene)platinum(1+)

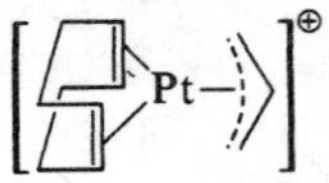

M 344.335 (ion)

Tetrafluoroborate: [62904-77-2].
$C_{11}H_{17}BF_4Pt$ M 431.139
Cryst. (CH_2Cl_2/Et_2O). Mp 191-6° dec.

Boag, N.M. *et al*, *J. Chem. Soc., Dalton Trans.*, 1980, 1200 (*synth, pmr, cmr*)

$C_{11}H_{20}IPPt$ Pt-00103

(η⁵-2,4-Cyclopentadien-1-yl)iodo(triethylphosphine)platinum, 10CI

[31760-66-4]

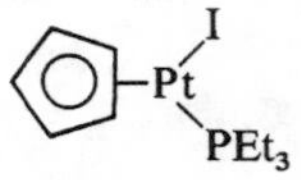

M 505.237

Orange cryst. (hexane). Mp 68-9°.

Cross, R.J. *et al*, *J. Chem. Soc. (A)*, 1971, 2000 (*synth, ir, pmr*)

$C_{12}H_8F_4N_2Pt$ Pt-00104

(2,2′-Bipyridine)(tetrafluoroethylene)platinum, 8CI

(2,2′-Bipyridine-N,N′)(η^2-tetrafluoroethene)platinum, 9CI

[33518-50-2]

$Pt(C_2F_4)(Bipy)$

M 451.282

Cryst. (Et_2O/hexane). Mp 225° dec.

Kemmitt, R.D.W. *et al, J. Chem. Soc. (A)*, 1971, 2472 (*synth, nmr*)

$C_{12}H_{10}O_2Pt_2$ Pt-00105

Dicarbonylbis(η^5-2,4-cyclopentadien-1-yl)diplatinum

Di(cyclopentadienyl)dicarbonyldiplatinum

M 576.370

Red cryst. (toluene). Mp 103° dec. (under N_2). Noncentrosymmetric struct.

Fischer, E.O. *et al, Z. Naturforsch., B*, 1963, **18**, 429 (*synth, ir, pmr*)

Fritz, H.P. *et al, Chem. Ber.*, 1963, **96**, 2008 (*pmr*)

$C_{12}H_{12}F_6Pt$ Pt-00106

[(1,2,5,6-η)-1,5-cyclooctadiene][(2,3-η)-1,1,1,4,4,4-hexafluoro-2-butyne]platinum, 9CI

Hexafluoro-2-butyne(1,5-cyclooctadiene)platinum

[66320-83-0]

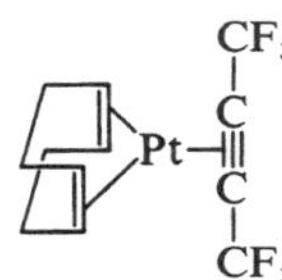

M 465.297

Cryst. (pet. ether).

Smart, L.E. *et al, J. Chem. Soc., Dalton Trans.*, 1977, 1777 (*synth, ir, pmr*)

$C_{12}H_{14}N_2Pt$ Pt-00107

(2,2′-Bipyridine-*N,N′*)dimethylplatinum, 9CI

Dimethyl(bipyridine)platinum. (Bipyridyl)-dimethylplatinum

[52594-52-2]

M 381.336

Used with C_2F_4 as a photoinitiator of free-radical polymerisation. Red air-stable cryst. (Me_2CO). Spar. sol. org. solvs. Reacts rapidly with MeOH, EtOH, chlorinated solvs. Mp 190-210° dec.

Chaudhury, N. *et al, J. Organomet. Chem.*, 1975, **84**, 105 (*synth, uv*)

Kuyper, J. *et al, Transition Met. Chem.*, 1976, **1**, 199 (*synth, nmr*)

$C_{12}H_{16}Br_2N_2Pt$ Pt-00108

Dibromodimethylbis(pyridine)platinum, 9CI

Dipyridinedibromodimethylplatinum. Dimethyldibromobis(pyridine)platinum

[32010-51-8]

M 543.160

Yellow cryst. ($CHCl_3$/EtOH).

Hall, J.R. *et al, J. Organomet. Chem.*, 1973, **56**, 419 (*pmr, ir*)

Reichart, B.E., *J. Organomet. Chem.*, 1974, **72**, 305 (*nmr*)

Kennedy, J.D. *et al, J. Chem. Soc., Dalton Trans.*, 1976, 874 (*nmr*)

Inorg. Synth., 1980, **20**, 185 (*synth*)

$C_{12}H_{16}N_2Pt$ Pt-00109

Dimethylbispyridineplatinum

Dipyridinedimethylplatinum

$PtMe_2Py_2$

M 383.352

Struct. not specified. Yellow cryst. (CH_2Cl_2/CCl_4). Mp 206-9° dec.

Kistner, C.R. *et al, Inorg. Chem.*, 1963, **2**, 1255.

$C_{12}H_{18}Br_2Pt$ Pt-00110

Dibromo[(2,3,5,6-η)-1,2,3,4,5,6-hexamethylbicyclo-[2.2.0]hexa-2,5-diene]platinum, 9CI

Dibromo(hexamethyldewarbenzene)platinum

[41619-36-7]

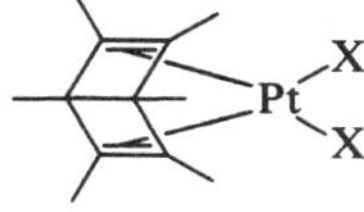

X = Br

M 517.162

Pale-yellow cryst. (CH_2Cl_2/MeOH). Dec. without melting at 120-7°.

Shaw, B.L. *et al, J. Chem. Soc., Dalton Trans.*, 1973, 264 (*synth, ir, pmr*)

$C_{12}H_{18}Cl_2Pt$ Pt-00111

Dichloro[(2,3,5,6-η)-1,2,3,4,5,6-hexamethylbicyclo-[2.2.0]hexa-2,5-diene]platinum, 9CI

(Hexamethyldewarbenzene)platinum chloride

[33309-74-9]

As Dibromo[(2,3,5,6-η)-1,2,3,4,5,6-hexamethylbicyclo-[2.2.0]hexa-2,5-diene]platinum, 9CI, Pt-00110 with

X = Cl

M 428.260

Cryst. ($CHCl_3/C_6H_6$). Dec. at 76°.

Balakrishnan, P.V. *et al, J. Chem. Soc. (A)*, 1971, 1715 (*synth, ir, pmr*)

Shaw, B.L. *et al, J. Chem. Soc., Dalton Trans.*, 1973, 264 (*synth, ir, pmr*)

$C_{12}H_{18}I_2Pt$ **Pt-00112**

[(2,3,5,6-η)-1,2,3,4,5,6-Hexamethylbicyclo[2.2.0]hexa-2,5-diene]diiodoplatinum, 9CI

(Hexamethyldewarbenzene)diiodoplatinum

[41619-37-8]

As Dibromo[(2,3,5,6-η)-1,2,3,4,5,6-hexamethylbicyclo[2.2.0]hexa-2,5-diene]platinum, Pt-00110 with

X = I

M 611.163

Yellow cryst. (CH_2Cl_2/MeOH). Dec. without melting at 105-12°.

Shaw, B.L. *et al*, *J. Chem. Soc., Dalton Trans.*, 1973, 264 (*synth, ir, pmr*)

$C_{12}H_{18}N_6Pt_2^{\oplus\oplus}$ **Pt-00113**

Hexakis(isocyanomethane)diplatinum(2+), 9CI

Hexakis(methyl isonitrile)diplatinum(2+)

[60021-76-3]

M 636.474 (ion)

Bis(hexafluorophosphate): [60767-36-4].
$C_{12}H_{18}F_{12}N_6P_2Pt_2$ M 926.403
Cryst. (MeCN/Et_2O). ir ν_{CN} 2240 cm^{-1}.

Bis(tetrafluoroborate): [60767-37-5].
$C_{12}H_{18}B_2F_8N_6Pt_2$ M 810.082
Cryst. (MeCN/Et_2O).

Boehm, J.R. *et al*, *J. Am. Chem. Soc.*, 1976, **98**, 4845 (*synth, ir, pmr*)

$C_{12}H_{20}Cl_4Pt_2$ **Pt-00114**

Di-μ-chlorodichlorobis[(1,2-η)-cyclohexene]diplatinum, 9CI

Tetrachlorobis(cyclohexene)diplatinum, 8CI

[12176-53-3]

M 696.262

Dimer. Hydrosilylation catalyst. Catalyses silicone rubber vulcanisations. Yellow cryst. ($CHCl_3$/pet. ether). Dec. at 150-5°.

Monomer: Dichloro(1,2-η-cyclohexene)platinum.
$C_6H_{10}Cl_2Pt$ M 348.131
Unknown.

Mann, B.E. *et al*, *J. Chem. Soc. (A)*, 1971, 3536 (*synth*)

$C_{12}H_{20}Pt$ **Pt-00115**

1,4-Butanediyl[(1,2,5,6-η)-1,5-cyclooctadiene]platinum, 9CI

(1,5-Cyclooctadiene)-1,4-tetramethyleneplatinum

[60161-34-4]

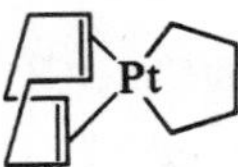

M 359.370

Cryst. (pet. ether). Mp 74°.

Brown, M.P. *et al*, *J. Chem. Soc., Dalton Trans.*, 1976, 786 (*synth, pmr*)
Young, G.B. *et al*, *J. Am. Chem. Soc.*, 1978, **100**, 5808 (*synth*)

$C_{12}H_{20}Pt_2$ **Pt-00116**

[μ-(1,2,5,6:3,4,7,8-η)-Cyclooctatetraene]tetramethyldiplatinum

μ-Cyclooctatetraenebis[dimethylplatinum]

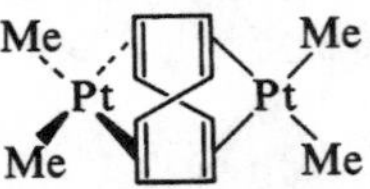

M 554.450

Yellow cryst. (CH_2Cl_2/hexane). Mp 168-71° dec.

Doyle, J.R. *et al*, *J. Am. Chem. Soc.*, 1961, **83**, 2768 (*synth*)
Kistner, C.R. *et al*, *Inorg. Chem.*, 1963, **2**, 1255 (*synth, pmr*)

$C_{12}H_{21}Cl_4NPtSn$ **Pt-00117**

Acetonitrilechloro[(3,4-η)-2,2,5,5-tetramethyl-3-hexyne](trichlorostannyl)platinum, 10CI

Acetonitrilechloro(di-tert-butylethyne)(trichlorostannyl)platinum

[75517-64-5]

$(Bu^tC\equiv CBu^t)PtCl(SnCl_3)(NCCH_3)$

M 634.887

Stereochem. unknown. Orange cryst. (CH_2Cl_2).

Moreto, J. *et al*, *J. Chem. Soc., Dalton Trans.*, 1980, 1368 (*synth, ir, nmr*)

$C_{12}H_{24}As_2Pt$ **Pt-00118**

Di-1-propynylbis(trimethylarsine)platinum, 10CI

Bis(methylethynyl)bis(trimethylarsine)platinum

$Pt(C\equiv CCH_3)_2(AsMe_3)_2$

M 513.245

trans-form [61483-32-7]

Cryst. (C_6H_6/pet. ether). Mp 146-8° dec.

Bell, R.A. *et al*, *Inorg. Chem.*, 1977, **16**, 677 (*synth, ir, nmr*)

$C_{12}H_{25}Cl_2PPt$ **Pt-00119**

Dichloro[(1,2-η)-1,2-propadiene](tripropylphosphine)platinum

Allenedichloro(tripropylphosphine)platinum

M 466.289

cis-form [77681-86-8]

Cryst. (CH_2Cl_2/pet. ether). Mp 123-8° dec.

Briggs, J.R. *et al*, *J. Chem. Soc., Dalton Trans.*, 1981, 121 (*synth, struct, nmr, ir*)

$C_{12}H_{30}Cl_4P_2PtSn$ Pt-00120

Chloro(trichlorostannyl)bis(triethylphosphine)platinum, 9CI
Chloro(trichlorotin)bis(triethylphosphine)platinum. (Trichlorotin)chlorobis(triethylphosphine)platinum

[PtCl(SnCl3)(PEt3)2]

M 691.899

trans-form [67619-49-2]
Yellow cryst. (hexane). Mp 92°. Disproportionates in Me_2CO. nmr $^1J(^{195}Pt—^{119}Sn)$ 28,954 Hz.

Pregosin, P.S. *et al*, *Helv. Chim. Acta*, 1978, **61**, 1848 (*synth, nmr*)
Butler, G. *et al*, *J. Organomet. Chem.*, 1979, **181**, 47 (*nmr*)
Ostoja Starzewski, K.-H.A. *et al*, *Angew. Chem., Int. Ed. Engl.*, 1980, **19**, 316 (*nmr*)
Koch, B.R. *et al*, *Inorg. Chim. Acta*, 1980, **45**, L51 (*nmr*)

$C_{12}H_{30}Cl_6P_2PtSn_2$ Pt-00121

Bis(trichlorostannyl)bis(triethylphosphine)platinum
Bis(trichlorotin)bis(triethylphosphine)platinum
[67619-50-5]

[Pt(SnCl3)2(PEt3)2]

M 881.495

trans-form
Orange cryst. (EtOH).

Pregosin, P.S. *et al*, *Helv. Chim. Acta*, 1978, **61**, 1848 (*nmr*)
Koch, B.R. *et al*, *Inorg. Chim. Acta*, 1980, **45**, L51 (*synth, nmr*)
Ostoja Starzewski, K.-H.A. *et al*, *Angew. Chem., Int. Ed. Engl.*, 1980, **19**, 316 (*nmr*)

$C_{12}H_{31}As_2BrPt$ Pt-00122

Bromohydrobis(triethylarsine)platinum
Bis(triethylarsine)platinum hydridobromide. Bromohydridobis(triethylarsine)platinum

H, AsEt3 / Pt / Et3As, Br

M 600.204

trans-form
Cryst. (MeOH). Mp 107-10°.

Chatt, J. *et al*, *J. Chem. Soc.*, 1962, 5075 (*synth, ir*)
Powell, J. *et al*, *J. Chem. Soc.*, 1965, 3879 (*pmr*)

$C_{12}H_{31}As_2ClPt$ Pt-00123

Chlorohydrobis(triethylarsine)platinum
Bis(triethylarsine)platinum hydridochloride. Chlorohydridobis(triethylarsine)platinum

H, AsEt3 / Pt / Et3As, Cl

M 555.753

trans-form
Cryst. (MeOH). Mp 91-3°.

Chatt, J. *et al*, *J. Chem. Soc.*, 1962, 5075 (*synth, ir*)
Powell, J. *et al*, *J. Chem. Soc.*, 1965, 3879 (*pmr*)

$C_{12}H_{31}As_2IPt$ Pt-00124

Hydroiodobis(triethylarsine)platinum
Bis(triethylarsine)platinum hydridoiodide. Hydridoiodobis(triethylarsine)platinum

H, AsEt3 / Pt / Et3As, I

M 647.205

trans-form
Cryst. (MeOH). Mp 109-12° dec.

Chatt, J. *et al*, *J. Chem. Soc.*, 1962, 5075 (*synth, ir*)
Powell, J. *et al*, *J. Chem. Soc.*, 1965, 3879 (*pmr*)

$C_{12}H_{31}BrP_2Pt$ Pt-00125

Bromohydrobis(triethylphosphine)platinum, 9CI, 8CI
Bis(triethylphosphine)platinum hydridobromide. Hydridobromobis(triethylphosphine)platinum
[20436-51-5]

H, PEt3 / Pt / Et3P, Br

M 512.308

trans-form [18660-33-8]
Cryst. (MeOH aq.). Sol. most org. solvs. Mp 94-7°. Dipole moment 4.45 D.

Chatt, J. *et al*, *J. Chem. Soc.*, 1962, 5075 (*synth, ir, pmr*)
Anderson, D.W.W. *et al*, *J. Chem. Soc., Dalton Trans.*, 1973, 854, 2370 (*nmr*)

$C_{12}H_{31}ClP_2Pt$ Pt-00126

Chlorohydrobis(triethylphosphine)platinum, 9CI, 8CI
Bis(triethylphosphine)platinum hydridochloride. Hydridochlorobis(triethylphosphine)platinum
[20436-52-6]

H, PEt3 / Pt / Et3P, Cl

M 467.857

trans-form [16842-17-4]
Methyl methacrylate polymerisation cocatalyst. Cryst. (MeOH). Sol. most org. solvs. Mp 81-2°. Reacts reversibly with C_2H_4 to yield Chloroethylbis(triethylphosphine)platinum, Pt-00167 Dipole moment 4.2 D. Reacts with halogenated hydrocarbons.

Chatt, J. *et al*, *J. Chem. Soc.*, 1962, 5075 (*synth, pmr, ir*)
Riggs, W.M., *Anal. Chem.*, 1972, **44**, 830 (*pe*)
Anderson, D.W.W. *et al*, *J. Chem. Soc., Dalton Trans.*, 1973, 854, 2370 (*nmr*)

$C_{12}H_{31}Cl_3P_2PtSn$ Pt-00127

Hydro(trichlorostannyl)bis(triethylphosphine)platinum

Hydrido(trichlorostannyl)bis(triethylphosphine)platinum. (Trichlorotin)hydridobis(triethylphosphine)-platinum

H PEt$_3$
Pt
Et$_3$P SnCl$_3$

M 657.453

trans-form [19662-51-2]

Catalyst for olefin hydrogenation. Cryst. (MeOH). Mp 100-1°.

Lindsey, R.V. *et al*, *J. Am. Chem. Soc.*, 1965, **87**, 658 (*synth*, *ir*, *pmr*)
Parish, R.V. *et al*, *J. Chem. Soc., Dalton Trans.*, 1973, 37 (*mossbauer*, *ir*)
Andersson, C. *et al*, *Chem. Scr.*, 1977, **11**, 140 (*pe*)
Butler, G. *et al*, *J. Organomet. Chem.*, 1979, **181**, 47 (*nmr*)
Ostoja, S. *et al*, *Angew. Chem.*, 1980, **92**, 323 (*nmr*)

$C_{12}H_{31}IP_2Pt$ Pt-00128

Hydroiodobis(triethylphosphine)platinum, 9CI, 8CI

Bis(triethylphosphine)platinum hydridoiodide. Hydridoiodobis(triethylphosphine)platinum

[19696-06-1]

H PEt$_3$
Pt
Et$_3$P I

M 559.309

trans-form [16971-06-5]

Cryst. (pet. ether). Mp 73-5°. Dipole moment 4.5 D.

Chatt, J. *et al*, *J. Chem. Soc.*, 1962, 5075 (*synth*, *ir*, *pmr*)
Anderson, D.W.W. *et al*, *J. Chem. Soc., Dalton Trans.*, 1973, 854, 2370 (*nmr*)
Dickinson, R.J. *et al*, *J. Chem. Soc., Dalton Trans.*, 1980, 895 (*mossbauer*)

$C_{12}H_{31}NO_2P_2Pt$ Pt-00129

Hydronitrobis(triethylphosphine)platinum, 8CI

Hydridonitrobis(triethylphosphine)platinum. Hydronitritobis(triethylphosphine)platinum, 8CI. Hydridonitritobis(triethylphosphine)platinum

[PtH(NO$_2$)(PEt$_3$)$_2$] (C$_{2v}$)

M 478.410

trans-form [21157-54-0]

Cryst. (pet. ether). Mp 95-97.5°. Dipole moment 5.8 D. The NO$_2$ ligand may be N-bonded (nitro) or O-bonded (nitrito).

Chatt, J. *et al*, *J. Chem. Soc.*, 1962, 5075 (*synth*, *ir*, *pmr*)
Powell, J. *et al*, *J. Chem. Soc.*, 1965, 3879 (*pmr*)
Dean, R.R. *et al*, *J. Chem. Soc. (A)*, 1968, 3047 (*nmr*)

$C_{12}H_{31}NO_3P_2Pt$ Pt-00130

Hydro(nitrato-*O*)bis(triethylphosphine)platinum, 9CI

Hydridobis(triethylphosphine)platinum nitrate. Hydridonitratobis(triethylphosphine)platinum

H PEt$_3$
Pt
Et$_3$P NO$_3$

M 494.409

trans-form [19582-28-6]

Catalyses hydrogenation of alkenes. Cryst. (pet. ether). Mp 47-9°.

Chatt, J. *et al*, *J. Chem. Soc.*, 1962, 5075 (*synth*, *ir*, *pmr*)
Powell, J. *et al*, *J. Chem. Soc.*, 1965, 3879 (*pmr*)
Dean, R.R. *et al*, *J. Chem. Soc. (A)*, 1968, 3047 (*nmr*)

$C_{12}H_{32}Cl_2P_2Pt$ Pt-00131

Dichlorodihydrobis(triethylphosphine)platinum

Dichlorodihydridobis(triethylphosphine)platinum. Dihydridodichlorobis(triethylphosphine)platinum

[40895-04-3]

H
Et$_3$P H
Pt
Cl PEt$_3$
Cl

M 504.318

Cryst. Reversibly loses HCl to generate Chlorohydrobis(triethylphosphine)platinum, Pt-00126 but slowly loses H$_2$ irreversibly in soln.

Chatt, J. *et al*, *J. Chem. Soc.*, 1962, 5075 (*synth*, *ir*)
Brooks, E.H. *et al*, *Inorg. Chim. Acta*, 1968, **2**, 17.
Anderson, D.W.W. *et al*, *J. Chem. Soc., Dalton Trans.*, 1973, 854, 2370 (*ir*, *raman*, *nmr*)

$C_{12}H_{32}P_2Pt$ Pt-00132

Dihydrobis(triethylphosphine)platinum

Bis(triethylphosphine)platinum dihydride

H PEt$_3$
Pt *cis-form*
H PEt$_3$

M 433.412

cis-form [80581-70-0]

Exists in soln. in equilibrium with *trans*-form, which is usually the predominant sp.

trans-form [62945-61-3]

Catalyses transformation of HCOOH to H$_2$ and CO$_2$. Cryst. (hexane), unstable above r.t. Can lose H$_2$ in soln., unless kept under hydrogen atmosphere.

Yoshida, T. *et al*, *J. Am. Chem. Soc.*, 1977, **99**, 2134 (*synth*, *nmr*, *ir*)
Paonessa, R.S. *et al*, *J. Am. Chem. Soc.*, 1982, **104**, 1138 (*synth*, *nmr*)
Paonessa, R.S. *et al*, *J. Am. Chem. Soc.*, 1982, **104**, 3529.

$C_{12}H_{42}B_8P_2Pt$ Pt-00133

[η^3-Dodecahydrooctaborato(2−)]bis(triethylphosphine)platinum, 9CI

[Octaborane(12)]bis(triethylphosphine)platinum, 8CI

[12563-57-4]

$[Pt(B_8H_{12})(PEt_3)_2]$

M 529.971

Photographic fogging agent.

Kane, A.R. *et al*, *J. Am. Chem. Soc.*, 1970, **92**, 2571.
Riggs, W.M., *Anal. Chem.*, 1972, **44**, 830.

$C_{12}H_{42}B_{10}P_2Pt$ Pt-00134

[(5,6,7,8,9,10-η)Dodecahydrodecaborato(2−)]bis(triethylphosphine)platinum, 9CI

[12375-22-3]

$[Pt(B_{10}H_{12})(PEt_3)_2]$

M 551.591

Possible developing agent for $AgNO_3$-based invisible inks. Yellow cryst. (MeCN), dec. >180°.

Klanberg, F. *et al*, *Inorg. Chem.*, 1968, **7**, 2072 (*synth, ir, nmr*)
Riggs, W.M., *Anal. Chem.*, 1972, **44**, 830 (*pe*)

$C_{12}Ni_3O_{12}Pt_3^{\ominus\ominus}$ Pt-00135

Dodecacarbonyltrinickelatetriplatinate(2−)

Tri-μ-carbonyltricarbonyl(tri-μ-carbonyltricarbonyltrinickelate)triplatinate(2−), 10CI

[72669-24-0]

$[Ni_3Pt_3(CO)_{12}]^{\ominus\ominus}$

M 1097.435 (ion)

Formed from mixt. of $[Pt_6(CO)_{12}]^{\ominus\ominus}$ and $[Ni_6(CO)_{12}]^{\ominus\ominus}$. Compd. not isol. in solid state. Sol. Me_2CO. Struct. is probably prismatic with Ni_3 and Pt_3 units retaining their identities.

Brown, C. *et al*, *J. Organomet. Chem.*, 1979, **181**, 233 (*nmr*)

$C_{12}O_{12}Pt_6^{\ominus\ominus}$ Pt-00136

Hexa-μ-carbonylhexacarbonylhexaplatinate(2−), 9CI

Bis[hexacarbonyltriplatinate](2−)

[52261-69-5]

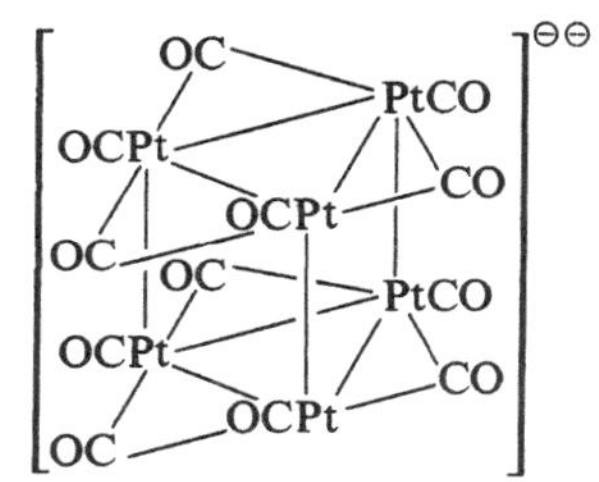

M 1506.605 (ion)

Orange-red soln. in THF.

Bis(tetraethylammonium) salt: [59473-02-8].
$C_{28}H_{40}N_2O_{12}Pt_6$ M 1767.110
Used in prep. of supported Pt aggregates; catalyses hydrocarbon synth. from H_2 + CO.

Calabrese, J.C. *et al*, *J. Am. Chem. Soc.*, 1974, **96**, 2614 (*synth, ir, struct*)
Ichikawa, M., *Chem. Lett.*, 1976, 335 (*use*)
Japan. Pat., 77 65 201, (*1977*); *CA*, **88**, 123625g (*use*)
Apai, G. *et al*, *J. Am. Chem. Soc.*, 1979, **101**, 6880 (*synth*)
Brown, C. *et al*, *J. Organomet. Chem.*, 1979, **181**, 233 (*nmr, cmr*)
Garin, F. *et al*, *Surf. Sci.*, 1981, **106**, 466 (*use*)

$C_{13}H_{16}Cl_2N_2Pt$ Pt-00137

Dichloro-1,3-propanediylbis(pyridine)platinum, 9CI

[12085-95-9]

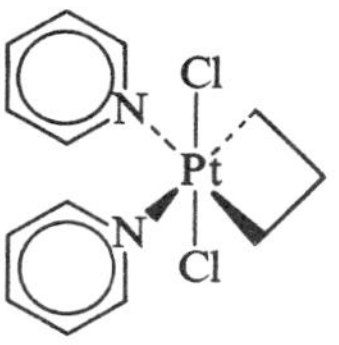

M 466.269

Cryst. ($CHCl_3$/pet. ether). Mp 145° dec.

Gillard, R.D. *et al*, *J. Organomet. Chem.*, 1971, **33**, 247 (*synth, pmr, ir, struct*)
Inorg. Synth., 1976, **16**, 113 (*synth, pmr*)

$C_{13}H_{17}IN_2Pt$ Pt-00138

(2,2′-Bipyridine-*N,N′*)iodotrimethylplatinum, 9CI

Trimethyliodo(bipyridine)platinum

[38194-05-7]

M 523.275

Cryst. (C_6H_6). Mp 273° dec.

Lile, W.J. *et al*, *J. Chem. Soc.*, 1949, 1168 (*synth*)
Clegg, D.E. *et al*, *J. Organomet. Chem.*, 1972, **38**, 403 (*synth, pmr, ir*)
Kuyper, J., *Inorg. Chem.*, 1977, **16**, 2171 (*pmr*)

$C_{13}H_{17}Pt^{\oplus}$ Pt-00139

[(1,2,5,6-η)-1,5-Cyclooctadiene][(η⁵-2,4-cyclopentadien-1-yl)]platinum(1+), 9CI

(π-Cyclopentadienyl)(1,5-cyclooctadiene)platinum(1+)

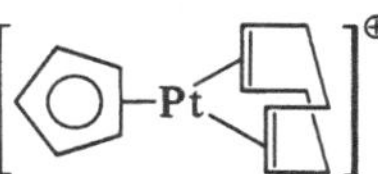

M 368.357 (ion)

Tetrafluoroborate: [31725-11-8].
$C_{13}H_{17}BF_4Pt$ M 455.161
Solid (CH_2Cl_2).

Chloride: [60767-00-2].
$C_{13}H_{17}ClPt$ M 403.810
Cryst. (Me_2CO). Mp 171°.

Hexafluorophosphate:
$C_{13}H_{17}F_6PPt$ M 513.321
Cryst. (CH_2Cl_2).

Johnson, B.F.G. *et al*, *J. Chem. Soc. (A)*, 1970, 1738.
Clark, H.C. *et al*, *Can. J. Chem.*, 1976, **54**, 2068 (*synth, pmr*)

$C_{13}H_{19}IN_2Pt$ Pt-00140

Iodotrimethylbis(pyridine)platinum, 9CI

Dipyridineiodotrimethylplatinum. Trimethyldipyridine-platinum iodide

[17362-77-5]

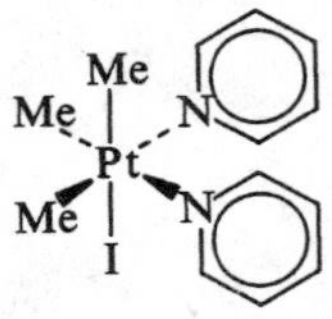

M 525.291

Cryst. (C_6H_6). Mp 168°.

Lile, W.J. *et al*, *J. Chem. Soc.*, 1949, 1168 (*synth*)
Hagnauer, H. *et al*, *J. Organomet. Chem.*, 1972, **46**, 179 (*raman, ir*)
Hall, J.R. *et al*, *J. Organomet. Chem.*, 1972, **42**, 479 (*synth, nmr*)
Kharchevnikov, V.M. *et al*, *Zh. Obshch. Khim.*, 1973, **43**, 817; *CA*, **79**, 42658g.
Kennedy, J.D. *et al*, *J. Chem. Soc., Dalton Trans.*, 1976, 874 (*nmr*)
Kuyper, J. *et al*, *Transition Met. Chem.*, 1976, **1**, 199 (*synth, nmr*)

$C_{13}H_{19}O_2Pt^{\oplus}$ Pt-00141

[(1,2,5,6-η)-1,5-Cyclooctadiene](2,4-pentanedionato-*O,O'*)platinum(1+), 9CI

(Acetylacetonato)(1,5-cyclooctadiene)platinum(1+)

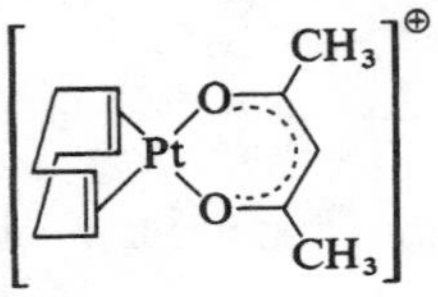

M 402.372 (ion)

Tetrafluoroborate: [31725-00-5].
$C_{13}H_{19}BF_4O_2Pt$ M 489.176
Cryst. (CH_2Cl_2/Et_2O), dec. >185°.

Johnson, B.F.G. *et al*, *J. Chem. Soc. (A)*, 1970, 1738.
White, D.A., *Synth. Inorg. Metal-Org. Chem.*, 1971, **1**, 133 (*synth*)
Inorg. Synth., 1972, **13**, 55 (*synth*)

$C_{13}H_{20}Cl_2NPPt$ Pt-00142

Dichloro(isocyanobenzene)(triethylphosphine)platinum, 9CI

Dichloro(phenylisocyanide)(triethylphosphine)platinum, 8CI. Dichloro(phenylisonitrile)(triethylphosphine)-platinum

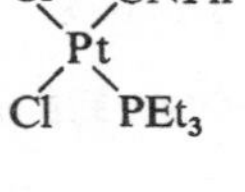

M 487.267

***cis*-form** [30376-90-0]
Cryst. (EtOH). Mp 163-4°.

Richards, R.L. *et al*, *J. Chem. Soc. (A)*, 1971, 21 (*synth, ir, pmr*)
Manojlović-Muir, L. *et al*, *J. Organomet. Chem.*, 1977, **142**, 265 (*struct*)
Crociani, B. *et al*, *J. Organomet. Chem.*, 1978, **144**, 85 (*cmr*)
Fehlhammer, W.P. *et al*, *J. Organomet. Chem.*, 1981, **209**, 57 (*synth*)

$C_{13}H_{30}ClOP_2Pt^{\oplus}$ Pt-00143

Carbonylchlorobis(triethylphosphine)platinum(1+), 9CI, 8CI

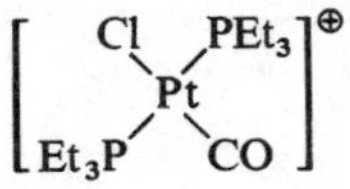

M 494.860 (ion)

***trans*-form** [20683-71-0]
Reacts with moisture or alcohols.

Pentafluorosilicate: [17192-41-5].
$C_{13}H_{30}ClF_5OP_2PtSi$ M 617.937
Cryst. (EtOAc). Mp 206-8°.

Tetrafluoroborate: [16743-82-1].
$C_{13}H_{30}BClF_4OP_2Pt$ M 581.664
Cryst. (EtOAc). Mp 168-71°.

Clark, H.C. *et al*, *J. Am. Chem. Soc.*, 1967, **89**, 3360 (*struct*)
Church, M.J. *et al*, *J. Chem. Soc. (A)*, 1968, 3074 (*synth, ir*)
Clark, H.C. *et al*, *J. Am. Chem. Soc.*, 1968, **90**, 2259 (*synth, ir*)
Clark, H.C. *et al*, *Inorg. Chem.*, 1970, **9**, 1229.
Crociani, B. *et al*, *J. Organomet. Chem.*, 1978, **144**, 85 (*cmr*)

$C_{13}H_{31}NP_2Pt$ Pt-00144

(Cyano-*C*)hydrobis(triethylphosphine)platinum, 9CI

Cyanohydridobis(triethylphosphine)platinum. Hydridocyanobis(triethylphosphine)platinum

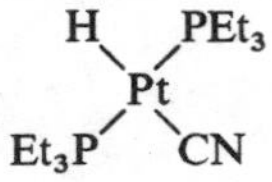

M 458.422

***trans*-form** [19528-87-1]
Cryst. (pet. ether). Mp 106-7°. Dipole moment 5.4 D.

Chatt, J. *et al*, *J. Chem. Soc.*, 1962, 5075 (*synth, ir, pmr*)
Powell, J. *et al*, *J. Chem. Soc.*, 1965, 3879 (*pmr*)
Dean, R.R. *et al*, *J. Chem. Soc. (A)*, 1968, 3047 (*nmr*)
Anderson, D.W.W. *et al*, *J. Chem. Soc., Dalton Trans.*, 1973, 2370 (*nmr*)

$C_{13}H_{31}OP_2Pt^{\oplus}$ Pt-00145

Carbonylhydrobis(triethylphosphine)platinum(1+), 9CI, 8CI

Hydridocarbonylbis(triethylphosphine)platinum(1+)

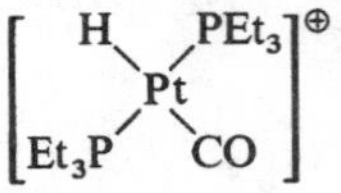

M 460.415 (ion)

***trans*-form**

Tetraphenylborate: [22276-39-7].
$C_{37}H_{51}BOP_2Pt$ M 779.647
Cryst. (Me_2CO/Et_2O). Mp 115-7° dec. (*in vacuo*).

Tetrafluoroborate: [33915-25-2].
$C_{31}H_{31}BF_4OP_2Pt$ M 763.416
Cryst. (C_6H_6). Sol. pet. ether, $CHCl_3$, MeOH, spar. sol. C_6H_6. Mp 168-71°.

Perchlorate: [19321-29-0].
$C_{13}H_{31}ClO_5P_2Pt$ M 559.865
Cryst. (Me_2CO/Et_2O).

Church, M.J. *et al*, *J. Chem. Soc. (A)*, 1968, 3074 (*synth, ir*)
Clark, H.C. *et al*, *J. Am. Chem. Soc.*, 1968, **90**, 2259; 1969, **91**, 596 (*synth, ir*)

Clark, H.C. *et al*, *Inorg. Chem.*, 1971, **10**, 2263.
Deeming, A.J. *et al*, *J. Chem. Soc., Dalton Trans.*, 1973, 1848 (*synth, ir, nmr*)
Cherwinski, W.J. *et al*, *J. Chem. Soc., Dalton Trans.*, 1975, 1156 (*cmr*)

$C_{13}H_{33}BrP_2Pt$ Pt-00146

Bromomethylbis(triethylphosphine)platinum, 9CI, 8CI
Methylbis(triethylphosphine)platinum bromide

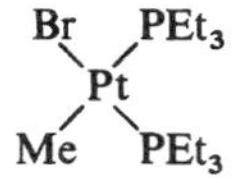

cis-form

M 526.335
cis-form [22289-47-0]
Cryst. Not obt. free of *trans*-form, to which it readily isomerises.
trans-form [15691-67-5]
Cryst. (MeOH). Mp 87-90°. Dipole moment 3.7 D.

Chatt, J. *et al*, *J. Chem. Soc.*, 1959, 705 (*synth*)
Allen, F.H. *et al*, *J. Chem. Soc. (A)*, 1968, 2700 (*synth, nmr*)
Roberts, D.A. *et al*, *Inorg. Chem.*, 1981, **20**, 789 (*uv*)

$C_{13}H_{33}ClP_2Pt$ Pt-00147

Chloromethylbis(triethylphosphine)platinum
Methylbis(triethylphosphine)platinum chloride

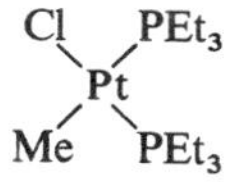

cis-form

M 481.884
cis-form [22289-46-9]
Mp 113-6° dec. Readily converted in soln. to *trans* isomer. Dipole moment 8.4D.
trans-form [13964-96-0]
Cryst. (pet. ether). Mp 99-100°. More stable isomer. Dipole moment 3.4D.

Chatt, J. *et al*, *J. Chem. Soc.*, 1959, 705 (*synth*)
Allen, F.H. *et al*, *J. Chem. Soc. (A)*, 1968, 2700 (*nmr*)
Riggs, W.M., *Anal. Chem.*, 1972, **44**, 830 (*pe*)
Kennedy, J.D. *et al*, *J. Chem. Soc., Dalton Trans.*, 1976, 874 (*nmr*)
Bardi, R. *et al*, *Cryst. Struct. Commun.*, 1981, **10**, 807 (*struct*)
Roberts, D.A. *et al*, *Inorg. Chem.*, 1981, **20**, 789 (*uv*)

$C_{13}H_{33}IP_2Pt$ Pt-00148

Iodomethylbis(triethylphosphine)platinum, 9CI, 8CI
Methylbis(triethylphosphine)platinum iodide
[29718-65-8]

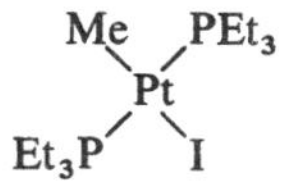

M 573.336
Catalyses carbonylation of alcohols.
trans-form [18974-13-5]
Cryst. (MeOH). Mp 71-71.5°. Dipole moment 4.1 D.

Chatt, J. *et al*, *J. Chem. Soc.*, 1959, 705 (*synth*)
Allen, F.H. *et al*, *J. Chem. Soc. (A)*, 1968, 2700 (*nmr*)
Kennedy, J.D. *et al*, *J. Chem. Soc., Dalton Trans.*, 1976, 874 (*nmr*)

$C_{13}H_{33}NO_2P_2Pt$ Pt-00149

Methylnitrobis(triethylphosphine)platinum
Nitro(methyl)bis(triethylphosphine)platinum

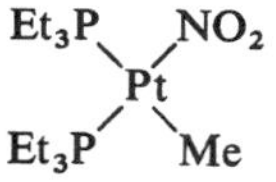

cis-form

M 492.437
cis-form [22289-33-4]
Not isol. Converts to *trans*-form in soln.
trans-form [22476-10-4]
Cryst. (pet. ether). Mp 102-4°. Dipole moment 3.75 D.

Adams, D.M. *et al*, *J. Chem. Soc.*, 1960, 2047 (*synth, ir*)
Allen, F.H. *et al*, *J. Chem. Soc. (A)*, 1968, 2700 (*synth, nmr*)

$C_{13}H_{33}NO_3P_2Pt$ Pt-00150

Methylnitratobis(triethylphosphine)platinum, 9CI
Methylbis(triethylphosphine)platinum nitrate

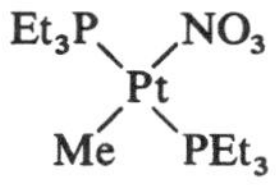

M 508.436
trans-form [22289-41-4]
Cryst. (pet. ether). Mp 56-8°. Dipole moment 6.0 D.

Chatt, J. *et al*, *J. Chem. Soc.*, 1959, 705 (*synth*)
Allen, F.H. *et al*, *J. Chem. Soc. (A)*, 1968, 2700 (*nmr*)

$C_{14}H_{10}Cl_2N_2Pt$ Pt-00151

Bis(benzonitrile)dichloroplatinum, 9CI, 8CI
Dichlorobis(cyanobenzene)platinum
[14873-63-3]

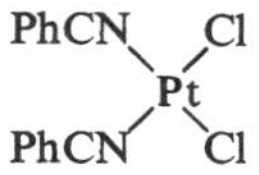

cis-form

M 472.232
Catalyst for hydroformylation of olefins and isomerisation of alkylamines. Versatile starting complex due to ease of replacement of PhCN ligands.
▷ATP-ase inhibitor
cis-form [15617-19-3]
Yellow cryst. Dipole moment 9.13 D, 11.63 D. Readily loses PhCN in soln.
▷TP2185000.
trans-form [51921-56-3]
Cryst. Less common form.

Walton, R.A. *et al*, *Spectrochim. Acta*, 1965, **21**, 1795 (*synth*)
Walton, R.A., *Can. J. Chem.*, 1968, **46**, 2347 (*ir, raman*)
Uchiyama, T. *et al*, *Bull. Chem. Soc. Jpn.*, 1981, **54**, 181 (*synth, ir, nmr*)

$C_{14}H_{10}Cl_3Pt^{\ominus}$ Pt-00152

Trichloro(diphenylacetylene)platinate(1−), 8CI
(Diphenylacetylene)trichloroplatinate(1−)

M 479.672 (ion)

Triethylammonium salt:
$C_{20}H_{26}Cl_3Pt$ M 567.864
Yellow cryst.

Bukhovets, S.V. *et al*, *Zh. Neorg. Khim.*, 1958, **3**, 1714 (*synth*)
Pukhova, N.K., *Zh. Neorg. Khim.*, 1969, **14**, 777; *Russ. J. Inorg. Chem.*, 1969, **14**, 406.

$C_{14}H_{10}O_2Pt$ Pt-00153

Dicarbonyldiphenylplatinum, 10CI
Diphenyldicarbonylplatinum
[76705-04-9]

$PtPh_2(CO)_2$

M 405.312
Observed in soln. and characterised spectroscopically.

Anderson, G.K. *et al*, *Inorg. Chem.*, 1981, **20**, 1636 (*synth, ir, nmr*)

$C_{14}H_{13}Cl_2OPPt$ Pt-00154

Carbonyldichloro(methyldiphenylphosphine)platinum
As Carbonyldichloro(triethylphosphine)platinum, Pt-00054 with

R^1 = Ph, R^2 = Me

M 494.216

cis-form [69109-32-6]
Cryst. ($CHCl_3$/hexane).

trans-form [73347-19-0]
Yellow solid; loses CO on heating. Readily isomerises to *cis*-form in soln.

Anderson, G.K. *et al*, *J. Chem. Res.*, 1979, M1601, S120 (*cmr*)
Anderson, G.K. *et al*, *J. Chem. Soc., Dalton Trans.*, 1980, 712 (*synth, ir*)
Anderson, G.K. *et al*, *J. Chem. Soc., Dalton Trans.*, 1980, 1988 (*synth, nmr, ir*)

$C_{14}H_{16}Cl_2N_2Pt$ Pt-00155

Dichloro(1,3-cyclobutanediyl)bis(pyridine)platinum, 9CI
[79789-89-2]

M 478.280
Cryst. Mp 160-2° dec. Solns. dec. above −25°.

Miyashita, A. *et al*, *J. Am. Chem. Soc.*, 1981, **103**, 6257.

$C_{14}H_{17}ClPt$ Pt-00156

Chloro[(1,2,5,6-η)-1,5-cyclooctadiene]phenylplatinum, 9CI
Phenylchloro(1,5-cyclooctadiene)platinum
[51177-65-2]

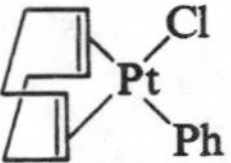

M 415.821
Cryst. (CH_2Cl_2/pentane). Mp 166-8°.

Clark, H.C. *et al*, *J. Organomet. Chem.*, 1973, **59**, 411 (*synth*)
Chisholm, M.H. *et al*, *J. Am. Chem. Soc.*, 1975, **97**, 721 (*cmr*)

$C_{14}H_{18}N_2Pt$ Pt-00157

(2,2′-Bipyridine-*N,N′*)diethylplatinum, 9CI
Diethyl(bipyridine)platinum
[52594-53-3]

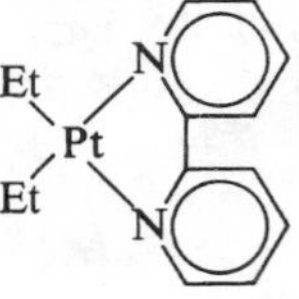

M 409.390
Red cryst. (Me_2CO). Mp 107-10° dec.

Chaudhury, N. *et al*, *J. Organomet. Chem.*, 1975, **84**, 105 (*synth, uv*)

$C_{14}H_{20}Pt$ Pt-00158

[(1,2,5,6-η)-1,5-Cyclooctadiene](2,4-cyclopentadien-1-yl-)methylplatinum, 9CI
(σ-Cyclopentadienyl)(1,5-cyclooctadiene)methylplatinum. Methyl(1,5-cyclooctadiene)(σ-cyclopentadienyl)-platinum
[56200-09-0]

M 383.392
Yellow cryst. (Et_2O). Mp 74-5°.

Clark, H.C. *et al*, *Can. J. Chem.*, 1976, **54**, 2068 (*synth, pmr*)
Day, C.S. *et al*, *Inorg. Chem.*, 1981, **20**, 2188 (*struct*)

$C_{14}H_{22}PtS_2$ Pt-00159

Bis(η^1-2,4-cyclopentadien-1-yl)bis(dimethyl sulfide)platinum
Dicyclopentadienylbis(methyl sulfide)platinum

cis-form

M 449.528
Obt. as *cis*- and *trans*-isomeric mixture. Unstable at r.t.

Fritz, H.P. *et al*, *J. Organomet. Chem.*, 1966, **5**, 103, 181 (*synth, pmr*)

$C_{14}H_{30}ClF_3P_2Pt$ Pt-00160

Chlorobis(triethylphosphine)(trifluorovinyl)platinum, 8CI

Chlorobis(triethylphosphine)(trifluoroethenyl)platinum, 10CI. *(Trifluorovinyl)bis(triethylphosphine)platinum chloride*

Cl, PEt_3 / Pt / Et_3P, $CF{=}CF_2$

M 547.867

trans-form [15318-27-1]

Cryst. (pentane/$CHCl_3$). Mp 61°.

Clark, H.C. *et al*, *J. Am. Chem. Soc.*, 1967, **89**, 529 (*synth*)
Clark, H.C. *et al*, *J. Am. Chem. Soc.*, 1967, **89**, 533 (*ir, nmr*)

$C_{14}H_{30}O_2P_2Pt$ Pt-00161

Dicarbonylbis(triethylphosphine)platinum, 10CI

[76125-09-2]

$[Pt(CO)_2(PEt_3)_2]$ (C_{2v})

M 487.417

Oil. Characterised spectroscopically, but not obt. pure. Sol. C_6H_6, Me_2CO. Eventually dec. to unidentified cluster compds.

Chini, P. *et al*, *J. Chem. Soc. (A)*, 1970, 1542 (*ir*)
Arnold, D.P. *et al*, *J. Organomet. Chem.*, 1980, **199**, C17 (*synth*)
Paonessa, R.S. *et al*, *Organometallics*, 1982, **1**, 768 (*synth*)

$C_{14}H_{33}ClOP_2Pt$ Pt-00162

Acetylchlorobis(triethylphosphine)platinum

Acetylbis(triethylphosphine)platinum chloride

Et_3P, $COCH_3$ / Pt / Cl, PEt_3

M 509.895

trans-form

Cryst. (pet. ether). Mp 70-1°. ir ν_{CO} 1629 cm^{-1}. Dipole moment 2.55D.

Booth, G. *et al*, *J. Chem. Soc. (A)*, 1966, 634 (*synth, ir*)

$C_{14}H_{33}ClO_2P_2Pt$ Pt-00163

Chloro(methoxycarbonyl)bis(triethylphosphine)platinum, 9CI

Chloro(methoxycarbonyl)bis(triethylphosphine)-platinum, 8CI

Et_3P, COOMe / Pt / Cl, PEt_3

M 525.894

trans-form [33915-46-7]

Oil.

Cherwinski, W.J. *et al*, *Inorg. Chem.*, 1971, **10**, 2263.

$C_{14}H_{33}IOP_2Pt$ Pt-00164

Acetyliodobis(triethylphosphine)platinum

Iodo(acetyl)bis(triethylphosphine)platinum

Et_3P, $COCH_3$ / Pt / I, PEt_3

M 601.346

trans-form

Cryst. (pet. ether). Mp 86-7°. Ir ν_{CO} 1635cm^{-1}. Dipole moment 3.6D.

Booth, G. *et al*, *J. Chem. Soc. (A)*, 1966, 634 (*synth, ir*)

$C_{14}H_{33}NP_2Pt$ Pt-00165

(Cyano-*C*)methylbis(triethylphosphine)platinum, 9CI

Methylbis(triethylphosphine)platinum cyanide

Me, PEt_3 / Pt / Et_3P, CN

M 472.449

trans-form [22289-45-8]

Cryst. (C_6H_6/pet. ether). Mp 84-6°, 118-20°.

Adams, D.M. *et al*, *J. Chem. Soc.*, 1960, 2047 (*synth, ir*)
Allen, F.H. *et al*, *J. Chem. Soc. (A)*, 1968, 2700 (*nmr*)
Treichel, P.M. *et al*, *Inorg. Chem.*, 1973, **12**, 1471 (*ir, pmr*)

$C_{14}H_{34}P_2Pt$ Pt-00166

Ethylenebis(triethylphosphine)platinum

Ethenebis(triethylphosphine)platinum

Et_3P, Et_3P / Pt–|| CH_2 = CH_2

M 459.450

Air-sensitive liq. Sol. org. solvs. Mp <–20°. Reacts with organic halides, but not with MeOH.

Paonessa, R.S. *et al*, *Organometallics*, 1982, **1**, 768 (*synth, nmr*)

$C_{14}H_{35}ClP_2Pt$ Pt-00167

Chloroethylbis(triethylphosphine)platinum, 9CI

Ethylbis(triethylphosphine)platinum chloride

Cl, PEt_3 / Pt / Et, PEt_3 *cis-form*

M 495.911

cis-form [61009-44-7]

Readily isom. to *trans* isomer in methanol.

trans-form

Cryst. (MeOH aq. or pet. ether). Mp 53-5°. Dipole moment 3.7D. Loses C_2H_4 on thermolysis to form Chlorohydrobis(triethylphosphine)platinum, Pt-00126 reversibly.

Chatt, J. *et al*, *J. Chem. Soc.*, 1959, 4020 (*synth*)
Romeo, R. *et al*, *Inorg. Chim. Acta*, 1976, **13**, L15.
Inorg. Synth., 1977, **17**, 132.
Bardi, R. *et al*, *Cryst. Struct. Commun.*, 1981, **10**, 333 (*struct*)
Roberts, D.A. *et al*, *Inorg. Chem.*, 1981, **20**, 789 (*uv*)

$C_{14}H_{35}P_2Pt^{\oplus}$ Pt-00168

Ethylene(hydrido)bis(triethylphosphine)platinum(1+)
(η^2-Ethene)hydrobis(triethylphosphine)platinum(1+), 9CI

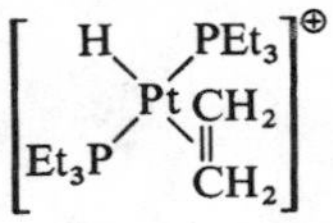

M 460.458 (ion)

trans-form

Treatment with $Cl^{\ominus}$ leads to mixt. of *trans*-$[PtHCl(PEt_3)_2]$ and *trans*-$[PtEtCl(PEt_3)_2]$.

Tetraphenylborate: [31781-38-1].
$C_{38}H_{55}BP_2Pt$ M 779.690
Cryst. (MeOH). Mp 78-80° (dec., gas evolution).

Hexafluorophosphate: [51794-48-0].
$C_{14}H_{35}F_6P_3Pt$ M 605.422
Observed in soln. only.

Deeming, A.J. *et al*, *J. Chem. Soc., Dalton Trans.*, 1973, 1848 (*synth, nmr*)
Clark, H.C. *et al*, *Inorg. Chem.*, 1974, **13**, 2213 (*synth, nmr*)

$C_{14}H_{36}Cl_2P_2Pt$ Pt-00169

Dichlorodimethylbis(triethylphosphine)platinum, 8CI
Dimethyldichlorobis(triethylphosphine)platinum

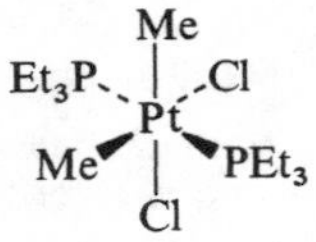

M 532.372
Cryst. (pet. ether). Mp 114-7°. Dipole moment 5.3D.

Chatt, J. *et al*, *J. Chem. Soc.*, 1959, 705 (*synth*)
Adams, D.M. *et al*, *J. Chem. Soc.*, 1960, 2047 (*ir*)
Allen, F.H. *et al*, *J. Chem. Soc. (A)*, 1968, 2700 (*nmr*)

$C_{14}H_{36}I_2P_2Pt$ Pt-00170

Diiododimethylbis(triethylphosphine)platinum, 8CI
Dimethyldiiodobis(triethylphosphine)platinum

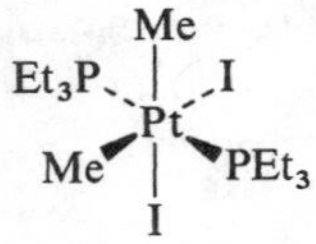

M 715.275
Cryst. (C_6H_6/pet. ether). Mp 101-3° dec. Dipole moment 5.85D.

Chatt, J. *et al*, *J. Chem. Soc.*, 1959, 705 (*synth*)
Adams, D.M. *et al*, *J. Chem. Soc.*, 1960, 2047 (*ir*)
Allen, F.H. *et al*, *J. Chem. Soc. (A)*, 1968, 2700 (*nmr*)

$C_{14}H_{36}P_2Pt$ Pt-00171

Dimethylbis(triethylphosphine)platinum, 9CI, 8CI
Bis(triethylphosphine)dimethylplatinum
[51607-32-0]

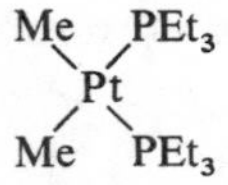

cis-form

M 461.466

cis-form [22289-34-5]
Cryst. (pet. ether). Mp 81-2°. $Bp_{0.0001}$ 85°. Dipole moment 5.65D. Subl. in air at 110°. More common isomer.

trans-form
Cryst. Mp 76-9°. Very difficult to obt. free of the *cis* isomer.

Chatt, J. *et al*, *J. Chem. Soc.*, 1959, 705 (*synth*)
Allen, F.H. *et al*, *J. Chem. Soc. (A)*, 1968, 2700 (*nmr*)
Riggs, W.M., *Anal. Chem.*, 1972, **44**, 830 (*pe*)
Glockling, F. *et al*, *Inorg. Chim. Acta*, 1974, **8**, 77 (*synth*)
Glockling, F. *et al*, *Inorg. Chim. Acta*, 1974, **8**, 81 (*ms*)
Roberts, D.A. *et al*, *Inorg. Chem.*, 1981, **20**, 789 (*uv*)

$C_{15}H_{11}ClF_6N_2Pt$ Pt-00172

(2,2′-Bipyridine-*N,N′*)chloro[(2,3-η)-1,1,1,4,4,4-hexafluoro-2-butyne]methylplatinum, 9CI
Methylchloro(hexafluoro-2-butyne)(bipyridine)platinum
[75764-69-1]

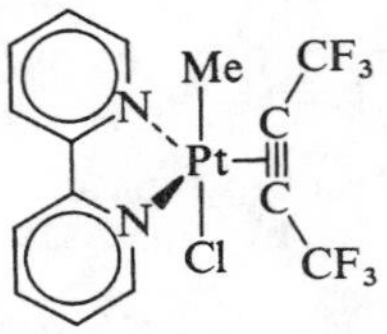

M 563.789
Cryst. (CH_2Cl_2). Mp 208-13°.

Chaudhury, N. *et al*, *Inorg. Chem.*, 1981, **20**, 467 (*synth, pmr, ir*)

$C_{15}H_{14}Cl_2Pt$ Pt-00173

Dichloro(1,2-diphenyl-1,3-propanediyl)platinum
(1,2-Diphenyl-1,3-propanediyl)dichloroplatinum
[60380-02-1]

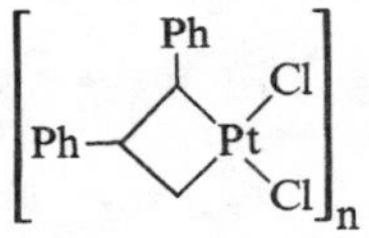

M 460.262
Chloride-bridged polymer. Pale-yellow solid. Insol. Mp 163° dec.

Inorg. Synth., 1976, **16**, 113 (*synth*)

$C_{15}H_{26}Cl_2NOPPt$ Pt-00174

Dichloro[ethoxy(phenylamino)methylene](triethylphosphine)-platinum, 9CI
(Anilinoethoxymethylene)dichloro(triethylphosphine)-platinum, 8CI. *Dichloro[ethoxy(phenylamino)carbene]-(triethylphosphine)platinum. (Anilinoethoxycarbene)-dichloro(triethylphosphine)platinum*
[25530-58-9]

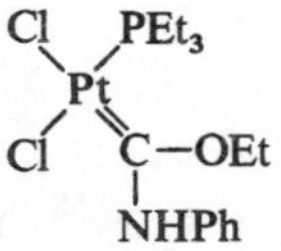

M 533.336

cis-form [30394-37-7]
Cryst. (EtOH). Mp 209-11°.

Richards, R.L. *et al*, *J. Chem. Soc. (A)*, 1971, 21 (*synth, ir, nmr*)
Crociani, B. *et al*, *J. Chem. Soc., Dalton Trans.*, 1974, 693 (*nmr*)
Baddley, E.M. *et al*, *J. Chem. Soc., Dalton Trans.*, 1976, 1930 (*struct*)

Inorg. Synth., 1979, **19**, 174 (*synth*)

$C_{15}H_{31}ClF_6P_2Pt$ Pt-00175

Chloro(1,1,1,3,3,3-hexafluoro-2-propyl)bis(triethylphosphine)platinum

Chlorobis(triethylphosphine)[2,2,2-trifluoro-1-(trifluoromethyl)ethyl]platinum, 8CI. *Chloro[2,2,2-trifluoro-1-(trifluoromethyl)ethyl]bis(triethylphosphine)platinum*

[18115-07-6]

Et_3P, $CH(CF_3)_2$, Pt, Et_3P, Cl — *cis-form*

M 617.881

cis-form [25482-36-4]

Yellow cryst. (hexane/CH_2Cl_2). Mp 97°.

trans-form [25482-37-5]

Cryst. (pentane/Et_2O). Mp 91°.

Cooke, J. *et al*, *J. Chem. Soc. (A)*, 1969, 1872 (*synth, ir, nmr*)

$C_{15}H_{35}BrP_2Pt$ Pt-00176

Bromo(2-propenyl)bis(triethylphosphine)platinum, 10CI

(*σ-Allyl*)*bromobis(triethylphosphine)platinum*

Br, PEt_3, Pt, Et_3P, $CH_2CH{=}CH_2$

M 552.373

trans-form [63324-94-7]

Cryst. (hexane). V. sol. most org. solvs. Mp 71-2° (*in vacuo*).

Huffman, J.C. *et al*, *Inorg. Chem.*, 1977, **16**, 2639 (*struct*)
Pearson, R.G. *et al*, *Isr. J. Chem.*, 1977, **15**, 243 (*synth, ir, nmr*)

$C_{15}H_{39}ClP_2PtSi$ Pt-00177

Chlorobis(triethylphosphine)(trimethylsilyl)platinum, 8CI

Trimethylsilylbis(triethylphosphine)platinum chloride

Cl, PEt_3, Pt, Et_3P, $SiMe_3$

M 540.039

trans-form [15559-62-3]

Pale-cream cryst. (pet. ether). Mp 42-3°.

Glockling, F. *et al*, *J. Chem. Soc. (A)*, 1967, 1066 (*synth, ir, pmr*)
Glockling, F. *et al*, *J. Chem. Soc. (A)*, 1968, 826.

$C_{16}H_{16}Cl_4Pt_2$ Pt-00178

Di-μ-chlorodichlorobis(styrene)diplatinum

Di-μ-chlorodichlorobis[(η²-ethenyl)benzene]diplatinum, 9CI. *Di-μ-chlorodichlorobis(phenylethene)diplatinum*

[12212-59-8]

Ph, Cl, Cl, Pt, Pt, Cl, Cl, Ph

M 740.274

Bridged dimer. Catalyses hydrosilylation of olefins, and cleavage of Si—C bonds.

Monomer: Dichloro(styrene)platinum.

$C_8H_8Cl_2Pt$ M 370.137

Unknown.

trans-form [60018-53-3]

Orange cryst. (C_6H_6). Mp 169-71° dec., 199-201°, 204°.

Joy, J.R. *et al*, *J. Am. Chem. Soc.*, 1959, **81**, 305 (*synth*)
Hupp, S.S. *et al*, *Inorg. Chem.*, 1976, **15**, 2349 (*synth*)
Busse, P. *et al*, *J. Organomet. Chem.*, 1977, **128**, 85 (*synth*)

$C_{16}H_{22}O_2PtS_2$ Pt-00179

Diphenylbis(dimethylsulfoxide)platinum

Diphenylbis[sulfinylbis[methane]-S]platinum, 10CI

As Dimethylbis(dimethylsulfoxide)platinum, Pt-00045 with

R = Ph

M 505.549

cis-form [70423-99-3]

Cryst. (CH_2Cl_2/Et_2O). Sol. C_6H_6, polar org. solvs., insol. H_2O. Dec. at 136°.

Eaborn, C. *et al*, *J. Chem. Soc., Dalton Trans.*, 1981, 933 (*synth, pmr, ir*)

$C_{16}H_{23}ClP_2Pt$ Pt-00180

Chlorohydrobis(dimethylphenylphosphine)platinum

Chlorobis(dimethylphenylphosphine)hydroplatinum, 9CI, 8CI. *Hydridochlorobis(dimethylphenylphosphine)-platinum*

Cl, PMe_2Ph, Pt, $PhMe_2P$, H

M 507.838

trans-form [12112-64-0]

Cocatalyst with $MeSO_3CF_3$ for olefin isomerisation. Cryst. (C_6H_6/pet. ether). Mp 102-4°. Reacts with C_2H_4 to yield Chlorobis(dimethylphenylphosphine)-ethylplatinum, Pt-00203 .

Chatt, J. *et al*, *J. Chem. Soc. (A)*, 1970, 1343 (*synth, ir, pmr*)

$C_{16}H_{24}Cl_4Pt_2$ Pt-00181

Di-μ-chlorodichlorobis[(1,2,3,4-η)-1,2,3,4-tetramethyl-1,3-cyclobutadiene]diplatinum, 10CI

[75517-61-2]

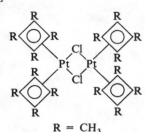

R = CH_3

M 748.338

Bridged dimer. Yellow cryst. (Me_2CO).

Monomer: Dichloro(tetramethylcyclobutadiene)-platinum.

$C_8H_{12}ClPt$ M 338.716

Unknown.

Moreto, J. *et al*, *J. Chem. Soc., Dalton Trans.*, 1980, 1368 (*synth, ir, nmr*)

$C_{16}H_{24}O_4Pt_2$ Pt-00182

Bis(2,4-pentanedionato-*O,O′*)bis[μ-[(1-η:2,3-η)-propenyl]]di-platinum, 9CI

Di-μ-allyldi(acetylacetonato)diplatinum

[33409-40-4]

M 670.523

Cryst. (CH_2Cl_2/pet. ether). Dec. at 155-61°.

McDonald, W.S. *et al*, *J. Chem. Soc., Chem. Commun.*, 1969, 1254.

Mann, B.E. *et al*, *J. Chem. Soc., Dalton Trans.*, 1971, 3536 (*synth, pmr*)

Raper, G. *et al*, *J. Chem. Soc., Dalton Trans.*, 1972, 265 (*struct*)

$C_{16}H_{24}Pt$ Pt-00183

Bis[(1,2,5,6-η)-1,5-cyclooctadiene]platinum, 9CI

[12130-66-4]

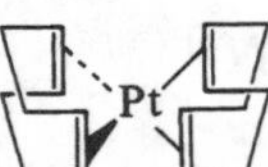

M 411.446

Versatile starting material for synthesis of platinum(0) and platinum(II) compds. Catalyst for telomerisation of butadiene and isoprene. Cryst. (pet. ether). Solid can be handled in air, but solns. are oxygen-sensitive.

Green, M. *et al*, *J. Chem. Soc., Dalton Trans.*, 1977, 271 (*synth, ir, nmr*)

Spencer, J.L., *Inorg. Synth.*, 1979, **19**, 213 (*synth*)

$C_{16}H_{30}F_6P_2Pt$ Pt-00184

[(2,3-η)-1,1,1,4,4,4-Hexafluoro-2-butyne]bis(triethylphosphine)platinum, 9CI

Bis(triethylphosphine)hexafluoro-2-butyneplatinum

[42029-75-4]

M 593.431

Cryst. (pet. ether). Mp 82-3° (subl. above 80°).

Browning, J. *et al*, *J. Chem. Soc., Dalton Trans.*, 1974, 97 (*synth, ir, nmr*)

Cherwinski, W.J. *et al*, *J. Chem. Soc., Dalton Trans.*, 1974, 1405 (*synth, ir, nmr*)

$C_{16}H_{31}ClF_6P_2Pt$ Pt-00185

Chloro[1,2-bis(trifluoromethyl)vinyl]bis(triethylphosphine)-platinum

Chlorobis(triethylphosphine)[3,3,3-trifluoro-1-(trifluoromethyl)-1-propenyl]platinum, 9CI. *[1,2-Bis(trifluoromethyl)vinyl]bis(triethylphosphine)platinum chloride*

[64397-36-0]

(E)-cis-form

M 629.892

(E)-cis-form [57173-43-0]

Cryst. (MeOH/Et_2O/hexane). Mp 132-4°.

(E)-trans-form [15389-52-3]

Cryst. (toluene/pet. ether). Mp 90-1°.

Clark, H.C. *et al*, *J. Am. Chem. Soc.*, 1967, **89**, 529 (*synth*)

Clark, H.C. *et al*, *J. Am. Chem. Soc.*, 1967, **89**, 533 (*ir, nmr*)

Attig, T.G. *et al*, *Can. J. Chem.*, 1977, **55**, 189 (*synth, nmr*)

$C_{16}H_{32}P_2Pt$ Pt-00186

Diethynylbis(triethylphosphine)platinum, 9CI

Bis(acetylide)bis(triethylphosphine)platinum. Bis-(triethylphosphine)diethynylplatinum

cis-form

M 481.456

cis-form [64396-20-9]

Cryst. (C_6H_6/hexane). Mp 130° dec. Slowly isom. to *trans*-form in soln.

trans-form [34230-58-5]

Cryst. (MeOH). Mp 62-3°. Dipole moment 0.7D.

Chatt, J. *et al*, *J. Chem. Soc.*, 1959, 4020 (*synth*)

Masai, H. *et al*, *Bull. Chem. Soc. Jpn.*, 1971, **44**, 2226 (*uv*)

Sonogashira, K. *et al*, *J. Organomet. Chem.*, 1978, **145**, 101 (*synth, ir*)

$C_{16}H_{37}P_2Pt^{\oplus}$ Pt-00187

[(1,2,3-η)-2-Butenyl]bis(triethylphosphine)platinum(1+), 9CI
(1-Methyl-π-allyl)bis(triethylphosphine)platinum(1+), 8CI. *(π-Crotyl)bis(triethylphosphine)platinum(1+)*
[31781-20-1]

M 486.496 (ion)
Hexafluorophosphate: [50726-35-7].
$C_{16}H_{37}F_6P_3Pt$ M 631.460
Cryst. (CH_2Cl_2/MeOH). Mp 219-22° dec.
Tetraphenylborate: [50726-34-6].
$C_{40}H_{57}BP_2Pt$ M 805.728
Cryst. (CH_2Cl_2/MeOH). Mp 148-50°.

Deeming, A.J. *et al*, *J. Chem. Soc., Dalton Trans.*, 1973, 1848 (*synth, pmr*)

$C_{16}H_{40}P_2Pt$ Pt-00188

Diethylbis(triethylphosphine)platinum, 9CI
Bis(triethylphosphine)diethylplatinum
[76189-28-1]

M 489.520
cis-form [75847-39-1]
Cryst. (MeOH). Mp 35-6°. Dipole moment 5.5 D.

Chatt, J. *et al*, *J. Chem. Soc.*, 1959, 4020 (*synth*)
McCarthy, T.J. *et al*, *J. Am. Chem. Soc.*, 1981, **103**, 3396.
Roberts, D.A. *et al*, *Inorg. Chem.*, 1981, **20**, 789 (*uv*)

$C_{16}H_{42}P_2Pt$ Pt-00189

Tetramethylbis(triethylphosphine)platinum
Bis(triethylphosphine)tetramethylplatinum

$Me_4Pt(PEt_3)_2$

M 491.535
cis-form [17567-57-6]
Cryst. (pet. ether). Mp 76-80°.

Ruddick, J.D. *et al*, *J. Chem. Soc. (A)*, 1969, 2801 (*synth, pmr, ir*)

$C_{17}H_{22}ClOP_2Pt^{\oplus}$ Pt-00190

Carbonylchlorobis(dimethylphenylphosphine)platinum(1+), 9CI, 8CI
Chlorocarbonylbis(dimethylphenylphosphine)-platinum(1+)

$R^1 = Me, R^2 = Ph$

M 534.841 (ion)
trans-form
Tetrafluoroborate: [33915-36-5].
$C_{17}H_{22}BClF_4OP_2Pt$ M 621.644
Colourless oil. ir ν_{CO} 2118 cm^{-1}.
Tetraphenylborate:
$C_{41}H_{42}BClOP_2Pt$ M 854.073
Cryst. (CH_2Cl_2/Et_2O). ir ν_{CO} 2093 cm^{-1}.
Perchlorate: [70739-07-0].
$C_{17}H_{22}Cl_2O_5P_2Pt$ M 634.291
Cryst. (Me_2CO). Mp 230-5° dec. ir ν_{CO} 2105 cm^{-1}.

Cherwinski, W.J. *et al*, *Inorg. Chem.*, 1971, **10**, 2263 (*synth, ir*)
Eaborn, C. *et al*, *J. Chem. Soc., Dalton Trans.*, 1979, 134 (*synth, ir, nmr*)

$C_{17}H_{25}BrP_2Pt$ Pt-00191

Bromobis(dimethylphenylphosphine)methylplatinum, 9CI
Bromo(methyl)bis(dimethylphenylphosphine)platinum. Methylbromobis(dimethylphenylphosphine)platinum

M 566.316
trans-form [24833-62-3]
Cryst. (MeOH). Mp 147.5-149.5°.

Ruddick, J.D. *et al*, *J. Chem. Soc. (A)*, 1969, 2801 (*synth, pmr, ir*)
Kennedy, J.D. *et al*, *J. Chem. Soc., Dalton Trans.*, 1976, 874 (*nmr*)
Behan, J. *et al*, *J. Chem. Soc., Chem. Commun.*, 1978, 444 (*pe*)

$C_{17}H_{25}ClP_2Pt$ Pt-00192

Chlorobis(dimethylphenylphosphine)methylplatinum, 9CI
Chloromethylbis(dimethylphenylphosphine)platinum. Methylbis(dimethylphenylphosphine)platinum chloride

cis-form

M 521.865
cis-form [30812-03-4]
Cryst. ($CHCl_3$/pet. ether). Mp 107-11°. Converts to *trans* isomer on melting or in soln. when treated with PMe_2Ph. Dipole moment 8.8D.
trans-form [24833-58-7]
Cryst. ($CHCl_3$). Mp 146-8°. Dipole moment 3.8D.

Ruddick, J.D. *et al*, *J. Chem. Soc. (A)*, 1969, 2801 (*synth, pmr, ir*)
Chisholm, M.H. *et al*, *J. Am. Chem. Soc.*, 1973, **95**, 8574 (*cmr*)
Kennedy, J.D. *et al*, *J. Chem. Soc., Dalton Trans.*, 1976, 874 (*nmr*)
Puddephatt, R.J. *et al*, *J. Organomet. Chem.*, 1976, **120**, C51 (*synth*)
Behan, J. *et al*, *J. Chem. Soc., Chem. Commun.*, 1978, 444 (*pe*)

$C_{17}H_{25}IP_2Pt$ Pt-00193

Bis(dimethylphenylphosphine)iodomethylplatinum, 9CI
Iodo(methyl)bis(dimethylphenylphosphine)platinum. Iodobis(dimethylphenylphosphine)methylplatinum. Methyliodobis(dimethylphenylphosphine)platinum

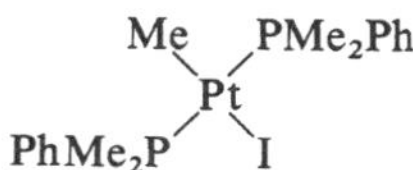

M 613.317

trans-form [24882-77-7]
Cryst. (MeOH). Mp 133-5°.

Ruddick, J.D. *et al*, *J. Chem. Soc. (A)*, 1969, 2801 (*synth*, *pmr*, *ir*)
Chisholm, M.H. *et al*, *J. Am. Chem. Soc.*, 1973, **95**, 8574 (*cmr*)
Bancroft, G. *et al*, *J. Am. Chem. Soc.*, 1974, **96**, 7208 (*möss-bauer*)
Kennedy, J.D. *et al*, *J. Chem. Soc., Dalton Trans.*, 1976, 874 (*nmr*)

$C_{17}H_{25}PPt$ Pt-00194

(η^5-2,4-Cyclopentadien-1-yl)phenyl(triethylphosphine)platinum, 10CI
Phenyl(cyclopentadienyl)(triethylphosphine)platinum
[31741-69-2]

$(C_5H_5)PtPh(PEt_3)_2$

M 455.438
Yellow liq. $Bp_{0.07}$ 60°.

Cross, R.J. *et al*, *J. Chem. Soc. (A)*, 1971, 2000 (*synth*, *ir*, *pmr*)

$C_{17}H_{27}Cl_2NPt$ Pt-00195

Dichloro(4-methylaniline)[(3,4-η)-2,2,5,5-tetramethyl-3-hexyne]platinum
Dichloro(2,2,5,5-tetramethyl-3-hexyne)(p-toluidine)-platinum, 8CI. *(1-Amino-4-methylbenzene)-dichloro[(3,4-η)-2,2,5,5-tetramethyl-3-hexyne)platinum]*. *(Di-tert-butylacetylene)dichloro(p-toluidine)-platinum*

M 511.393
trans-form [31742-08-2]
Yellow cryst. (C_6H_6/pet. ether). Mp 189-93° dec.

Chatt, J. *et al*, *J. Chem. Soc.*, 1961, 827 (*synth*)
Davies, G.R. *et al*, *J. Chem. Soc. (A)*, 1970, 1873 (*struct*)

$C_{17}H_{35}P_2Pt^{\oplus}$ Pt-00196

(η^5-2,4-Cyclopentadien-1-yl)bis(triethylphosphine)platinum(1+), 10CI

M 496.491 (ion)
Chloride: [34850-24-3].
$C_{17}H_{35}ClP_2Pt$ M 531.944
Not isol. Unstable in soln.
Perchlorate: [34850-25-4].
$C_{17}H_{35}ClO_4P_2Pt$ M 595.942
Red-brown cryst. ($CHCl_3$). Mp 180-2° dec.

Cross, R.J. *et al*, *J. Chem. Soc. (A)*, 1971, 2000 (*synth*, *ir*, *pmr*)

$C_{17}H_{40}P_2Pt$ Pt-00197

(2,2-Dimethyl-1,3-propanediyl)bis(triethylphosphine)platinium, 10CI
Bis(triethylphosphine)-3,3-dimethylplatinacyclobutane
[70620-74-5]

M 501.531
Cryst. (MeOH/Et_2O). Mp 41.3-42.5°.

Foley, P. *et al*, *J. Am. Chem. Soc.*, 1980, **102**, 6713 (*synth*, *pmr*, *ms*)
DiCosimo, R. *et al*, *J. Am. Chem. Soc.*, 1982, **104**, 3601.

$C_{18}H_{18}Cl_2Pt_2$ Pt-00198

Di-μ-chlorobis(η^3-1-phenyl-2-propenyl)diplatinum
Di-μ-chlorobis(1-phenyl-π-allyl)diplatinum, 8CI

M 695.406
No details reported.

Irwin, W.J. *et al*, *Tetrahedron Lett.*, 1968, 1937 (*synth*)

$C_{18}H_{18}F_{18}P_2Pt$ Pt-00199

[1,2,3,4,5,6-Hexakis(trifluoromethyl)-1,3,5-hexatriene-1,6-diyl]bis(trimethylphosphine)platinum, 9CI
[57545-92-3]

M 833.339
Formed by Pt-induced ring opening of hexakis(trifluoromethyl)benzene.

Browning, J. *et al*, *J. Chem. Soc., Chem. Commun.*, 1975, 723 (*synth*, *nmr*)

$C_{18}H_{22}F_4P_2Pt$ Pt-00200

Bis(dimethylphenylphosphine)(η^2-tetrafluoroethene)platinum, 9CI
Bis(dimethylphenylphosphine)(tetrafluoroethylene)platinum, 8CI
[33518-46-6]

$Pt(C_2F_4)(PMe_2Ph)_2$

M 571.393
Cryst. (CH_2Cl_2/hexane). Mp 127-9°.

Kemmitt, R.D.W. *et al*, *J. Chem. Soc. (A)*, 1971, 2472 (*synth*, *nmr*)
Kemmitt, R.D.W. *et al*, *J. Organomet. Chem.*, 1972, **44**, 403.

$C_{18}H_{24}PtS_2$ Pt-00201

[1,2-Bis(ethylthio)ethane-*S*,*S'*]diphenylplatinum, 9CI, 8CI
[Ethylenebis[ethylsulfide]]diphenylplatinum. *(3,6-Dithiaoctane)diphenylplatinum*

[33572-97-3]
As [1,2-Bis(ethylthio)ethane-*S*,*S'*]dimethylplatinum, Pt-00075 with

R = Ph

M 499.588
Cryst.

Cross, R.J. *et al*, *J. Chem. Soc., Dalton Trans.*, 1972, 992 (*nmr*)

$C_{18}H_{25}ClOP_2Pt$ Pt-00202

Acetylchlorobis(dimethylphenylphosphine)platinum, 9CI
Chlorobis(dimethylphenylphosphine)ethionylplatinum

Cl, PMe_2Ph, Pt, $PhMe_2P$, $COCH_3$

M 549.875

trans-form [30180-03-1]
Cryst. (MeOH). Mp 153-7° dec.

Clark, H.C. *et al*, *Inorg. Chem.*, 1970, **9**, 2670 (*synth, pmr*)
Chisholm, M.H. *et al*, *Inorg. Chem.*, 1975, **14**, 900 (*synth*)

$C_{18}H_{27}ClP_2Pt$ Pt-00203

Chlorobis(dimethylphenylphosphine)ethylplatinum, 9CI
Chloro(ethyl)bis(dimethylphenylphosphine)platinum. Ethylchlorobis(dimethylphenylphosphine)platinum

Cl, PMe_2Ph, Pt, $PhMe_2P$, Et

M 535.892

trans-form [38832-88-1]
Cryst. (C_6H_6/pentane). Mp 114-5° (106-8°).

Clark, H.C. *et al*, *Inorg. Chem.*, 1972, **11**, 1275 (*synth*)
Hall, T.L. *et al*, *J. Chem. Soc., Dalton Trans.*, 1980, 1448 (*synth*)

$C_{18}H_{28}Br_2P_2Pt$ Pt-00204

Dibromobis(dimethylphenylphosphine)dimethylplatinum, 9CI
Dibromodimethylbis(dimethylphenylphosphine)platinum. Dimethyldibromobis(dimethylphenylphosphine)platinum

[a]Br, Me_2PhP[e], [b]Br, Pt, [d]Me, [c]PMe_2Ph, [f]Me — *ab*-dibromo-*ce*-diphosphine-*df*-dimethyl-*form*

M 661.255

ab-dibromo-ce-diphosphine-df-dimethyl-form [60133-79-1]
Cryst. (C_6H_6/pet. ether). Mp 184-6° dec. (182-3°).

af-dibromo-bc-diphosphine-de-dimethyl-form [24882-68-6]
Yellow cryst. (MeOH). Mp 135-40° dec.

Ruddick, J.D. *et al*, *J. Chem. Soc. (A)*, 1969, 2801 (*synth, pmr, ir*)
Kennedy, J.D. *et al*, *J. Chem. Soc., Dalton Trans.*, 1976, 874 (*nmr*)
Puddephatt, R.J. *et al*, *J. Organomet. Chem.*, 1976, **117**, 395 (*synth, pmr*)

$C_{18}H_{28}Cl_2P_2Pt$ Pt-00205

Dichlorobis(dimethylphenylphosphine)dimethylplatinum, 9CI
Dichlorodimethylbis(dimethylphenylphosphine)platinum. Dimethyldichlorobis(dimethylphenylphosphine)platinum

[a]Cl, [e]$PhMe_2P$, [b]Cl, Pt, [d]Me, [c]PMe_2Ph, [f]Me — *ab*-dichloro-*ce*-diphosphine-*df*-dimethyl-*form*

M 572.353

ab-dichloro-ce-diphosphine-df-dimethyl-form [27072-44-2]
Cryst. (C_6H_6). Mp 184-90° dec. Dipole moment 5.3D.

af-dichloro-bc-diphosphine-de-dimethyl-form [24833-66-7]
Yellow cryst. (C_6H_6/pet. ether). Dipole moment 5.9D.

Ruddick, J.D. *et al*, *J. Chem. Soc. (A)*, 1969, 2801 (*synth, pmr, ir*)
Kennedy, J.D. *et al*, *J. Chem. Soc., Dalton Trans.*, 1976, 874 (*nmr*)
Puddephatt, R.J. *et al*, *J. Organomet. Chem.*, 1976, **117**, 395 (*synth, pmr*)

$C_{18}H_{28}I_2P_2Pt$ Pt-00206

Bis(dimethylphenylphosphine)diiododimethylplatinum, 9CI
Diiododimethylbis(dimethylphenylphosphine)platinum. Dimethyldiiodobis(dimethylphenylphosphine)platinum

[a]PMe_2Ph, [e]Me, I^b, Pt, [d]Me, I^c, [f]PMe_2Ph — *af*-diphosphine-*bc*-diiodo-*de*-dimethyl-*form*

M 755.256

af-diphosphine-bc-diiodo-de-dimethyl-form [42402-13-1]
Cryst. (C_6H_6/pet. ether). Mp 174-7° dec. More stable isomer.

ab-diphosphine-ce-diiodo-df-dimethyl-form [61848-71-3]
Orange cryst. (Et_2O). Mp 154-8° dec. Isomerises in solution.

Ruddick, J.D. *et al*, *J. Chem. Soc. (A)*, 1969, 2801 (*synth, pmr, ir*)
Kennedy, J.D. *et al*, *J. Chem. Soc., Dalton Trans.*, 1976, 874 (*nmr*)
Puddephatt, R.J. *et al*, *J. Organomet. Chem.*, 1979, **166**, 251 (*synth, pmr*)

$C_{18}H_{28}PPt^{\ominus}$ Pt-00207

(Methyldiphenylphosphine)pentamethylplatinate(1−)
Pentamethyl(methyldiphenylphosphine)platinate(1−)

$[PtMe_5(PMePh_2)]^{\ominus}$

M 470.473 (ion)

Li salt: [58675-86-8].
$C_{18}H_{28}LiPPt$ M 477.414
Air-sensitive soln. in Et_2O.

Rice, G.W. *et al*, *J. Am. Chem. Soc.*, 1977, **99**, 2141 (*synth, pmr*)

$C_{18}H_{28}P_2Pt$ Pt-00208

Bis(dimethylphenylphosphine)dimethylplatinum, 9CI
Dimethylbis(dimethylphenylphosphine)platinum

Me PMe₂Ph / Pt / Me PMe₂Ph

M 501.447

cis-form [24917-48-4]
Cryst. (C_6H_6/Et_2O). Mp 79-81°. Dipole moment 5.5D. Reacts with *cis*- [$PtCl_2(PMe_2Ph)_2$] to produce Chlorobis(dimethylphenylphosphine)methylplatinum, Pt-00192 .

Ruddick, J.D. *et al*, *J. Chem. Soc. (A)*, 1969, 2801 (*synth*, *pmr*, *ir*)
Clark, H.C. *et al*, *Can. J. Chem.*, 1974, **52**, 1165 (*cmr*)
Kennedy, J.D. *et al*, *J. Chem. Soc., Dalton Trans.*, 1976, 874 (*nmr*)
Puddephatt, R.J. *et al*, *J. Organomet. Chem.*, 1976, **120**, C51.
Behan, J. *et al*, *J. Chem. Soc., Chem. Commun.*, 1978, 444 (*pe*)

$C_{18}H_{30}ClF_5P_2Pt$ Pt-00209

Chloro(pentafluorophenyl)bis(triethylphosphine)platinum, 9CI
(Pentafluorophenyl)bis(triethylphosphine)platinum chloride

cis-form

M 633.908

cis-form [14494-02-1]
Cryst. (MeOH). Mp 144-6°. $Bp_{0.1}$ 160° subl. Converts to *trans*-form when heated at 230°/0.6 mm.

trans-form
Cryst. (MeOH aq.). Mp 119-20°.

Rosevear, D.T. *et al*, *J. Chem. Soc.*, 1965, 5275 (*synth*)
Goggin, P.L. *et al*, *J. Chem. Soc. (A)*, 1966, 1462 (*ir*)
Crocker, C. *et al*, *J. Chem. Soc., Dalton Trans.*, 1977, 1449 (*nmr*)
Bresciani-Pahor, N. *et al*, *Inorg. Chim. Acta*, 1978, **31**, 171 (*struct*)

$C_{18}H_{30}Cl_3F_5P_2Pt$ Pt-00210

Trichloro(pentafluorophenyl)bis(triethylphosphine)platinum, 9CI
Pentafluorophenyltrichlorobis(triethylphosphine)platinum
[52970-55-5]

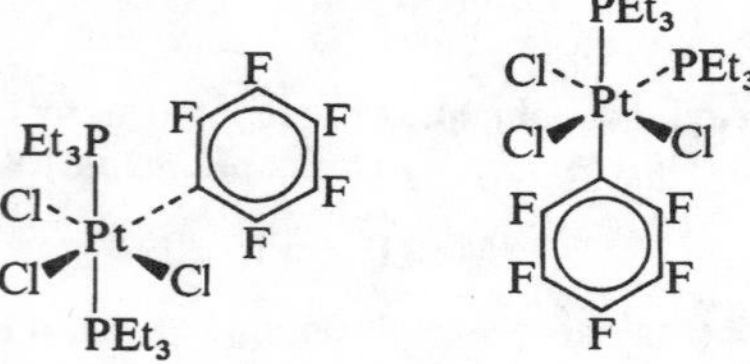

mer-trans-form *mer-cis-form*

M 704.814

mer-cis-form
Obt. from Cl_2 and *cis*-[$PtCl(C_6F_5)(PEt_3)_2$]. Yellow cryst. ($EtOH/CHCl_3$). Mp 151-2°. Dipole moment 9.5 D.

mer-trans-form
Obt. from Cl_2 and *trans*-[$PtCl(C_6F_5)(PEt_3)_2$]. Yellow cryst. ($EtOH/CHCl_3$). Mp 110-5°. Dipole moment 2.3 D.

Usón, R. *et al*, *CA*, 1974, **81**, 49793x (*synth*)
Crocker, C. *et al*, *J. Chem. Soc., Dalton Trans.*, 1977, 1448 (*nmr*)

$C_{18}H_{32}Cl_2NOPPt$ Pt-00211

Dichloro[ethoxy(phenylamino)methylene](tripropylphosphine)platinum, 9CI
(Anilinoethoxymethylene)dichloro(tripropylphosphine)platinum, 8CI. [Ethoxy(phenylamino)carbene]dichloro(tripropylphosphine)platinum

M 575.417

cis-form [30394-40-2]
Cryst. (EtOH). Mp 196-8°.

Bradley, E.M. *et al*, *J. Chem. Soc. (A)*, 1971, 21 (*synth*)
Busetto, L. *et al*, *J. Chem. Soc., Dalton Trans.*, 1972, 1800 (*pmr*)
Crociani, B. *et al*, *J. Chem. Soc., Dalton Trans.*, 1974, 693 (*pmr*)

$C_{18}H_{35}ClP_2Pt$ Pt-00212

Chlorophenylbis(triethylphosphine)platinum, 9CI
Phenylbis(triethylphosphine)platinum chloride

cis-form

M 543.955

cis-form [15702-92-8]
Cryst. (pet. ether). Mp 133-6° dec. Dipole moment 9.05D. Readily isom. to *trans*-form, catalysed by PEt_3.

trans-form [13938-93-7]
Cryst. (pet. ether). Mp 105-7°. Dipole moment 2.6D.

Chatt, J. *et al*, *J. Chem. Soc.*, 1959, 4020 (*synth*)
Adams, D.M. *et al*, *J. Chem. Soc.*, 1964, 734 (*ir*)
Parshall, G.W., *J. Am. Chem. Soc.*, 1965, **87**, 2133 (*synth*)
Goggin, P.L. *et al*, *J. Chem. Soc. (A)*, 1966, 1462 (*ir*)
Coulson, D.R., *J. Am. Chem. Soc.*, 1976, **98**, 3111 (*cmr*)

$C_{18}H_{35}Cl_3P_2Pt$ Pt-00213

Trichlorophenylbis(triethylphosphine)platinum, 9CI
Phenylbis(triethylphosphine)trichloroplatinum
[51351-70-3]

M 614.861

Yellow cryst. (CCl_4). Mp 102-102.5°. Converted to [PEt_3Ph][$PtCl_3(PEt_3)$] on heating in polar solvs.

Coulson, D.R., *J. Chem. Soc., Dalton Trans.*, 1973, 2459 (*synth*, *nmr*)

$C_{18}H_{35}Cl_3P_2PtSn$ Pt-00214

Phenyl(trichlorostannyl)bis(triethylphosphine)platinum, 9CI
Phenyl(trichlorotin)bis(triethylphosphine)platinum

M 733.551

trans-form [21773-69-3]
Cryst. (C_6H_6/hexane). Mp 186-8° dec.

Parshall, G.W., *J. Am. Chem. Soc.*, 1966, **88**, 704 (*synth*)
Coulson, D.R., *J. Am. Chem. Soc.*, 1976, **98**, 3111 (*cmr*)
Butler, G. *et al*, *J. Organomet. Chem.*, 1979, **181**, 47 (*nmr*)
Koch, B.R. *et al*, *Inorg. Chim. Acta*, 1980, **45**, L51 (*nmr*)

$C_{18}H_{35}IP_2Pt$ Pt-00215

Iodo(phenyl)bis(triethylphosphine)platinum, 9CI
Phenyliodobis(triethylphosphine)platinum

cis-form

M 635.407

cis-form [56553-44-7]
Isomerisation to *trans*-form well documented, but no physical data reported.

trans-form [15559-63-4]
Cryst. (pet. ether). Mp 122°. Dipole moment 3.25D.

Booth, G. *et al*, *J. Chem. Soc. (A)*, 1966, 635 (*synth*)
Coulson, D., *J. Am. Chem. Soc.*, 1976, **98**, 3111 (*cmr*)
Louw, W.J. *et al*, *Inorg. Chem.*, 1979, **19**, 2878 (*isom*)
Rieke, R.D. *et al*, *J. Org. Chem.*, 1979, **44**, 3069 (*synth*)

$C_{18}H_{36}Cl_4O_2Pt_2$ Pt-00216

Di-μ-chlorodichlorobis[3,3-dimethyl-1-(1-methylethoxy-)butylidene]diplatinum, 10CI
Di-μ-chlorodichlorobis[(2,2-dimethylpropyl)(1-methylethoxy)methylene]diplatinum. Di-μ-chlorodichlorobis[neopentyl(isopropoxy)methylene]diplatinum. Tetrachlorobis[3,3-dimethyl-1-(1-methylethoxy)butylidene]-diplatinum
[71514-51-7]

M 816.453
Bridged dimer. Cryst. (hexane/Et_2O).
Monomer: Dichloro[3,3-dimethyl-1-(1-methylethoxy)-butylidene]platinum.
$C_9H_{18}Cl_2OPt$ M 408.227
Unknown.

Pukhnarevich, V.B. *et al*, *J. Gen. Chem. USSR*, 1972, **42**, 2677 (*synth*)
Struchkov, Yu.T. *et al*, *J. Organomet. Chem.*, 1979, **172**, 269 (*struct*)

$C_{18}H_{36}P_2Pt$ Pt-00217

Di(1-propynyl)bis(triethylphosphine)platinum, 9CI
Bis(methylethynyl)bis(triethylphosphine)platinum. Bis-(methylacetylide)bis(triethylphosphine)platinum. Bis-(triethylphosphine)dipropynylplatinum

M 509.510

trans-form [34230-61-0]
Cryst. (pet. ether). Mp 93-95.5°.

Chatt, J. *et al*, *J. Chem. Soc.*, 1959, 4020 (*synth*)
Masai, H. *et al*, *Bull. Chem. Soc. Jpn.*, 1971, **44**, 2226 (*uv*)

$C_{18}H_{40}N_2O_4Pt_2$ Pt-00218

(μ-Ethylenediamine)hexamethylbis(2,4-pentanedionato)diplatinum, 8CI
Bis(acetylacetonato)(μ-ethylenediamine)hexamethyldiplatinum. (μ-1,2-Diaminoethane-N:N′)-hexamethylbis(2,4-pentanedionato-O,O′]diplatinum
[17375-22-3]

M 738.685
Cryst.

Robson, A. *et al*, *J. Chem. Soc.*, 1965, 630 (*struct*)
Kite, K. *et al*, *J. Chem. Soc. (A)*, 1966, 1744 (*pmr*)
Kite, K. *et al*, *J. Chem. Soc. (A)*, 1968, 934 (*ir, uv*)

$C_{18}H_{45}P_3Pt$ Pt-00219

Tris(triethylphosphine)platinum, 9CI
[39045-37-9]

$[Pt(PEt_3)_3]$

M 549.555
Catalyses water-gas shift reaction and photolysis of water. Viscous orange-red oil, extremely air-sensitive. Sol. saturated hydrocarbons. Reacts with halocarbons. Reversibly adds water to give $[PtH(PEt_3)_3]OH$.

Inorg. Synth., 1979, **19**, 107 (*synth*)
Yoshida, T. *et al*, *J. Am. Chem. Soc.*, 1979, **101**, 2027 (*use*)
Mann, B.E. *et al*, *J. Chem. Soc., Dalton Trans.*, 1980, 776 (*nmr*)

$C_{18}H_{46}P_3Pt^{\oplus}$ Pt-00220

Hydrotris(triethylphosphine)platinum(1+), 9CI, 8CI
Hydridotris(triethylphosphine)platinum(1+)
[48074-87-9]

$[PtH(PEt_3)_3]^{\oplus}$ (C_{2v})

M 550.563 (ion)
Catalyses alkene hydroformylation.
Perchlorate: [22653-44-7].

$C_{18}H_{46}ClO_4P_3Pt$ M 650.013
Cryst. (CH_2Cl_2/hexane). Mp 158-60°.
Tetraphenylborate: [22276-37-5].
$C_{42}H_{66}BP_3Pt$ M 869.795
Cryst. (Me_2CO/Et_2O). Mp 133-4°.

Church, M.J. *et al*, *J. Chem. Soc. (A)*, 1968, 3074 (*synth, ir*)
Clark, H.C. *et al*, *J. Am. Chem. Soc.*, 1969, **91**, 596 (*synth, ir*)
Giustiniani, M. *et al*, *J. Chem. Soc. (A)*, 1969, 2046 (*synth, props*)
Cetinkaya, B. *et al*, *J. Chem. Soc., Dalton Trans.*, 1973, 906 (*pmr*)
Dingle, T.W. *et al*, *Inorg. Chem.*, 1974, **13**, 846 (*nmr*)
Russell, D.R. *et al*, *J. Chem. Soc., Dalton Trans.*, 1980, 1737 (*struct*)

$C_{18}O_{18}Pt_9^{\ominus\ominus}$ Pt-00221

Nona-μ-carbonylnonacarbonylnonaplatinate(2−), 9CI
Tris[hexacarbonyltriplatinate](2−)
[52399-67-4]

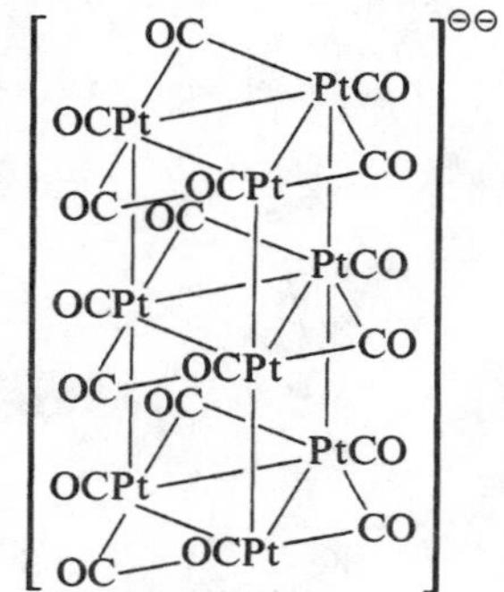

M 2259.907 (ion)
Used in prep. of alumina-supported Pt catalyst for hexane isomerization. Red-violet soln. in THF.
Bis(tetraethylammonium) salt: [59451-61-5].
$C_{34}H_{40}N_2O_{18}Pt_9$ M 2520.413
Catalyses hydrocarbon and methanol synthesis; used for prep. of silica-supported Pt catalyst for low-temp. hydrocarbon hydrogenolysis.

Calabrese, J.C. *et al*, *J. Am. Chem. Soc.*, 1974, **96**, 2614 (*synth, ir, struct*)
Ichikawa, M., *Bull. Chem. Soc. Jpn.*, 1978, **51**, 2268 (*use*)
Apai, G. *et al*, *J. Am. Chem. Soc.*, 1979, **101**, 6880 (*synth*)
Brown, C. *et al*, *J. Organomet. Chem.*, 1979, **181**, 233 (*cmr, nmr*)
Garin, F. *et al*, *Surf. Sci.*, 1981, **106**, 466 (*use*)
Simpson, A.F. *et al*, *J. Organomet. Chem.*, 1981, **213**, 157 (*use*)

$C_{19}H_{15}AsCl_2OPt$ Pt-00222

Carbonyldichloro(triphenylarsine)platinum
Dichlorocarbonyl(triphenylarsine)platinum

Cl AsPh$_3$ / Pt / Cl CO *cis-form*

M 600.235
***cis*-form** [71600-57-2]
Cryst.
***trans*-form** [73347-22-5]
Obt. only in soln. Hydroformylation catalyst with $SnCl_2$. Yellow. Readily isom. to *cis*-form, catalysed by CO.

Anderson, G.K. *et al*, *J. Chem. Res. (S)*, 1979, 120; *J. Chem. Res. (M)*, 1601 (*nmr, ir*)
Anderson, G.K. *et al*, *J. Chem. Soc., Dalton Trans.*, 1980, 1988 (*synth, ir*)

$C_{19}H_{15}Cl_2OPPt$ Pt-00223

Carbonyldichloro(triphenylphosphine)platinum, 8CI
[22585-09-7]
As Carbonyldichloro(triethylphosphine)platinum, Pt-00054 with

$$R^1 = R^2 = Ph$$

M 556.287
***cis*-form** [19618-78-1]
Cryst. (EtOH). Mp 220-30° dec. Dipole moment 9.65 D.
***trans*-form** [73347-20-3]
Yellow solid; loses CO on heating. Readily isom. in soln. to *cis*-form.

Smithies, A.C. *et al*, *J. Organomet. Chem.*, 1968, **12**, 199 (*synth, ir*)
Klassen, K.L. *et al*, *J. Inorg. Nucl. Chem.*, 1973, **35**, 2602 (*ir, ms*)
Manojlović-Muir, L. *et al*, *J. Chem. Soc., Dalton Trans.*, 1976, 1279 (*struct*)
Anderson, G.K. *et al*, *J. Chem. Res.*, 1979, M1601, S120 (*cmr*)
Anderson, G.K. *et al*, *J. Chem. Soc., Dalton Trans.*, 1980, 1988 (*synth, nmr, ir*)

$C_{19}H_{16}Pt$ Pt-00224

[(2,3,5,6-η)-Bicyclo[2.2.1]hepta-2,5-diene](1,1′-biphenyl-2,2′-diyl)platinum, 9CI
Norbornadiene(1,1′-biphenyl-2,2′-diyl)platinum. 5,5-Norbornadienedibenzoplatinide
[51112-50-6]

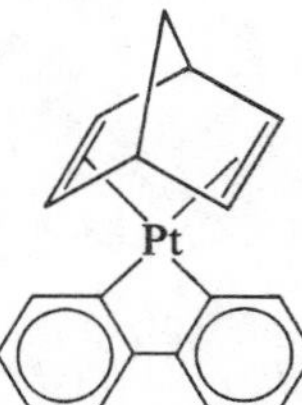

M 439.415
Brown cryst. (C_6H_6/hexane). Mp 200-2°.

Gardner, S.A. *et al*, *J. Organomet. Chem.*, 1973, **60**, 179.

$C_{19}H_{18}Pt$ Pt-00225

[(2,3,5,6-η)-Bicyclo[2.2.1]hepta-2,5-diene]diphenylplatinum, 9CI
2,5-Norbornadienediphenylplatinum, 8CI. Diphenyl(2,5-norbornadiene)platinum
[32966-32-8]

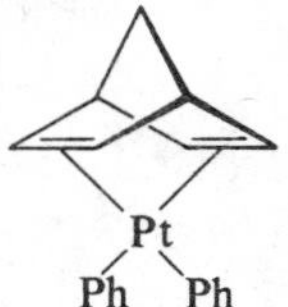

M 441.431
Catalyses hydrosilylation of alkenes. Cryst. (hexane). Mp 146-52°.

Kistner, C. *et al*, *Inorg. Chem.*, 1963, **2**, 1255 (*synth*)
Seguitz, A. *et al*, *J. Organomet. Chem.*, 1977, **124**, 113 (*synth*)

$C_{19}H_{20}Cl_2N_2Pt$ Pt-00226

Dichloro(2-phenyl-1,3-propanediyl)bis(pyridine)platinum, 9CI
Dichlorobis(pyridine)(2-phenyl-1,3-propanediyl)platinum
[38889-63-3]

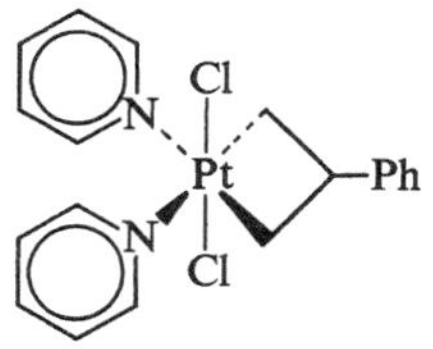

M 542.366
Cryst. (EtOH). Mp 130° dec.

McQuillin, F.J. *et al*, *J. Chem. Soc., Dalton Trans.*, 1972, 2123 (*synth, ir*)
Inorg. Synth., 1976, **16**, 113 (*synth*)

$C_{19}H_{24}F_6OPt_2$ Pt-00227

Bis[(1,2,5,6-η)-1,5-cyclooctadiene][μ-[(1,1,1,3,3,3-hexafluoro-2-propanolato(2−)-C^2,O]diplatinum, 9CI
Bis(1,5-cyclooctadiene)(μ-hexafluoroacetone)diplatinum
[57197-50-9]

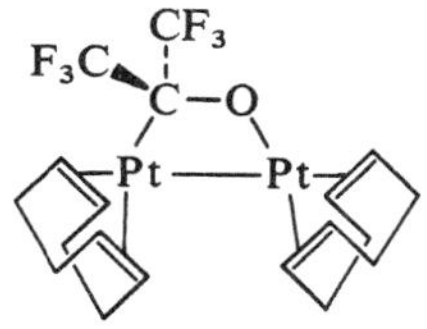

M 772.548
Yellow cryst. (Et_2O). Mp 180° dec.

Green, M. *et al*, *J. Chem. Soc., Dalton Trans.*, 1977, 278 (*synth, ir, nmr, struct*)

$C_{19}H_{27}ClP_2Pt$ Pt-00228

Chloro(cyclopropyl)bis(dimethylphenylphosphine)platinum, 9CI
Cyclopropyl(chloro)bis(dimethylphenylphosphine)platinum. Bis(dimethylphenylphosphine)-chloro(cyclopropyl)platinum

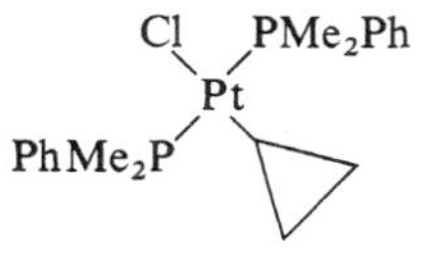

M 547.903
trans-form [64522-78-7]
Cryst. (C_6H_6/pet. ether). Mp 156°.

Phillips, R.L. *et al*, *J. Chem. Soc., Dalton Trans.*, 1978, 1732.

$C_{19}H_{27}Cl_2N_2PPt$ Pt-00229

Dichloro[bis(phenylamino)methylene](triethylphosphine)platinum
Dichloro[bis(phenylamino)carbene](triethylphosphine)-platinum. Dichloro(dianilinomethylene)(triethylphosphine)platinum, 8CI

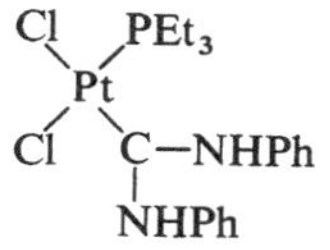

M 580.395
cis-form
Cryst. (EtOH). Mp 235-6°.

Richards, R.L. *et al*, *J. Chem. Soc. (A)*, 1971, 21 (*synth, ir, pmr*)
Inorg. Synth., 1979, **19**, 174 (*synth*)

$C_{19}H_{27}P_2Pt^{\oplus}$ Pt-00230

Bis(dimethylphenylphosphine)(η^3-2-propenyl)platinum(1+), 9CI
(π-Allyl)bis(dimethylphenylphosphine)platinum(1+). Bis(dimethylphenylphosphine)(π-enyl)platinum(1+)

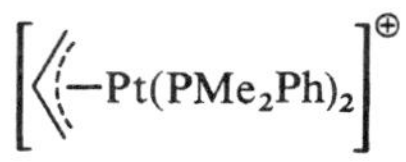

M 512.450 (ion)
Hexafluorophosphate: [37668-23-8].
$C_{19}H_{27}F_6P_3Pt$ M 657.414
Cryst. (CH_2Cl_2/pentane). Mp 158-60°.

Clark, H.C. *et al*, *Inorg. Chem.*, 1972, **11**, 1275 (*synth, pmr*)
Phillips, R.L. *et al*, *J. Organomet. Chem.*, 1977, **136**, C52.

$C_{19}H_{29}As_2IPt$ Pt-00231

[1,2-Ethanediylbis(methylphenylarsine)-*As,As'*]iodotrimethylplatinum, 9CI
[Ethylenebis(methylphenylarsine)]iodotrimethylplatinum

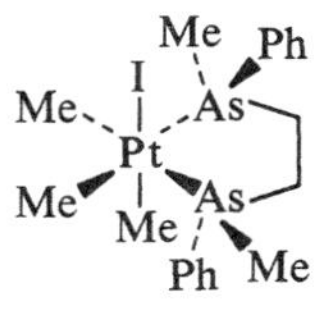

(±)-*form*

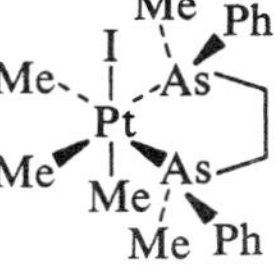

meso-form

M 729.266
(±)-form [50701-18-3]
Pale-yellow cryst. (C_6H_6/pet. ether). Mp 162-9° dec.
meso-form [36670-15-2]
Pale-yellow cryst. (EtOH). Mp 186-92° dec.

Cheney, A.J. *et al*, *J. Chem. Soc. (A)*, 1971, 3549 (*synth, pmr, ir*)
Casalone, G. *et al*, *Inorg. Chim. Acta*, 1973, **7**, 429 (*struct*)

$C_{19}H_{31}IP_2Pt$ Pt-00232

Bis(dimethylphenylphosphine)iodotrimethylplatinum, 9CI

Iodotrimethylbis(dimethylphenylphosphine)platinum. Trimethyliodobis(dimethylphenylphosphine)platinum

[40894-89-1]

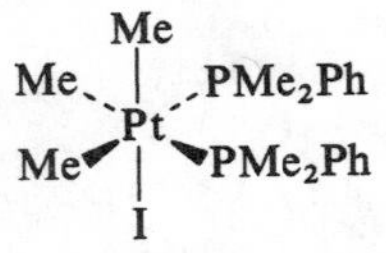

M 643.386

Yellow cryst. (C_6H_6/pet. ether). Mp 144-6°, 155-60° dec. Dipole moment 7.4D.

Ruddick, J.D. *et al*, *J. Chem. Soc. (A)*, 1969, 2801 (*synth*, *pmr*, *ir*)
Treichel, P.M. *et al*, *J. Organomet. Chem.*, 1973, **61**, 415 (*synth*, *ir*)
King, R.B. *et al*, *J. Am. Chem. Soc.*, 1974, **96**, 1338 (*synth*, *struct*)
Seddon, K.R. *et al*, *J. Chem. Soc., Dalton Trans.*, 1974, 2415 (*ir*, *raman*)

$C_{19}H_{33}Cl_2OPPt$ Pt-00233

Carbonyldichloro(tricyclohexylphosphine)platinum

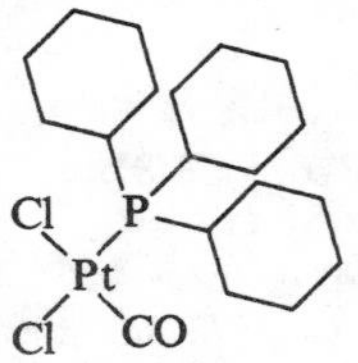

cis-form

M 574.429

cis-form [19618-81-6]

Cocatalyst with $SnCl_2$ for hydroformylation reaction. Cryst. ($CHCl_3$/Et_2O).

trans-form [76189-24-7]

Not isol. ir ν_{CO} 2125 cm^{-1}. Isom. in soln. to *cis*-form.

Anderson, G.K. *et al*, *J. Chem. Soc., Dalton Trans.*, 1980, 712 (*synth*)
Anderson, G.K. *et al*, *Inorg. Chem.*, 1981, **20**, 944 (*synth*)
Anderson, G.K. *et al*, *Inorg. Chem.*, 1981, **20**, 1636.

$C_{19}H_{33}F_5P_2Pt$ Pt-00234

Methyl(pentafluorophenyl)bis(triethylphosphine)platinum, 9CI

Bis(triethylphosphine)methyl(pentafluorophenyl)platinum. (Pentafluorophenyl)methylbis(triethylphosphine)-platinum

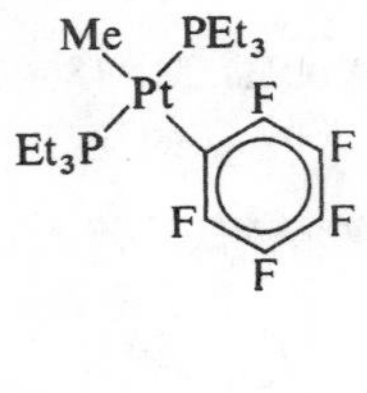

M 613.489

trans-form [15697-56-0]

Cryst. (MeOH). Mp 101-2°.

Hopton, F.J. *et al*, *J. Chem. Soc. (A)*, 1966, 1326 (*synth*, *nmr*)
Goggin, P.L. *et al*, *J. Chem. Soc. (A)*, 1966, 1462 (*ir*)

$C_{19}H_{35}NP_2Pt$ Pt-00235

(Cyano-*C*)phenylbis(triethylphosphine)platinum, 9CI

Phenylcyanobis(triethylphosphine)platinum

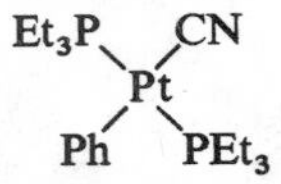

M 534.520

trans-form [33914-65-7]

Cryst. (hexane). Mp 127-8° (113-9°).

Gerlach, D.H. *et al*, *J. Am. Chem. Soc.*, 1971, **93**, 3543 (*synth*)
Coulson, D.R., *J. Am. Chem. Soc.*, 1976, **98**, 3111 (*cmr*)
Rieke, R.D. *et al*, *J. Org. Chem.*, 1979, **44**, 3069 (*synth*)

$C_{19}H_{37}ClP_2Pt$ Pt-00236

Chloro(4-methylphenyl)bis(triethylphosphine)platinum, 9CI

(p-*Tolyl*)*chlorobis(triethylphosphine)platinum*

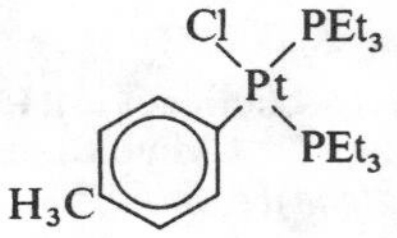

M 557.982

cis-form [69176-04-1]

Cryst. (C_6H_6/pet. ether). Mp 130-8° dec. Dipole moment 8.95D.

Chatt, J. *et al*, *J. Chem. Soc.*, 1959, 4020 (*synth*)
Bresciani-Pahor, N. *et al*, *Inorg. Chim. Acta*, 1978, **31**, 171 (*struct*)

$C_{19}H_{37}ClP_2Pt$ Pt-00237

Chloro(2-methylphenyl)bis(triethylphosphine)platinum, 10CI, 9CI

Chloro(o-*tolyl*)*bis(triethylphosphine)platinum*, *8CI*

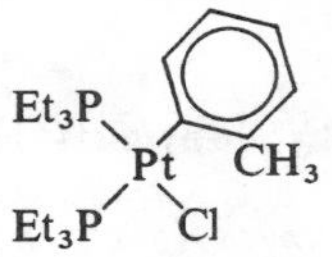

cis-form

M 557.982

Substitution and isomerisation reactions extensively examined.

cis-form [33395-88-9]

Cryst. (C_6H_6/pet. ether). Mp 153-7°. Dipole moment 9.15D. Spontaneously converts to *trans*-form in MeOH or EtOH.

trans-form [29961-88-4]

Cryst. (Et_2O). Sol. org. solvs. Mp 104-5°. Dipole moment 2.35D.

Chatt, J. *et al*, *J. Chem. Soc.*, 1959, 4020 (*synth*)
Basolo, F. *et al*, *J. Chem. Soc.*, 1961, 2207 (*synth*)

$C_{19}H_{37}ClP_2Pt$ Pt-00238

Chloro(3-methylphenyl)bis(triethylphosphine)platinum, 10CI

Chloro(m-*tolyl*)*bis(triethylphosphine)platinum*

[74824-29-6]

M 557.982

cis-form [70445-93-1]

Cryst. (C_6H_6/Et_2O). Mp 122-5°.

trans-form

Cryst. (pet. ether). Mp 82-4°.

Romeo, R. *et al*, *Inorg. Chem.*, 1979, **18**, 2362; 1980, **19**, 3663 (*synth, ir, pmr*)

$C_{19}H_{43}OP_2Pt^{\oplus}$ Pt-00239

Carbonyl(hydrido)bis(triisopropylphosphine)platinum(1+)

Carbonyl(hydro)bis[tris(1-methylethyl)phosphine]platinum(1+)

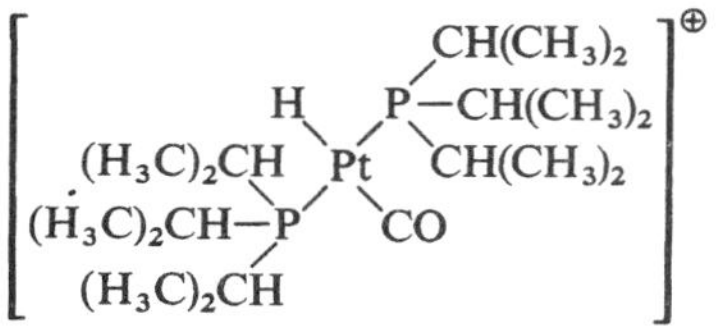

[H, CO, Pt, P–CH(CH₃)₂ ...]$^{\oplus}$ *trans-form*

M 544.576 (ion)

Catalyses water-gas shift reaction.

trans-form

Hydroxide:

$C_{19}H_{44}O_2P_2Pt$ M 561.583

Not isol. Intermed. in water-gas shift reaction.

Tetraphenylborate:

$C_{43}H_{63}BOP_2Pt$ M 863.808

Solid. ir ν_{PtH} 2178cm^{-1} ν_{CO} 2058cm^{-1}.

Yoshida, T. *et al*, *J. Am. Chem. Soc.*, 1978, **100**, 3941 (*synth, ir, pmr*)

$C_{19}H_{45}OP_3Pt$ Pt-00240

Carbonyltris(triethylphosphine)platinum

$Pt(CO)(PEt_3)_3$ (C_{3v})

M 577.565

Not isol. Should be manipulated under CO atm.

Chini, P. *et al*, *J. Chem. Soc. (A)*, 1970, 1542 (*ir*)

$C_{19}H_{46}P_2Pt$ Pt-00241

Hydridomethylbis(triisopropylphosphine)platinum

Hydromethylbis[tris(1-methylethyl)phosphine]platinum, 10CI. *Methylhydridobis[tris(1-methylethyl)phosphine]platinum*

[76125-04-7]

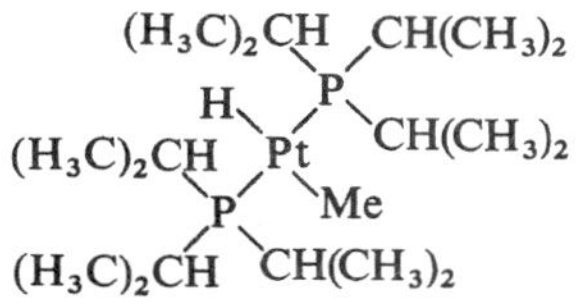

M 531.600

Cryst. (toluene/MeOH).

Abis, L. *et al*, *J. Organomet. Chem.*, 1981, **215**, 263 (*synth, pmr, ir*)

$C_{20}H_{17}AsCl_2Pt$ Pt-00242

Dichloro[[2-(η^2-ethenyl)phenyl]diphenylarsine-*As*]platinum, 9CI

Dichloro[(2-vinylphenyl)diphenylarsine]platinum

[56845-26-2]

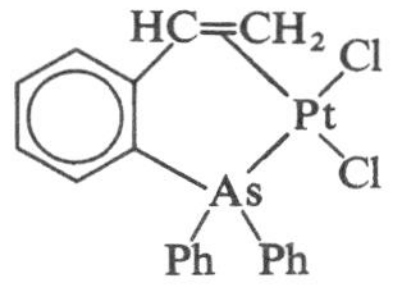

M 598.262

Yellow cryst. ($CHCl_3$/EtOH). Mp 260° dec.

Cooper, M.K. *et al*, *J. Organomet. Chem.*, 1975, **91**, 117 (*synth, pmr*)

Cooper, M.K. *et al*, *J. Chem. Soc., Dalton Trans.*, 1980, 349 (*struct*)

$C_{20}H_{18}Cl_2NPPt$ Pt-00243

Dichloro(isocyanomethane)(triphenylphosphine)platinum, 9CI

Dichloro(methyl isocyanide)(triphenylphosphine)platinum, 8CI. *Dichloro(methylisonitrile)(triphenylphosphine)platinum*

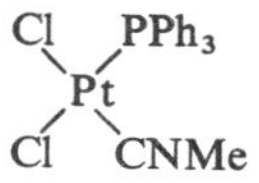

M 569.329

cis-form [33989-94-5]

Cryst. (C_6H_6). Mp 264-7°.

Treichel, P.M. *et al*, *J. Am. Chem. Soc.*, 1971, **93**, 5424 (*synth, ir, pmr*)

Fehlhammer, W.P. *et al*, *Angew. Chem., Int. Ed. Engl.*, 1975, **14**, 757.

$C_{20}H_{18}IOPPt$ Pt-00244

Carbonyl(iodo)methyl(triphenylphosphine)platinum, 9CI

Methyl(triphenylphosphine)carbonylplatinum iodide

[52348-99-9]

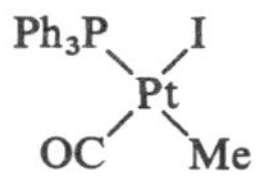

M 627.320

Yellow cryst.

Wilson, C.J. *et al*, *J. Chem. Soc., Dalton Trans.*, 1974, 421, 1293 (*synth, ir, pmr*)

$C_{20}H_{19}AsCl_2Pt$ Pt-00245

Dichloro(ethylene)(triphenylarsine)platinum

Dichloro(η^2-ethene)(triphenylarsine)platinum, 10CI

[38498-13-4]

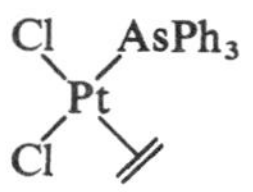

M 600.278

Cryst. ($CHCl_3$). Dec. without melting at 100° to lose C_2H_4.

Ashley-Smith, J. *et al*, *J. Chem. Soc., Dalton Trans.*, 1972, 1776 (*ir, nmr*)

De Renzi, A. *et al*, *Gazz. Chim. Ital.*, 1972, **102**, 413 (*synth, ir, pmr*)

$C_{20}H_{19}Cl_2PPt$ Pt-00246

Dichloro(ethylene)(triphenylphosphine)platinum, 8CI

Dichloro(η^2-ethene)(triphenylphosphine)platinum, 9CI

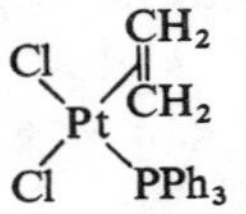

M 556.330

Catalyses cleavage of organosilicon bonds.

cis-form [38095-87-3]

Cryst. ($CHCl_3$/toluene). Loses C_2H_4 above 100° to form $[Pt_2Cl_4(PPh_3)_2]$.

Panunzi, A. *et al*, *J. Am. Chem. Soc.*, 1969, **91**, 3879 (*synth*)
De Renzi, A. *et al*, *Gazz. Chim. Ital.*, 1972, **102**, 413.

$C_{20}H_{22}Pt$ Pt-00247

[(1,2,5,6-η)-1,5-Cyclooctadiene]diphenylplatinum, 9CI

Diphenyl(1,5-cyclooctadiene)platinum

[12277-88-2]

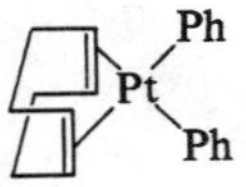

M 457.474

Catalyses hydrosilylation of alkenes. Cryst. (C_6H_6). Mp 52° dec.

Kistner, C.R. *et al*, *Inorg. Chem.*, 1963, **2**, 1255 (*synth*)
Eaborn, C. *et al*, *J. Chem. Soc., Dalton Trans.*, 1978, 357 (*ir, nmr*)
Anderson, G.K. *et al*, *Inorg. Chem.*, 1981, **20**, 1636.

$C_{20}H_{26}Cl_2P_2Pt$ Pt-00248

Bis(1-chloroethenyl)bis(dimethylphenylphosphine)platinum, 9CI

Bis(1-chlorovinyl)bis(dimethylphenylphosphine)platinum

$(H_2C{=}CCl)_2Pt(PMe_2Ph)_2$

M 594.359

trans-form [60293-84-7]

Cryst. (toluene/pet. ether). Mp 130°. Dec. >130° to C_2H_2 + *trans*-$PtCl(CCl{=}CH_2)(PMe_2Ph)_2$.

Bell, R.A. *et al*, *J. Am. Chem. Soc.*, 1976, **98**, 6046 (*synth, struct, pmr*)
Bell, R.A. *et al*, *Inorg. Chem.*, 1977, **16**, 677, 687 (*synth, pmr*)

$C_{20}H_{26}F_6N_2O_4Pt_2$ Pt-00249

Tetramethylbis(4-methylpyridine)bis[μ-(trifluoroacetate-*O,O'*)]diplatinum, 9CI

Tetramethylbis(4-picoline)bis[μ-(trifluoroacetato-O:O')]diplatinum

[63056-61-1]

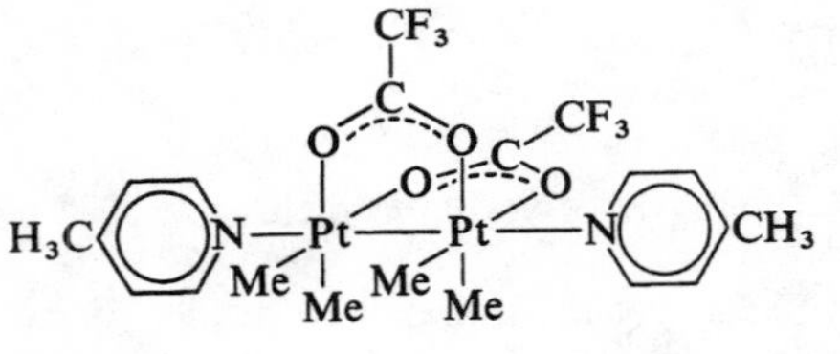

M 862.587

Yellow cryst.

Kuyper, J. *et al*, *Transition Met. Chem.*, 1976, **1**, 208 (*synth, pmr, cmr*)
Schagen, J.D. *et al*, *Inorg. Chem.*, 1978, **17**, 1938 (*struct*)

$C_{20}H_{28}Cl_4P_2Pt_2$ Pt-00250

μ-[(1,2:3,4-η)Butadiene]tetrachlorobis(dimethylphenylphosphine)diplatinum

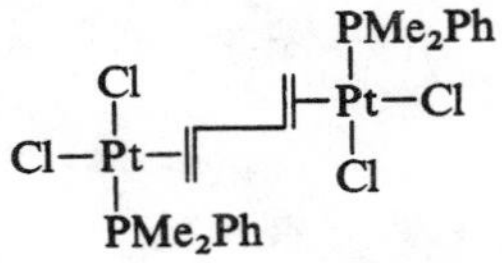

M 862.361

Cryst. (Me_2CO), dec. >130°. *meso* isomer.

Briggs, J.R. *et al*, *J. Chem. Soc., Dalton Trans.*, 1982, 457 (*synth, nmr, struct*)

$C_{20}H_{28}P_2Pt$ Pt-00251

(Diphenylacetylene)bis(trimethylphosphine)platinum

[1,1'-(η^2-1,2-Ethynediyl)bis[benzene]]bis(trimethylphosphine)platinum, 10CI. *Diphenylethynebis(trimethylphosphine)platinum*

[75982-99-9]

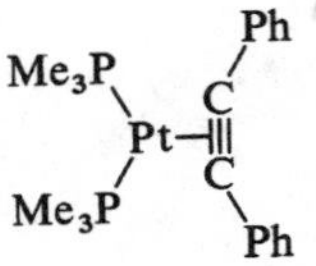

M 525.469

Cryst. (pet. ether).

Boag, N.M. *et al*, *J. Chem. Soc., Dalton Trans.*, 1980, 2171 (*synth, ir, nmr*)

$C_{20}H_{30}I_2P_2Pt$ Pt-00252

1,4-Butanediylbis(dimethylphenylphosphine)diiodoplatinum, 9CI

(1,4-Butanediyl)diiodobis(dimethylphenylphosphine)platinum

[59991-49-0]

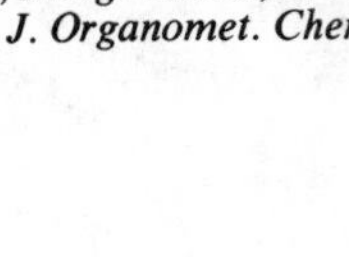

M 781.294

Orange-red cryst. (CH_2Cl_2/MeOH). Mp 214° dec.

Brown, M.P. *et al*, *J. Chem. Soc., Dalton Trans.*, 1976, 786 (*synth, pmr*)
Cheetham, A.K. *et al*, *Inorg. Chem.*, 1976, **15**, 2997 (*struct*)
Perkins, D.C.L. *et al*, *J. Organomet. Chem.*, 1978, **154**, C16.

$C_{20}H_{31}OP_2Pt^{\oplus}$ Pt-00253

Bis(dimethylphenylphosphine)methyl[methyl(methoxy)methylene]platinum(1+)

Bis(dimethylphenylphosphine)(1-methoxyethylidene)methylplatinum(1+), 9CI, 8CI. *Bis(dimethylphenylphosphine)[methoxy(methyl)carbene]methylplatinum(1+)*

Me, PMe_2Ph, Pt, CH_3, $PhMe_2P$, C, OMe ($\oplus$)

M 544.492 (ion)

trans-form

Hexafluorophosphate: [27776-75-6].
$C_{20}H_{31}F_6OP_3Pt$ M 689.456
Cryst. ($MeOH/Et_2O$). Mp 148-50° dec.

Chisholm, M.H. *et al*, *Inorg. Chem.*, 1971, **10**, 1711 (*synth*)
Stepaniak, R.F. *et al*, *J. Organomet. Chem.*, 1973, **57**, 213 (*struct*)
Chisholm, M.H. *et al*, *Inorg. Chem.*, 1975, **14**, 900.
Bell, R.A. *et al*, *Inorg. Chem.*, 1977, **16**, 677.

$C_{20}H_{33}ClP_2PtSi$ Pt-00254

Chlorobis(dimethylphenylphosphine)(trimethylsilylmethyl)platinum, 9CI

(Trimethylsilylmethyl)chlorobis(dimethylphenylphosphine)platinum

Cl, PMe_2Ph, Pt, Me_3SiH_2C, PMe_2Ph *cis-form*

M 594.047

cis-form [33937-92-7]

Converts in soln. to mixt. of *cis-* and *trans-*forms, catalysed by traces of PMe_2Ph.

Collier, M.R. *et al*, *J. Chem. Soc., Chem. Commun.*, 1972, 613 (*synth*)
Jovanović, B. *et al*, *J. Chem. Soc., Dalton Trans.*, 1974, 195 (*struct*)

$C_{20}H_{34}As_2Pt$ Pt-00255

Bis(dimethylphenylarsine)tetramethylplatinum, 8CI

Tetramethylbis(dimethylphenylarsine)platinum

$Me_4Pt(AsMe_2Ph)_2$

M 619.412

cis-form [17567-55-4]

Cryst. (Et_2O/pet. ether). Mp 95-101°. Dipole moment 5.4D.

Ruddick, J.D. *et al*, *J. Chem. Soc. (A)*, 1969, 2965 (*synth, pmr, ir*)

$C_{20}H_{34}P_2Pt$ Pt-00256

Bis(dimethylphenylphosphine)tetramethylplatinum, 8CI

Tetramethylbis(dimethylphenylphosphine)platinum

$Me_4Pt(PMe_2Ph)_2$

M 531.516

cis-form [17567-56-5]

Cryst. (pet. ether). Mp 123-9° dec. Dipole moment 5.75D.

Ruddick, J.D. *et al*, *J. Chem. Soc. (A)*, 1969, 2801 (*synth, pmr, ir*)

$C_{20}H_{36}Cl_4Pt_2$ Pt-00257

Di-μ-chlorodichlorobis[(3,4-η)-2,2,5,5-tetramethyl-3-hexyne]diplatinum

*Di-μ-chlorodichlorobis[di(*tert*-butyl)acetylene]diplatinum*

$C(CH_3)_3$, C, Cl, Cl, $C(CH_3)_3$, C, Pt, Pt, $(H_3C)_3C$, Cl, Cl, C, C, $C(CH_3)_3$

M 808.476

Bridged dimer. Red cryst. (pet. ether). Mp 184-7° dec.

Monomer: Dichloro(2,2,5,5-tetramethyl-3-hexyne)platinum.
$C_{10}H_{18}Cl_2Pt$ M 404.238
Unknown.

Chatt, J. *et al*, *J. Chem. Soc.*, 1961, 827 (*synth*)

$C_{20}H_{36}Cl_8Pt_2Sn_2$ Pt-00258

Di-μ-chlorobis[(3,4-η)-2,2,5,5-tetramethyl-3-hexyne]bis(trichlorostannyl)diplatinum, 10CI

*Di-μ-chlorobis(di-*tert*-butylethyne)bis(trichlorostannyl)diplatinum*

[75525-41-6]

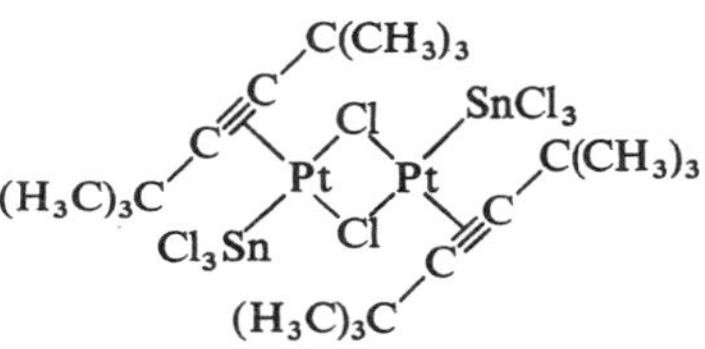

M 1187.668

Bridged dimer. Orange cryst. (chlorobenzene).

Monomer: Chloro(2,2,5,5-tetramethyl-3-hexyne)(trichlorostannyl)platinum.
$C_{10}H_{18}Cl_4PtSn$ M 593.834
Unknown.

Moreto, J. *et al*, *J. Chem. Soc., Dalton Trans.*, 1980, 1368 (*synth, ir, nmr*)

$C_{20}H_{36}O_4Pt_2$ Pt-00259

Di-μ-methoxobis[(1,4,5-η)-8-methoxy-4-cycloocten-1-yl]diplatinum

Di-μ-methoxybis[(1,4,5-η)-8-methoxy-4-cycloocten-1-yl]diplatinum, 9CI

[75534-44-0]

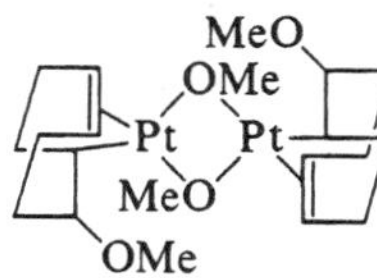

M 730.662

Cryst. (C_6H_6/MeOH). Mp 140-50° dec. Originally incompletely characterised as an "α-dimethoxide", $[C_8H_{12}Pt(OMe)_2]_n$.

Chatt, J. *et al*, *J. Chem. Soc.*, 1957, 2496.
Goel, A.B. *et al*, *Inorg. Chim. Acta*, 1981, **54**, L169 (*synth, struct*)

$C_{21}H_{15}O_3PPt$ Pt-00260

Tricarbonyl(triphenylphosphine)platinum, 9CI

[51455-30-2]

$Pt(CO)_3(PPh_3)$ (C_{3v})

M 541.401

Obt. only in soln. and under high pressure of CO.

Inglis, T. *et al*, *Nature* (*London*) Phys. Sci., 1972, **239**, 13 (*synth*, *ir*)
Whyman, R., *J. Organomet. Chem.*, 1973, **63**, 467 (*synth*, *ir*)

$C_{21}H_{20}AsClOPt$ Pt-00261

Carbonylchloro(ethyl)(triphenylarsine)platinum, 8CI
(Triphenylarsine)ethylchlorocarbonylplatinum
[32409-21-5]

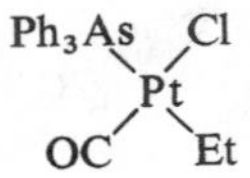

Ph_3As, Cl, Pt, OC, Et

M 593.843
Yellow cryst. (CH_2Cl_2/pet. ether).

Mawby, R.J. *et al*, *Inorg. Chem.*, 1971, **10**, 854 (*synth*, *ir*, *pmr*)

$C_{21}H_{20}ClPPt$ Pt-00262

Chloro(η^3-2-propenyl)(triphenylphosphine)platinum, 9CI
Allylchloro(triphenylphosphine)platinum
[35770-09-3]

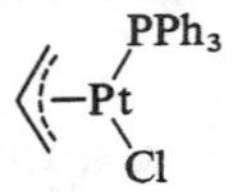

PPh_3, Pt, Cl

M 533.896
Cryst. Reacts with PPh_3 to generate (η^3-2-Propenyl)-bis(triphenylphosphine)platinum(1+), Pt-00398 (chloride).

Mann, B.E. *et al*, *J. Chem. Soc.* (*A*), 1971, 3536 (*synth*, *pmr*)
Carturan, G. *et al*, *J. Organomet. Chem.*, 1979, **172**, 91 (*nmr*)

$C_{21}H_{31}OP_2Pt^{\oplus}$ Pt-00263

[Dihydro-2(3*H*)-furanylidene]bis(dimethylphenylphosphine)-methylplatinum(1+), 9CI, 8CI
Methyl(2-oxacyclopentylidene)bis(dimethylphenyl-phosphine)platinum(1+)

$[PhMe_2P$, Me–Pt, $PhMe_2P]^{\oplus}$, O

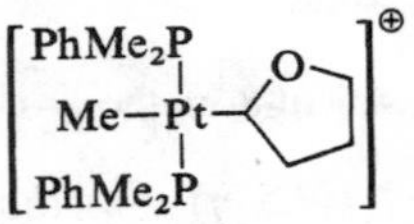

M 556.503 (ion)
Hexafluorophosphate: [27776-78-9].
$C_{21}H_{31}F_6OP_3Pt$ M 701.467
Cryst. (MeOH/Et_2O). Mp 155°.

Chisholm, M.H. *et al*, *Inorg. Chem.*, 1971, **10**, 1711.
Chisholm, M.H. *et al*, *J. Am. Chem. Soc.*, 1973, **95**, 8574 (*cmr*)
Stepaniak, R.F. *et al*, *J. Organomet. Chem.*, 1974, **72**, 453 (*struct*)
Chisholm, M.H. *et al*, *Inorg. Chem.*, 1975, **14**, 893, 900 (*cmr*, *pmr*)

$C_{21}H_{31}P_2Pt^{\oplus}$ Pt-00264

[(2,3-η)-2-Butyne]bis(dimethylphenylphosphine)methylplatinum(1+), 9CI
(Dimethylacetylene)bis(dimethylphenylphosphine)methylplatinum(1+). Methyl(2-butyne)-bis(dimethylphenylphosphine)platinum(1+)

$[PtMe(CH_3C{\equiv}CCH_3)(PMe_2Ph)_2]^{\oplus}$

M 540.503 (ion)

***trans*-form**
Hexafluorophosphate: [35797-58-1].
$C_{21}H_{31}F_6P_3Pt$ M 685.468
Cryst. (CH_2Cl_2/Et_2O). Mp 150° dec.

Chisholm, M.H. *et al*, *Inorg. Chem.*, 1971, **10**, 2557 (*synth*, *ir*, *pmr*)
Chisholm, M.H. *et al*, *J. Am. Chem. Soc.*, 1973, **95**, 8574 (*cmr*)
Davies, B.W. *et al*, *Can. J. Chem.*, 1973, **51**, 3477 (*struct*)

$C_{21}H_{34}NP_2Pt^{\oplus}$ Pt-00265

[(Dimethylamino)ethylidene]bis(dimethylphenylphosphine)-methylplatinum(1+), 9CI
[Dimethylamino(methyl)methylene]methylbis(dimethylphenylphosphine)platinum(1+). Methyl[N,N-dimethylamino(methyl)carbene]bis(dimethylphenyl-phosphine)platinum(1+)

[Me, PMe_2Ph, Pt, CH_3, $PhMe_2P$, C, $NMe_2]^{\oplus}$

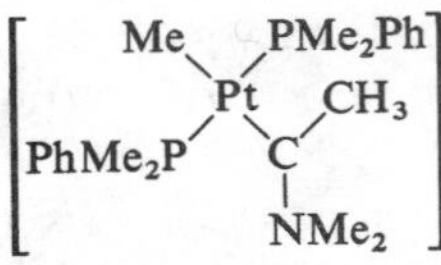

M 557.534 (ion)

***trans*-form**
Hexafluorophosphate: [49631-76-7].
$C_{21}H_{34}F_6NP_3Pt$ M 702.498
Cryst. (CH_2Cl_2). Mp 160°.

Stepaniak, R.F. *et al*, *Inorg. Chem.*, 1974, **13**, 797 (*struct*)
Chisholm, M.H. *et al*, *Inorg. Chem.*, 1975, **14**, 893, 900 (*pmr*, *cmr*)

$C_{21}H_{38}ClPPt$ Pt-00266

Chloro(η^3-2-propenyl)(tricyclohexylphosphine)platinum
Allylchloro(tricyclohexylphosphine)platinum
[71035-50-2]

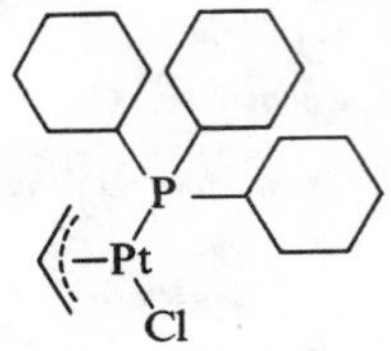

P, Pt, Cl

M 552.038
Cryst. (CH_2Cl_2/Et_2O). Mp 187°.

Carturan, G. *et al*, *J. Organomet. Chem.*, 1979, **172**, 91 (*synth*, *nmr*)

$C_{21}H_{41}BrP_2Pt$ Pt-00267

Bromobis(triethylphosphine)(2,4,6-trimethylphenyl)platinum, 9CI
Bromo(mesityl)bis(triethylphosphine)platinum. Bromo(2,4,6-trimethylphenyl)bis(triethylphosphine)-platinum. Mesitylbromobis(triethylphosphine)platinum

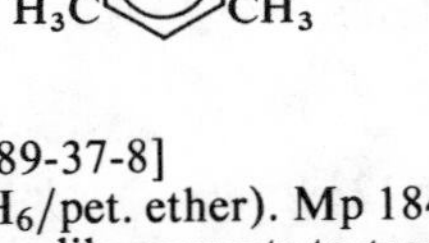

Br, PEt_3, H_3C, Pt, PEt_3, H_3C, CH_3 *cis-form*

M 630.486

***cis*-form** [22289-37-8]
Cryst. (C_6H_6/pet. ether). Mp 184-6°. Dipole moment 9.15D. Readily converts to *trans*-isomer in methanol.

trans-form [68681-91-4]
Cryst. (pet. ether). Mp 185.5-187° subl. Dipole moment 3.15D.

Chatt, J. *et al*, *J. Chem. Soc.*, 1959, 4020 (*synth*)
Basolo, F. *et al*, *J. Chem. Soc.*, 1961, 2207 (*synth*)
Romeo, R. *et al*, *Inorg. Chem.*, 1976, **15**, 1134.

$C_{21}H_{41}ClP_2Pt$ Pt-00268

Chlorobis(triethylphosphine)(2,4,6-trimethylphenyl)platinum, 9CI
Chloromesitylbis(triethylphosphine)platinum, 8CI.
(2,4,6-Trimethylphenyl)chlorobis(triethylphosphine)-platinum
[52021-49-5]

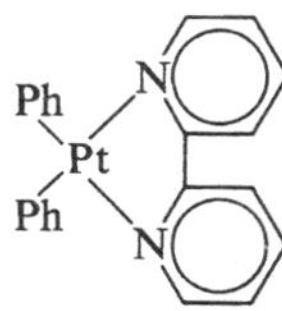

M 586.035
trans-form [25513-00-2]
Cryst. (pet. ether). Mp 196.5-197.5°. Subl. on melting. Dipole moment 2.45D.

Basolo, F. *et al*, *J. Chem. Soc.*, 1961, 2207 (*synth*)

$C_{22}H_{18}N_2Pt$ Pt-00269

(2,2′-Bipyridine-*N,N′*)diphenylplatinum, 9CI
Diphenyl(2,2′-bipyridine)platinum
[54891-36-0]

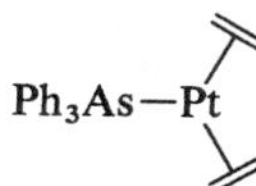

M 505.478
Yellow cryst. (CH_2Cl_2/Et_2O). Mp 290-300° dec.

Chaudhury, N. *et al*, *J. Organomet. Chem.*, 1975, **84**, 105 (*synth, uv*)
Usón, R. *et al Synth. React. Inorg. Met.-Org. Chem.*, 1977, **7**, 211 (*synth, ir*)

$C_{22}H_{20}N_2Pt$ Pt-00270

Diphenylbis(pyridine)platinum
Dipyridinediphenylplatinum

$PtPh_2Py_2$

M 507.493
Cryst. (CH_2Cl_2). Mp 157-65° dec.

Doyle, J.R. *et al*, *J. Am. Chem. Soc.*, 1961, **83**, 2768 (*synth*)
Kistner, C.R. *et al*, *Inorg. Chem.*, 1963, **2**, 1255 (*synth*)

$C_{22}H_{23}AsPt$ Pt-00271

Bis(ethylene)(triphenylarsine)platinum
Bis(η^2-ethene)(triphenylarsine)platinum, 10CI
[69134-56-1]

Ph₃As—Pt

M 557.425
Cryst. (pet. ether). Mp 82-6° dec.

Harrison, N.C. *et al*, *J. Chem. Soc., Dalton Trans.*, 1978, 1337 (*synth, ir, nmr*)

$C_{22}H_{23}PPt$ Pt-00272

Bis(ethylene)(triphenylphosphine)platinum
Bis(η^2-ethene)(triphenylphosphine)platinum, 9CI
[60038-75-7]

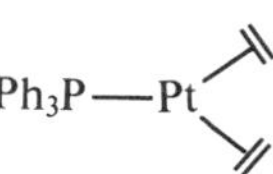

M 513.477
Cryst. (pet. ether). Mp 82-5° dec.

Harrison, N.C. *et al*, *J. Chem. Soc., Dalton Trans.*, 1978, 1337 (*synth, nmr*)

$C_{22}H_{30}Cl_2O_2Pt_2$ Pt-00273

Di-μ-chlorobis[(2,3,5-η)-3*a*,4,5,6,7,7*a*-hexahydro-6-methoxy-4,7-methano-1*H*-inden-5-yl]diplatinum, 9CI
Di-μ-chlorobis(methoxydicyclopentadiene)diplatinum.
Bis(dicyclopentadiene methoxide)-$\mu\mu'$-dichlorodiplatinum
[12156-15-9]

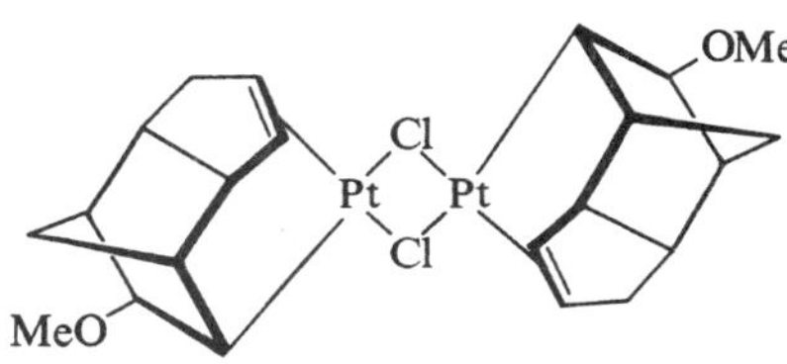

M 787.544
Bridged dimer. Vulcanisation accelerator for silicone rubber. Cryst. ($CHCl_3/Et_2O$). Mp 210-20° dec.
Monomer: Chloro(8-methoxytricyclo[5.2.1.0^{2,6}]dec-3-ene)platinum.
$C_{11}H_{15}ClOPt$ M 393.772
Unknown.

Chatt, J. *et al*, *J. Chem. Soc.*, 1957, 2496 (*synth*)
Stille, J.K. *et al*, *J. Am. Chem. Soc.*, 1966, **88**, 5135 (*synth, nmr*)

$C_{22}H_{33}ClP_2Pt$ Pt-00274

Chlorobis(diethylphenylphosphine)ethenylplatinum
Chlorobis(diethylphenylphosphine)vinylplatinum.
Vinylchlorobis(diethylphenylphosphine)platinum

$PtCl(CH{=}CH_2)(PEt_2Ph)_2$

M 589.983
trans-form [51466-64-9]
Cryst. (Me_2CO). Mp 108°.

Cardin, C.J. *et al*, *J. Chem. Soc., Dalton Trans.*, 1977, 767 (*synth, ir, nmr*)
Cardin, C.J. *et al*, *J. Chem. Soc., Dalton Trans.*, 1977, 1593 (*struct*)

$C_{22}H_{35}ClNOP_2Pt^{\oplus}$ Pt-00275

Chloro[dimethylamino(3-hydroxypropyl)methylene]bis(dimethylphenylphosphine)platinum(1+)

*Chloro(3-hydroxypropyl-*N,N*-dimethylaminocarbene)-bis(dimethylphenylphosphine)platinum(1+). Chloro[1-(dimethylamino)-4-hydroxybutylidene]bis(dimethylphenylphosphine)platinum(1+)*

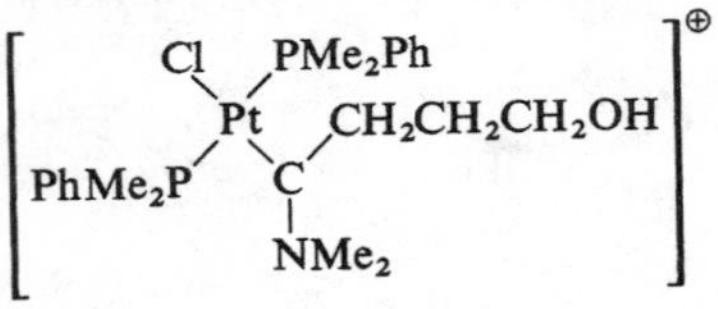

M 622.005 (ion)

trans-form

Hexafluorophosphate: [67352-53-8].
$C_{22}H_{35}ClF_6NOP_3Pt$ M 766.969
Cryst. (CH_2Cl_2/Et_2O).

Stepaniak, R.F., *Can. J. Chem.*, 1978, **56**, 1602 (*struct*)

$C_{22}H_{36}P_2Pt$ Pt-00276

Biscyclopropylbis(dimethylphenylphosphine)platinum

Dicyclopropylbis(dimethylphenylphosphine)platinum. Bis(dimethylphenylphosphine)dicyclopropylplatinum

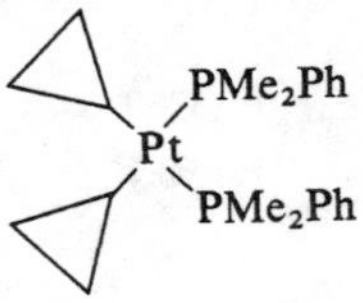

M 557.554

cis-form [64522-77-6]
Cryst. (pet. ether), dec. at 120°. Mp 104°.

Phillips, R.L. *et al*, *J. Chem. Soc., Dalton Trans.*, 1978, 1732 (*synth, pmr*)
Jones, N.L. *et al*, *Organometallics*, 1982, **1**, 326 (*struct*)

$C_{22}H_{41}PPt$ Pt-00277

Bis(ethylene)(tricyclohexylphosphine)platinum

Bis(η^2-ethene)(tricyclohexylphosphine)platinum, 9CI
[57158-83-5]

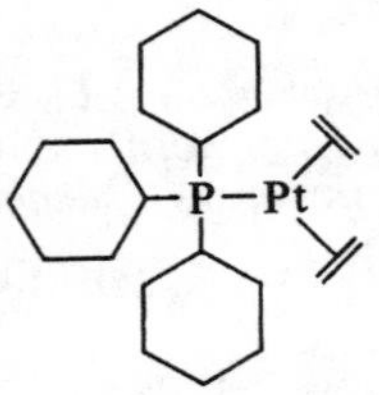

M 531.620

Catalyses hydrosilylation of olefins. Cryst. (pet. ether). Sol. aromatic solvs. Mp 135-40° dec. Can be handled in air, but should be stored under N_2.

Harrison, N.C. *et al*, *J. Chem. Soc., Dalton Trans.*, 1978, 1337 (*synth, nmr*)
Inorg. Synth., 1979, **19**, 213 (*synth*)

$C_{22}O_{22}Pt_{19}^{\ominus\ominus\ominus\ominus}$ Pt-00278

Deca-μ-carbonyldodecacarbonylnonadecaplatinate(4−), 9CI

Docosacarbonylnonadecaplatinate(4−)
[71966-26-2]

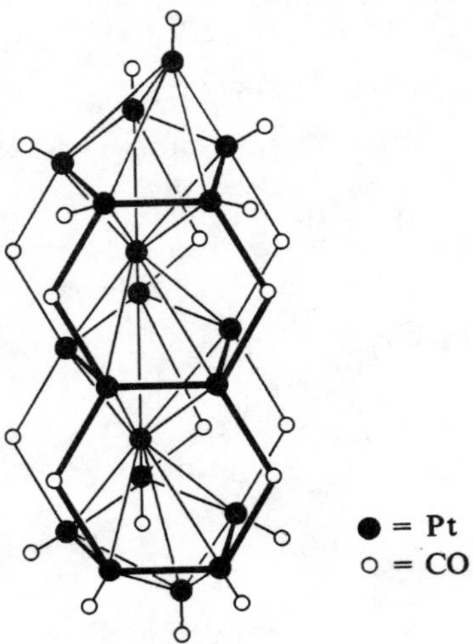

M 4322.749 (ion)

Tetrakis(tetraphenylphosphonium) salt: [72026-46-1].
$C_{118}H_{80}O_{22}P_4Pt_{19}$ M 5680.332
Brown cryst. + 4MeCN. Subject to cryst. decay.

Tetrakis(tetrabutylammonium) salt: [72026-40-5].
$C_{86}H_{144}N_4O_{22}Pt_{19}$ M 5292.617
Brown cryst. Subject to cryst. decay.

Washecheck, D.M. *et al*, *J. Am. Chem. Soc.*, 1979, **101**, 6110 (*synth, struct, ir, cmr, stereochem*)

$C_{23}H_{21}IN_2Pt$ Pt-00279

(2,2′-Bipyridine-*N,N′*)iodomethyldiphenylplatinum

Methyldiphenyliodo(bipyridine)platinum. Diphenylmethyliodo(bipyridine)platinum
[58411-19-1]

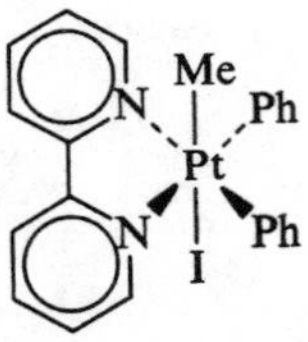

M 647.417

Cryst. (CH_2Cl_2/Et_2O). Mp 245° dec.

Usón, R. *et al*, *J. Organomet. Chem.*, 1976, **105**, C25 (*synth*)
Jawad, J.K. *et al*, *J. Organomet. Chem.*, 1976, **117**, 297 (*synth*)
Usón, R. *et al*, *Synth. React. Inorg. Met.-Org. Chem.*, 1977, **7**, 211 (*synth, ir*)

$C_{24}H_{20}ClOPPt$ Pt-00280

Carbonylchloro(η^1-2,4-cyclopentadien-1-yl)(triphenylphosphine)platinum, 8CI

σ-Cyclopentadienyl(carbonyl)chloro(triphenylphosphine)platinum

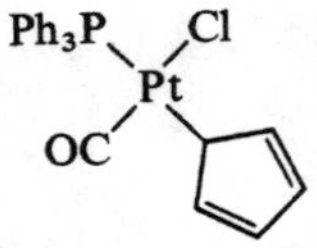

M 585.928

Orange powder. Mp 106-8°.

Cross, R.J. *et al*, *J. Chem. Soc. (A)*, 1971, 2000 (*synth, pmr, ir*)
Cross, R.J. *et al*, *J. Chem. Soc., Dalton Trans.*, 1983, 359 (*synth, nmr*)

$C_{24}H_{20}OPPt^{\oplus}$ Pt-00281

Carbonyl(η^5-2,4-cyclopentadien-1-yl)(triphenylphosphine)platinum(1+), 9CI
Cyclopentadienyl(carbonyl)(triphenylphosphine)platinum(1+)

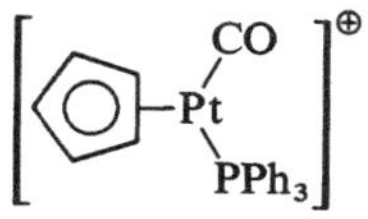

M 550.475 (ion)
Perchlorate: [64040-94-4].
$C_{24}H_{20}ClO_5PPt$ M 649.926
Orange cryst. (CH_2Cl_2/Et_2O). Mp 195° dec.
▷Potentially explosive

Kurosawa, H. *et al*, *J. Am. Chem. Soc.*, 1980, **102**, 6996 (*synth, pmr, ir*)

$C_{24}H_{22}O_2Pt$ Pt-00282

Acetylacetonato(η^3-triphenylmethyl)platinum
[η^3-6-(Diphenylmethylene)-2,4-cyclohexadien-1-yl]-(2,4-pentanedionato-O,O′)-platinum, 9CI
[56050-89-6]

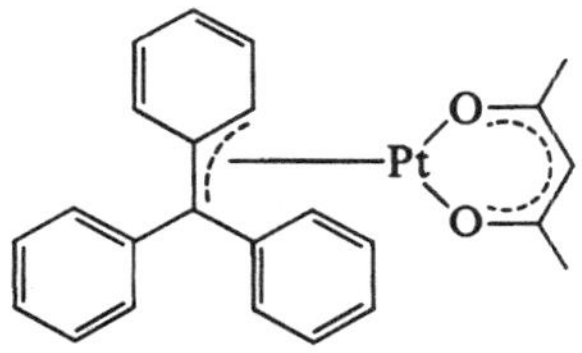

M 537.517
Yellow cryst. (C_6H_6/pet. ether). Mp 175-8° dec.

Mann, B.E. *et al*, *J. Chem. Soc., Dalton Trans.*, 1979, 338 (*nmr, synth*)
Sonoda, A. *et al*, *J. Chem. Soc., Dalton Trans.*, 1979, 346 (*struct*)

$C_{24}H_{26}ClPPt$ Pt-00283

Chloro(η^3-2-propenyl)[tris(4-methylphenyl)phosphine]platinum, 10CI
Allylchloro(tri-p-tolylphosphine)platinum

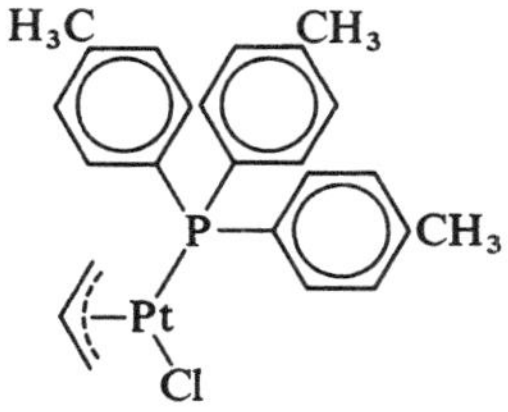

M 575.976
Cryst. (CH_2Cl_2/Et_2O). Mp 175-7°.

Carturan, G. *et al*, *J. Organomet. Chem.*, 1979, **172**, 91 (*synth, ir, nmr*)
Del Pra, A. *et al*, *Inorg. Chim. Acta*, 1979, **33**, L137.

$C_{24}H_{29}PPtSn$ Pt-00284

(η^3-2-Propenyl)(trimethylstannyl)(triphenylphosphine)platinum, 9CI
Allyl(trimethylstannyl)(triphenylphosphine)platinum.
π-Allyl(trimethyltin)(triphenylphosphine)platinum
[72110-51-1]

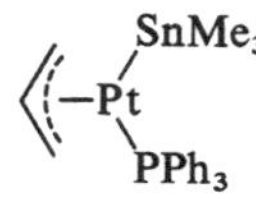

M 662.237
Yellow cryst. (hexane). Mp 122-6° dec.

Christofides, A. *et al*, *J. Organomet. Chem.*, 1979, **178**, 273 (*synth, ir, nmr*)

$C_{24}H_{30}Cl_2F_{10}P_2Pt$ Pt-00285

Dichlorobis(pentafluorophenyl)bis(triethylphosphine)platinum, 9CI
Bis(pentafluorophenyl)dichlorobis(triethylphosphine)-platinum
[52970-61-3]

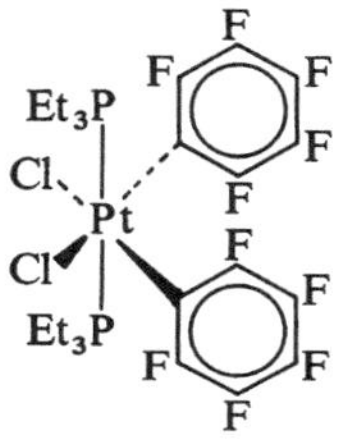

M 836.419
Cryst. ($EtOH/CHCl_3$). Mp 192-4°. Dipole moment 4.6 D.

Usón, R. *et al*, *CA*, 1974, **81**, 49793x (*synth*)
Crocker, C. *et al*, *J. Chem. Soc., Dalton Trans.*, 1977, 1448 (*nmr*)

$C_{24}H_{30}F_{10}P_2Pt$ Pt-00286

Bis(pentafluorophenyl)bis(triethylphosphine)platinum, 9CI
Bis(triethylphosphine)bis(pentafluorophenyl)platinum

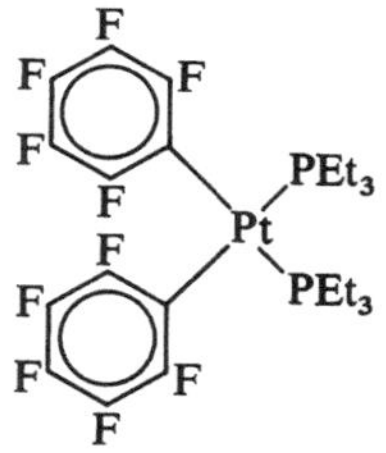

cis-form

M 765.513
cis-form [14283-95-5]
Cryst. (MeOH). Mp 160-1°. Converted to *trans*-form when heated with benzene + I_2 in sealed tube.
trans-form [14840-51-8]
Cryst. (C_6H_6/MeOH). Mp 228-9°.

Rosevear, D.T. *et al*, *J. Chem. Soc.*, 1965, 5275 (*synth*)
Goggin, P.L. *et al*, *J. Chem. Soc. (A)*, 1966, 1462 (*ir*)
Crocker, C. *et al*, *J. Chem. Soc., Dalton Trans.*, 1977, 1448 (*nmr*)

$C_{24}H_{30}F_{18}P_2Pt$ Pt-00287

[(1,2-η)-Hexakis(trifluoromethyl)benzene]bis(triethylphosphine)platinum, 9CI

[40982-03-4]

M 917.500

Orange cryst. (Et_2O). Mp 203°.

Browning, J. *et al*, *J. Chem. Soc., Dalton Trans.*, 1974, 97 (*synth, ir, nmr*)
Browning, J. *et al*, *J. Cryst. Mol. Struct.*, 1974, **4**, 335 (*struct*)

$C_{24}H_{34}Br_2Pt_2$ Pt-00288

Di-μ-bromobis(η^3-1,2,4,5,6-pentamethyl-3-methylenebicyclo[2.2.0]hex-5-en-2-yl)diplatinum, 9CI

Di-μ-bromobis(α,2,3-η-pentamethylbicyclo[2.2.0]hexa-2,5-dien-2-ylmethyl)diplatinum

[41702-08-3]

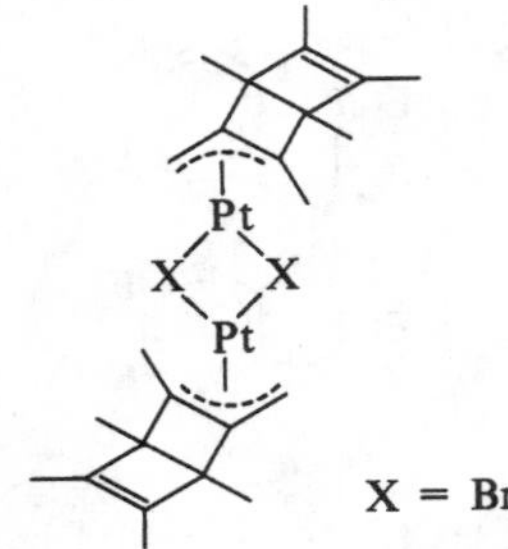

X = Br

M 872.501

Bridged dimer. Yellow cryst. (CH_2Cl_2/MeOH). Dec. without melting at 145-9°.

Monomer: Bromo(1,2,4,5,6-pentamethyl-3-methylene-bicyclo[2.2.0]hex-5-en-2-yl)platinum.
$C_{12}H_{17}BrPt$ M 436.250
Unknown.

Shaw, B.L. *et al*, *J. Chem. Soc., Dalton Trans.*, 1973, 264 (*synth, ir, nmr*)

$C_{24}H_{34}Cl_2Pt_2$ Pt-00289

Dichlorobis[μ-[η,η^4-(1,3,4,5,6-pentamethylbicyclo[2.2.0]-hexa-2,5-dien-2-yl)methyl]]diplatinum, 9CI

Dichloro-di-μ-(pentamethylbicyclo[2.2.0]hexa-2,5-di-ene-2-yl-methyl)diplatinum

[32994-04-0]

M 783.599

Yellow cryst. (CH_2Cl_2/MeOH). Mp 175-202° dec.

Mason, R. *et al*, *J. Chem. Soc. (A)*, 1970, 535 (*struct*)
Shaw, B.L. *et al*, *J. Chem. Soc., Dalton Trans.*, 1973, 264 (*synth, ir, pmr*)

$C_{24}H_{34}Cl_2Pt_2$ Pt-00290

Di-μ-chlorobis(η^3-1,2,4,5,6-pentamethyl-3-methylenebicyclo[2.2.0]hex-5-en-1-yl)diplatinum, 9CI

Di-μ-chlorobis(α,2,3-η-pentamethylbicyclo[2.2.0]hexa-2,5-dien-2-ylmethyl)diplatinum

[41572-71-8]

As Di-μ-bromobis(η^3-1,2,4,5,6-pentamethyl-3-methylenebicyclo ex-5-en-2-yl)diplatinum, Pt-00288 with

X = Cl

M 783.599

Bridged dimer. Pale-yellow cryst. (CH_2Cl_2/MeOH). Dec. at 157-63°.

Monomer: Chloro(1,2,4,5,6-pentamethyl-3-methylene-bicyclo[2.2.0]hex-5-en-1-yl)platinum.
$C_{12}H_{17}ClPt$ M 391.799
Unknown.

Shaw, B.L. *et al*, *J. Chem. Soc., Dalton Trans.*, 1973, 264.

$C_{24}H_{36}Cl_6Pt_3Sn_2$ Pt-00291

Tris[(1,2,5,6-η)-1,5-cyclooctadiene]bis(μ_3-trichlorostannyl-)triplatinum, 9CI

Bis(μ_3-trichlorotin)tris(1,5-cyclooctadiene)triplatinum

[12204-04-5]

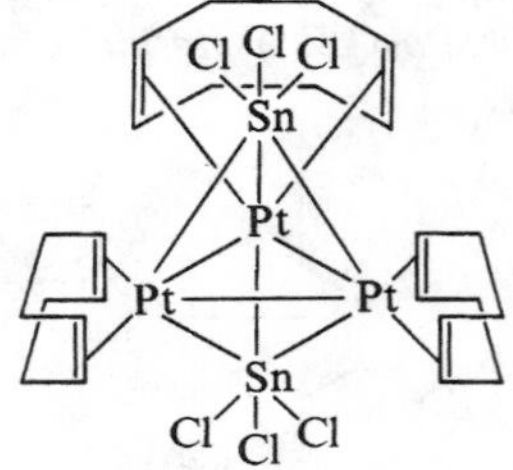

M 1359.886

Hydrogenation catalyst. Orange cryst. (CH_2Cl_2/$MeNO_2$).

Lindsey, R.V. *et al*, *Inorg. Chem.*, 1966, **5**, 109 (*synth*)
Guggenberger, L.J., *J. Chem. Soc., Chem. Commun.*, 1968, 512 (*struct*)
Terzis, A. *et al*, *Inorg. Chem.*, 1971, **11**, 2617 (*ir, raman*)
Riggs, W.M., *Anal. Chem.*, 1972, **44**, 830 (*pe*)

$C_{24}H_{36}O_2P_2Pt$ Pt-00292

Bis(dimethylphenylphosphine)bis(3-methoxy-1-propenyl)platinum, 9CI

Bis(3-methoxy-1-propenyl)bis(dimethylphenylphosphine)platinum

$(MeOCH_2CH{=}CH)_2Pt(PMe_2Ph)_2$

M 613.575

trans-form [57145-95-6]

Cryst. (C_6H_6/hexane). Mp 104-6°.

Empsall, H.D. *et al*, *J. Organomet. Chem.*, 1975, **96**, 461 (*synth, nmr*)
O'Flynn, K.H.P. *et al*, *Acta Crystallogr., Sect. B*, 1976, **32**, 1596 (*struct*)

$C_{24}H_{38}N_2OP_2Pt^{\oplus\oplus}$ Pt-00293

Bis(dimethylphenylphosphine)[ethoxy(ethylamino)methylene]-(isocyanoethane)platinum(2+), 9CI

Bis(dimethylphenylphosphine)[ethylamino(ethoxy)methylene](ethylisocyanide)platinum(2+). Bis(dimethylphenylphosphine)[ethoxy(ethylamino)carbene](isocyanoethane)platinum(2+)

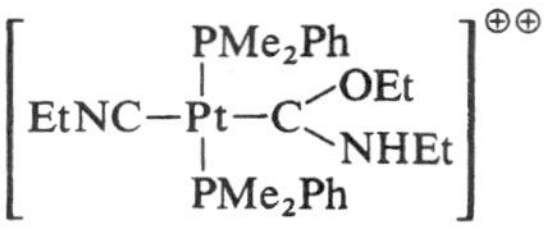

M 627.605 (ion)

Bishexafluorophosphate: [33661-17-5].
$C_{24}H_{38}F_{12}N_2OP_4Pt$ M 917.533
Cryst. (Et_2O/MeOH). Mp 165° dec.

Clark, H.C. *et al*, *Inorg. Chem.*, 1972, **11**, 503 (*synth, pmr, ir*)

$C_{24}H_{40}I_2P_2Pt$ Pt-00294

Diiododiphenylbis(triethylphosphine)platinum, 8CI

Bis(triethylphosphine)diiododiphenylplatinum. Diphenyldiiodobis(triethylphosphine)platinum

[22622-41-9]

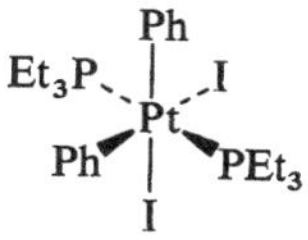

M 839.417

Yellow cryst. (EtOH). Mp 149-52°. Dipole moment 4.95D.

Chatt, J. *et al*, *J. Chem. Soc.*, 1959, 4020 (*synth*)
Ettorre, R., *Inorg. Nucl. Chem. Lett.*, 1969, **5**, 45.

$C_{24}H_{40}P_2Pt$ Pt-00295

Diphenylbis(triethylphosphine)platinum

Bis(triethylphosphine)diphenylplatinum

[16787-10-3]

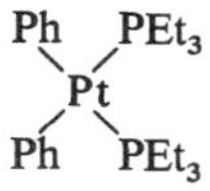

cis-form

M 585.608

cis-form [15638-50-3]
Cryst. (pet. ether). Mp 151-4° dec. Dipole moment 7.2D.

trans-form [15293-16-0]
Cryst. (EtOH). Mp 176-80°. Dipole moment ~0D. Less common isomer.

Chatt, J. *et al*, *J. Chem. Soc.*, 1959, 4020 (*synth*)
Goggin, P.L. *et al*, *J. Chem. Soc. (A)*, 1966, 1462 (*ir*)
Heaton, B.T. *et al*, *J. Organomet. Chem.*, 1968, **14**, 235 (*nmr*)
Riggs, W.M., *Anal. Chem.*, 1972, **44**, 830 (*pe*)
Glockling, F. *et al*, *Inorg. Chim. Acta*, 1974, **8**, 81 (*ms*)
Coulson, D.R., *J. Am. Chem. Soc.*, 1976, **98**, 3111 (*cmr*)
Eaborn, C. *et al*, *J. Chem. Soc., Dalton Trans.*, 1981, 933 (*synth*)

Handle all chemicals with care

$C_{24}H_{46}P_2Pt$ Pt-00296

Dihydro[[1,2-phenylenebis(methylene)]bis[bis(1,1-dimethylethyl)phosphine]-*P,P'*]platinum, 9CI

[60446-99-3]

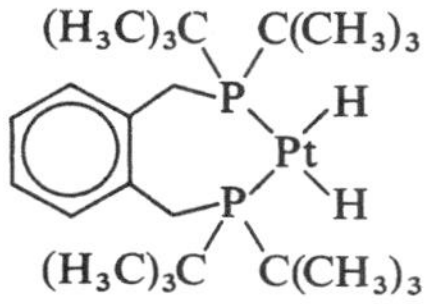

M 591.655

No details available.

Moulton, C.J. *et al*, *J. Chem. Soc., Chem. Commun.*, 1976, 365.

$C_{24}H_{48}Cl_4Pt_2$ Pt-00297

Di-μ-chlorodichlorobis(1-dodecene)diplatinum

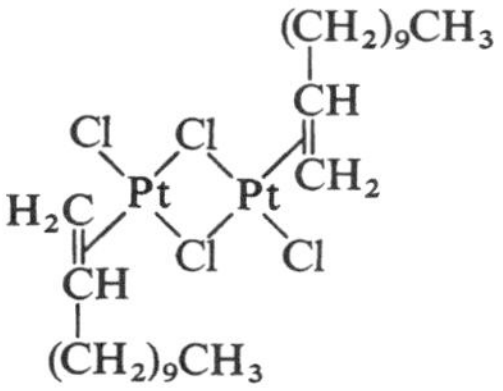

M 868.615

Bridged dimer. Orange solid. Sol. Me_2CO, Et_2O, THF, alcohols; less sol. halogenated hydrocarbons. Mp 73°.

Monomer: Dichloro-1-dodeceneplatinum.
$C_{12}H_{24}Cl_2Pt$ M 434.308
Unknown.

Joy, J.R. *et al*, *J. Am. Chem. Soc.*, 1959, **81**, 305.
Inorg. Synth., 1980, **20**, 181 (*synth*)

$C_{24}H_{52}Cl_2P_2Pt_2$ Pt-00298

Bis[2-(di-*tert*-butylphosphino)-2-methylpropyl-*C,P*]di-μ-chlorodiplatinum

*Bis[2-[bis(1,1-dimethylethyl)phosphino]-2-methylpropyl-*C,P*]di-μ-chlorodiplatinum, 9CI. Di-μ-chlorobis-[2-(di-*tert*-butylphosphino)-2-methylpropyl-*C,P*]diplatinum. Bis[2-[bis(1,1-dimethylethyl)phosphine]-2,2-dimethylethyl-*C,P*]di-μ-chlorodiplatinum*

[74523-69-6]

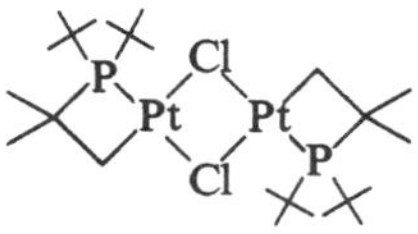

M 863.688

Cryst. (C_6H_6/hexane). Mp 212-5°.

Clark, H.C. *et al*, *Inorg. Chem.*, 1980, **19**, 3220 (*synth*)
Goel, A.B. *et al*, *Inorg. Chim. Acta*, 1981, **54**, L267 (*struct*)

$C_{24}H_{54}Cl_2P_2Pt$ Pt-00299

Dichlorobis(tributylphosphine)platinum, 9CI

Bis(tributylphosphine)platinum(II) chloride

[15076-72-9]

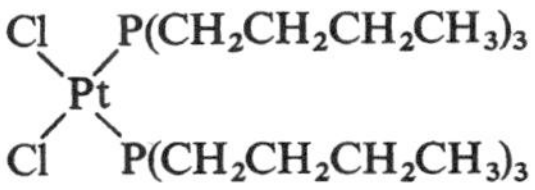

cis-form

M 670.624

Cocatalyst with $SnCl_2$ for hydroformylation reaction, and for carboxylation of olefins.

cis-form [15390-92-8]
Cryst. (pet. ether). Sl. sol. H_2O. Sol. in C_6H_6, CS_2, EtOH. Mp 144-144.5°. Dipole moment 11.5 D. Readily isom. in presence of free phosphine.
trans-form [15391-01-2]
Yellow cryst. (EtOH). Insol. H_2O, sol. most org. solvs. Mp 65-6°. Zero dipole moment.

Inorg. Synth., 1963, **7**, 245 (*synth*)
Balimann, G. *et al*, *J. Magn. Reson.*, 1976, **22**, 235 (*nmr*)

$C_{24}H_{54}Cl_4P_2Pt_2$ Pt-00300

Di-μ-chlorodichlorobis(tributylphosphine)diplatinum, 9CI, 8CI
Tetrachlorobis(tributylphosphine)diplatinum. Bistributylphosphinedichloro-μ,μ'-dichlorodiplatinum
[15670-38-9]

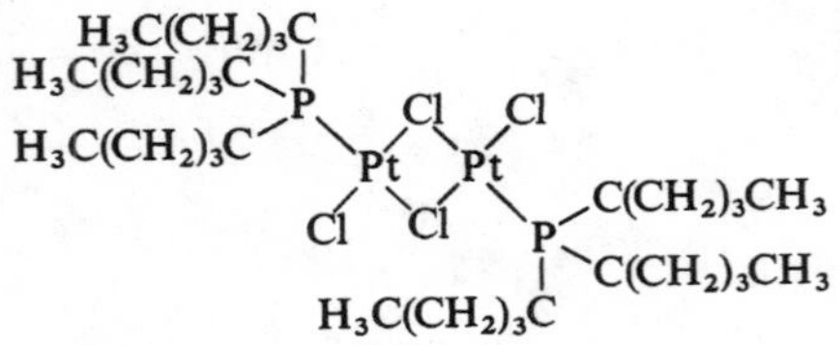

M 936.610
Bridged dimer. Catalyses cleavage of C-Si bonds in organosilanes. Selective hydroformylation catalyst.
trans-form [15282-39-0]
Yellow-orange cryst. (Me_2CO). Mp 143-4°.
Monomer: Dichloro(tributylphosphine)platinum.
$C_{12}H_{27}Cl_2PPt$ M 468.305
Unknown.

Chatt, J. *et al*, *J. Chem. Soc.*, 1955, 2787 (*synth*)
Pidcock, A. *et al*, *J. Chem. Soc. (A)*, 1966, 1707 (*nmr*)
Balimann, G. *et al*, *J. Magn. Reson.*, 1976, **22**, 235 (*nmr*)

$C_{24}H_{54}P_2Pt$ Pt-00301

Bis(tri-*tert*-butylphosphine)platinum
Bis[tris(1,1-dimethylethyl)phosphine]platinum, 9CI
[60648-70-6]

$[(H_3C)_3C]_3PPtP[C(CH_3)_3]_3$

M 599.718
Cryst. (hexane). Mp 237° dec. Reacts with $CHCl_3$ to form Bis[2-(di-*tert*-butylphosphino)-2-methylpropyl-*C,P*]di-μ-chlorodiplatinum, Pt-00298 .

Otsuka, S. *et al*, *J. Am. Chem. Soc.*, 1976, **98**, 5850 (*synth, struct, ms, pmr*)
Moynihan, K.J. *et al*, *Acta Crystallogr., Sect. B*, 1979, **35**, 3060 (*struct*)
Goel, R.G. *et al*, *Angew. Chem.*, 1981, **93**, 715 (*synth*)
Goel, R.G. *et al*, *J. Organomet. Chem.*, 1981, **214**, 405 (*synth, pmr, nmr*)

$C_{24}H_{55}P_2Pt^{\oplus}$ Pt-00302

Hydrobis(tri-*tert*-butylphosphine)platinum(1+)
Hydridobis[tris-(1,1-dimethylethyl)phosphine]platinum(1+)

$[(H_3C)_3C]_3PPtHP[C(CH_3)_3]_3^{\oplus}$

M 600.726 (ion)
ir ν_{PtH} 2645 cm^{-1}.

Hexafluorophosphate:
$C_{24}H_{55}F_6P_3Pt$ M 745.690
Yellow cryst. (Me_2CO or MeOH).

Goel, R.G. *et al*, *J. Organomet. Chem.*, 1981, **204**, C13 (*synth, ir, nmr*)

$C_{24}H_{56}As_2Pt$ Pt-00303

Dihydrobis(tri-*tert*-butylarsine)platinum
Dihydrobis[tris(1,1-dimethylethyl)arsine]platinum. Dihydridobis(tri-tert-butylarsine)platinum

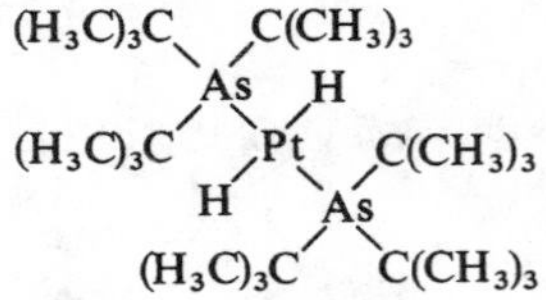

M 689.630
Cryst. (hexane). Mp 173° dec. ir ν_{PtH} 1775cm^{-1}.

Goel, R.G. *et al*, *Inorg. Chem.*, 1982, **21**, 1627 (*synth, ir, pmr*)

$C_{24}H_{56}P_2Pt$ Pt-00304

Dihydrobis(tri-*tert*-butylphosphine)platinum
Dihydrobis[tris(1,1-dimethylethyl)phosphine]platinum, 10CI. Bis(tri-tert-butylphosphine)platinum dihydride
[67870-05-7]

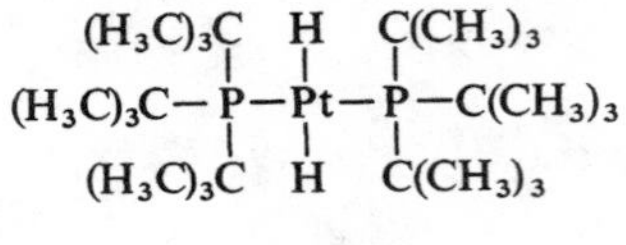

M 601.734
Cryst. (EtOH). ir ν_{PtH} 1820cm^{-1}.

Clark, H.C. *et al*, *J. Organomet. Chem.*, 1978, **157**, C16 (*synth*)
Ferguson, G. *et al*, *J. Chem. Res. (S)*, 1979, 362; *J. Chem. Res. (M)*, 1979, 4337 (*struct*)

$C_{24}H_{60}O_{12}P_4Pt$ Pt-00305

Tetrakis(triethylphosphite-*P*)platinum, 9CI
Tetrakis(phosphorous acid)platinum dodecaethyl ester
[23066-15-1]

$Pt[P(OEt)_3]_4$ (T_d)

M 859.706
Catalyses telomerisation of isoprene with NH_3, and silicone rubber vulcanisation. Cryst. (MeOH aq.). Insol. H_2O, sl. sol. MeOH, v. sol. hydrocarbons. Mp 114°. Can be handled briefly in air, but should be stored in a vacuum.

Inorg. Synth., 1972, **13**, 112 (*synth*)
Pregosin, P.S. *et al*, *Helv. Chim. Acta*, 1977, **60**, 1371 (*nmr*)

$C_{24}H_{60}P_4Pt$ Pt-00306

Tetrakis(triethylphosphine)platinum, 9CI
[33937-26-7]

$[Pt(PEt_3)_4]$ (T_d)

M 667.713
Air-sensitive cryst. (hexane). Sol. hydrocarbons. Mp 47-8° (under N_2). Readily dissociates to $[Pt(PEt_3)_3]$.

Schunn, R.A., *Inorg. Chem.*, 1976, **15**, 208 (*synth*)
Inorg. Synth., 1979, **19**, 110 (*synth*)
Yoshida, T. *et al*, *J. Am. Chem. Soc.*, 1979, **101**, 2027 (*use*)

Mann, B.E. *et al*, *J. Chem. Soc., Dalton Trans.*, 1980, 776 (*nmr*)

$C_{24}H_{63}P_4Pt_2^{\oplus}$ **Pt-00307**

Di-μ-hydrohydrotetrakis(triethylphosphine)diplatinum(1+)

Di-μ-hydridohydridotetrakis(triethylphosphine)diplatinum(1+). Tetrakis(triethylphosphine)-trihydridodiplatinum(1+)

[H–$Pt(PEt_3)_2(\mu$-$H)_2Pt(PEt_3)_2]^{\oplus}$

M 865.817 (ion)

Tetraphenylborate: [81800-05-7].
$C_{48}H_{83}BP_4Pt_2$ M 1185.049
Yellow air stable cryst.

Formate: [81800-04-6].
$C_{25}H_{64}O_2P_4Pt_2$ M 910.834
Not isol. Formed by treating $[PtH_2(PEt_3)_2]$ with CO_2.

Paonessa, R.S. *et al*, *J. Am. Chem. Soc.*, 1982, **104**, 3529.

$C_{24}H_{64}P_5Pt_2^{\oplus}$ **Pt-00308**

Dihydro-μ-phosphinotetrakis(triethylphosphine)diplatinum(1+), 9CI

μ-Phosphidobis[hydridobis(triethylphosphine)platinum](1+)

$[Et_3P$–$Pt(PEt_3)(H)$–PH_2–$Pt(PEt_3)_2$–$H]^{\oplus}$ *cis,trans-form*

M 897.798 (ion)

cis-trans-form

Chloride: [67145-29-3].
$C_{24}H_{64}ClP_5Pt_2$ M 933.251
Observed in soln. only.

trans-trans-form

Converts to *cis-trans*-form in soln.
Chloride: [62906-17-6]. Yellow solid, dec. >85°.

Ebsworth, E.A.V., *Angew. Chem., Int. Ed. Engl.*, 1977, **16**, 482 (*synth, nmr*)
Ebsworth, E.A.V., *J. Chem. Soc., Dalton Trans.*, 1978, 272 (*synth, nmr*)

$C_{24}H_{65}Cl_2P_5Pt_2^{\oplus}$ **Pt-00309**

Chlorotrihydro-μ-phosphinotetrakis(triethylphosphine)diplatinum(1+), 9CI

[62990-74-3]

$[H$–$Pt(PEt_3)_2$–PH_2–$Pt(Et_3P)(H)(Cl)(PEt_3)$–$H]^{\oplus}$

M 969.712 (ion)
Obt. in soln. by treating Pt-00308 (as chloride) with HCl.

Ebsworth, E.A.V. *et al*, *Angew. Chem., Int. Ed. Engl.*, 1977, **16**, 482 (*synth, nmr*)

$C_{24}H_{66}Cl_2P_5Pt_2^{\oplus}$ **Pt-00310**

Dichlorotetrahydro-μ-phosphinotetrakis(triethylphosphine)diplatinum(1+), 9CI

[62906-16-5]

$[H$–$Pt(Et_3P)(H)(Cl)(PEt_3)$–H_2P–$Pt(Et_3P)(H)(Cl)(PEt_3)$–$H]^{\oplus}$

M 970.720 (ion)
Obt. in soln. by treating Pt-00308 (as chloride) with HCl.

Ebsworth, E.A.V. *et al*, *Angew. Chem., Int. Ed. Engl.*, 1977, **16**, 482 (*synth, nmr*)

$C_{24}O_{24}Pt_{12}^{\ominus\ominus}$ **Pt-00311**

Dodeca-μ-carbonyldodecacarbonyldodecaplatinate(2−), 9CI

Tetrakis[hexacarbonyltriplatinate](2−)

[52349-77-6]

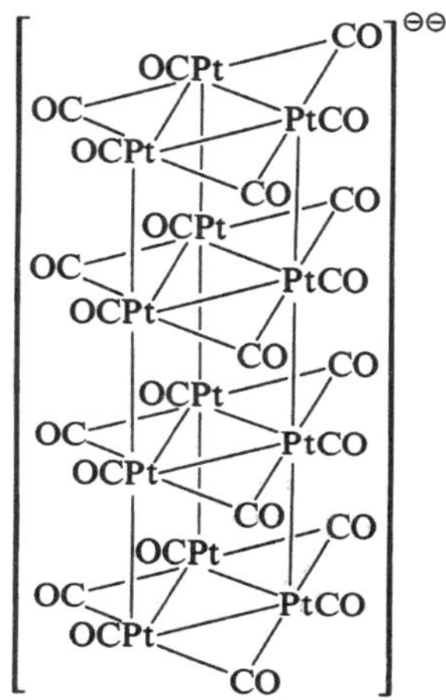

M 3013.210 (ion)
Used in prep. of Pt catalyst for hexane isomerization. Blue-green soln. in THF.

Bis(tetrabutylammonium) salt:
$C_{56}H_{72}N_2O_{24}Pt_{12}$ M 3498.144
Blue-green cryst.

Calabrese, J.C. *et al*, *J. Am. Chem. Soc.*, 1974, **96**, 2614 (*synth, ir, struct*)
Japan. Pat., 77 65 201, (*1977*); *CA*, **88**, 123625g (*use*)
Chini, P. *et al*, *Chim. Ind.* (*Milan*), 1978, **60**, 989; *CA*, **91**, 150386y (*struct*)
Apai, G. *et al*, *J. Am. Chem. Soc.*, 1979, **101**, 6880 (*synth*)
Brown, C. *et al*, *J. Organomet. Chem.*, 1979, **181**, 233 (*cmr, nmr*)
Garin, F. *et al*, *Surf. Sci.*, 1981, **106**, 466 (*use*)

$C_{25}H_{20}Cl_2NPPt$ **Pt-00312**

Dichloro(isocyanobenzene)(triphenylphosphine)platinum, 9CI

Dichloro(phenylisonitrile)(triphenylphosphine)platinum. Dichloro(phenyl isocyanide)(triphenylphosphine)-platinum

[54712-93-5]

$Pt(Cl)_2(PPh_3)(CNPh)$

M 631.399

cis-form [41101-20-6]
Cryst. Mp 248-55°.

Chatt, J. *et al*, *Inorg. Chim. Acta*, 1972, **6**, 669 (*synth, ir*)
Fehlhammer, W.P., *Angew. Chem., Int. Ed. Engl.*, 1975, **14**, 369 (*synth*)

$C_{25}H_{24}Cl_2N_2Pt$ Pt-00313

Dichloro(1,2-diphenyl-1,3-propanediyl)bis(pyridine)platinum
Dichlorobis(pyridine)(1,2-diphenyl-1,3-propanediyl)-platinum
[38889-66-6]

M 618.464
Cryst. (EtOH). Mp 116°.

McQuillin, F.J. *et al*, *J. Chem. Soc., Dalton Trans.*, 1972, 2123 (*synth, ir*)
McGinnety, J.A. *et al*, *J. Organomet. Chem.*, 1973, **59**, 429 (*struct*)
Inorg. Synth., 1976, **16**, 113 (*synth*)

$C_{25}H_{24}PPt^{\oplus}$ Pt-00314

Cyclopentadienyl(ethylene)(triphenylphosphine)platinum(1+)
(η^5*-2,4-Cyclopentadien-1-yl*)(η^2*-ethene*)(*triphenylphosphine*)*platinum*(*1*+), 9CI. *Ethylene*(*cyclopentadienyl*)-(*triphenylphosphine*)*platinum*(*1*+)

M 550.518 (ion)
Perchlorate: [64040-96-6].
$C_{25}H_{24}ClO_4PPt$ M 649.969
Orange cryst. (CH_2Cl_2/Et_2O). Mp 170° dec.
▷Potentially explosive

Kurosawa, H. *et al*, *J. Am. Chem. Soc.*, 1980, **102**, 6996 (*synth, pmr, ir*)

$C_{25}H_{62}NP_4Pt_2^{\oplus}$ Pt-00315

[μ-(Cyano-*C:N*)]dihydrotetrakis(triethylphosphine)diplatinum(1+), 9CI
Dihydrido-μ-cyanotetrakis(triethylphosphine)diplatinum(1+)

M 890.827 (ion)
Hexafluorophosphate: [60594-96-9].
$C_{25}H_{62}F_6NP_5Pt_2$ M 1035.791
Cryst. (MeOH).

Manzer, L.E. *et al*, *Inorg. Chem.*, 1976, **15**, 3114 (*synth, nmr*)

$C_{26}H_{27}AsClPt^{\oplus}$ Pt-00316

Chloro[(1,2,5,6-η)-1,5-cyclooctadiene](triphenylarsine)platinum(1+), 9CI
(1,5-Cyclooctadiene)chloro(triphenylarsine)platinum

M 644.954 (ion)
Tetrafluoroborate: [31940-97-3].
$C_{26}H_{27}AsBClF_4Pt$ M 731.758
Solid.

Inorg. Synth., 1972, **13**, 55.

$C_{26}H_{35}OP_2Pt^{\oplus}$ Pt-00317

Bis(dimethylphenylphosphine)methyl[methoxy(phenylmethyl)-methylene]platinum(1+)
Bis(dimethylphenylphosphine)(α-methoxyphenethylidene)methylplatinum(1+), 9CI. *[Benzyl(methoxy)carbene]bis(dimethylphenylphosphine)-methylplatinum(1+)*

M 620.589 (ion)
trans-form
Hexafluorophosphate: [27776-77-8].
$C_{26}H_{35}F_6O_2P_3Pt$ M 781.553
Mp 185-90° dec.

Chisholm, M.H. *et al*, *Inorg. Chem.*, 1971, **10**, 1711.

$C_{26}H_{44}P_2Pt$ Pt-00318

Bis(2-methylphenyl)bis(triethylphosphine)platinum
Di-o-tolylbis(triethylphosphine)platinum

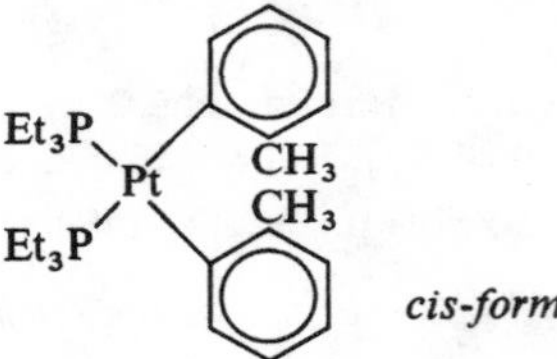

M 613.661
cis-form
Cryst. (pet. ether). Mp 176-80° dec. Dipole moment 7.5 D.
trans-form
Cryst. Mp 192-6°. Dipole moment zero.

Chatt, J. *et al*, *J. Chem. Soc.*, 1959, 4020 (*synth*)

$C_{26}H_{44}P_2Pt$ Pt-00319

Dibenzylbis(triethylphosphine)platinum
Bis(phenylmethyl)bis(triethylphosphine)platinum, 9CI
[65391-83-5]

M 613.661

cis-form [42167-76-0]
Cryst. (MeOH). Mp 103-4°. Dipole moment 6.7 D.

Chatt, J. *et al*, *J. Chem. Soc.*, 1959, 4020 (*synth*)
Cardin, D.J. *et al*, *J. Chem. Soc., Chem. Commun.*, 1973, 350.
Van Leeuwen, P.W.N.M. *et al*, *J. Organomet. Chem.*, 1977, **142**, 233.

$C_{26}H_{56}Cl_2P_2Pt_2$ Pt-00320

Bis[3-(di-*tert*-butylphosphino)-2,2-dimethylpropyl-*C,P*]di-μ-chlorodiplatinum

*Bis[3-[bis(1,1-dimethylethyl)phosphino]-2,2-dimethylpropyl-*C,P*]di-μ-chlorodiplatinum*, 9CI. *Di-μ-chlorobis-[3-(di-*tert*-butylphosphino)-2,2-dimethylpropyl-*C,P*]-diplatinum*

[60767-62-6]

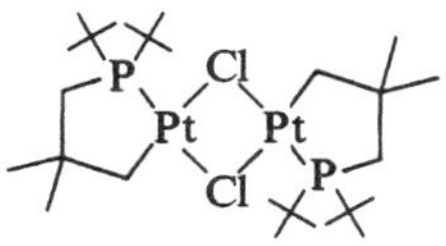

M 891.742
Cryst. (CH_2Cl_2).

Mason, R. *et al*, *J. Chem. Soc., Chem. Commun.*, 1976, 292 (*synth, struct*)

$C_{27}H_{20}F_5PPt$ Pt-00321

Pentafluorophenyl(η^3-2-propenyl)(triphenylphosphine)platinum, 10CI

π-Allyl(pentafluorophenyl)(triphenylphosphine)platinum

[62415-32-1]

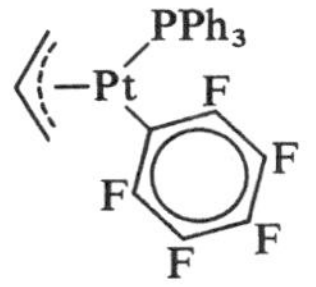

M 665.501
Yellow cryst. (C_6H_6/MeOH). Mp 133°.

Numata, S. *et al*, *Inorg. Chem.*, 1977, **16**, 1737 (*synth*)

$C_{27}H_{26}ClF_3P_2Pt$ Pt-00322

Chlorobis(methyldiphenylphosphine)(trifluoromethyl)platinum

Bis(methyldiphenylphosphine)(trifluoromethyl)platinum chloride. (Trifluoromethyl)-chlorobis(methyldiphenylphosphine)platinum

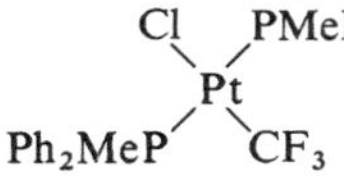

M 699.978

trans-form [68914-98-7]
Cryst. (CH_2Cl_2/EtOH). Mp 168-70°.

Bennett, M.A. *et al*, *Inorg. Chem.*, 1979, **18**, 1061 (*synth, struct*)

$C_{27}H_{27}ClP_2Pt$ Pt-00323

Chloro[ethylenebis[diphenylphosphine]]methylplatinum, 8CI

Chloro[1,2-ethanediylbis[diphenylphosphine]-P,P′]-methylplatinum, 9CI

[27711-50-8]

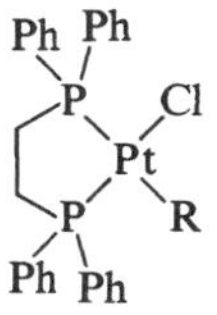

R = Me

M 643.991
Cryst. (CH_2Cl_2/Et_2O). Mp 265-7°.

Clarke, H.C. *et al*, *Inorg. Chem.*, 1975, **14**, 1518 (*synth, ir*)
Appleton, T.G. *et al*, *Inorg. Chem.*, 1978, **17**, 738 (*nmr*)

$C_{27}H_{28}OP_2Pt$ Pt-00324

[1,2-Ethanediylbis(diphenylphosphine)-*P,P′*]hydroxy-(methyl)platinum, 9CI

[Ethylenebis(diphenylphosphine)]hydroxo(methyl)platinum

[43210-95-3]

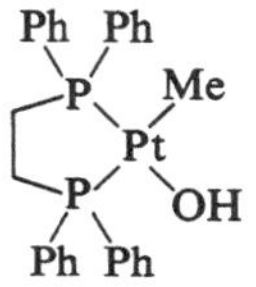

M 625.545
Cryst. ($CHCl_3$/hexane). Mp 160° dec.

Appleton, T.G. *et al*, *Inorg. Chem.*, 1978, **17**, 738 (*synth, nmr*)
Arnold, D.P. *et al*, *J. Organomet. Chem.*, 1980, **199**, C17.

$C_{27}H_{28}P_2Pt$ Pt-00325

[Bis(diphenylphosphino)methane]dimethylplatinum

Dimethyl[methylenebis(diphenylphosphine)-P,P′]platinum, 9CI

[52595-90-1]

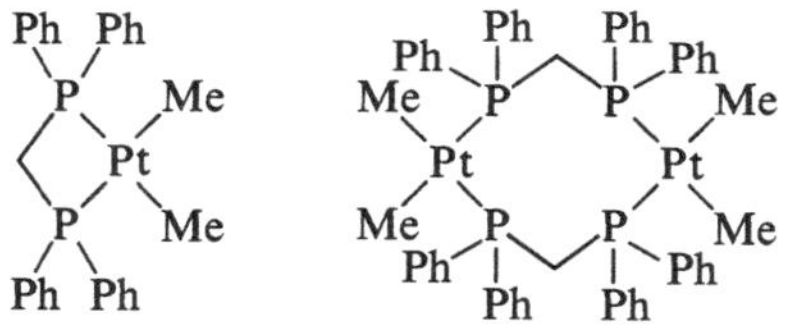

monomer dimer

M 609.546
Cryst. (C_6H_6/hexane). Mp 157-9° dec. Reacts with $Ph_2PCH_2PPh_2$ to form Dimethylbis[methylenebis(diphenylphosphine)-*P*]platinum, Pt-00446 .

Dimer: [79870-63-6]. *Bis[μ-[methylenebis[diphenylphosphine]-P:P′]]tetramethyldiplatinum*, 10CI. *Tetramethylbis-μ-[(diphenylphosphino)methane]diplatinum.*
$C_{54}H_{56}P_4Pt_2$ M 1219.091
Cryst. The dimer is less stable thermodynamically than the monomer, but is less likely to undergo oxidative addition reactions.

Appleton, T.G. *et al*, *J. Chem. Soc., Dalton Trans.*, 1976, 439 (*synth, nmr*)
Cooper, S.J. *et al*, *Inorg. Chem.*, 1981, **20**, 1374 (*synth*)
Puddephatt, R.J. *et al*, *J. Chem. Soc., Chem. Commun.*, 1981, 805 (*synth, nmr, struct*)

Pringle, P.G. *et al*, *J. Chem. Soc., Chem. Commun.*, 1982, 1313.

$C_{27}H_{29}ClP_2Pt$ Pt-00326

Chloro(methyl)bis(methyldiphenylphosphine)platinum

Bis(methyldiphenylphosphine)methylplatinum chloride. Methylchlorobis(methyldiphenylphosphine)platinum

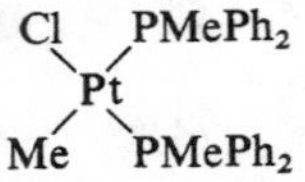

Cl PMePh₂ / Pt / Me PMePh₂ *cis-form*

M 646.007

cis-form [24833-59-8]

Cryst. ($CHCl_3$/pet. ether). Mp 135-40°. Converts to *trans* isomer in soln.

trans-form [24833-61-2]

Cryst. ($CHCl_3$/EtOH). Mp 162-3° dec., 178-80°.

Ruddick, J.D. *et al*, *J. Chem. Soc. (A)*, 1969, 2801 (*synth, pmr, ir*)
Appleton, T.G. *et al*, *J. Chem. Soc., Dalton Trans.*, 1976, 439 (*pmr*)
Bennett, M.A. *et al*, *Inorg. Chem.*, 1979, **18**, 1061 (*struct*)

$C_{27}H_{63}P_3Pt$ Pt-00327

Tris(triisopropylphosphine)platinum

Tris[tris(1-methylethyl)phosphine]platinum, 9CI
[60648-72-8]

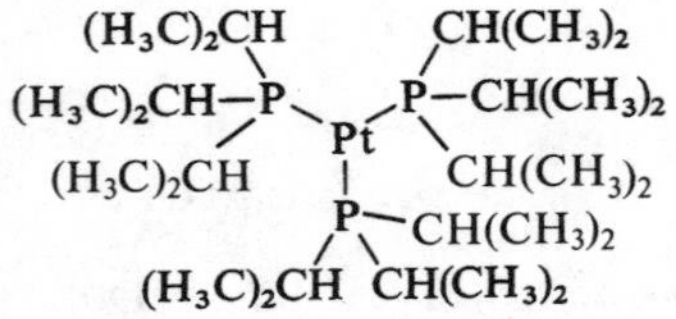

$Pt[P(CH(CH_3)_2)_3]_3$

M 675.796

Catalyses water-gas shift reaction. Air-sensitive, pale-yellow cryst. (pentane). Sol. hydrocarbons. Mp 60-2° (sealed tube under N_2). Reacts with weak protic acids (e.g. EtOH).

Inorg. Synth., 1979, **19**, 107 (*synth*)

$C_{28}H_{20}Pt$ Pt-00328

Bis(diphenylacetylene)platinum

Bis[1,1'-(η^2-1,2-ethynediyl)bis[benzene]]platinum, 10CI. *Bis(diphenylethyne)platinum*
[61771-08-2]

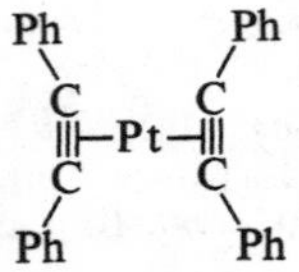

$(PhC{\equiv}CPh)_2Pt$

M 551.546

Cryst. (pet. ether). Mp 140-5° dec.

Boag, N.M. *et al*, *J. Chem. Soc., Dalton Trans.*, 1980, 2170 (*synth, struct, ir, nmr*)

$C_{28}H_{26}ClF_5P_2Pt$ Pt-00329

Chlorobis(methyldiphenylphosphine)(pentafluoroethyl)platinum

Bis(methyldiphenylphosphine)(pentafluoroethyl)platinum chloride. (Pentafluoroethyl)-chlorobis(methyldiphenylphosphine)platinum

Cl PMePh₂ / Pt / Ph₂MeP CF₂CF₃

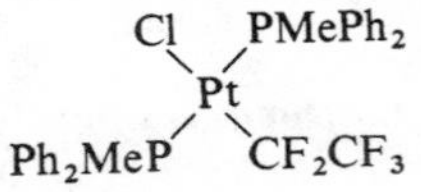

M 749.986

trans-form [68908-21-4]

Cryst. Mp 123-6°.

Bennett, M.A. *et al*, *Inorg. Chem.*, 1979, **18**, 1061 (*synth, struct*)

$C_{28}H_{29}ClP_2Pt$ Pt-00330

Chloroethyl[ethylenebis[diphenylphosphine]]platinum

Chloro[1,2-ethanediylbis[diphenylphosphine]-P,P']ethylplatinum, 9CI. *Ethylchloro[1,2-bis(diphenylphosphino)ethane]platinum*
[65098-10-4]

As Chloro[ethylenebis[diphenylphosphine]]-methylplatinum, Pt-00323 with

R = Et

M 658.018

Cryst. (CH_2Cl_2/Et_2O). Mp 180° dec., 190-200°.

Slack, D.A. *et al*, *Inorg. Chim. Acta*, 1977, **24**, 277 (*synth, nmr, ir*)
Appleton, T.G. *et al*, *Inorg. Chem.*, 1978, **17**, 738 (*synth, nmr*)

$C_{28}H_{30}P_2Pt$ Pt-00331

[Ethylenebis[diphenylphosphine]]dimethylplatinum, 8CI

[1,2-Ethanediylbis[diphenylphosphine]-P,P']dimethylplatinum, 9CI. *Dimethyl[1,2-bis(diphenylphosphino)-ethane]platinum*
[15630-18-9]

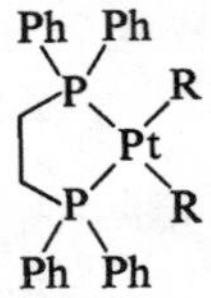

$(Ph_2PCH_2CH_2PPh_2)PtR_2$

R = Me

M 623.573

Cryst. (Me_2CO). Mp 221-3° dec.

Hooton, K.A., *J. Chem. Soc. (A)*, 1970, 1896 (*synth*)
Appleton, T.G. *et al*, *J. Chem. Soc., Dalton Trans.*, 1976, 439 (*synth, nmr*)
Hietkamp, S. *et al*, *J. Organomet. Chem.*, 1979, **169**, 107.

$C_{28}H_{31}ClP_2Pt$ Pt-00332

Chlorohydrobis(ethyldiphenylphosphine)platinum

Chlorobis(ethyldiphenylphosphine)hydroplatinum, 10CI. *Hydridochlorobis(ethyldiphenylphosphine)platinum*

H PEtPh₂ / Pt / Ph₂EtP Cl

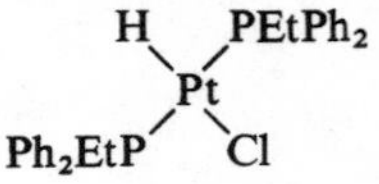

M 660.033

***trans*-form** [67336-53-2]
Cryst. (MeOH). Mp 131-132.5°.

Chatt, J. *et al*, *J. Chem. Soc.*, 1962, 5075 (*synth, ir*)
Eisenberg, R. *et al*, *Inorg. Chem.*, 1965, **4**, 773 (*struct*)
Andersson, C. *et al*, *Chem. Scr.*, 1977, **11**, 140 (*pe*)

$C_{28}H_{32}P_2Pt$ Pt-00333

Dimethylbis(methyldiphenylphosphine)platinum, 9CI
Bis(methyldiphenylphosphine)dimethylplatinum

Me, $PMePh_2$ / Pt / Me, $PMePh_2$ *cis-form*

M 625.588

***cis*-form** [24917-50-8]
Cryst. (pet. ether). Mp 145-50°, 157-60°.

Ruddick, J.D. *et al*, *J. Chem. Soc. (A)*, 1969, 2801 (*synth, pmr, ir*)
Treichel, P.M. *et al*, *J. Organomet. Chem.*, 1973, **61**, 415.
Appleton, T.G. *et al*, *J. Chem. Soc., Dalton Trans.*, 1976, 439 (*nmr*)
Kennedy, J.D. *et al*, *J. Chem. Soc., Dalton Trans.*, 1976, 874 (*nmr*)
Bennett, M.A., *Inorg. Chem.*, 1979, **18**, 1061 (*synth*)

$C_{28}H_{35}ClP_2Pt$ Pt-00334

Chlorobis(diethylphenylphosphine)(phenylethynyl)platinum, 9CI
Chlorobis(diethylphenylphosphine)(phenylacetylide)-platinum.
Phenylethynylchlorobis(diethylphenylphosphine)platinum

$PtCl(C{\equiv}CPh)(PEt_2Ph)_2$

M 664.065

***trans*-form** [51466-65-0]
Cryst. (hexane). Mp 108°.

Cardin, C.J. *et al*, *J. Chem. Soc., Dalton Trans.*, 1977, 767 (*synth, ir*)
Cardin, C.J. *et al*, *J. Chem. Soc., Dalton Trans.*, 1978, 46 (*struct*)

$C_{28}H_{40}As_2Pt$ Pt-00335

Bis(phenylethynyl)bis(triethylarsine)platinum
Bis(phenylacetylide)bis(triethylarsine)platinum

$Pt(C{\equiv}CPh)_2(AsEt_3)_2$

M 721.547

***trans*-form**
Yellow cryst. (pet. ether or EtOH). Mp 178-81° dec. Dipole moment 1.3 D.

Chatt, J. *et al*, *J. Chem. Soc.*, 1959, 4020 (*synth, ir*)

$C_{28}H_{40}P_2Pt$ Pt-00336

Bis(phenylethynyl)bis(triethylphosphine)platinum, 9CI
Bis(phenylacetylide)bis(triethylphosphine)platinum

Et_3P, $C{\equiv}CPh$ / Pt / Et_3P, $C{\equiv}CPh$ *cis-form*

M 633.652

***cis*-form**
Cryst. (C_6H_6/hexane). Mp 138-9° dec. Slowly isom. to *trans*-form in soln.

***trans*-form** [15927-86-3]
Cryst. (pet. ether). Mp 186-7° dec. Dipole moment 0.9D.

Chatt, J. *et al*, *J. Chem. Soc.*, 1959, 4020 (*synth*)
Masai, H. *et al*, *Bull. Chem. Soc. Jpn.*, 1971, **44**, 2226 (*uv*)
Masai, H. *et al*, *J. Organomet. Chem.*, 1971, **26**, 271 (*ir*)
Sonogashira, K. *et al*, *J. Organomet. Chem.*, 1978, **145**, 101 (*synth, ir*)

$C_{28}H_{46}P_2Pt$ Pt-00337

Bis(di-*tert*-butylphenylphosphine)platinum
Bis[bis-(1,1-dimethylethyl)phenylphosphine]platinum, 10CI
[59765-06-9]

$Ph{-}P(C(CH_3)_3)_2{-}Pt{-}P(C(CH_3)_3)_2{-}Ph$

M 639.699
Linear. Pale-yellow cryst. (pentane); air-sensitive.

Inorg. Synth., 1979, **19**, 101 (*synth, nmr*)
Mann, B.E. *et al*, *J. Chem. Soc., Dalton Trans.*, 1980, 776 (*synth, nmr*)

$C_{29}H_{25}BrNPPt$ Pt-00338

Bromo[1-(8-quinolinyl)ethyl-*C,N*]triphenylphosphineplatinum, 9CI
[59645-01-1]

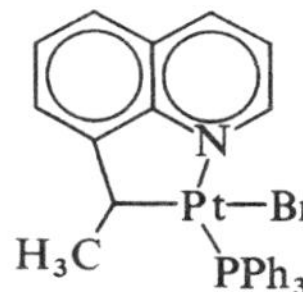

M 693.481
Prepd. from 8-(α-bromoethyl)quinoline and $[Pt(PPh_3)_3]$ with retention of configuration.

Sokolov, V.I., *Inorg. Chim. Acta*, 1976, **18**, L9.

$C_{30}H_{30}O_2P_2Pt$ Pt-00339

Dicarbonylbis(ethyldiphenylphosphine)platinum
Bis(ethyldiphenylphosphine)dicarbonylplatinum
[36608-09-0]

$Pt(CO)_2(PPh_2Et)_2$ (C_{2v})

M 679.593
Yellow cryst. Mp 95-7° dec.

Chini, P. *et al*, *J. Chem. Soc. (A)*, 1970, 1542 (*synth*)
Albano, V.G. *et al*, *J. Organomet. Chem.*, 1972, **35**, 423 (*struct*)

$C_{30}H_{31}P_2Pt^{\oplus}$ Pt-00340

[1,2-Ethanediylbis(diphenylphosphine)-*P,P'*](1,2,3-η)-2-methyl-2-propenyl]platinum(1+), 9CI

2-Methylallyl[ethylenebis(diphenylphosphine)]platinum(1+)

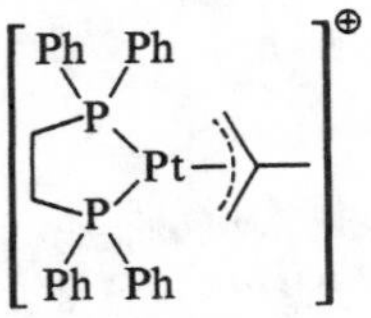

M 648.602 (ion)

Hexafluorophosphate: [54788-65-7].
$C_{30}H_{31}F_6P_3Pt$ M 793.567
Cryst. ($CHCl_2/Et_2O$). Mp 208-9°.

Clark, H.C. *et al*, *Inorg. Chem.*, 1975, **14**, 1518 (*synth, nmr, ir*)

$C_{30}H_{34}P_2Pt$ Pt-00341

Diethyl[ethylenebis[diphenylphosphine]]platinum

[1,2-Ethanediylbis[diphenylphosphine]-P,P']diethylplatinum, 9CI. *Diethyl[1,2-bis(diphenylphosphino)-ethane]platinum*

[52621-10-0]

As [Ethylenebis[diphenylphosphine]]dimethylplatinum, Pt-00331 with

R = Et

M 651.626
Cryst. (CH_2Cl_2/Et_2O). Mp 198-200° dec.

Glockling, F. *et al*, *Inorg. Chim. Acta*, 1974, **8**, 81 (*ms*)
Slack, D.A. *et al*, *Inorg. Chim. Acta*, 1977, **24**, 277 (*synth, nmr*)

$C_{30}H_{38}P_2Pt$ Pt-00342

Tetramethylbis(methyldiphenylphosphine)platinum, 9CI

Bis(methyldiphenylphosphine)tetramethylplatinum

[62742-25-0]

$Me_4Pt(PMePh_2)_2$

M 655.658
Cryst. (hexane). Mp 120° dec. Reacts in chloroform to eliminate ethane and form *trans*-[$PtMeCl(PMePh_2)_2$].

Rice, G.W. *et al*, *J. Am. Chem. Soc.*, 1977, **99**, 2141 (*synth, pmr, ir*)

$C_{30}H_{52}Br_2P_2Pt_2$ Pt-00343

Di-μ-bromodiphenylbis(tripropylphosphine)diplatinum

Diphenyldibromobis(tripropylphosphine)diplatinum

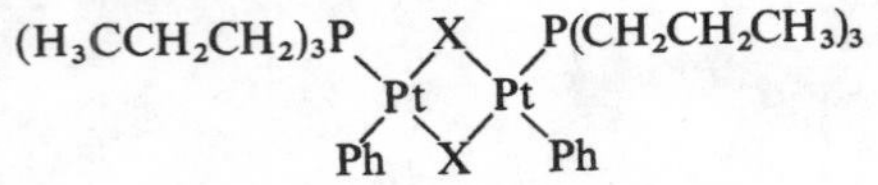

X = Br

M 1024.656
Bridged dimer. Cryst. (C_6H_6). Mp 209°. Dipole moment 4.05D.

Monomer: Bromophenyl(tripropylphosphine)platinum.
$C_{15}H_{26}BrPPt$ M 512.328
Unknown.

Chatt, J. *et al*, *J. Chem. Soc.*, 1964, 2433 (*synth*)

$C_{30}H_{52}I_2P_2Pt_2$ Pt-00344

Di-μ-iododiphenylbis(tripropylphosphine)diplatinum

Diphenyldiiodobis(tripropylphosphine)diplatinum

As Di-μ-bromodiphenylbis(tripropylphosphine)diplatinum, Pt-00343 with

X = I

M 1118.657
Bridged dimer. Orange cryst. (Me_2CO). Mp 186°. Dipole moment 4.15D.

Monomer: Iodophenyl(tripropylphosphine)platinum.
$C_{15}H_{26}IPPt$ M 559.329
Unknown.

Chatt, J. *et al*, *J. Chem. Soc.*, 1964, 2433 (*synth*)

$C_{30}H_{54}N_6Pt_3$ Pt-00345

Tris-μ-(2-isocyano-2-methylpropane)tris(2-isocyano-2-methylpropane)triplatinum, 9CI

Tris-μ-(tert-butylisonitrile)tris(tert-butylisonitrile)triplatinum. Hexakis(2-isocyano-2-methylpropane)triplatinum. Hexakis(tert-butylisonitrile)triplatinum

[55664-26-1]

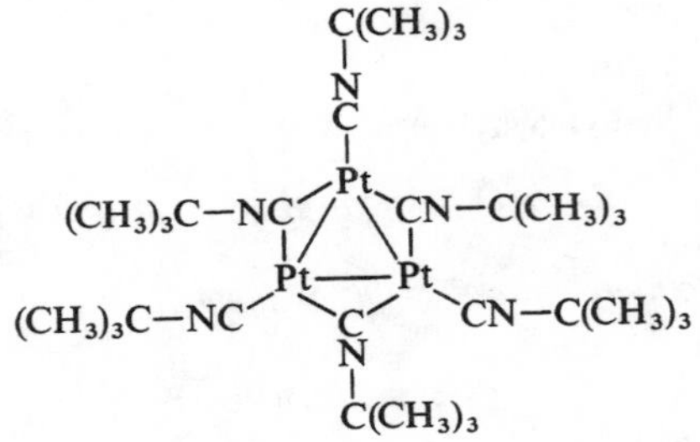

M 1084.037
Orange-red solid (pentane). Dec. at 125-45°.

Green, M. *et al*, *J. Chem. Soc., Chem. Commun.*, 1975, 3 (*struct, ir*)
Goel, R.G. *et al*, *J. Organomet. Chem.*, 1981, **214**, 405 (*synth, pmr, ir*)
Goel, R.G. *et al*, *Organometallics*, 1982, **1**, 819 (*synth, ir*)

$C_{30}H_{67}P_4Pt_2^{\oplus}$ Pt-00346

μ-Hydrohydrophenyltetrakis(triethylphosphine)diplatinum(1+)

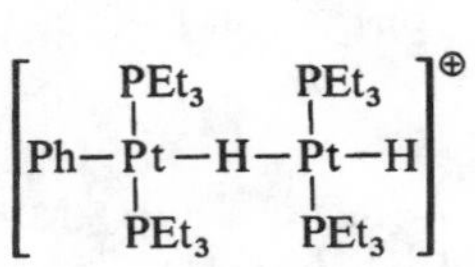

M 941.914 (ion)

Tetraphenylborate: [67891-25-2].
$C_{54}H_{87}BP_4Pt_2$ M 1261.146
Air stable solid, slowly dec. in soln. ($CHCl_3$/MeOH).

Hexafluorophosphate:
$C_{30}H_{67}F_6P_5Pt_2$ M 1086.879
Air stable solid, slowly dec. in soln. (CH_2Cl_2/MeOH).

Bracher, G. *et al*, *Angew. Chem., Int. Ed. Engl.*, 1978, **17**, 778 (*synth, nmr, struct*)

$C_{30}O_{30}Pt_{15}^{\ominus\ominus}$ Pt-00347

Pentadeca-μ-carbonylpentadecacarbonylpentadecaplatinate(2−)

Pentakis[hexacarbonyltriplatinate](2−)

[52349-90-3]

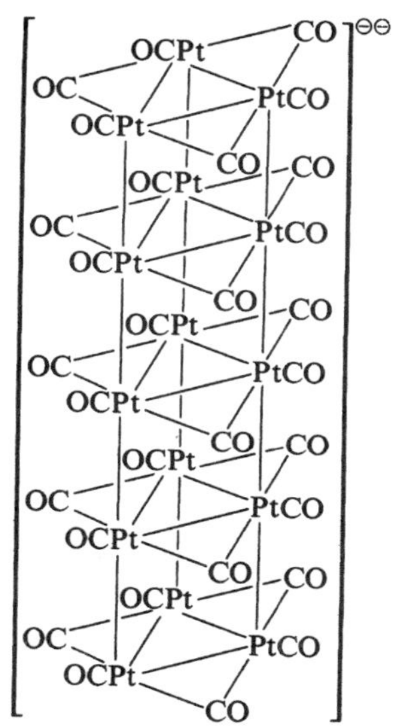

M 3766.512 (ion)

Yellow-green soln. in THF.

Bis(tetrabutylammonium) salt: [61215-55-2].
$C_{62}H_{72}N_2O_{30}Pt_{15}$ M 4251.446
Catalyses hydroformylation and water-gas shift reactions and reduction of aromatic nitro compounds; used for prep. of Pt catalyst for hexane isomerization.

Bis(tetraethylammonium) salt: [59451-62-6].
$C_{46}H_{40}N_2O_{30}Pt_{15}$ M 4027.017
Catalyses hydrocarbon synthesis and methanol synthesis from hydrogen and carbon monoxide.

Calabrese, J.C. *et al*, *J. Am. Chem. Soc.*, 1974, **96**, 2614 (*synth, ir, struct*)
Kang, H.C. *et al*, *J. Am. Chem. Soc.*, 1977, **99**, 8323 (*use*)
Cann, K. *et al*, *J. Am. Chem. Soc.*, 1978, **100**, 3969 (*use*)
Ichikawa, M., *Bull. Chem. Soc. Jpn.*, 1978, **51**, 2268 (*use*)
Apai, G. *et al*, *J. Am. Chem. Soc.*, 1979, **101**, 6880 (*synth*)
Brown, C. *et al*, *J. Organomet. Chem.*, 1979, **181**, 233 (*cmr, nmr*)
Garin, F. *et al*, *Surf. Sci.*, 1981, **106**, 466 (*use*)

$C_{31}H_{34}AsClO_2Pt$ Pt-00348

[8-(1-Acetyl-2-oxopropyl)-4-cycloocten-1-yl]chloro(triphenylarsine)platinum, 9CI

Chloro[(1,4,5-η)-8-(1-acetylacetonyl)-4-cycloocten-1-yl]triphenylarsineplatinum. [8-(1-Acetylacetonyl)-4-cycloocten-1-yl]chloro(triphenylarsine)platinum

[11141-96-1]

COCH₃
CH
COCH₃
PtCl(AsPh₃)

M 744.063

Cryst. ($CHCl_3/Et_2O$). Mp 204-5°.

Johnson, B.F.G. *et al*, *J. Chem. Soc.* (*A*), 1968, 1993.
Inorg. Synth., 1972, **13**, 55 (*synth*)

$C_{32}H_{28}Pt_2$ Pt-00349

[μ-[(1,2,5,6-η:3,4,7,8-η)-Cyclooctatetraene]]tetraphenyldiplatinum

μ-Cyclooctatetraenebis(diphenylplatinum)

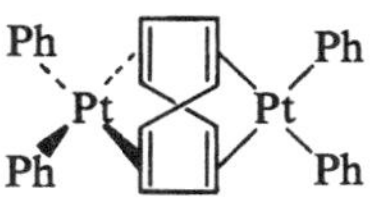

M 802.733

Green cryst. (CH_2Cl_2/hexane) or pale-yellow cryst. Mp 155-65° dec.

Doyle, J.R. *et al*, *J. Am. Chem. Soc.*, 1961, **83**, 2768 (*synth*)
Kistner, C.R. *et al*, *Inorg. Chem.*, 1963, **2**, 1255 (*synth, pmr*)

$C_{32}H_{29}ClP_2Pt$ Pt-00350

Chloro[ethylenebis(diphenylphosphine)]phenylplatinum, 8CI

Chloro[1,2-ethanediylbis[diphenylphosphine]-P,P′]-phenylplatinum, 9CI. Phenyl[1,2-bis(diphenylphosphino)-ethane]chloroplatinum

[27711-51-9]

As Chloro[ethylenebis[diphenylphosphine]]-methylplatinum, Pt-00323 with

R = Ph

M 706.062

Cryst. (C_6H_6). Mp 279-80°.

Hooton, K.A., *J. Chem. Soc.* (*A*), 1970, 1896 (*synth*)
Eaborn, C. *et al*, *J. Chem. Soc., Dalton Trans.*, 1978, 357 (*nmr, synth*)
Anderson, G.K. *et al*, *Inorg. Chem.*, 1981, **20**, 3607 (*nmr*)

$C_{32}H_{31}ClP_2Pt$ Pt-00351

Chlorobis(methyldiphenylphosphine)phenylplatinum, 9CI

Bis(methyldiphenylphosphine)phenylplatinum(II) chloride. Phenylchlorobis(methyldiphenylphosphine)-platinum

Ph PMePh₂
Pt
Ph₂MeP Cl

M 708.077

***trans*-form** [60772-01-2]

Cryst. (C_6H_6/pet. ether). Mp 185° (182-3°).

Garrou, P.E. *et al*, *J. Am. Chem. Soc.*, 1976, **98**, 4115 (*nmr*)
Anderson, G.K. *et al*, *J. Chem. Soc., Dalton Trans.*, 1979, 1246 (*synth*)

$C_{32}H_{32}P_2Pt$ Pt-00352

Bis(dimethylphenylphosphine)bis(phenylethynyl)platinum, 9CI

Bis(phenylethynyl)bis(dimethylphenylphosphine)platinum. Bis(phenylacetylide)-bis(dimethylphenylphosphine)platinum

$[Pt(C{\equiv}CPh)_2(PMe_2Ph)_2](D_{2h})$

M 673.632

***trans*-form** [28775-98-6]

Yellow cryst. (C_6H_6/pet. ether). Mp 191-2° (177°).

Chatt, J. *et al*, *J. Organomet. Chem.*, 1970, **23**, 109 (*synth*)
Almeida, J.F. *et al*, *J. Organomet. Chem.*, 1981, **209**, 415 (*synth, nmr*)

$C_{34}H_{28}O_2Pt$ Pt-00353

Bis[(C^3,O^3-η)-1,5-diphenyl-1,4-pentadien-3-one]platinum, 9CI

Bis(dibenzylideneacetone)platinum

[33677-56-4]

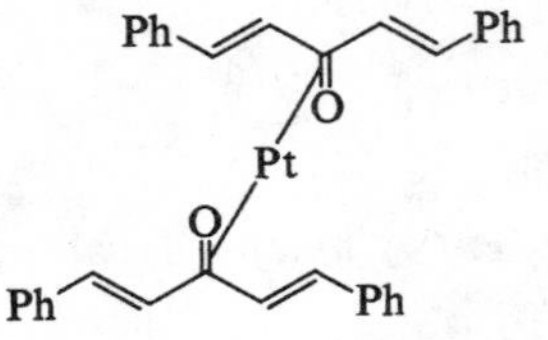

M 663.674

Probably bonded to ketone group as shown, though olefinic bonding has been postulated. Catalyses oligomerisation of acetylenes. Air-stable, dark-purple cryst. (Me_2CO). Sol. MeOH. Dec. above 170° to Pt and dibenzylideneacetone.

Moseley, K. *et al*, *J. Chem. Soc., Chem. Commun.*, 1971, 982 (*synth, pmr, ir*)
Cherwinski, W.J. *et al*, *J. Chem. Soc., Dalton Trans.*, 1974, 1405 (*synth*)

$C_{34}H_{38}P_2Pt_2$ Pt-00354

Bis(diphenylacetylene)bis(trimethylphosphine)diplatinum

[μ-[1,1'-($η^2$:$η^2$-1,2-Ethynediyl)bis[benzene]]][1,1'-(η-^{2}-1,2-ethynediyl)bis[benzene]]bis(trimethylphosphine)-diplatinum, 10CI

[61823-50-5]

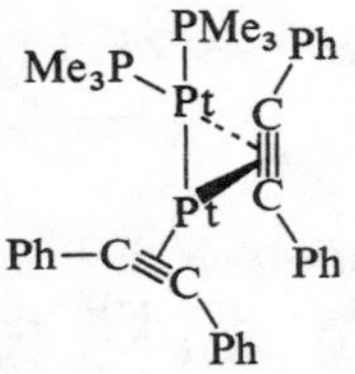

M 898.782

Orange-yellow cryst. (Et_2O).

Green, M. *et al*, *J. Chem. Soc., Chem. Commun.*, 1976, 759 (*synth, struct, ir, nmr*)
Boag, N.M. *et al*, *J. Chem. Res. (S)*, 1978, 228; *J. Chem. Res. (M)*, 2962 (*nmr*)

$C_{36}H_{30}Cl_2P_2Pt$ Pt-00355

Dichlorobis(triphenylphosphine)platinum, 9CI, 8CI

Bis(triphenylphosphine)platinum dichloride. Bis(triphenylphosphine)dichloroplatinum

[10199-34-5]

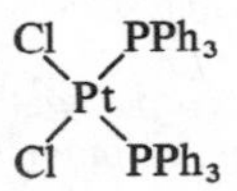

cis-form

M 790.567

Catalyst, often with added $SnCl_2$, for hydrogenation and hydroformylation reactions. Catalyses hydrosilylation and carboxylation of olefins, isomerisation and polymerisation of alkenes and alkynes.

▷ATPase inhibitor

cis-form [15604-36-1]

V. pale-yellow cryst. ($CHCl_3$). Mp 310-2°.

trans-form [14056-88-3]

Yellow cryst. (C_6H_6). Mp 307-10°.

Allen, A.D. *et al*, *Chem. Ind. (London)*, 1965, 139 (*synth*)
Bailar, J.C. *et al*, *Inorg. Chem.*, 1965, **4**, 1618 (*synth*)
Mastin, S.H., *J. Am. Chem. Soc.*, 1971, **93**, 6823 (*synth*)
Gillard, R.D. *et al*, *J. Chem. Soc., Dalton Trans.*, 1974, 2320 (*synth*)
Mastin, S.H., *Inorg. Chem.*, 1974, **13**, 1003 (*ir, raman*)
Goel, R.G., *Inorg. Nucl. Chem. Lett.*, 1979, **15**, 437 (*nmr*)

$C_{36}H_{30}O_2P_2Pt$ Pt-00356

(Dioxygen)bis(triphenylphosphine)platinum, 9CI, 8CI

Peroxybis(triphenylphosphine)platinum, 9CI, 8CI. Dioxobis(triphenylphosphine)platinum, 8CI. Bis(triphenylphosphine)oxygenoplatinum

[15614-67-2]

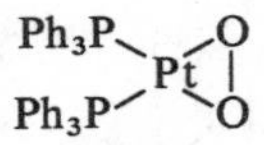

M 751.659

Catalyst for oxidn. of alkenes, aldehydes and phosphines. Orange cryst. (C_6H_6). Mp 135-6°. Frequently cryst. with a solv. mol. in lattice.

Nyman, C.J. *et al*, *J. Chem. Soc. (A)*, 1968, 561 (*synth*)
Cheng, P.T. *et al*, *Can. J. Chem.*, 1971, **49**, 3772 (*struct*)
Mastin, M.H. *et al*, *Inorg. Chem.*, 1974, **13**, 1003 (*ir*)
Sen, A. *et al*, *Inorg. Chem.*, 1980, **19**, 1073 (*nmr*)

$C_{36}H_{31}ClP_2Pt$ Pt-00357

Chlorohydrobis(triphenylphosphine)platinum, 9CI, 8CI

Chlorohydridobis(triphenylphosphine)platinum. Bis(triphenylphosphine)platinum hydridochloride

[16902-93-5]

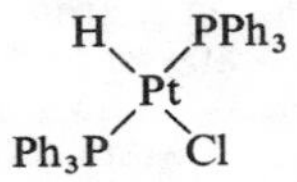

M 756.121

cis-form [25879-12-3]

The compound originally designated *cis* geometry appears to be a different crystallographic form of the *trans* isomer.

trans-form [16841-99-9]

Catalyst for alkene isomerisation, hydrogenation, and for PhC≡CH polymerisation. Cocatalyst with $SnCl_2$ for hydroformylation and hydrosilylation. Cryst. (C_6H_6/MeOH). Mp 215-20° dec. Dipole moment 4.4 D.

▷ATP-ase inhibitor

Chatt, J. *et al*, *J. Chem. Soc.*, 1962, 5075 (*synth, ir*)
Clemmit, A. *et al*, *J. Chem. Soc. (A)*, 1969, 2163 (*ir, pmr*)
Darensbourg, D.J. *et al*, *J. Chem. Phys.*, 1973, **59**, 3869 (*ir*)
McFarlane, W., *J. Chem. Soc., Dalton Trans.*, 1974, 324 (*nmr*)
Balimann, G. *et al*, *J. Magn. Reson.*, 1976, **22**, 235 (*nmr*)
Andersson, C. *et al*, *Chem. Scr.*, 1977, **11**, 140 (*ir, pe*)

$C_{36}H_{31}Cl_3P_2PtSn$ Pt-00358

Hydro(trichlorostannyl)bis(triphenylphosphine)platinum, 9CI

Hydrido(trichlorostannyl)bis(triphenylphosphine)platinum. (Trichlorotin)hydridobis(triphenylphosphine)-platinum

[18041-19-5]

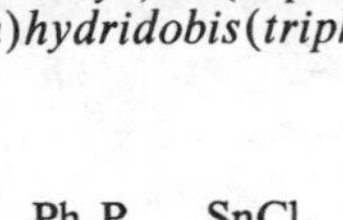

M 945.717

Catalyst for hydroformylation and isomerisation of olefins.

trans-form [18117-31-2]

Yellow-orange solid. Mp 130-5° dec., 172-3° dec.

Baird, M.C., *J. Inorg. Nucl. Chem.*, 1967, **29**, 367 (*synth*)
Hsu, C.-Y. *et al*, *J. Am. Chem. Soc.*, 1975, **97**, 3553 (*synth*)
Antonov, P.G. *et al*, *Zh. Neorg. Khim.*, 1979, **24**, 1008; *CA*, **91**, 12956h (*ir*, *pmr*, *nqr*)
Starzewski, K.A.O. *et al*, *Inorg. Chim. Acta*, 1979, **36**, L445 (*nmr*)

$C_{36}H_{52}P_4Pt_2$ Pt-00359

Dihydrobis-μ-(diphenylphosphino)bis(triethylphosphine)diplatinum

Dihydridobis-μ-(diphenylphosphino)bis(triethylphosphine)diplatinum

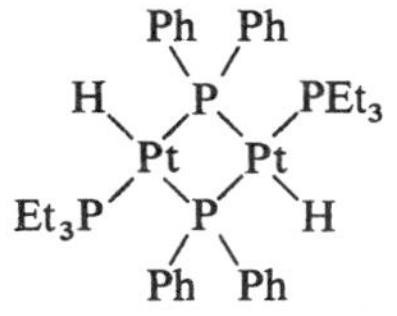

M 998.862

Cryst. ($CHCl_3$/MeOH). ir ν(PtH)2005 cm^{-1}.

Chatt, J. *et al*, *J. Chem. Soc.*, 1964, 2433 (*synth*, *ir*)

$C_{36}H_{66}P_2Pt$ Pt-00360

Bis(tricyclohexylphosphine)platinum, 9CI

[55664-33-0]

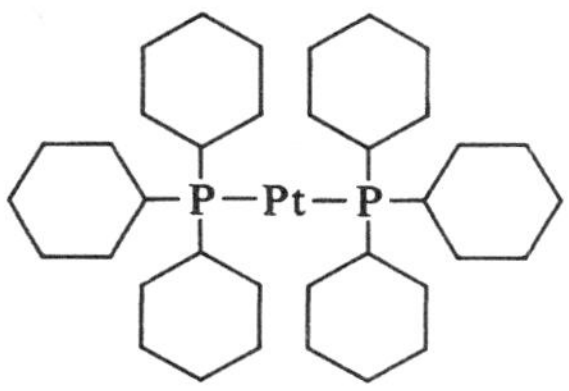

M 755.945

Near-linear struct. Catalyses nitrile hydration reactions. Air-sensitive cryst. (hexane). Sol. C_6H_6, hexane. Mp 204-8° (sealed tube under N_2). Reacts readily with weak protic acids (e.g. EtOH).

Immirzi, A. *et al*, *Inorg. Chim. Acta*, 1975, **13**, L13 (*struct*)
Inorg. Synth., 1979, **19**, 101 (*synth*)
Mann, B.E. *et al*, *J. Chem. Soc., Dalton Trans.*, 1980, 776 (*synth*, *nmr*)

$C_{36}H_{68}P_2Pt$ Pt-00361

Dihydrobis(tricyclohexylphosphine)platinum

Bis(tricyclohexylphosphine)platinum dihydride

[42764-83-0]

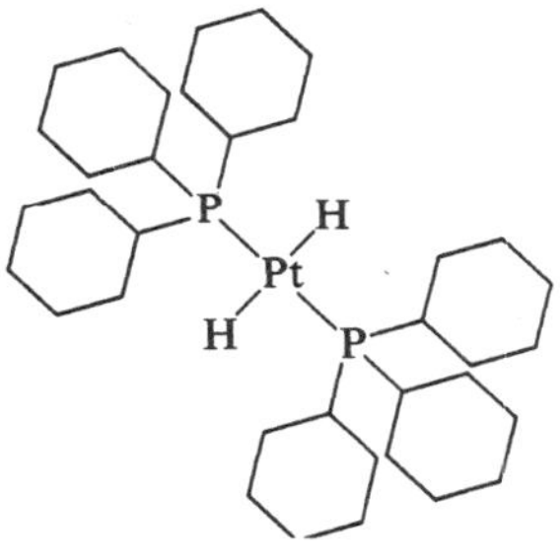

M 757.961

Cryst. (toluene) or pale-yellow cryst. (hexane).

Immirzi, A. *et al*, *Inorg. Chim. Acta*, 1975, **12**, L23 (*synth*, *struct*)
Albinati, A. *et al*, *Inorg. Chim. Acta*, 1976, **18**, 219.
Immirzi, A. *et al*, *Inorg. Chim. Acta*, 1977, **22**, L35.
Clark, H.C. *et al*, *J. Organomet. Chem.*, 1978, **152**, C45 (*synth*)

$C_{36}H_{70}P_2Pt_2$ Pt-00362

Di-μ-hydrodihydrobis(tricyclohexylphosphine)diplatinum, 10CI

Di-μ-hydridodihydridobis(tricyclohexylphosphine)diplatinum

[61502-11-2]

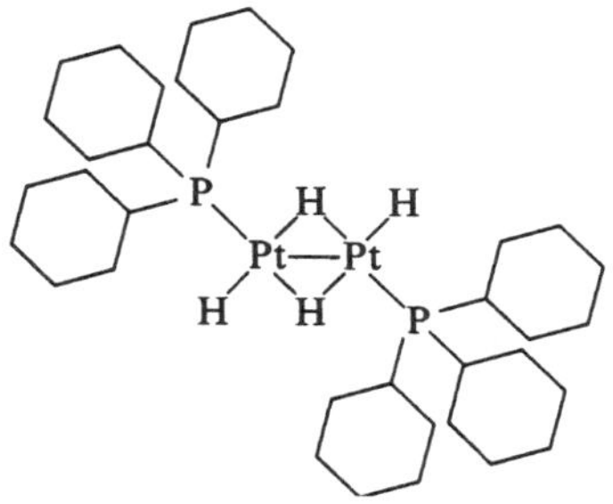

M 955.057

Possible hydrosilylation catalyst.

Green, M. *et al*, *J. Chem. Soc., Chem. Commun.*, 1976, 671.

$C_{36}H_{87}P_3Pt_3$ Pt-00363

Tri-μ-hydrotrihydrotris(tri-*tert*-butylphosphine)triplatinum

Tri-μ-hydridotrihydridotris[tris-(1,1-dimethylethyl-)phosphine]triplatinum

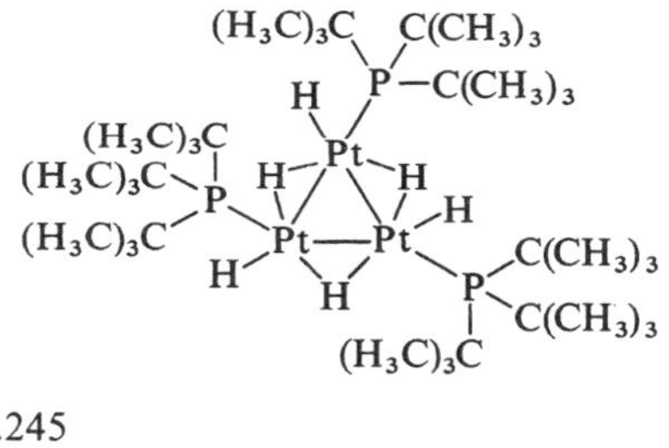

M 1198.245

Yellow cryst. (pet. ether).

Frost, P.W. *et al*, *J. Chem. Soc., Chem. Commun.*, 1981, 1104 (*synth*, *struct*)

$C_{36}O_{36}Pt_{18}^{\ominus\ominus}$ Pt-00364

Octadeca-μ-carbonyloctadecacarbonyloctadecaplatinate(2−), 9CI
Hexakis[hexacarbonyltriplatinate](2−)
[61162-90-1]

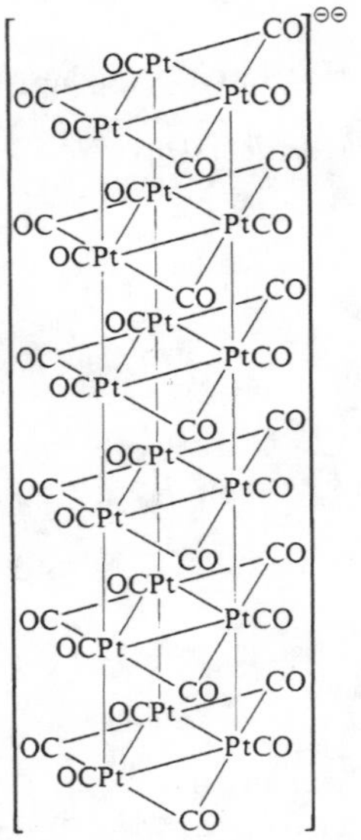

M 4519.814 (ion)
Bis(tetraphenylphosphonium) salt: [61251-07-8].
$C_{84}H_{40}O_{36}P_2Pt_{18}$ M 5198.606
Deposits Pt on Al_2O_3 or SiO_2 to form heterogeneous catalysts. Olive-green cryst. (2-propanol).

Longoni, G. *et al*, *J. Am. Chem. Soc.*, 1976, **98**, 7225 (*synth*, *ir*)
Watters, K.L., *SIA*, *Surf. Interface Anal.*, 1981, **3**, 55; *CA*, **94**, 163159p.

$C_{37}H_{30}ClOP_2Pt^{\oplus}$ Pt-00365

Carbonylchlorobis(triphenylphosphine)platinum(1+), 9CI, 8CI
Chlorocarbonylbis(triphenylphosphine)platinum(1+)
[32424-72-9]
As Carbonylchlorobis(dimethylphenylphosphine)-platinum(1+), Pt-00190 with

$$R^1 = R^2 = Ph$$

M 783.124 (ion)
Cocatalyst with $SnCl_2$ for olefin hydroformylation.
***trans*-form** [20683-70-9]
Reacts with boiling water to form Chlorohydrobis(dimethylphenylphosphine)platinum, Pt-00180 .
Tetrafluoroborate: [19184-24-8].
$C_{37}H_{30}BClF_4OP_2Pt$ M 869.928
Cryst. (C_6H_6). Insol. pet. ether, sol. $CHCl_3$, MeOH. Mp 282° dec. (270°).
Perchlorate: [53203-81-9].
$C_{37}H_{30}Cl_2O_5P_2Pt$ M 882.575
Solid.

Clark, H.C. *et al*, *J. Am. Chem. Soc.*, 1968, **90**, 2259 (*synth*, *ir*)
Cherwinski, W.J. *et al*, *J. Chem. Soc., Dalton Trans.*, 1975, 1156 (*cmr*)
Kurosawa, H., *Inorg. Chem.*, 1975, **14**, 2148 (*synth*)

$C_{37}H_{30}F_3IP_2Pt$ Pt-00366

Iodo(trifluoromethyl)bis(triphenylphosphine)platinum, 8CI
(Trifluoromethyl)bis(triphenylphosphine)platinum iodide. Bis(triphenylphosphine)-perfluoromethyliodoplatinum
[23868-36-2]

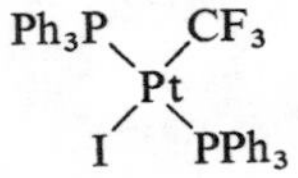

M 915.571
***trans*-form** [19469-54-6]
Orange cryst. (C_6H_6/MeOH). Mp 302°.

Rosevear, D.T. *et al*, *J. Chem. Soc. (A)*, 1968, 164 (*synth*, *ir*)
Appleton, T.G. *et al*, *J. Organomet. Chem.*, 1978, **154**, 369 (*nmr*)

$C_{37}H_{30}OP_2PtS$ Pt-00367

(Carbon oxysulfide)bis(triphenylphosphine)platinum
(Monocarbon monooxide monosulfide)bis(triphenylphosphine)platinum, 10CI. (Carbonyl sulfide)bis(triphenylphosphine)platinum, 8CI
[10210-51-2]

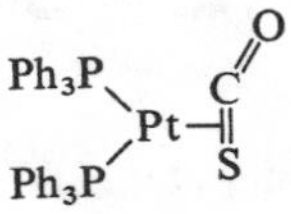

M 779.731
Tangerine-pink solid. Dec. in CH_2Cl_2 or $CHCl_3$ to $[Pt_2S(CO)_2(PPh_3)_3]$.

Baird, M.C. *et al*, *J. Chem. Soc. (A)*, 1967, 865 (*synth*)
Poddar, R.K. *et al*, *J. Coord. Chem.*, 1977, **6**, 207.

$C_{37}H_{30}P_2PtS_2$ Pt-00368

(Carbon disulfide-*C*,*S*)bis(triphenylphosphine)platinum, 9CI
(Carbon disulfide-S)bis(triphenylphosphine)platinum, 9CI. Dithiocarboxylatobis(triphenylphosphosphine)platinum, 8CI
[15308-68-6]

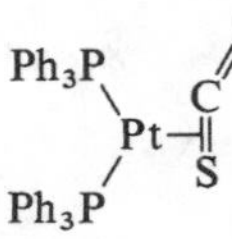

M 795.792
Orange, air-stable cryst. (CH_2Cl_2/Et_2O). Mp 145-65° dec.

Baird, M.C. *et al*, *J. Chem. Soc. (A)*, 1967, 865 (*synth*, *ir*)
Mason, R. *et al*, *J. Chem. Soc. (A)*, 1970, 1767 (*struct*)
Cherwinski, W.J. *et al*, *J. Chem. Soc., Dalton Trans.*, 1974, 1405 (*synth*)
Vergamini, P.J. *et al*, *Inorg. Chim. Acta*, 1979, **34**, L291 (*nmr*)

$C_{37}H_{30}P_2PtSe_2$ Pt-00369

[(*C,Se*-η)-Carbondiselenide]bis(triphenylphosphine)platinum, 9CI

Bis(triphenylphosphine)(carbon diselenide)platinum

[51976-65-9]

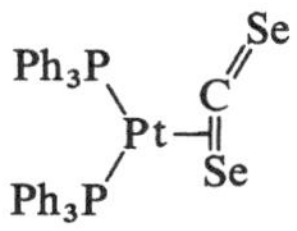

M 889.592

Green or brown solid. Sol. C_6H_6, CH_2Cl_2, insol. EtOH, Et_2O. Mp 158-63° dec., 120-2° dec.

Jensen, K.A. *et al*, *Acta Chem. Scand.*, 1973, **27**, 3605 (*synth*)
Kawakami, K. *et al*, *J. Organomet. Chem.*, 1974, **69**, 151 (*synth*)

$C_{37}H_{31}F_3P_2Pt$ Pt-00370

Hydro(trifluoromethyl)bis(triphenylphosphine)platinum

(Trifluoromethyl)hydridobis(triphenylphosphine)platinum

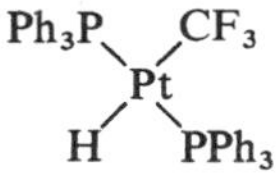

M 789.675

trans-form [64933-37-5]

Cryst. (EtOH). Sol. C_6H_6, CH_2Cl_2, sl. sol. alcohols.

Michelin, R.A. *et al*, *Inorg. Chim. Acta*, 1977, **24**, L33 (*synth, nmr*)
Del Pra, A. *et al*, *Cryst. Struct. Commun.*, 1979, **8**, 729 (*struct*)

$C_{37}H_{31}OP_2Pt^{\oplus}$ Pt-00371

Carbonylhydrobis(triphenylphosphine)platinum(1+)

Hydridocarbonylbis(triphenylphosphine)platinum(1+)

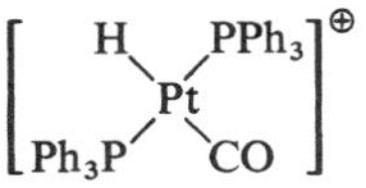

M 748.679 (ion)

trans-form

Perchlorate: [32109-32-3].
$C_{37}H_{31}ClO_5P_2Pt$ M 848.129
Hydrosilylation catalyst. Cryst. (Me_2CO/pet. ether).

Trichlorostannate: [56231-80-2].
$C_{37}H_{31}Cl_3OP_2PtSn$ M 973.728
Hydroformylation catalyst. Green-yellow cryst. (C_6H_6). Mp 93-5° dec. The trichlorostannate might coordinate to give a 5-coordinate complex.

Tetrafluoroborate: [33915-37-6].
$C_{37}H_{31}BF_4OP_2Pt$ M 835.482
Amber oil (CH_2Cl_2).

Gavrilova, I.V. *et al*, *Zh. Neorg. Khim.*, 1971, **16**, 1124; *Russ. J. Inorg. Chem. (Engl. Transl.)*, **16**, 596 (*synth, ir*)
Cherwinski, W.J. *et al*, *Inorg. Chem.*, 1971, **10**, 2263 (*synth, ir*)
Hsu, C.-Y. *et al*, *J. Am. Chem. Soc.*, 1975, **97**, 3553 (*synth, use*)

$C_{37}H_{33}BrP_2Pt$ Pt-00372

Bromo(methyl)bis(triphenylphosphine)platinum, 9CI, 8CI

Methylbis(triphenylphosphine)platinum bromide

[15276-80-9]

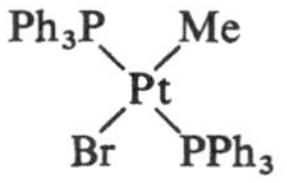

trans-form

M 814.599

cis-(?)-form [41620-25-1]

Yellow cryst.

trans-form [28850-20-6]

Cryst. (MeOH). Mp 275-7°.

Clark, H.C. *et al*, *Inorg. Chem.*, 1970, **9**, 2670 (*synth, ir, nmr*)
Crociani, B. *et al*, *J. Organomet. Chem.*, 1973, **49**, 249 (*synth*)

$C_{37}H_{33}ClP_2Pt$ Pt-00373

Chloromethylbis(triphenylphosphine)platinum, 9CI, 8CI

Methylbis(triphenylphosphine)platinum chloride

[15278-39-4]

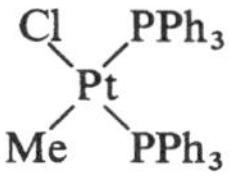

cis-form

M 770.148

cis-form [52193-96-1]

Observed in soln. but not isol.

trans-form [28850-21-7]

Cryst. (C_6H_6). Mp 273-8° dec.

Cook, C.D. *et al*, *Can. J. Chem.*, 1967, **45**, 301 (*synth*)
Cook, C.D., *J. Am. Chem. Soc.*, 1970, **92**, 2595 (*nmr*)
Petrosyan, V.S. *et al*, *J. Organomet. Chem.*, 1974, **65**, C7 (*synth*)
Eaborn, C. *et al*, *J. Chem. Soc., Dalton Trans.*, 1978, 357 (*nmr*)
Bardi, R. *et al*, *Inorg. Chim. Acta*, 1981, **47**, 249 (*struct*)

$C_{37}H_{33}IP_2Pt$ Pt-00374

Iodomethylbis(triphenylphosphine)platinum, 9CI, 8CI

Methylbis(triphenylphosphine)platinum iodide

[39697-58-0]

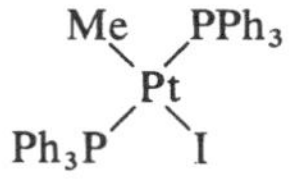

M 861.600

trans-form [28850-19-3]

Cryst. (C_6H_6). Mp 273-5°.

Chatt, J. *et al*, *J. Chem. Soc.*, 1959, 705 (*synth*)
Kistner, C.R. *et al*, *Inorg. Chem.*, 1963, **2**, 1255 (*synth*)
Cook, C.D., *J. Am. Chem. Soc.*, 1970, **92**, 2595 (*nmr*)
Gynane, M.J.S. *et al*, *J. Chem. Soc., Chem. Commun.*, 1978, 192 (*synth*)

$C_{37}H_{33}I_3P_2Pt$ Pt-00375

Triiodo(methyl)bis(triphenylphosphine)platinum

Methyltriiodobis(triphenylphosphine)platinum

$PtI_3Me(PPh_3)_2$

M 1115.409

Red cryst. (C_6H_6). Mp 215° dec.

Kistner, C.R. *et al*, *Inorg. Chem.*, 1963, **2**, 1255 (*synth*)

$C_{37}H_{44}O_5P_4Pt_4$ Pt-00376

Penta-μ-carbonyltetrakis(dimethylphenylphosphine)tetraplatinum, 8CI

[23336-33-6]

PMe₂Ph
OC—Pt—CO
Me₂PhP—Pt CO Pt—PMe₂Ph
OC—Pt—CO
PMe₂Ph

M 1472.967

Brown cryst. (MeOH under CO). Mp 101-4° dec.

Vranka, R.G. *et al*, *J. Am. Chem. Soc.*, 1969, **91**, 1574 (*struct*)
Chatt, J. *et al*, *J. Chem. Soc.* (*A*), 1970, 1538 (*synth, ir, pmr*)

$C_{37}H_{70}P_2Pt$ Pt-00377

Hydromethylbis(tricyclohexylphosphine)platinum, 10CI

Methylhydridobis(tricyclohexylphosphine)platinum

[79452-65-6]

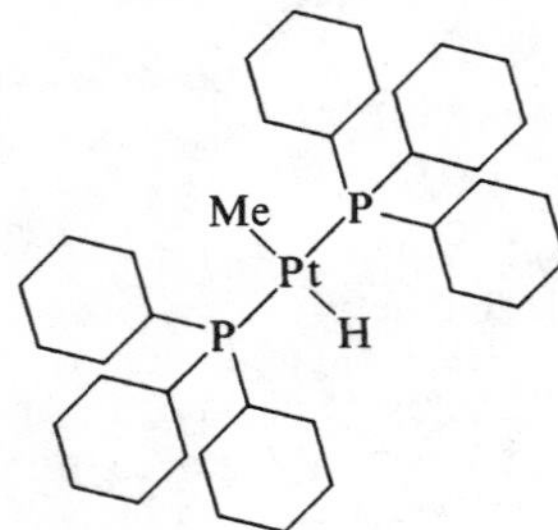

M 771.988

Cryst. (toluene/MeOH). ir ν_{PtH} 1925cm^{-1}.

Abis, L. *et al*, *J. Organomet. Chem.*, 1981, **215**, 263 (*synth, nmr, ir*)

$C_{38}H_{30}As_2F_4Pt$ Pt-00378

(Tetrafluoroethylene)bis(triphenylarsine)platinum

(η^2-*Tetrafluoroethene*)*bis*(*triphenylarsine*)*platinum*, 9CI

[33518-44-4]

Ph₃As CF₂
Pt—‖
Ph₃As CF₂

M 907.572

Cryst. (C_6H_6/pet. ether or CH_2Cl_2/EtOH). Mp 179-81°.

Kemmitt, R.D.W. *et al*, *J. Chem. Soc.* (*A*), 1971, 2472 (*synth, nmr*)
Russell, D.R. *et al*, *J. Chem. Soc., Dalton Trans.*, 1975, 1752 (*struct*)

$C_{38}H_{30}Cl_4P_2Pt$ Pt-00379

(Tetrachloroethylene)bis(triphenylphosphine)platinum, 8CI

(η^2-*Tetrachloroethene*)*bis*(*triphenylphosphine*)*platinum*, 9CI

[15793-10-9]

As (Tetrafluoroethylene)bis(triphenylphosphine)platinum, Pt-00381 with

X = Cl

M 885.495

Cryst. (C_6H_6). Mp 190° dec. Isomerises to [PtCl(C_2Cl_3)(PPh_3)$_2$].

Bland, W.J. *et al*, *J. Chem. Soc.* (*A*), 1968, 1278 (*synth, ir*)
Francis, J.N. *et al*, *J. Organomet. Chem.*, 1971, **29**, 131 (*struct*)
Mason, R. *et al*, *J. Chem. Soc., Dalton Trans.*, 1972, 1729 (*pe*)

$C_{38}H_{30}F_3NP_2Pt$ Pt-00380

[(*N*,1-η)-Trifluoroacetonitrile]bis(triphenylphosphine)platinum, 9CI

(*Trifluoromethyl cyanide*)*bis*(*triphenylphosphine*)*platinum*

[42535-16-0]

CF₃
Ph₃P C
Pt—‖‖
Ph₃P N

M 814.684

Yellow solid. Mp 130-3° dec. Near planar coordination about Pt.

Bland, W.J. *et al*, *J. Chem. Soc., Dalton Trans.*, 1973, 1292 (*synth, ir, nmr*)

$C_{38}H_{30}F_4P_2Pt$ Pt-00381

(Tetrafluoroethylene)bis(triphenylphosphine)platinum, 8CI

(η^2-*Tetrafluoroethene*)*bis*(*triphenylphosphine*)*platinum*, 9CI

[15747-38-3]

Ph₃P CX₂
Pt—‖
Ph₃P CX₂

X = F

M 819.676

Cryst. (CH_2Cl_2/MeOH). Sol. C_6H_6, CH_2Cl_2, $CHCl_3$, insol. MeOH, pet. ether. Mp 200° dec., 218-20°.

Bland, W.J. *et al*, *J. Chem. Soc.* (*A*), 1968, 1278 (*synth, ir*)
Mason, R. *et al*, *J. Chem. Soc., Dalton Trans.*, 1972, 1729 (*pe*)
Kennedy, J.D. *et al*, *J. Chem. Soc., Dalton Trans.*, 1976, 847 (*nmr*)
Kennedy, J.D. *et al*, *J. Organomet. Chem.*, 1979, **172**, 479 (*nmr*)

$C_{38}H_{30}F_5IP_2Pt$ Pt-00382

Iodo(pentafluoroethyl)bis(triphenylphosphine)platinum

Pentafluoroethylbis(triphenylphosphine)platinum iodide. Bis(triphenylphosphine)iodo(pentafluoroethyl)platinum

Ph₃P R
Pt
I PPh₃

R = —CF₂CF₃

M 965.579

***trans*-form** [19469-55-7]

Orange cryst. (C_6H_6). Mp 311°.

Rosevear, D.T. *et al*, *J. Chem. Soc.* (*A*), 1968, 164 (*synth, ir*)

$C_{38}H_{30}O_2P_2Pt$ Pt-00383

Dicarbonylbis(triphenylphosphine)platinum, 9CI, 8CI

[15377-00-1]

$Pt(CO)_2(PPh_3)_2$ (C_{2v})

M 775.681

Pale-cream cryst. (Me_2CO under CO). Mp 105° dec.

Chini, P. *et al*, *J. Chem. Soc. (A)*, 1970, 1542 (*synth*, *ir*)
Sen, A. *et al*, *Inorg. Chem.*, 1980, **19**, 1073 (*nmr*)

$C_{38}H_{32}ClNP_2Pt$ Pt-00384

Chloro(cyanomethyl)bis(triphenylphosphine)platinum, 9CI

(Cyanomethyl)chlorobis(triphenylphosphine)platinum

Ph_3P, CH_2CN / Pt / Ph_3P, CH_2CN *cis-form*

M 795.158

cis-form [53702-17-3]

Cryst. ($CHCl_3/Me_2CO$). Mp 176°. Readily converted to *trans* isomer in soln. with trace of free Ph_3P.

trans-form [42481-62-9]

Cryst. (CH_2Cl_2/MeOH). Mp 292-5° dec.

Bland, W.J. *et al*, *J. Chem. Soc., Dalton Trans.*, 1973, 1292 (*synth*)
Suzuki, K. *et al*, *J. Organomet. Chem.*, 1974, **73**, 131 (*synth*, *ir*, *pmr*)
Roz, R. *et al*, *Helv. Chim. Acta*, 1975, **58**, 133 (*synth*, *nmr*)
Pra, A.D. *et al*, *Inorg. Chim. Acta*, 1979, **36**, 121 (*struct*)
Favez, R. *et al*, *Inorg. Chem.*, 1980, **19**, 1356.
Almeida, J.F. *et al*, *J. Organomet. Chem.*, 1981, **209**, 415 (*synth*, *nmr*)

$C_{38}H_{32}P_2Pt$ Pt-00385

Acetylenebis(triphenylphosphine)platinum

(η^2-Ethyne)bis(triphenylphosphine)platinum, 9CI

[24507-93-5]

$(Ph_3P)_2Pt$–$HC{\equiv}CH$

M 745.698

Koie, Y. *et al*, *J. Chem. Soc., Dalton Trans.*, 1981, 1082 (*nmr*)

$C_{38}H_{33}NP_2Pt$ Pt-00386

Cyanomethylhydrobis(triphenylphosphine)platinum, 9CI

Hydrido(cyanomethyl)bis(triphenylphosphine)platinum

Ph_3P, CH_2CN / Pt / H, PPh_3

M 760.713

trans-form [61344-61-4]

Cryst. (C_6H_6/MeOH). Mp 164-5°.

Ros, R. *et al*, *J. Organomet. Chem.*, 1977, **139**, 355 (*synth*, *nmr*)
Del Pra, A. *et al*, *J. Chem. Soc., Dalton Trans.*, 1979, 1862 (*struct*)

$C_{38}H_{34}P_2Pt$ Pt-00387

[1,2-Ethanediylbis[diphenylphosphine]-*P,P'*]diphenylplatinum, 9CI

[Ethylenebis[diphenylphosphine]]diphenylplatinum

[52595-92-3]

As [Ethylenebis[diphenylphosphine]]dimethylplatinum, Pt-00331 with

R = Ph

M 747.714

Cryst. (C_6H_6). Mp 207-12° dec.

Glockling, F. *et al*, *Inorg. Chim. Acta*, 1974, **8**, 77 (*synth*)
Glockling, F. *et al*, *Inorg. Chim. Acta*, 1974, **8**, 81 (*ms*)
Appleton, T.G. *et al*, *Inorg. Chem.*, 1978, **17**, 738 (*synth*)
Eaborn, C. *et al*, *J. Chem. Soc., Dalton Trans.*, 1978, 357 (*nmr*)

$C_{38}H_{34}P_2Pt$ Pt-00388

Ethylenebis(triphenylphosphine)platinum

Ethenebis(triphenylphosphine)platinum, 9CI

[12120-15-9]

$(Ph_3P)_2Pt$–$CH_2{=}CH_2$

M 747.714

Extensively used in oxidative addition reactions to Pt. On polymer or membrane can be used to separate mono- and di-olefins. White solid. Sol. C_6H_6, CH_2Cl_2, insol. alcohols. Mp 126-8° dec. Can be briefly handled in air and stored indefinitely under N_2.

Cheng, P.-T. *et al*, *Can. J. Chem.*, 1972, **50**, 912 (*struct*)
Hall, P.W. *et al*, *J. Organomet. Chem.*, 1974, **71**, 145 (*nmr*)
Kennedy, J.D. *et al*, *J. Chem. Soc., Dalton Trans.*, 1976, 874 (*nmr*)
Inorg. Synth., 1978, **18**, 120 (*synth*)

$C_{38}H_{36}P_2Pt$ Pt-00389

Dimethylbis(triphenylphosphine)platinum, 9CI, 8CI

Bis(triphenylphosphine)dimethylplatinum

[15692-56-5]

Me, PPh_3 / Pt / Me, PPh_3 *cis-form*

M 749.730

Catalyses formn. of poly(dimethylsilylmethylene).

cis-form [17567-35-0]

Cryst. (C_6H_6). Mp 235-7° (206-9°) dec. Dipole moment 5.45D.

trans-form [33677-20-2]

No details on synth. or phys. props.

Chatt, J. *et al*, *J. Chem. Soc.*, 1959, 705 (*synth*)
Kistner, C.R. *et al*, *Inorg. Chem.*, 1963, **2**, 1255 (*synth*)
Greaves, E.O. *et al*, *J. Chem. Soc., Chem. Commun.*, 1967, 860 (*pmr*)
Clark, D.T. *et al*, *J. Chem. Soc., Chem. Commun.*, 1971, 602 (*pe*)
Morrow, B.A. *et al*, *Can. J. Chem.*, 1971, **49**, 2921 (*ir*)
Glockling, F. *et al*, *Inorg. Chim. Acta*, 1974, **8**, 81 (*ms*)

$C_{38}H_{84}P_4Pt_2$ **Pt-00390**

Bis[bis(di-*tert*-butylphosphino)propane]diplatinum

Bis[1,3-propanediylbis[bis(1,1-dimethylethyl)phosphine]-P,P′]diplatinum, 9CI

[66467-51-4]

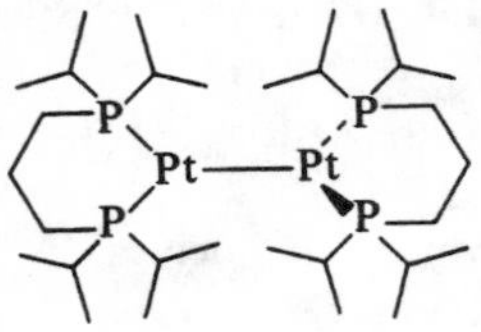

M 1055.137

Red-orange cryst. (toluene). Mp 234° (dec., under N_2).

Yoshida, T. *et al*, *J. Am. Chem. Soc.*, 1978, **100**, 2063 (*synth, struct*)

Tulip, H. *et al*, *Inorg. Chem.*, 1979, **18**, 2239.

$C_{38}H_{87}P_4Pt_2^{\oplus}$ **Pt-00391**

μ-Hydrodihydrobis[1,3-propanediylbis[bis(1,1-dimethylethylphosphine]-*P,P′*]diplatinum(1+), 9CI

*μ-Hydridodihydridobis[bis(di-*tert*-butylphosphino)propane]diplatinum*

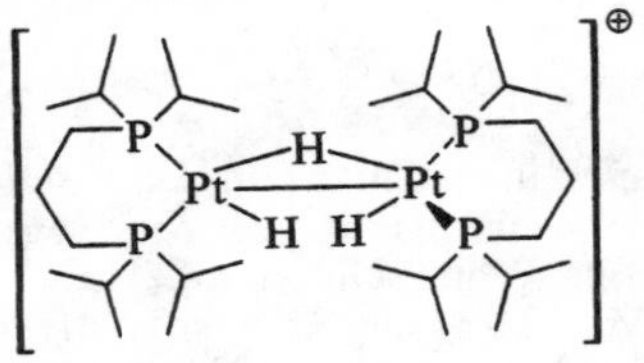

M 1058.160 (ion)

Methoxide: [70095-71-5].

$C_{39}H_{90}OP_4Pt_2$ M 1089.194

Not isol., pale-brown soln. in MeOH.

Tetraphenylborate: [70072-47-8].

$C_{62}H_{107}BP_4Pt_2$ M 1377.392

Cryst. (EtOH). Mp 225° (dec., under N_2).

Tulip, H. *et al*, *Inorg. Chem.*, 1979, **18**, 2239 (*synth, struct, nmr*)

$C_{39}H_{30}F_6OP_2Pt$ **Pt-00392**

[Oxy[trifluoro-1-(trifluoromethyl)ethylidene]]bis(triphenylphosphine)platinum, 8CI

(Hexafluoroacetone)bis(triphenylphosphine)platinum

[19554-14-4]

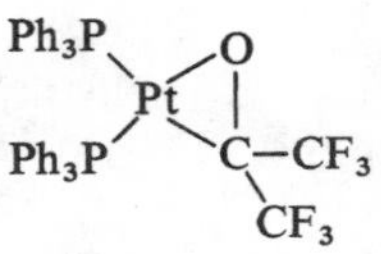

M 885.683

Cryst. (C_6H_6/pet. ether). Mp 216-8° (*in vacuo*).

Clarke, B. *et al*, *J. Chem. Soc. (A)*, 1968, 167 (*synth, ir, nmr*)

Ashley-Smith, J. *et al*, *J. Chem. Soc. (A)*, 1970, 3161.

$C_{39}H_{30}F_7IP_2Pt$ **Pt-00393**

Iodo(heptafluoropropyl)bis(triphenylphosphine)platinum

Heptafluoropropylbis(triphenylphosphine)platinum iodide

As Iodo(pentafluoroethyl)bis(triphenylphosphine)platinum, Pt-00382 with

R = —$CF_2CF_2CF_3$

M 1015.587

***trans*-form** [19469-56-8]

Orange cryst. (C_6H_6/pet. ether). Mp 309°.

Rosevear, D.T. *et al*, *J. Chem. Soc. (A)*, 1968, 164 (*synth, ir*)

$C_{39}H_{31}F_6NP_2Pt$ **Pt-00394**

[(*N*,2-η)-1,1,1,3,3,3-Hexafluoro-2-propanimine]bis(triphenylphosphine)platinum, 9CI

[Bis(trifluoromethyl)methyleneamine]bis(triphenylphosphine)platinum

[50768-96-2]

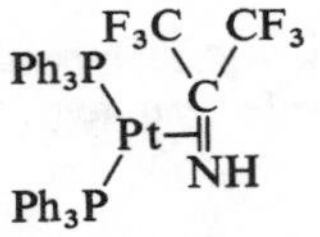

M 884.699

Cryst. (C_6H_6 or CH_2Cl_2). Mp 175-80°, 196°.

Ashley-Smith, J. *et al*, *J. Chem. Soc. (A)*, 1970, 3161 (*synth*)

Cetinkaya, B. *et al*, *J. Chem. Soc., Dalton Trans.*, 1973, 1975 (*synth, ir, nmr*)

$C_{39}H_{31}F_7P_2Pt$ **Pt-00395**

(1,1,1,3,3,3-Hexafluoro-2-propyl)fluorobis(triphenylphosphine)platinum

Fluoro[2.2.2-trifluoro-1-(trifluoromethyl)ethyl]bis(triphenylphosphine)platinum, 9CI

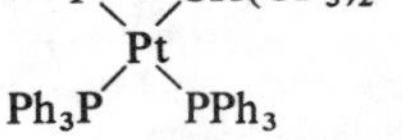

cis-form

M 889.690

***cis*-form** [50701-17-2]

Cryst. (C_6H_6). Mp 272° dec.

***trans*-form** [50701-21-8]

Cryst. (C_6H_6). Mp 215-6° dec. Converts to the *cis*-form in refluxing benzene.

Clemens, J. *et al*, *J. Chem. Soc., Dalton Trans.*, 1973, 1620 (*synth, nmr*)

Howard, J. *et al*, *J. Chem. Soc., Dalton Trans.*, 1973, 1840 (*struct*)

$C_{39}H_{34}P_2Pt$ **Pt-00396**

[(1,2-η)-1,2-Propadiene]bis(triphenylphosphine)platinum, 9CI

(Methyleneethylene)bis(triphenylphosphine)platinum, 8CI. Allenebis(triphenylphosphine)platinum

[21205-49-2]

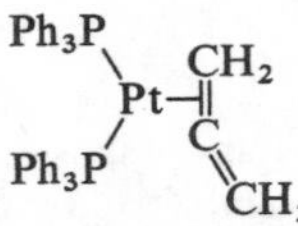

M 759.725

Cryst. (EtOH). Mp 152-4° dec.

Otsuka, S. *et al*, *J. Organomet. Chem.*, 1968, **14**, P30 (*synth, pmr*)

Kadonaga, M. *et al*, *J. Chem. Soc., Chem. Commun.*, 1971, 1597 (*struct*)

Otsuka, S. *et al*, *J. Chem. Soc., Dalton Trans.*, 1973, 2491 (*nmr*)

$C_{39}H_{35}ClP_2Pt$ Pt-00397

Chloro-2-propenylbis(triphenylphosphine)platinum, 9CI
(σ-Allyl)chlorobis(triphenylphosphine)platinum

Cl PPh₃
Pt
Ph_3P $CH_2CH{=}CH_2$

M 796.186

***trans*-form** [61374-44-5]
Cryst. (C_6H_6/pentane). Prepd. and isol. along with $[Pt(\eta^3\text{-}C_3H_5)(PPh_3)_2]Cl$.

Kaduk, J.A. *et al*, *J. Organomet. Chem.*, 1977, **139**, 199 (*synth, struct*)

$C_{39}H_{35}P_2Pt^{\oplus}$ Pt-00398

(η^3-2-Propenyl)bis(triphenylphosphine)platinum(1+), 9CI
Allylbis(triphenylphosphine)platinum(1+)

$[(\eta^3\text{-allyl})Pt(PPh_3)_2]^{\oplus}$

M 760.733 (ion)
Hydrosilylation catalyst.

Chloride: [12246-65-0].
$C_{39}H_{35}ClP_2Pt$ M 796.186
Cryst. ($CHCl_3/Et_2O$). Sol. MeOH, CH_2Cl_2, $CHCl_3$, sl. sol. Me_2CO, $MeNO_2$, insol. Et_2O. Mp 180-4° dec., 194-8° dec. Chloride can attack Pt to cause $\eta^3 \rightarrow \eta^1$ conversion in soln. and can eliminate PPh_3 to generate Chloro(η^3-2-propenyl)(triphenylphosphine)platinum, Pt-00262 .

Perchlorate: [36484-05-6].
$C_{39}H_{35}ClO_4P_2Pt$ M 860.184
Not fully descr.

Tetrafluoroborate: [36484-04-5].
$C_{39}H_{35}BF_4P_2Pt$ M 847.537
Cryst.

Hexafluorophosphate: [37668-21-6].
$C_{39}H_{35}F_6P_3Pt$ M 905.697
Cryst. (CH_2Cl_2/pentane). Mp 247-50° dec.

Trichlorostannate: [32679-54-4].
$C_{39}H_{35}Cl_3P_2PtSn$ M 985.782
Yellow cryst. (C_6H_6/pet. ether). Mp 165° dec. Can lose PPh_3 in sol. to leave orange $[Pt(\eta^3\text{-}C_3H_5)(SnCl_3)(PPh_3)]$.

Baird, M.C. *et al*, *J. Chem. Soc. (A)*, 1967, 865 (*synth*)
Crosby, J.N. *et al*, *J. Organomet. Chem.*, 1971, **26**, 277 (*synth*)
Clark, H.C. *et al*, *Inorg. Chem.*, 1972, **11**, 1275 (*synth*)
Clark, H.C. *et al*, *Inorg. Chem.*, 1973, **12**, 356 (*pmr*)
Yoshida, G. *et al*, *Chem. Lett.*, 1976, 705.
Nesmeyanov, A.N. *et al*, *J. Organomet. Chem.*, 1979, **164**, 259 (*synth*)

$C_{39}H_{39}ClP_2PbPt$ Pt-00399

Chloro(trimethylplumbyl)bis(triphenylphosphine)platinum
Bis(triphenylphosphine)(trimethylplumbyl)chloroplatinum

Me_3Pb PPh_3
Pt *trans-form*
Ph_3P Cl

M 1007.418
Not isol. Both *cis* and *trans* (major) isomers formed.

Al-Allaf, T.A.K. *et al*, *J. Organomet. Chem.*, 1980, **188**, 335.

$C_{39}H_{39}ClP_2PtSn$ Pt-00400

(Chlorodimethylstannyl)methylbis(triphenylphosphine)platinum, 9CI
Methyl(chlorodimethyltin)bis(triphenylphosphine)platinum

Ph_3P $SnClMe_2$
Pt
Ph_3P Me

M 918.908
This compound was previously formulated as $[PtCl(SnMe_3)(PPh_3)_2]$.

***cis*-form** [59991-61-6]
Cryst. (CH_2Cl_2/EtOH). Mp 240-2° dec.

Eaborn, C. *et al*, *J. Chem. Soc., Dalton Trans.*, 1976, 767 (*synth, nmr, ir*)
Butler, G. *et al*, *J. Organomet. Chem.*, 1980, **185**, 367 (*nmr, synth*)

$C_{39}H_{71}P_2Pt^{\oplus}$ Pt-00401

(η^3-2-Propenyl)bis(tricyclohexylphosphine)platinum(1+), 9CI
Allylbis(tricyclohexylphosphine)platinum(1+)

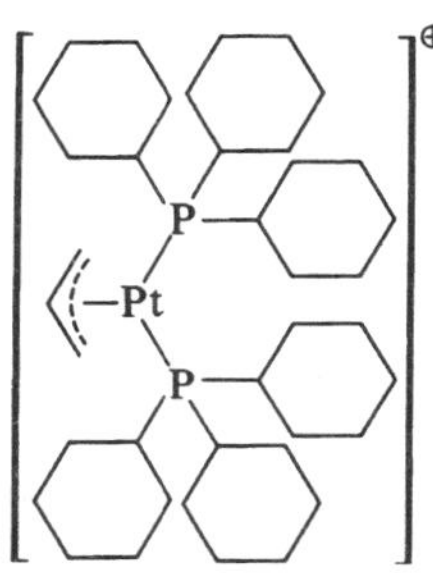

M 797.017 (ion)

Hexafluorophosphate: [55927-91-8].
$C_{39}H_{71}F_6P_3Pt$ M 941.982
Cryst. (CH_2Cl_2/toluene).

Attig, T.G. *et al*, *J. Organomet. Chem.*, 1975, **94**, C49 (*synth*)
Smith, J.D. *et al*, *Inorg. Chem.*, 1978, **17**, 2585 (*struct*)

$C_{39}H_{81}O_3P_3Pt_3$ Pt-00402

Tricarbonyltris(tri-*tert*-butylphosphine)triplatinum
Tricarbonyltris[tris(1,1-dimethylethyl)phosphine]triplatinum
[79138-89-9]

$[Pt(\mu\text{-}CO)(P(C(CH_3)_3)_3)]_3$ (Pt₃ triangle, bridging CO)

M 1276.228
Dark-orange cryst. (hexane/C_6H_6). Sol. C_6H_6, $CHCl_3$. Dec. at 155-70°.

Goel, R.G. *et al*, *J. Organomet. Chem.*, 1981, **214**, 405 (*synth, ir, pmr*)
Goel, R.G. *et al*, *Organometallics*, 1982, **1**, 819 (*synth, ir*)

$C_{40}H_{30}Cl_2N_2P_2Pt$ Pt-00403

(Dichlorodicyanoethylene)bis(triphenylphosphine)platinum

(1,1-Dichloro-2,2-dicyanoethene)bis(triphenylphosphine)platinum. [(Dichloromethylene)propanedinitrile]-bis(triphenylphosphine)platinum

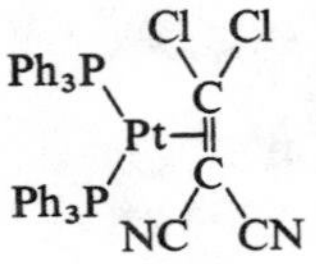

M 866.624

Cryst. (Me_2CO aq.). Partial melting and resolidification at 150° accompanies isomerisation to a vinyl complex, Mp 310-2°.

McAdam, A. *et al*, *J. Organomet. Chem.*, 1971, **29**, 149 (*synth, ir, struct*)

$C_{40}H_{30}F_6P_2Pt$ Pt-00404

[(2,3-η)-1,1,1,4,4,4-Hexafluoro-2-butyne]bis(triphenylphosphine)platinum, 9CI

(Bistrifluoromethylethyne)bis(triphenylphosphine)platinum

[23626-16-6]

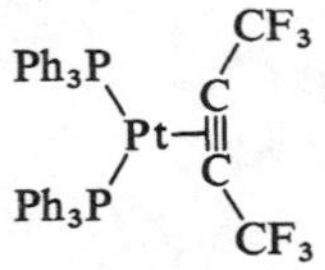

M 881.695

Cryst. (Et_2O). Readily sol. common org. solvs. Mp 215-6°.

Boston, J.L. *et al*, *J. Chem. Soc.*, 1963, 3468 (*synth, ir*)
Davies, B.W. *et al*, *Inorg. Chem.*, 1974, **13**, 1848 (*struct*)
Kennedy, J.D. *et al*, *J. Chem. Soc., Dalton Trans.*, 1976, 847 (*nmr*)
Van Gaal, H.L.M. *et al*, *J. Organomet. Chem.*, 1977, **131**, 453 (*ir*)
Koie, Y. *et al*, *J. Chem. Soc., Dalton Trans.*, 1981, 1082 (*nmr*)

$C_{40}H_{30}F_8P_2Pt$ Pt-00405

[(2,3-η)-1,1,1,2,3,4,4,4-Octafluoro-2-butene]bis(triphenylphosphine)platinum, 9CI

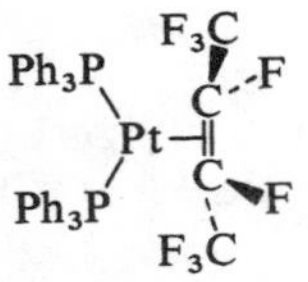

M 919.692

trans-form [51371-70-1]

Air-stable cryst. (CH_2Cl_2/MeOH).

Roundhill, D.M. *et al*, *J. Chem. Soc. (A)*, 1968, 506 (*synth, ir*)
Baraban, J.M. *et al*, *J. Am. Chem. Soc.*, 1975, **97**, 4232 (*struct, synth*)

$C_{40}H_{30}N_2P_2Pt$ Pt-00406

[(2,3-η)-2-Butynedinitrile]bis(triphenylphosphine)platinum, 10CI

(Acetylenedicarbonitrile)bis(triphenylphosphine)platinum, 8CI. (Dicyanoacetylene)bis(triphenylphosphine)-platinum. (Dicyanoethyne)bis(triphenylphosphine)-platinum

[29012-89-3]

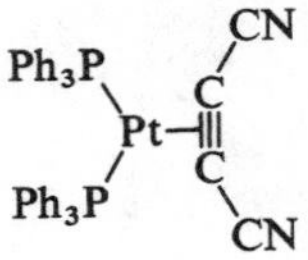

M 795.718

Orange cryst. (C_6H_6/hexane). Mp 233-5° dec. Isomerises photochemically to $[Pt(CN)(C{\equiv}CC{\equiv}N)(PPh_3)_2]$.

McClure, G.L. *et al*, *J. Organomet. Chem.*, 1970, **25**, 261 (*synth, ir*)
Baddley, W.H. *et al*, *J. Am. Chem. Soc.*, 1971, **93**, 5590.
Koie, Y. *et al*, *J. Chem. Soc., Dalton Trans.*, 1981, 1082 (*nmr*)

$C_{40}H_{36}P_2Pt$ Pt-00407

[(1,2-η)-3-Methylcyclopropene]bis(triphenylphosphine)platinum, 9CI

[40982-14-7]

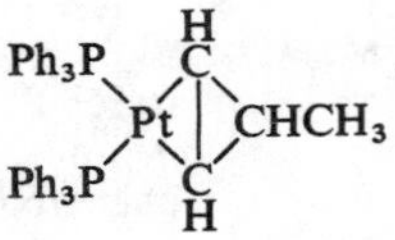

M 773.752

Cryst. (toluene/EtOH).

Visser, J.P. *et al*, *J. Organomet. Chem.*, 1973, **47**, 433 (*synth, pmr*)
de Boer, J.J. *et al*, *J. Chem. Soc., Dalton Trans.*, 1975, 662 (*struct*)

$C_{40}H_{37}P_2Pt^{\oplus}$ Pt-00408

[(1,2,3-η)-2-Methyl-2-propenyl]bis(triphenylphosphine)platinum(1+), 9CI

(2-Methylallyl)bis(triphenylphosphine)platinum(1+)

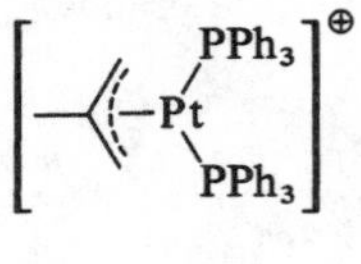

M 774.760 (ion)

Chloride: [60977-22-2].
$C_{40}H_{37}ClP_2Pt$ M 810.213
Cryst. + $CHCl_3$($CHCl_3$). Mp 290-5° dec. In soln., Cl^- can coordinate to Pt causing $\eta^3{\rightarrow}\eta^1$ conversion of the allyl and displacement of PPh_3.

Perchlorate: [37036-84-3].
$C_{40}H_{37}ClO_4P_2Pt$ M 874.210
Not fully descr.

Tetraphenylborate: [35770-41-3].
$C_{64}H_{57}BP_2Pt$ M 1093.992
Cryst. (MeOH). Mp 187-90° dec.

Hexafluorophosphate: [69456-13-9].
$C_{40}H_{37}F_6P_3Pt$ M 919.724
Cryst. (MeOH).

Mann, B.E. *et al*, *J. Chem. Soc. (A)*, 1971, 3536 (*synth, pmr*)
Clark, H.C. *et al*, *Inorg. Chem.*, 1973, **12**, 357 (*synth, pmr*)

Kurosawa, H., *J. Organomet. Chem.*, 1976, **112**, 369 (*synth*)
Yoshida, G. *et al*, *Chem. Lett.*, 1976, 705.
Nesmeyanov, A.N. *et al*, *J. Organomet. Chem.*, 1978, **164**, 259 (*synth*)
Phillips, R.L. *et al*, *J. Chem. Soc., Dalton Trans.*, 1978, 1736 (*synth*)

$C_{40}H_{40}P_2Pt$ Pt-00409

Diethylbis(triphenylphosphine)platinum, 9CI, 8CI
Bis(triphenylphosphine)diethylplatinum
[28855-35-8]

$Et_2Pt(PPh_3)_2$

M 777.784

cis-form [43097-18-3]
Cryst. ($EtOH/CH_2Cl_2$). Mp 153-4° (147-8°).

Morrow, B.A., *Can. J. Chem.*, 1970, **48**, 2192 (*ir*)
McDermott, J.X. *et al*, *J. Am. Chem. Soc.*, 1976, **98**, 6521 (*synth*)
Slack, D.A. *et al*, *Inorg. Chim. Acta*, 1977, **24**, 277 (*ir, nmr*)

$C_{40}H_{42}P_2PbPt$ Pt-00410

Methyl(trimethylplumbyl)bis(triphenylphosphine)platinum, 9CI
Bis(triphenylphosphine)(trimethylplumbyl)methylplatinum
[41620-22-8]

$Me_3PbPtMe(PPh_3)_2$

M 986.999
Pale-yellow microcryst. Mp 130-2° dec.

Crociani, B. *et al*, *J. Organomet. Chem.*, 1973, **49**, 249.

$C_{40}H_{66}F_6P_2Pt$ Pt-00411

[(2,3-η)-1,1,1,4,4,4-Hexafluoro-2-butyne]bis(tricyclohexylphosphine)platinum, 10CI
[65400-05-7]

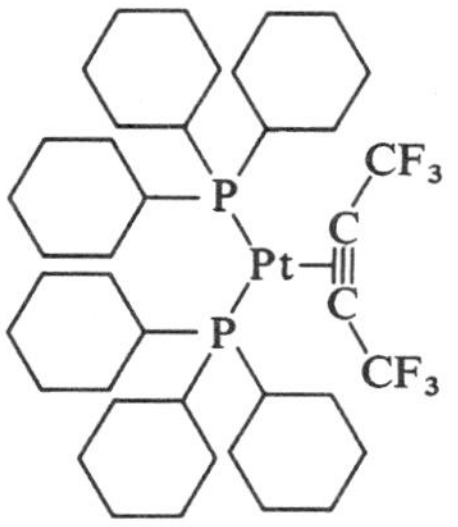

M 917.979
Cryst. ($CH_2Cl_2/MeOH$).

Attig, T.G. *et al*, *Can. J. Chem.*, 1977, **55**, 189 (*synth, nmr*)
Richardson, J.F. *et al*, *Can. J. Chem.*, 1977, **55**, 3203 (*struct*)

$C_{41}H_{38}P_2Pt$ Pt-00412

[(1,2-η)-1,2-Dimethylcyclopropene]bis(triphenylphosphine)platinum, 9CI
[35768-61-7]

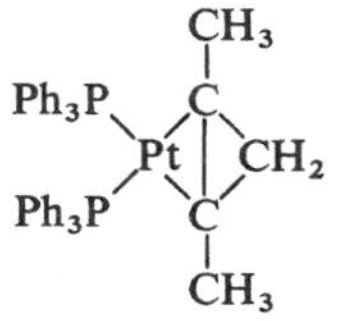

M 787.779
Cryst. (toluene/EtOH).

Visser, J.P. *et al*, *J. Organomet. Chem.*, 1973, **47**, 433 (*synth, pmr*)
de Boer, J.J. *et al*, *J. Chem. Soc., Dalton Trans.*, 1975, 662 (*struct*)

$C_{42}H_{30}N_4P_2Pt$ Pt-00413

(Tetracyanoethylene)bis(triphenylphosphine)platinum
(Tetracyanoethene)bis(triphenylphosphine)platinum, 8CI. (Ethanetetracarbonitrile)bis(triphenylphosphine)platinum, 8CI
[15711-22-5]

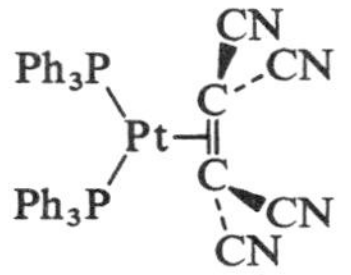

M 847.753
Cryst. ($C_6H_6/EtOH$ or $CH_2Cl_2/EtOH$).

Baddley, W.H. *et al*, *Inorg. Chem.*, 1966, **5**, 33 (*synth, ir*)
Bombieri, G. *et al*, *J. Chem. Soc. (A)*, 1970, 1313 (*struct*)

$C_{42}H_{32}ClN_3O_6P_2Pt$ Pt-00414

Chloro(2,4,6-trinitrophenyl)bis(triphenylphosphine)platinum
Chloropicrylbis(triphenylphosphine)platinum, 8CI

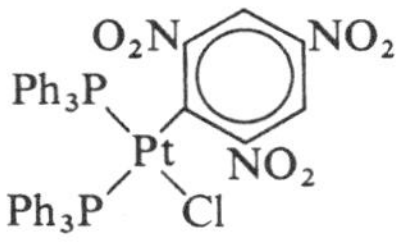

M 967.212
Mp 264-5° dec.

cis-form [25066-81-3]
Orange-yellow cryst. ($C_6H_6/EtOH$). Mp 264-5° dec.

Norris, A.R. *et al*, *Can. J. Chem.*, 1969, **47**, 3003.

$C_{42}H_{35}BrP_2Pt$ Pt-00415

Bromo(phenyl)bis(triphenylphosphine)platinum, 9CI
Phenylbis(triphenylphosphine)platinum bromide
[57694-39-0]

As Chloro(phenyl)bis(triphenylphosphine)platinum, Pt-00416 with

X = Br

M 876.670

cis-form [67087-65-4]
No physical data available.
trans-form [41620-24-0]
Pale-yellow cryst. (CCl_4/Et_2O). Mp >250°.

Crociani, B. *et al*, *J. Organomet. Chem.*, 1973, **49**, 249 (*synth*)
Garrou, P.E. *et al*, *J. Am. Chem. Soc.*, 1976, **98**, 4115 (*synth*)
Gynane, M.J.S. *et al*, *J. Chem. Soc., Chem. Commun.*, 1978, 192 (*synth*)
Eaborn, C. *et al*, *J. Chem. Soc., Dalton Trans.*, 1981, 933 (*nmr*)

$C_{42}H_{35}ClP_2Pt$ Pt-00416

Chlorophenylbis(triphenylphosphine)platinum, 9CI, 8CI
Phenylchlorobis(triphenylphosphine)platinum. Bis(triphenylphosphine)phenylplatinum chloride
[16744-25-5]

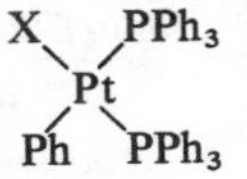

X PPh₃ / Pt / Ph PPh₃ *cis-form*

X = Cl

M 832.219
cis-form [60019-01-4]
Obt. in soln. alongside *trans*-form.
trans-form [18421-49-3]
Cryst. ($CHCl_3/MeOH$). Mp 287-90° dec.

Baird, M.C., *J. Inorg. Nucl. Chem.*, 1967, **29**, 367 (*synth*)
Eaborn, C. *et al*, *J. Chem. Soc., Dalton Trans.*, 1976, 767; 1978, 357 (*nmr*)

$C_{42}H_{35}IP_2Pt$ Pt-00417

Iodophenylbis(triphenylphosphine)platinum, 9CI
Phenylbis(triphenylphosphine)platinum iodide
[67254-04-0]
As Chlorophenylbis(triphenylphosphine)platinum, Pt-00416 with

X = I

M 923.671
Catalyses acylation of PhI by CO and $Sn(CH_2CH_2CH_2CH_3)_4$.
trans-form [53424-01-4]
Cryst. Mp >250° dec.

Katawa, N. *et al*, *Bull. Chem. Soc. Jpn.*, 1974, **47**, 1807 (*synth, nmr*)
Garrou, P.E. *et al*, *J. Am. Chem. Soc.*, 1976, **98**, 4115 (*synth, nmr*)
Anderson, G.K. *et al*, *J. Chem. Soc., Dalton Trans.*, 1980, 1434 (*nmr*)
Eaborn, C. *et al*, *J. Chem. Soc., Dalton Trans.*, 1981, 933 (*synth, nmr*)

$C_{42}H_{38}P_2Pt$ Pt-00418

[(1,4-η)-Bicyclo[2.2.0]hex-1(4)-ene]bis(triphenylphosphine)platinum, 9CI
Bis(triphenylphosphine)(bicyclo[2.2.0]hex-1(4)-ene)platinum
[54071-60-2]

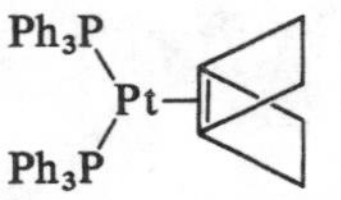

Ph₃P / Pt / Ph₃P

M 799.790
Pale-yellow air-stable cryst. (toluene/Et_2O).

Jason, M.E. *et al*, *J. Am. Chem. Soc.*, 1974, **96**, 6531 (*synth, struct*)
Jason, M.E. *et al*, *Inorg. Chem.*, 1975, **14**, 3025 (*struct*)

$C_{42}H_{38}P_2Pt$ Pt-00419

[(1,2-η)-Cyclohexyne]bis(triphenylphosphine)platinum, 9CI
[34872-50-9]

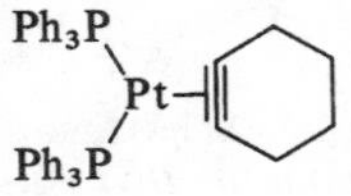

Ph₃P / Pt / Ph₃P

M 799.790
Catalyses hydration of nitriles. Cryst. (THF or $C_6H_6/EtOH$). Mp 157-9°.

Bennett, M.A. *et al*, *J. Am. Chem. Soc.*, 1971, **93**, 3797 (*synth, ir, nmr*)
Robertson, G.B. *et al*, *J. Am. Chem. Soc.*, 1975, **97**, 1051 (*struct*)
Bennett, M.A. *et al*, *J. Am. Chem. Soc.*, 1978, **100** 1750 (*synth, ir, nmr*)

$C_{42}H_{43}ClP_2Pt$ Pt-00420

Chlorohydrobis(tribenzylphosphine)platinum
Chlorohydrobis[tris(phenylmethyl)phosphine]platinum, 10CI. Chlorohydridobis[tris(phenylmethyl)phosphine]platinum. Hydridochlorobis(tribenzylphosphine)platinum

H P(CH₂Ph)₃ / Pt / (PhCH₂)₃P Cl

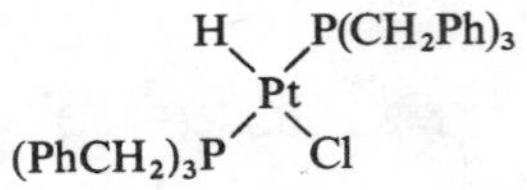

M 840.282
trans-form [59690-17-4]
Cryst. (C_6H_6/hexane). Mp 161-3°.

Miyamoto, T., *J. Organomet. Chem.*, 1977, **134**, 335 (*synth, ir, nmr*)

$C_{42}H_{62}AsBrP_2Pt_2$ Pt-00421

μ-Bromo-μ-(diphenylarsino)diphenylbis(tripropylphosphine)diplatinum
Diphenyl-μ-bromo-μ-(diphenylarsino)bis(tripropylphosphine)platinum

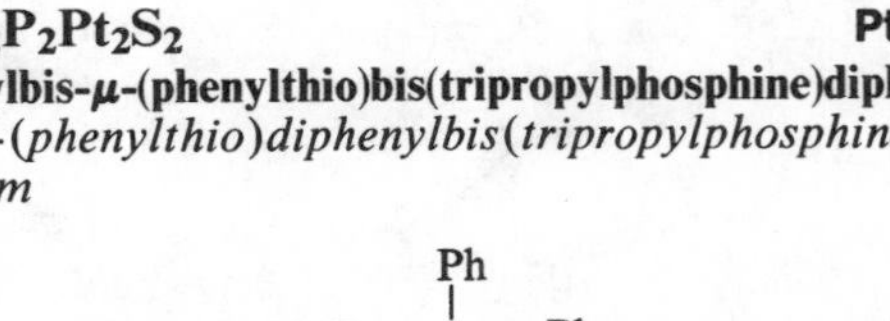

(H₃CCH₂CH₂)₃P Br P(CH₂CH₂CH₃)₃ / Pt Pt / Ph As Ph / Ph Ph

M 1173.885
Cryst. (EtOH). Mp 151°. Dipole moment 5.1D.

Chatt, J. *et al*, *J. Chem. Soc.*, 1964, 2433 (*synth*)

$C_{42}H_{62}P_2Pt_2S_2$ Pt-00422

Diphenylbis-μ-(phenylthio)bis(tripropylphosphine)diplatinum
Di-μ-(phenylthio)diphenylbis(tripropylphosphine)diplatinum

Ph / (H₃CCH₂CH₂)₃P S Ph / Pt Pt / Ph S P(CH₂CH₂CH₃)₃ / Ph

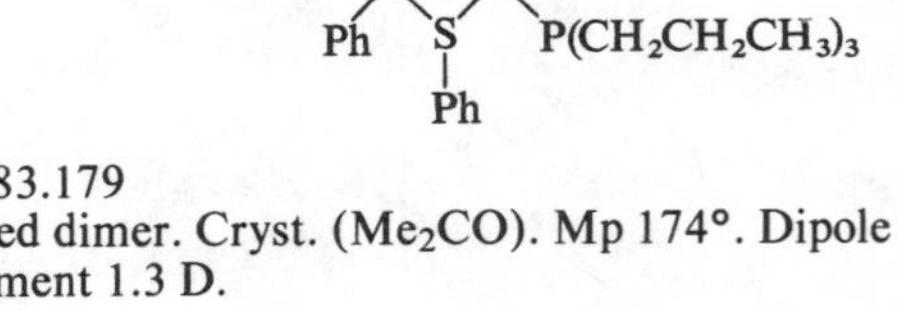

M 1083.179
Bridged dimer. Cryst. (Me_2CO). Mp 174°. Dipole moment 1.3 D.

Monomer: Phenyl(phenylthio)(tripropylphosphine)-platinum.
$C_{21}H_{31}PPtS$ M 541.590
Unknown.

Chatt, J. *et al*, *J. Chem. Soc.*, 1964, 2433 (*synth*)

$C_{43}H_{40}P_2Pt$ Pt-00423

[(1,2-η)-Cycloheptyne]bis(triphenylphosphine)platinum, 9CI
[34872-49-6]

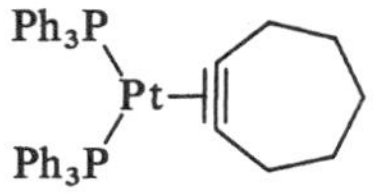

M 813.817
Cryst. (THF or C_6H_6/EtOH). Mp 163-6°.

Bennett, M.A. *et al*, *J. Am. Chem. Soc.*, 1971, **93**, 3797 (*synth, ir, nmr*)
Robertson, G.B. *et al*, *J. Am. Chem. Soc.*, 1975, **97**, 1051 (*struct*)
Bennett, M.A. *et al*, *J. Am. Chem. Soc.*, 1978, **100**, 1750 (*synth, ir, nmr*)

$C_{44}H_{35}ClP_2Pt$ Pt-00424

[[Benzo[*c*]phenanthrene-2,11-diylbis(methylene)]bis[diphenylphosphine]-*P,P'*]chlorohydroplatinum, 9CI
[55758-63-9]

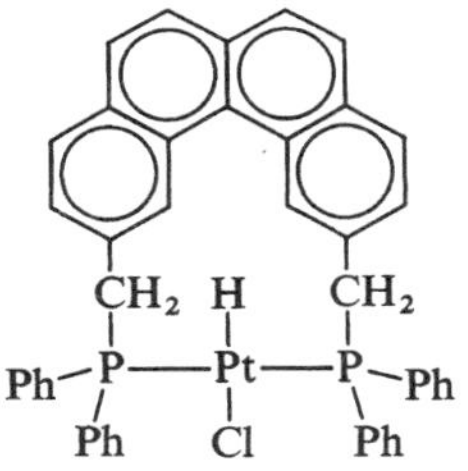

M 856.241
Solid.

Bracher, G. *et al*, *Angew. Chem., Int. Ed. Engl.*, 1975, **14**, 563.

$C_{44}H_{36}P_2Pt$ Pt-00425

(Phenylacetylene)bis(triphenylphosphine)platinum
(η^2-Ethynylbenzene)bis(triphenylphosphine)platinum, 9CI. *(Phenylethyne)bis(triphenylphosphine)platinum*
[14640-28-9]

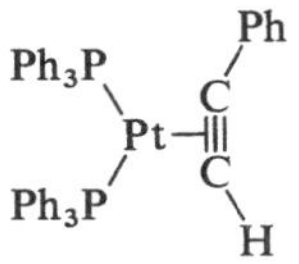

M 821.796
Catalyses polymerisation of phenylacetylene. Cryst. (C_6H_6/EtOH). Mp 153-5°.

Clark, D.T. *et al*, *J. Chem. Soc., Dalton Trans.*, 1971, 602 (*pe*)
Furlani, A. *et al*, *J. Organomet. Chem.*, 1974, **67**, 315 (*synth, ir*)
Koie, Y. *et al*, *J. Chem. Soc., Dalton Trans.*, 1981, 1082 (*nmr*)

$C_{44}H_{42}P_2Pt$ Pt-00426

[(1,2-η)-Cyclooctyne]bis(triphenylphosphine)platinum, 9CI
[20692-56-2]

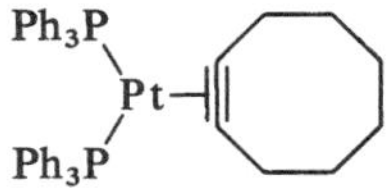

M 827.843
Cryst. (C_6H_6/EtOH). Mp 180-2° dec., 205-7° dec.

Bennett, M.A. *et al*, *J. Am. Chem. Soc.*, 1978, **100**, 1750 (*synth, ir, nmr*)
Manojlović-Muir, L. *et al*, *Acta Crystallogr., Sect. B*, 1979, **35**, 2416 (*struct*)

$C_{44}H_{48}P_2Pt$ Pt-00427

Dibutylbis(triphenylphosphine)platinum, 9CI
Bis(triphenylphosphine)dibutylplatinum
[28855-38-1]

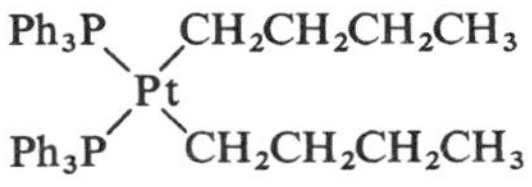

M 833.891

cis-form [38192-85-7]
Cryst. (CH_2Cl_2). Mp 132-4° (125° dec.).

Morrow, B.A., *Can. J. Chem.*, 1970, **48**, 2192 (*synth*)
Whitesides, G.M. *et al*, *J. Organomet. Chem.*, 1971, **33**, 241 (*nmr*)
Whitesides, G.M. *et al*, *J. Am. Chem. Soc.*, 1972, **94**, 5258 (*synth, ir, pmr*)

$C_{45}H_{35}F_5P_2Pt$ Pt-00428

(Pentafluorophenyl)-2-propenylbis(triphenylphosphine)platinum, 10CI
σ-Allyl(pentafluorophenyl)bis(triphenylphosphine)platinum
[62415-37-6]

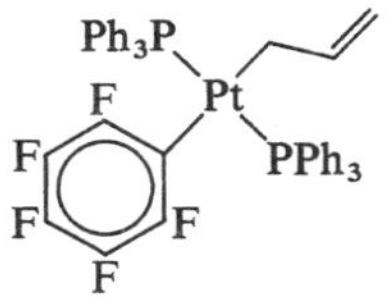

M 927.791
Unusually stable σ-allyl complex. Pale-yellow cryst. (CH_2Cl_2/hexane). Mp 194-5°.

Numata, S. *et al*, *Inorg. Chem.*, 1977, **16**, 1737 (*synth, pmr*)

$C_{47}H_{38}O_2P_2Pt$ Pt-00429

[(3,4-η)-3-Methyl-4-phenyl-3-cyclobutene-1,2-dione]bis(triphenylphosphine)platinum, 9CI
(1-Methyl-2-phenylcyclobutenedione)bis(triphenylphosphine)platinum
[55622-77-0]

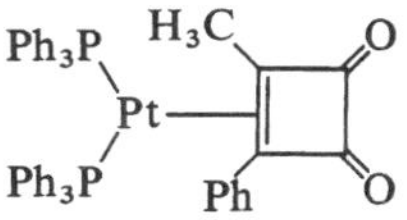

M 891.844
Pale-yellow cryst. ($CHCl_3$/pet. ether).

Hamner, E.R. *et al*, *J. Chem. Soc., Chem. Commun.*, 1974, 841 (*synth, ir, pmr*)
Russell, D.R. *et al*, *J. Chem. Soc., Dalton Trans.*, 1976, 2181 (*struct*)

$C_{47}H_{38}P_2Pt$ Pt-00430

(Methylene-1,8-naphthalenediyl)bis(triphenylphosphine)platinum, 9CI

[52563-99-2]

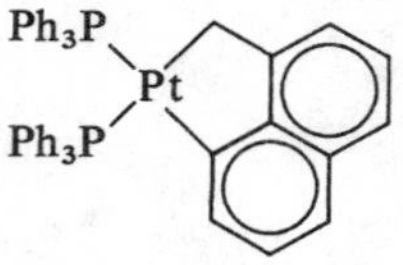

M 859.845

Cryst. (C_6H_6/heptane). Mp 238-40°.

Duff, J.A. *et al*, *J. Organomet. Chem.*, 1974, **66**, C18 (*synth*)

$C_{48}H_{30}F_{10}P_2Pt$ Pt-00431

Bis(pentafluorophenyl)bis(triphenylphosphine)platinum, 8CI

$(Ph_3P)_2Pt(C_6F_6)_2$

M 1053.777

***cis*-form** [14638-96-1]

Cryst. (C_6H_6). Mp 243-50° (resolidifies to *trans*-form).

***trans*-form**

Cryst. Mp 315-6°.

Rosevear, D.T. *et al*, *J. Chem. Soc.*, 1965, 5275 (*synth*)

$C_{48}H_{40}P_2Pt$ Pt-00432

Diphenylbis(triphenylphosphine)platinum, 9CI

Bis(triphenylphosphine)diphenylplatinum

[50988-66-4]

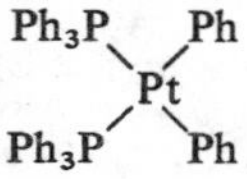

M 873.872

***cis*-form** [58073-72-6]

Cryst. (C_6H_6/pet. ether). Mp 146° dec. Dipole moment 7.2 (7.0) D. Thermal decomposition (by reductive elimination) is accelerated by free phosphine.

Chatt, J. *et al*, *J. Chem. Soc.*, 1959, 4020 (*synth*)

Braterman, P.S. *et al*, *J. Chem. Soc., Dalton Trans.*, 1976, 1306, 1310.

Eaborn, C. *et al*, *J. Chem. Soc., Dalton Trans.*, 1978, 357; 1981, 933 (*nmr*)

$C_{48}H_{60}Ge_2P_2Pt$ Pt-00433

Bis(triethylphosphine)bis(triphenylgermyl)platinum

$Pt(GePh_3)_2(PEt_3)_2$

M 1039.210

Yellow cryst. (methylcyclohexane). Spar. sol. org. solvs. Mp 160° dec.

Cross, R.J. *et al*, *J. Chem. Soc.*, 1965, 5422 (*synth*)

$C_{48}H_{60}P_2Pb_2Pt$ Pt-00434

Bis(triethylphosphine)bis(triphenyllead)platinum

Bis(triethylphosphine)bis(triphenylplumbyl)platinum, 9CI, 8CI

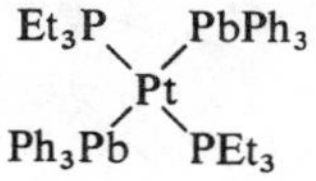

M 1308.430

***trans*-form** [22722-56-1]

Yellow solid. Mp 178-80° dec.

Deganello, G. *et al*, *J. Chem. Soc. (A)*, 1968, 2873 (*synth, ir*)

Al-Allaf, T.A.K. *et al*, *J. Organomet. Chem.*, 1980, **188**, 335 (*nmr*)

$C_{48}H_{60}P_2PtSn_2$ Pt-00435

Bis(triethylphosphine)bis(triphenylstannyl)platinum, 9CI

Bis(triphenyltin)bis(triethylphosphine)platinum

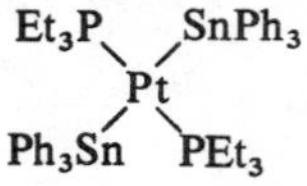

M 1131.410

***trans*-form** [56995-59-6]

Solid. Mp 175°.

Eaborn, C. *et al*, *J. Chem. Soc., Dalton Trans.*, 1975, 809 (*synth, nmr*)

$C_{48}H_{84}P_4Pt_4$ Pt-00436

Octahydrotetrakis(phenyldiisopropylphosphine)tetraplatinum

Octahydridotetrakis[phenylbis(1-methylethyl)phosphine]tetraplatinum

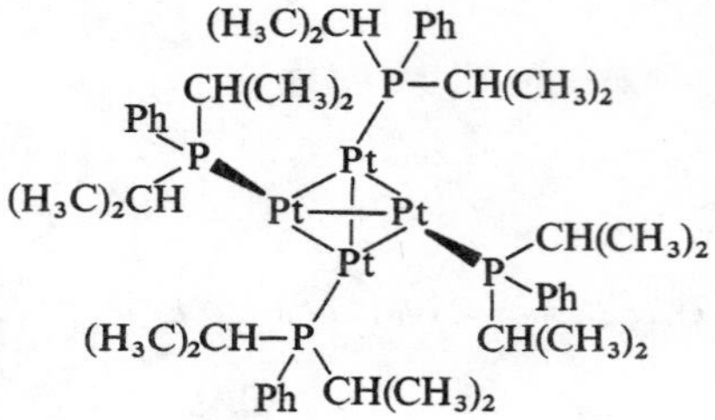

M 1565.407

H atoms on Pt not shown; they are fluxional and not detected crystallographically. Orange cryst. (pet. ether). ir ν_{PtH} 2100 and 1550 cm^{-1}.

Frost, P.W. *et al*, *J. Chem. Soc., Chem. Commun.*, 1981, 1104 (*synth, struct*)

$C_{48}H_{110}P_4Pt_4$ Pt-00437

Dihydrotetrakis(tri-*tert*-butylphosphine)tetraplatinum

Dihydridotetrakis[tris-(1,1-dimethylethyl)phosphine]-tetraplatinum

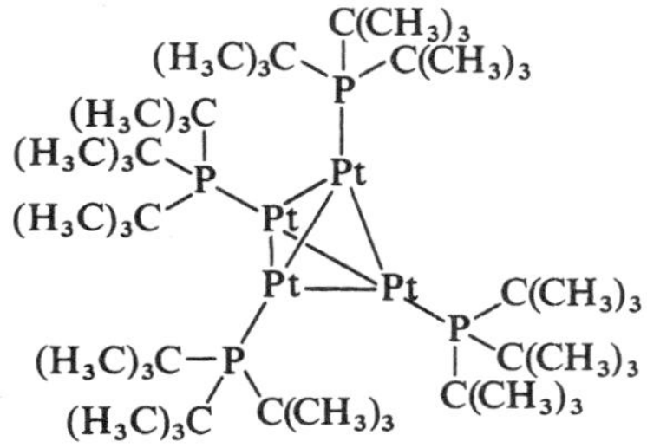

M 1591.612

2 Fluxional H atoms not shown. Dark-red cryst. (toluene).

Frost, P.W. *et al*, *J. Chem. Soc., Chem. Commun.*, 1981, 1104 (*synth, struct*)

$C_{50}H_{40}P_2Pt$ Pt-00438

(Diphenylacetylene)bis(triphenylphosphine)platinum, 8CI

[1,1′-(η²-1,2-Ethynediyl)bis[benzene]]bis(triphenylphosphine)platinum, 9CI. (Diphenylethyne)bis(triphenylphosphine)platinum

[15308-61-9]

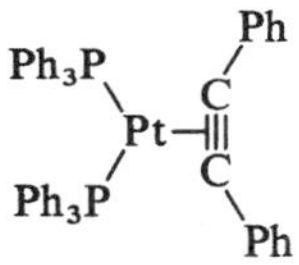

M 897.894

Air-stable solid (EtOH). Sol. $CHCl_3$, CH_2Cl_2, C_6H_6, insol. Et_2O. Mp 160-5° dec.

Glanville, J.O. *et al*, *J. Organomet. Chem.*, 1967, **7**, P9 (*struct*)
Cook, C.J. *et al*, *J. Am. Chem. Soc.*, 1971, **93**, 1904 (*pe*)
Van Gaal, H.L.M. *et al*, *J. Organomet. Chem.*, 1977, **131**, 453 (*ir*)
Inorg. Synth., 1978, **18**, 120 (*synth*)
Koie, Y. *et al*, *J. Chem. Soc., Dalton Trans.*, 1981, 1082 (*nmr*)

$C_{50}H_{47}P_4Pt_2^{\oplus}$ Pt-00439

μ-Hydrodihydrobis[μ-[methylenebis[diphenylphosphine]-*P*:*P*′]diplatinum(1+), 9CI

Bis-μ-bis(diphenylphosphino)methane-μ-hydridobis[hydridoplatinum](1+). μ-Hydridodihydridobis[μ-[methylenebis(diphenylphosphine)-P,P′]]diplatinum(1+)

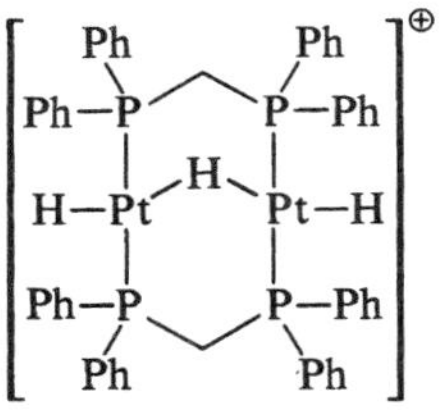

M 1161.976 (ion)

Hexafluorophosphate: [63911-00-2].
$C_{50}H_{47}F_6P_5Pt_2$ M 1306.941
Cryst. (MeOH). Mp 180-5° dec.
Chloride: [63910-98-5].
$C_{50}H_{47}ClP_4Pt_2$ M 1197.429
Cryst. (MeOH). Mp 210-4° dec.

Brown, M.P. *et al*, *J. Chem. Soc., Dalton Trans.*, 1978, 516 (*synth, nmr*)
Brown, M.P. *et al*, *Inorg. Chem.*, 1981, **20**, 3516 (*nmr*)
Foley, H.C. *et al*, *J. Am. Chem. Soc.*, 1981, **103**, 7337 (*uv*)

$C_{51}H_{43}OP_2Pt^{\oplus}$ Pt-00440

[(1,2,3-η)-6-Ethoxy-1*H*-phenalen-1-yl]bis(triphenylphosphine)platinum, 10CI

[(4,5,6-η)-1-Ethoxyphenalenyl]bis(triphenylphosphine)platinum(1+)

[67483-95-8]

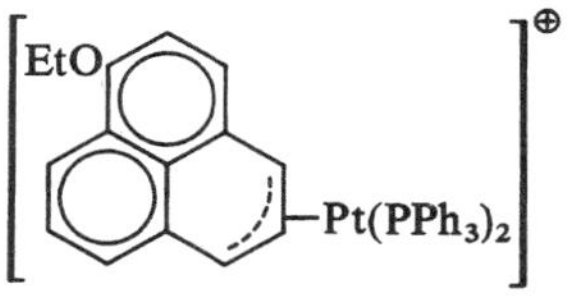

M 928.928 (ion)

Tetrafluoroborate:
$C_{51}H_{43}BF_4OP_2Pt$ M 1015.731
Yellow cryst. + $1CH_2Cl_2$ (CH_2Cl_2/hexane).

Keasey, A. *et al*, *J. Chem. Soc., Chem. Commun.*, 1978, 142 (*synth, struct, nmr*)

$C_{51}H_{46}Cl_2P_4Pt_2$ Pt-00441

Dichloro-μ-methylenebis[μ-[methylenebis[diphenylphosphine]-*P*:*P*′]]diplatinum, 9CI

Dichloro-μ-methylenebis-μ-[bis(diphenylphosphino)methane]diplatinum

[68851-49-0]

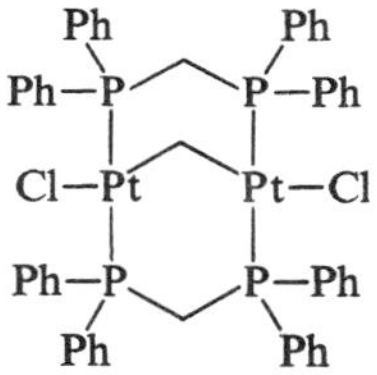

M 1243.885

Lemon-yellow cryst. (CH_2Cl_2).

Brown, M.P. *et al*, *Inorg. Chem.*, 1979, **18**, 2808 (*synth, nmr*)

$C_{51}H_{49}P_4Pt_2^{\oplus}$ Pt-00442

μ-Hydrohydromethylbis[μ-[methylenebis(diphenylphosphine)-*P*:*P*′]]diplatinum(1+)

Methyl-μ-hydridehydridobis[μ-bis(diphenylphosphino)methane]diplatinum(1+)

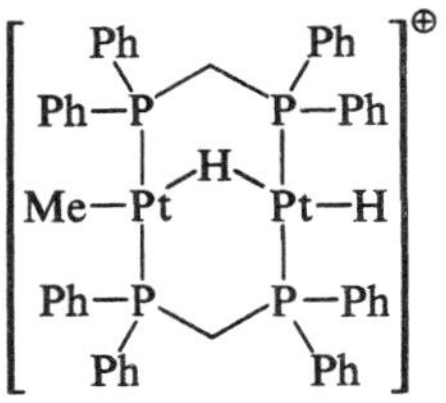

M 1176.003 (ion)

Hexafluoroantimonate:
$C_5H_{49}F_6P_4Pt_2Sb$ M 859.238
No phys. props. reported.

Azam, K.A., *J. Organomet. Chem.*, 1982, **234**, C31.

$C_{52}H_{40}P_2Pt$ **Pt-00443**

Bis(phenylethynyl)bis(triphenylphosphine)platinum, 9CI
Bis(phenylacetylide)bis(triphenylphosphine)platinum.
Bis(triphenylphosphine)bis(phenylethynyl)platinum

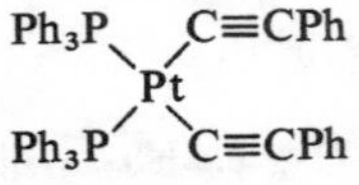

cis-form

M 921.916
Catalyses polymerisation of phenylacetylene.

cis-form [23318-76-5]
Cryst. ($CHCl_3$/hexane or Me_2CO). Mp 206-8° dec. Dipole moment 7.1 D.

trans-form [23318-77-6]
Yellow cryst. (C_6H_6). Sol. CH_2Cl_2, $CHCl_3$, C_6H_6. Insol. MeOH, hexane. Mp 220-2° dec.

Collimati, I. *et al*, *J. Organomet. Chem.*, 1969, **17**, 457 (*synth*)
Furlani, A. *et al*, *J. Organomet. Chem.*, 1976, **116**, 113 (*ir, pmr*)
Bonamico, M. *et al*, *Cryst. Struct. Commun.*, 1977, **6**, 39 (*struct*)
Furlani, A. *et al*, *Ann. Chim.* (*Rome*), 1979, **69**, 101 (*ms*)

$C_{52}H_{44}O_2P_4Pt_2^{\oplus\oplus}$ **Pt-00444**

Dicarbonylbis[μ-[methylenebis[diphenylphosphine]-*P*:*P'*]]-diplatinum(2+)

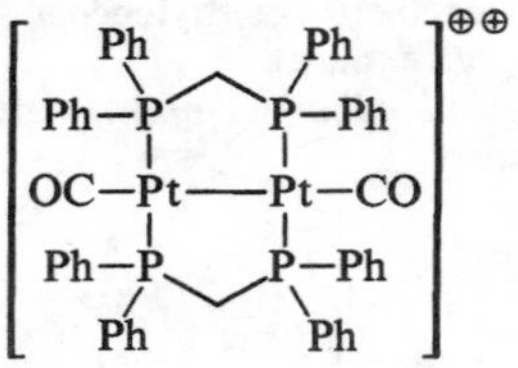

M 1214.973 (ion)
Bis(hexafluorophosphate): [68851-46-7].
$C_{52}H_{44}F_{12}O_2P_6Pt_2$ M 1504.902
Pale-yellow cryst. (Me_2CO/propanol) or white solid (CH_2Cl_2/hexane).

Brown, M.P. *et al*, *J. Organomet. Chem.*, 1979, **178**, 281 (*synth, ir, nmr*)
Fisher, J.R. *et al*, *Organometallics*, 1982, **1**, 1421 (*struct*)

$C_{52}H_{50}ClP_4Pt_2^{\oplus}$ **Pt-00445**

μ-Chlorodimethylbis[μ-[methylenebis[diphenylphosphine]-*P*:*P'*]]diplatinum(1+), 9CI
Dimethyl-μ-chlorobis-μ-[bis(diphenylphosphino)methane]diplatinum(1+)

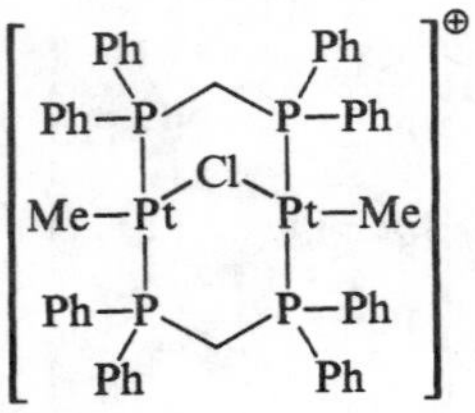

M 1224.475 (ion)
Chloride: [76648-80-1].
$C_{52}H_{50}Cl_2P_4Pt_2$ M 1259.928
Cryst. (CH_2Cl_2/hexane).
Hexafluorophosphate: [75862-29-2].
$C_{52}H_{50}ClF_6P_5Pt_2$ M 1369.439
Cryst. (CH_2Cl_2/hexane).

Cooper, S.J. *et al*, *Inorg. Chem.*, 1981, **20**, 1374 (*synth, nmr*)

$C_{52}H_{50}P_4Pt$ **Pt-00446**

Dimethylbis[methylenebis(diphenylphosphine)-*P*]platinum

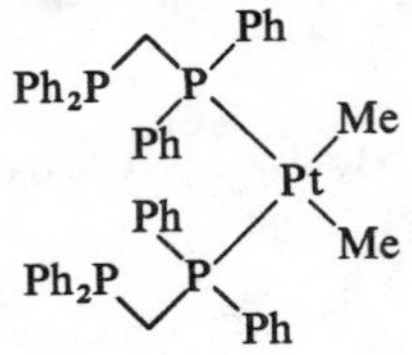

M 993.942
Dissociates in solution to equiibrate with [Bis(diphenylphosphino)methane]dimethylplatinum, Pt-00325 .

Pringle, P.G. *et al*, *J. Chem. Soc., Chem. Commun.*, 1982, 1313.

$C_{52}H_{51}P_4Pt_2^{\oplus}$ **Pt-00447**

Di-μ-hydrodimethylbis[μ-[methylenebis[diphenylphosphine]-*P*:*P'*]]diplatinum(1+), 10CI
Dimethyldi-μ-hydridobis-μ-[bis(diphenylphosphino)methane]diplatinum(1+)

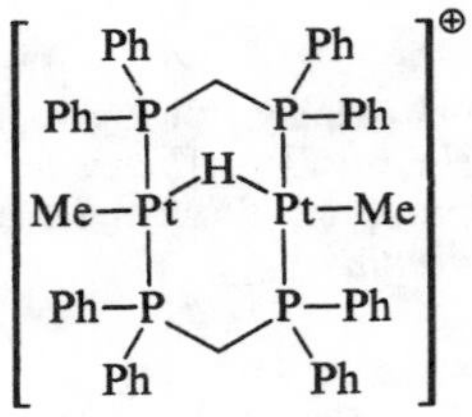

M 1190.030 (ion)
Hexafluorophosphate: [75862-27-0].
$C_{52}H_{51}F_6P_5Pt_2$ M 1334.994
Cryst. (CH_2Cl_2/hexane). Stable as solid up to 170°, but tends to dec. in soln.

Bancroft, G.M. *et al*, *Inorg. Chim. Acta*, 1981, **53**, L119 (*pe*)
Brown, M.P. *et al*, *J. Chem. Soc., Dalton Trans.*, 1982, 299 (*synth, struct, nmr*)

$C_{52}H_{54}P_2PtSn_2$ **Pt-00448**

Bis(dimethylphenylphosphine)dihydridobis(triphenyltin)platinum
Bis(dimethylphenylphosphine)dihydrobis(triphenylstannyl)platinum, 9CI. Bis(triphenyltin)dihydridobis(dimethylphenylphosphine)platinum
[56995-62-1]

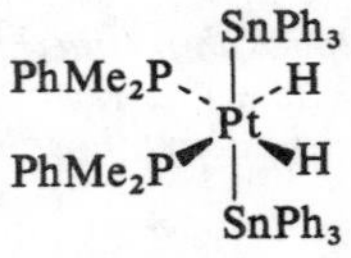

M 1173.406
Solid. Mp 176-7°. Reversibly eliminates H_2 in C_6H_6 soln.

Eaborn, C. *et al*, *J. Chem. Soc., Dalton Trans.*, 1975, 809 (*synth, nmr*)

$C_{52}H_{64}P_2Pt$ Pt-00449

Dioctylbis(triphenylphosphine)platinum

Bis(triphenylphosphine)dioctylplatinum

[65337-71-5]

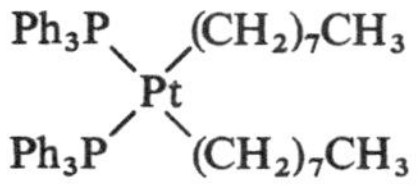

Ph_3P $(CH_2)_7CH_3$ Pt Ph_3P $(CH_2)_7CH_3$

M 946.105

cis-form [38192-86-8]

Cryst. (Me_2CO). Mp 76° dec.

Whitesides, G.M. *et al*, *J. Am. Chem. Soc.*, 1972, **94**, 5258 (*synth, ir*)

Van Leeuwen, P.W.N.M. *et al*, *J. Organomet. Chem.*, 1977, **142**, 233.

$C_{52}H_{80}P_4Pt_3$ Pt-00450

Bis(μ-diphenylacetylene)tetrakis(triethylphosphine)triplatinum

Bis[μ-[1,1′-(η^2:η^2-1,2-ethynediyl)bis[benzene]]]tetrakis(triethylphosphine)triplatinum, 9CI

[66916-62-9]

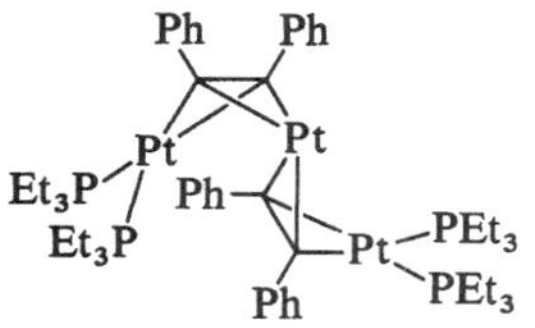

M 1414.339

Orange-red cryst. (pet. ether). Mp 143-8° dec.

Boag, N.M. *et al*, *J. Chem. Soc., Dalton Trans.*, 1980, 2170, 2182 (*synth, ir, pmr, struct*)

$C_{53}H_{53}P_4Pt_2^{\oplus}$ Pt-00451

Trimethylbis[μ-[methylenebis[diphenylphosphine]-*P*:*P′*]]diplatinum(1+), 9CI

Trimethylbis-μ-[bis(diphenylphosphino)methane]diplatinum(1+)

[75583-11-8]

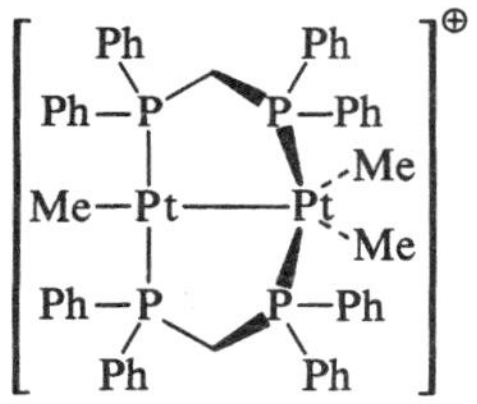

M 1204.057 (ion)

Hexafluorophosphate: [75583-12-9].

$C_{53}H_{53}F_6P_5Pt_2$ M 1349.021

Yellow cryst. (CH_2Cl_2/hexane).

Hexafluoroantimonate: [76600-28-7].

$C_{53}H_{53}F_6P_4Pt_2Sb$ M 1439.797

Yellow cryst. (CH_2Cl_2/hexane).

Perchlorate: [73464-61-6].

$C_{53}H_{53}ClO_4P_4Pt_2$ M 1303.507

Yellow cryst. (Me_2CO).

Frew, A.A. *et al*, *J. Chem. Soc., Chem. Commun.*, 1980, 624 (*struct*)

Brown, M.P. *et al*, *Inorg. Chem.*, 1981, **20**, 1500 (*synth*)

Puddephatt, R.J. *et al*, *J. Chem. Soc., Chem. Commun.*, 1981, 805.

$C_{54}H_{45}P_3Pt$ Pt-00452

Tris(triphenylphosphine)platinum

[13517-35-6]

$Pt(PPh_3)_3$

M 981.951

Catalyses water-gas shift reaction, oxidn. of ketones and cleavage of Si-C bonds. Yellow air-sensitive cryst. (EtOH). Sol. C_6H_6 with slight dissociation. Mp 205-6° (*in vacuo*). Reacts with CCl_4.

Inorg. Synth., 1968, **11**, 105 (*synth, ir*)

$C_{54}H_{46}P_3Pt^{\oplus}$ Pt-00453

Hydrotris(triphenylphosphine)platinum(1+), 9CI

Hydridotris(triphenylphosphine)platinum(1+)

[47899-53-6]

$[PtH(PPh_3)_3]^{\oplus}$ (C_{2v})

M 982.959 (ion)

Hydroformylation catalyst.

Perchlorate: [19568-66-2].

$C_{54}H_{46}ClO_4P_3Pt$ M 1082.409

Solid.

Tetraphenylborate: [17347-88-5].

$C_{78}H_{66}BP_3Pt$ M 1302.191

Cryst.

Hydridobis(trifluoroacetate): [39047-31-9].

$C_{58}H_{47}F_6O_4P_3Pt$ M 1209.999

Cryst. (CH_2Cl_2). Mp 132° dec.

Clark, H.C. *et al*, *J. Am. Chem. Soc.*, 1969, **91**, 596 (*synth*)

Gavrilova, I.V. *et al*, *Zh. Neorg. Khim.*, 1971, **16**, 1124; *Russ. J. Inorg. Chem. (Engl. Transl.)*, **16**, 596 (*synth, nmr*)

Thomas, K. *et al*, *Inorg. Chem.*, 1972, **11**, 1795 (*synth, pmr*)

Bracher, G. *et al*, *Helv. Chim. Acta*, 1980, **63**, 2519 (*nmr*)

$C_{54}H_{72}P_4Pt_2$ Pt-00454

Bis-μ-(diphenylphosphido)diphenylbis(tripropylphosphine)diplatinum

Diphenyldi-μ-(diphenylphosphido)bis(tripropylphosphine)diplatinum

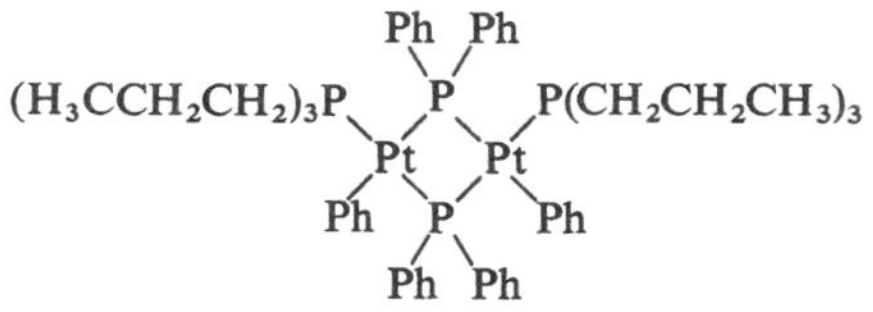

M 1235.218

cis-form

Cryst. (C_6H_6/EtOH). Mp 198° (resolidifies as *trans*-form). Dipole moment 6.35D.

trans-form

Cryst. (C_6H_6). Mp 275°. Dipole moment 0.25D.

Chatt, J. *et al*, *J. Chem. Soc.*, 1964, 2433 (*synth*)

The first digit of the Entry number defines the Supplement in which the Entry is found. 0 indicates the Main Work

$C_{54}H_{82}P_3Pt^{\oplus}$ Pt-00455

Hydrobis(tricyclohexylphosphine)(triphenylphosphine)platinum(1+), 10CI

Hydridobis(tricyclohexylphosphine)(triphenylphosphine)platinum(1+)

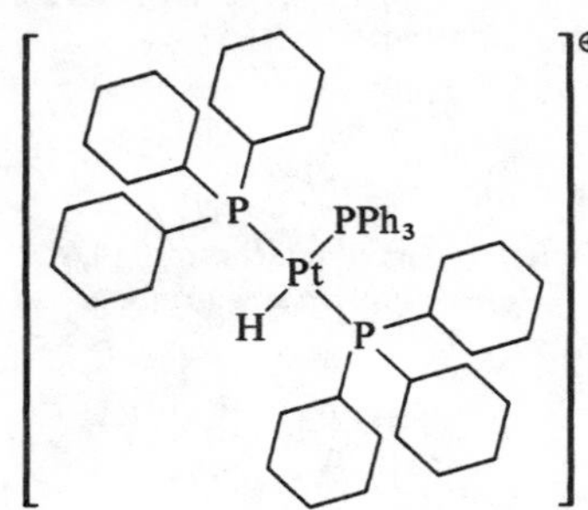

M 1019.243 (ion)

trans-form

Hexafluorophosphate: [67551-89-7].
$C_{54}H_{82}F_6P_4Pt$ M 1164.207
Air-stable cryst. (CH_2Cl_2).

Clark, H.C. *et al*, *J. Organomet. Chem.*, 1978, **154**, C40 (*synth, struct*)

$C_{54}H_{94}P_2Pt_2Si_2$ Pt-00456

Di-μ-hydrobis(benzyldimethylsilyl)bis(tricyclohexylphosphine)diplatinum

Bis[dimethyl(phenylmethyl)silyl]di-μ-hydrobis(tricyclohexylphosphine)diplatinum, 10CI. Di-μ-hydridobis-[dimethyl(phenylmethyl)silyl]bis(tricyclohexylphosphine)diplatinum

[68249-74-1]

M 1251.615

Hydrosilylation catalyst. Yellow, air-stable cryst. Mp 136-9° dec.

Ciriano, M. *et al*, *J. Chem. Soc., Dalton Trans.*, 1978, 801 (*synth, nmr*)
Tsipsis, C.A., *J. Organomet. Chem.*, 1980, **187**, 427; **188**, 53 (*use*)

$C_{55}H_{45}OP_3Pt$ Pt-00457

Carbonyltris(triphenylphosphine)platinum, 9CI

[15376-99-5]

$Pt(CO)(PPh_3)_3$ (C_{3v})

M 1009.961

Colourless-form

Colourless cryst. (Me_2CO under CO). Mp 100° dec. ir ν_{CO} 1908 cm^{-1} (nujol). More stable form.

Yellow-form

Pale-yellow cryst. (C_6H_6/hexane, under CO). Sol. Me_2CO, C_6H_6, insol. hexane. Mp 120° dec.

Albana, V.G. *et al*, *Inorg. Chem.*, 1969, **8**, 2109 (*struct*)
Chini, P. *et al*, *J. Chem. Soc.* (*A*), 1970, 1542 (*synth, ir*)
Sen, A. *et al*, *Inorg. Chem.*, 1980, **19**, 1073 (*nmr*)

$C_{55}H_{45}OP_3Pt_2S$ Pt-00458

Carbonyl(μ-sulfido)tris(triphenylphosphine)diplatinum

Carbonyl-μ-thioxotris(triphenylphosphine)diplatinum, 9CI, 8CI. μ-Sulfidocarbonyltris(triphenylphosphine)diplatinum. μ-Sulfidocyclo[bis(triphenylphosphine)platinumcarbonyltriphenylphosphineplatinum]

[27664-43-3]

M 1237.101

Yellow plates ($CHCl_3/Me_2CO$ or C_6H_6/MeOH). Mp 210-2° dec.

Skapski, A.C. *et al*, *J. Chem. Soc.* (*A*), 1969, 2772 (*synth, struct*)
Podder, R.K. *et al*, *J. Coord. Chem.*, 1977, **6**, 207 (*synth*)
Hunt, C.T. *et al*, *Inorg. Chem.*, 1981, **20**, 2270 (*nmr, synth, struct*)

$C_{55}H_{48}P_3Pt^{\oplus}$ Pt-00459

Methyltris(triphenylphosphine)platinum(1+), 9CI

$(Ph_3P)_3PtMe^{\oplus}$ (C_{2v})

M 996.985 (ion)

Tetrafluoroborate: [74679-77-9].
$C_{55}H_{48}BF_4P_3Pt$ M 1083.789
No phys. props. reported.

Fluorosulfonate: [50726-58-4].
$C_{55}H_{48}FO_3P_3PtS$ M 1096.042
Cryst. (Me_2CO/C_6H_6).

Peterson, J.L. *et al*, *J. Am. Chem. Soc.*, 1973, **95**, 8195 (*synth, ir, nmr*)
Pregosin, P.S. *et al*, *Inorg. Chim. Acta*, 1980, **45**, L7 (*nmr*)

$C_{55}H_{52}O_3P_4Pt_3$ Pt-00460

Tri-μ-carbonyltetrakis(methyldiphenylphosphine)triplatinum, 8CI

[27518-11-2]

M 1470.149

Violet-red cryst. (C_6H_6/hexane under N_2). Sol. Me_2CO. Mp 139-42° dec.

Chatt, J. *et al*, *J. Chem. Soc.* (*A*), 1970, 1538 (*synth, ir, pmr*)

$C_{56}H_{40}Cl_4Pt_2$ Pt-00461

Di-μ-chlorodichlorobis[1,2,3,4-tetraphenyl-1,3-cyclobutadiene]diplatinum, 8CI

[33010-79-6]

As Di-μ-chlorodichlorobis[(1,2,3,4-η)-1,2,3,4-tetramethyl-1,3-cyclobutadiene]diplatinum, Pt-00181 with

R = Ph

M 1244.904

Bridged dimer. Orange cryst. (Me_2CO). Sl. sol. $CHCl_3$, Me_2CO, insol. other org. solvs. Mp 300° dec.

Monomer: Dichloro(tetraphenylcyclobutadiene)-platinum.
$C_{28}H_{20}Cl_2Pt$ M 622.452
Unknown.

Canziani, F. *et al*, *J. Organomet. Chem.*, 1971, **26**, 285 (*synth, ir*)

$C_{56}H_{50}P_3Pt^{\oplus}$ Pt-00462

Ethyltris(triphenylphosphine)platinum(1+), 9CI

$(Ph_3P)_3PtEt^{\oplus}$ (C_{2v})

M 1011.012 (ion)

Tetrafluoroborate: [74679-79-1].
$C_{56}H_{50}BF_4P_3Pt$ M 1097.816
No phys. props. reported.

Pregosin, P.S. *et al*, *Inorg. Chim. Acta*, 1980, **45**, L7 (*nmr*)

$C_{57}H_{45}P_2Pt^{\oplus}$ Pt-00463

[(2,3-η)-1,2,3-Triphenyl-2-cyclopropen-1-ylium]bis(triphenylphosphine)platinum(1+), 9CI

M 987.010 (ion)

One Pt-C bond is longer than the other two.

Hexfluorophosphate: [42012-03-3].
$C_{57}H_{45}F_6P_3Pt$ M 1131.974
Cryst. + $1C_6H_6$ (C_6H_6).

McClure, M.D. *et al*, *J. Organomet. Chem.*, 1973, **54**, C59 (*synth, struct*)

$C_{60}H_{50}P_2PbPt$ Pt-00464

Phenylbis(triphenylphosphine)triphenylplumbylplatinum, 9CI

Phenyl(triphenylplumbyl)bis(triphenylphosphine)platinum. (Triphenyllead)phenylbis(triphenylphosphine)-platinum

M 1235.283

cis-form [65877-85-2]

Off-white cryst. ($MeOH/CH_2Cl_2$). Mp 168° dec.

Crociani, B. *et al*, *J. Organomet. Chem.*, 1973, **49**, 249 (*synth, struct*)
Al-Allaf, T.A.K. *et al*, *J. Organomet. Chem.*, 1980, **188**, 335 (*synth, nmr*)
Carr, S. *et al*, *J. Organomet. Chem.*, 1982, **240**, 143 (*nmr*)

$C_{61}H_{52}P_3Pt^{\oplus}$ Pt-00465

Benzyltris(triphenylphosphine)platinum(1+)

(Phenylmethyl)tris(triphenylphosphine)platinum(1+), 9CI

$(Ph_3P)_3PtCH_2Ph^{\oplus}$ (C_{2v})

M 1073.083 (ion)

Tetrafluoroborate: [74679-83-7].
$C_{61}H_{52}BF_4P_3Pt$ M 1159.887
No phys. props. reported.

Pregosin, P.S. *et al*, *Inorg. Chim. Acta.*, 1980, **45**, L7 (*nmr*)

$C_{62}H_{56}P_4Pt_2$ Pt-00466

Bis[μ-[methylenebis[diphenylphosphine]-*P:P'*]]tetrapropyne-1-yldiplatinum

Bis-μ-[bis(diphenylphosphino)methane]bis[di(methylethynyl)platinum]

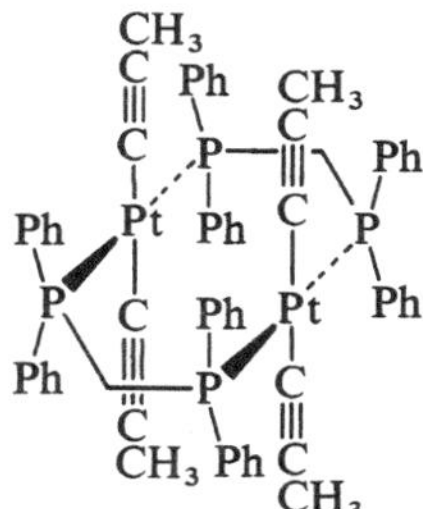

M 1315.179

Cryst. ($CHCl_2/EtOH$).

Puddephatt, R.J. *et al*, *J. Organomet. Chem.*, 1982, **238**, 231 (*synth*)

$C_{62}H_{58}P_2PtSn_2$ Pt-00467

Dihydrobis(methyldiphenylphosphine)bis(triphenylstannyl)-platinum, 9CI

Bis(triphenyltin)dihydridobis(methyldiphenylphosphine)platinum

[57048-81-4]

M 1297.548

Solid. Mp 125°.

Eaborn, C. *et al*, *J. Chem. Soc., Dalton Trans.*, 1975, 809 (*synth, nmr*)

$C_{72}H_{60}O_2P_4Pt_3S$ Pt-00468

[μ-(Diphenylphosphino)]-μ-phenyl-μ-sulfonyltris(triphenylphosphine)triplatinum, 9CI

(μ-Diphenylphosphino)(μ-phenyl)(μ-sulfur dioxide)-tris[triphenylphosphine platinum]

[77649-70-8]

M 1698.460

Red cryst. ($C_6H_6/MeOH$).

Evans, G.D. *et al*, *J. Chem. Soc., Chem. Commun.*, 1980, 1255 (*synth, struct*)

$C_{72}H_{60}O_{12}P_4Pt$ Pt-00469

Tetrakis(triphenylphosphite-*P*)platinum, 9CI

Tetrakis(phosphorous acid)platinum dodecaphenyl ester, 8CI

[22372-53-8]

$Pt[P(OPh)_3]_4$ (T_d)

M 1436.234
Catalyses silicone rubber vulcanisation, hydrosilylation, polysiloxane formn. Cryst. (C_6H_6/hexane). Mp 148-54°. Air-stable for significant periods.

Inorg. Synth., 1972, **13**, 105 (*synth*)
Pregosin, P.S. *et al*, *Helv. Chim. Acta*, 1977, **60**, 1371 (*nmr*)

$C_{72}H_{60}P_2Pb_2Pt$ Pt-00470

Bis(triphenylphosphine)bis(triphenylplumbyl)platinum, 9CI
[41705-72-0]

$(Ph_3Pb)_2Pt(PPh_3)_2$

M 1596.694
Yellowish microcryst. Mp 155-60° dec.

Crociani, B. *et al*, *J. Organomet. Chem.*, 1973, **49**, 249.

$C_{72}H_{60}P_4Pt$ Pt-00471

Tetrakis(triphenylphosphine)platinum
[14221-02-4]

$Pt(PPh_3)_4$ (T_d)

M 1244.241
Catalyses hydrosilylation of olefins, cleavage of Si-C bonds, vulcanisation of silicone rubbers, carbonylation, hydrogenation and isom. of olefins, and oxidations of organomercurials. Yellow air-sensitive solid. Mp 159-60° (*in vacuo*). Dissociates in C_6H_6, giving Tris(triphenylphosphine)platinum, Pt-00452 Reacts with CCl_4.

McAvoy, J. *et al*, *J. Chem. Soc.*, 1965, 1376 (*nmr*)
Inorg. Synth., 1968, **11**, 105 (*synth, ir*)
Adams, D.M. *et al*, *J. Chem. Soc. (A)*, 1969, 588 (*ir*)
Riggs, W.M., *Anal. Chem.*, 1972, **44**, 830 (*pe*)

$C_{75}H_{60}O_3P_4Pt_3$ Pt-00472

Tri-μ-carbonyltetrakis(triphenylphosphine)triplatinum, 9CI
[16222-02-9]

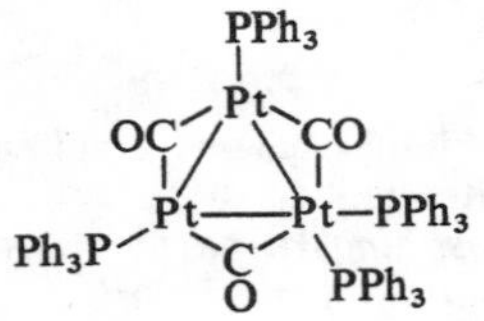

PPh₃ / Pt / OC CO / Ph₃P–Pt——Pt–PPh₃ / C / O PPh₃

M 1718.432
Orange-red cryst. (Me_2CO). Mp 179-82° dec.

Vranka, R.G. *et al*, *J. Am. Chem. Soc.*, 1969, **91**, 1579 (*struct*)
Chatt, J. *et al*, *J. Chem. Soc. (A)*, 1970, 1538 (*synth, ir*)

$C_{75}H_{66}P_6Pt_2$ Pt-00473

Tris[methylenebis(diphenylphosphine)]diplatinum, 9CI
Tris-μ-[bis(diphenyphosphino)methane]diplatinum
[37266-96-9]

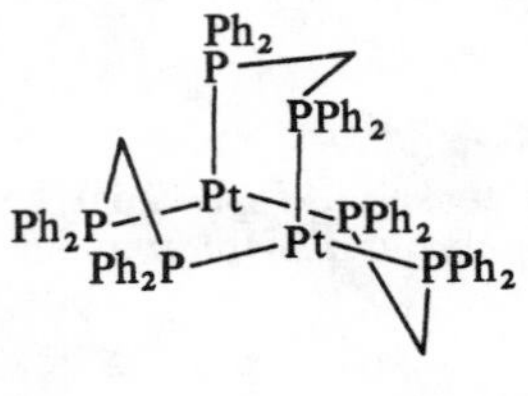

M 1543.349

Catalyses reduction of NO and O_2 by CO. Red cryst. (C_6H_6/propanol). Probably little Pt-Pt interaction (3.023Å).

Chin, C.-S. *et al*, *Inorg. Chim. Acta*, 1978, **31**, L443 (*use*)
Grossel, M.C. *et al*, *J. Organomet. Chem.*, 1982, **232**, C13 (*synth, pmr, nmr*)
Manojlovic-Muir, L. *et al*, *J. Chem. Soc., Chem. Commun.*, 1982, 1155 (*struct*)

$Cl_8PtSn_2^{\ominus\ominus}$ Pt-00474

Dichlorobis(trichlorostannyl)platinate(2−), 9CI
Dichlorobis(trichlorotin)platinate(2−). Bis(trichlorostannyl)dichloroplatinate(2−)
[44967-93-3]

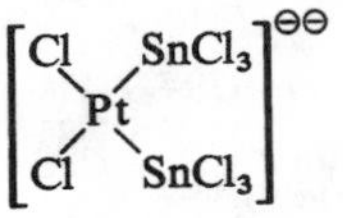

$[PtCl_2(SnCl_3)_2]^{\ominus\ominus}$

M 716.084 (ion)
Catalyses hydrogenation of diphenylacetylene.

Bis(triphenylmethylphosphonium) salt:
$C_{38}H_{36}Cl_8P_2PtSn_2$ M 1270.734
Yellow cryst. (MeOH). Mp 142-3°.

Bis(triphenylbenzylphosphonium) salt: [41071-60-7].
$C_{50}H_{44}P_2PtSn_2$ M 1139.305
Yellow cryst. (Me_2CO/hexane). Mp 182-6° dec.

Cramer, R.D. *et al*, *J. Am. Chem. Soc.*, 1963, **85**, 1691 (*synth*)
Parish, R.V. *et al*, *J. Chem. Soc., Dalton Trans.*, 1973, 37 (*mössbauer*)
Nelson, J.H. *et al*, *Inorg. Nucl. Chem. Lett.*, 1980, **16**, 263 (*nmr*)
Alcock, N.W. *et al*, *J. Chem. Soc., Dalton Trans.*, 1982, 2415 (*struct, synth*)

$Cl_{12}HPtSn_4^{\ominus\ominus\ominus}$ Pt-00475

Hydrotetrakis(trichlorostannyl)platinate(3−)
Hydridotetrakis(trichlorostannyl)platinate(3−)

$[PtH(SnCl_3)_4]^{\ominus\ominus\ominus}$

M 1096.284 (ion)
Catalyst for olefin hydrogenation, isomerisation, hydroformylation, and carboalkoxylation.

Tris(tetramethylammonium) salt:
$C_{12}H_{37}Cl_{12}N_3PtSn_4$ M 1318.720
ν_{PtH} 2072 cm^{-1}.

Tris(tetraethylammonium) salt: [41127-49-5].
$C_{24}H_{61}Cl_{12}N_3PtSn_4$ M 1487.042
No phys. props. reported.

Cramer, R.D. *et al*, *J. Am. Chem. Soc.*, 1965, **87**, 658 (*synth*)
Parshall, G.W., *J. Am. Chem. Soc.*, 1972, **94**, 8716.

$Cl_{15}PtSn_5^{\ominus\ominus\ominus}$ Pt-00476

Pentakis(trichlorostannyl)platinate(3−)
[40770-13-6]

$Pt(SnCl_3)_5^{\ominus\ominus\ominus}$

M 1320.325 (ion)
Catalyst for olefin isomerisation, hydrogenation and hydrogen exchange.

Tris(tetramethylammonium) salt: [41071-62-9].
$C_{12}H_{36}Cl_{15}N_3PtSn_5$ M 1542.762
Not fully descr.

Tris(triphenylmethylphosphonium) salt:
$C_{57}H_{54}Cl_{15}P_3PtSn_5$ M 2152.300
Red cryst. Sol. Me_2CO, $MeNO_2$.

Tris(tetraethylammonium) salt: [24328-97-0].
$C_{24}H_{60}Cl_{15}N_3PtSn_5$ M 1711.083
Not fully descr.

Cramer, R.D. *et al*, *J. Am. Chem. Soc.*, 1963, **85**, 1691 (*synth*)
Cramer, R.D. *et al*, *J. Am. Chem. Soc.*, 1965, **87**, 658 (*struct*)
Riggs, W.M., *Anal. Chem.*, 1972, **44**, 830 (*pe*)
Varnek, V.A. *et al*, *Koord. Khim.*, 1975, **1**, 161 (*mössbauer*)
Yurchenko, E.N. *et al*, *Koord. Khim.*, 1976, **2**, 1632 (*ir, nmr*)
Nelson, J.H., *Inorg. Nucl. Chem. Lett.*, 1980, **16**, 263 (*nmr*)

$F_{12}P_4Pt$ Pt-00477

Tetrakis(trifluorophosphine)platinum

Tetrakis(phosphorous trifluoride)platinum, 9CI, 8CI
[19529-53-4]

$Pt(PF_3)_4$ (T_d)

M 546.956
Colourless liq. Mp −15°. Bp_{730} 86°. Dec. at 90°, but can be distilled under N_2 at 1 atm.

Kruck, Th. *et al*, *Angew. Chem.*, 1965, **77**, 505 (*synth, ir*)
Bassett, P.J. *et al*, *J. Chem. Soc., Dalton Trans.*, 1974, 2316 (*pe*)
Ritz, C.L., *J. Mol. Struct.*, 1976, **31**, 73 (*struct*)

Name Index

Acetato(π-allyl)triphenylphosphinenickel, *see* Ni-00219
(Acetato-O,O')copper, Cu-00006
[μ-(Acetato-O:O')][μ-[1-η:2,3-η)-2,4-cyclopentadien-1-yl]]-bis[tris(1-methylethyl)phosphine]dipalladium, *see* Pd-00219
Acetato(cyclopentadienyl)triisopropylphosphinepalladium, Pd-00129
(Acetato-O)(η^5-2,4-cyclopentadien-1-yl)[tris(1-methylethyl)phosphine]palladium, *see* Pd-00129
(Acetato)(6,6-dimethyl-2-methylenebicyclo[3.3.1]hept-3-yl)palladium, *in* Pd-00205
(Acetato-O)(η^3-2-propenyl)(triphenylphosphine)nickel, Ni-00219
(Acetato)silver, Ag-00006
Acetonitrilechloro(di-*tert*-butylethyne)(trichlorostannyl)platinum, *see* Pt-00117
Acetonitrilechloro[(3,4-η)-2,2,5,5-tetramethyl-3-hexyne]-(trichlorostannyl)platinum, Pt-00117
Acetonitrilehydrotris(triphenylphosphine)nickel(1+), Ni-00368
Acetonitriletrichlorogold, Au-00006
Acetoxy(3,2,10-η-pinene)palladium, *in* Pd-00205
Acetylacetonatoacetylacetonyltriphenylphosphinepalladium, *see* Pd-00227
Acetylacetonato(acetyl)(trimethylphosphine)nickel, *see* Ni-00076
(Acetylacetonato)(allyl)palladium, *see* Pd-00039
Acetylacetonato(benzoyl)(triphenylphosphine)nickel, *see* Ni-00277
(Acetylacetonato)(2-butene)chloroplatinum, *see* Pt-00085
(Acetylacetonato)(1,5-cyclooctadiene)palladium(1+), *see* Pd-00087
(Acetylacetonato)(1,5-cyclooctadiene)platinum(1+), *see* Pt-00141
Acetylacetonato(2,4-cyclooctadienyl)palladium, *see* Pd-00086
(Acetylacetonato)[(1,4,5-η)-4-cycloocten-1-yl]nickel, *see* Ni-00105
Acetylacetonato[2-[(dimethylamino)methyl]ferrocenyl]palladium, *see* Pd-00147
(Acetylacetonato)ethyl(triphenylphosphine)nickel, *see* Ni-00244
(Acetylacetonato)methyltricyclohexylphosphinenickel, *see* Ni-00238
Acetylacetonato(methyl)(trimethylphosphine)nickel, *see* Ni-00066
Acetylacetonato(methyl)(triphenylphosphine)nickel, *see* Ni-00232
(Acetylacetonato)(norbornadiene)palladium(1+), *see* Pd-00073
Acetylacetonato-(1,3,4,5,6-pentamethylbicyclo[2.2.0]hexa-2,5-diene-2-methen-1-yl)palladium, *see* Pd-00134
(Acetylacetonato)phenyl(triphenylphosphine)nickel, *see* Ni-00273
(Acetylacetonato)trimethylplatinum, Pt-00072
Acetylacetonato(triphenylmethyl)palladium, *see* Pd-00199
Acetylacetonato(η^3-triphenylmethyl)platinum, Pt-00282
(Acetylacetonato)triphenylphosphine gold, *see* Au-00079
(1-Acetylacetonyl)chloro(2,4-pentanedionato)platinate(1−), *see* Pt-00091
[8-(1-Acetylacetonyl)-4-cycloocten-1-yl]-chloro(triphenylarsine)platinum, *see* Pt-00348
[8-(1-Acetylacetonyl)-π-4-cycloocten-1-yl](2,4-pentanedionato)palladium, Pd-00150
Acetylbis(triethylphosphine)platinum chloride, *see* Pt-00162
Acetylcarbonyl(η^5-2,4-cyclopentadien-1-yl)nickel, Ni-00045
Acetylchlorobis(dimethylphenylphosphine)platinum, Pt-00202
Acetylchlorobis(triethylphosphine)palladium, Pd-00107
Acetylchlorobis(triethylphosphine)platinum, Pt-00162
Acetylchlorobis(trimethylphosphine)nickel, Ni-00059
Acetylchlorobis(triphenylphosphine)palladium, Pd-00275
Acetyl(π-cyclopentadienyl)carbonylnickel, *see* Ni-00045
Acetyl(η^5-2,4-cyclopentadien-1-yl)ethylmethylplatinum, Pt-00094
Acetylenebis(triphenylphosphine)platinum, Pt-00385
(Acetylenedicarbonitrile)bis(triphenylphosphine)platinum, *see* Pt-00406
(1-Acetyl-4-ethylidenepiperidinyl)chloropalladium, *in* Pd-00151
Acetyliodobis(triethylphosphine)platinum, Pt-00164
Acetyliodobis(trimethylphosphine)palladium, Pd-00044
(1-Acetyl-2-oxopropyl)chloro(2,4-pentanedionato-O,O')platinate(1−), Pt-00091
[8-(1-Acetyl-2-oxopropyl)-4-cycloocten-1-yl]-chloro(triphenylarsine)platinum, Pt-00348
(1-Acetyl-2-oxopropyl)(2,4-pentanedionato-O,O')-(triphenylphosphine)palladium, Pd-00227
(1-Acetyl-2-oxopropyl)(triphenylphosphine)gold, Au-00079
[η^3-2-[2-(Acetyloxy)ethylidene]-6-methyl-5-heptenyl]chloropalladium, *in* Pd-00206
Acetyl(2,4-pentanedionato-O,O')(trimethylphosphine)nickel, Ni-00076
Acetyltris(trimethylphosphine)palladium(1+), Pd-00070
Acrylonitrilebis(triphenylphosphine)nickel, *see* Ni-00324
Ag(fod), *see* Ag-00026
Allenebis(triphenylphosphine)platinum, *see* Pt-00396
(Allene)dichloro(dimethylphenylphosphine)platinum, *see* Pt-00100
Allenedichloro(tripropylphosphine)platinum, *see* Pt-00119
(Allyl alcohol)trichloroplatinate(1−), *see* Pt-00016
π-Allylbis(dimethylphenylphosphine)palladium(1+), *see* Pd-00164
(π-Allyl)bis(dimethylphenylphosphine)platinum(1+), *see* Pt-00230
(π-Allyl)bis(thiourea)nickel(1+), *see* Ni-00020
Allylbis(tricyclohexylphosphine)platinum(1+), *see* Pt-00401
π-Allylbis(triethylphosphine)palladium(1+), *see* Pd-00112
(π-Allyl)bis(triphenylphosphine)palladium(1+), *see* Pd-00282
Allylbis(triphenylphosphine)platinum(1+), *see* Pt-00398
Allyl(bromo)bis(triethylphosphine)palladium, *see* Pd-00111
(σ-Allyl)bromobis(triethylphosphine)platinum, *see* Pt-00176
Allylbromonickel, *in* Ni-00029
Allylbromopalladium, *in* Pd-00019
Allylbromo(tricyclohexylphosphine)nickel, *see* Ni-00201
(π-Allyl)bromo(triethylphosphine)palladium, *see* Pd-00049
Allylbromo(triphenylphosphine)nickel, *see* Ni-00197
Allylchloro(benzonitrile)palladium, *see* Pd-00051
π-Allylchlorobis(triethylphosphine)palladium, *in* Pd-00112
(σ-Allyl)chlorobis(triphenylphosphine)platinum, *see* Pt-00397
Allylchloronickel, *in* Ni-00030
Allylchloropalladium, *in* Pd-00022
Allylchloroplatinum, *see* Pt-00014
Allylchloro(tricyclohexylphosphine)platinum, *see* Pt-00266
Allylchloro(trimethylphosphine)nickel, *see* Ni-00035
Allylchloro(trimethylphosphine)platinum, *see* Pt-00042
(π-Allyl)chlorotriphenylphosphinenickel, *see* Ni-00198
Allylchloro(triphenylphosphine)platinum, *see* Pt-00262
Allylchloro(tri-*p*-tolylphosphine)platinum, *see* Pt-00283
Allyl(1,5-cyclooctadiene)palladium(1+), *see* Pd-00065
(π-Allyl)(1,5-cyclooctadiene)platinum(1+), *see* Pt-00102
(μ-π-Allyl)(μ-π-cyclopentadienyl)bis(triphenylphosphine)dipalladium, *see* Pd-00312
π-Allyl-π-cyclopentadienylnickel, *see* Ni-00046
π-Allyl-π-cyclopentadienylpalladium, *see* Pd-00032

(2,2′-Bipyridine)(tetrafluoroethylene)platinum, Pt-00104
(2,2′-Bipyridine-*N,N′*)[(1,2,3,4-η)-1,2,3,4-tetramethyl-1,3-cyclobutadiene]nickel, Ni-00163
(2,2′-Bipyridine)tetramethylenenickel, *see* Ni-00114
(2,2′-Bipyridine-*N,N′*)trichloro(pentafluorophenyl)palladium, Pd-00117
Bipyridyl(dimethyl)palladium, *see* Pd-00072
(Bipyridyl)dimethylplatinum, *see* Pt-00107
Bis-μ-acetatobis[(7,1,2-η)-pinene]dipalladium, *see* Pd-00205
Bis[μ-(acetato-*O:O′*)]bis(η^3-2-propenyl)dipalladium, Pd-00055
Bis(acetato-*O*)bis(triphenylphosphine)palladium, Pd-00286
Bis(μ-acetato)di-π-allyldipalladium, *see* Pd-00055
Bis[μ-(acetato-*O:O*)](η^3-6,6-dimethyl-2-methylenebicyclo[3.1.1]hept-3-yl)dipalladium, Pd-00205
Bis[μ-(acetato-*O:O′*)]disilver, *in* Ag-00006
Bis(acetonitrile)dichloroplatinum, Pt-00023
Bis(acetonitrile)gold(1+), Au-00021
Bis(acetonitrile)silver(1+), Ag-00010
Bis[acetoxy(3,2,10-η-pinene)palladium], *see* Pd-00205
Bis(acetylacetonato)bis(triphenylcyclopropenyl)tripalladium, *see* Pd-00325
Bis(acetylacetonato)chloroplatinate(1−), *see* Pt-00091
Bis(acetylacetonato)(μ-ethylenediamine)hexamethyldiplatinum, *see* Pt-00218
▷Bis(acetylacetonato)nickel, *see* Ni-00072
Bis(acetylacetonato)palladium, *see* Pd-00053
Bis(acetylacetonato)platinum, *see* Pt-00092
Bis(acetylacetonato)(triphenylphosphine)palladium, *see* Pd-00227
Bis[μ-(1-acetylacetonyl)]hexamethyldiplatinum, *in* Pt-00072
Bis(η^3-1-acetyl-4-ethylidenepiperidinyl)di-μ-chlorodipalladium, Pd-00151
Bis(acetylide)bis(triethylphosphine)platinum, *see* Pt-00186
Bis[η^3-2-[2-(acetyloxy)ethylidene]-6-methyl-5-heptenyl]-di-μ-chlorodipalladium, Pd-00206
Bis[(16,17-20-η)-(3β)-3-(acetyloxy)-pregna-5,16-dien-20-yl]di-μ-chlorodipalladium, Pd-00316
Bis(acrylonitrile)(2,2′-bipyridine)nickel, *see* Ni-00142
▷Bis(acrylonitrile)nickel, *see* Ni-00025
▷Bis(acrylonitrile)triphenylphosphinenickel, *see* Ni-00229
Bisallylbis(trifluoroacetato)dinickel, *see* Ni-00067
Bis(allylchloronickel), *see* Ni-00030
▷Bis(allylchloropalladium), *see* Pd-00022
Bis(π-allyl)di-μ-bromodinickel, *see* Ni-00029
Bisallyldi-μ-bromodipalladium, *see* Pd-00019
Bis(allyl)diiododinickel, *see* Ni-00031
Bis(π-allyl)di-μ-iododiplatinum, *see* Pt-00039
Bis(allyl)dimethyldinickel, *in* Ni-00007
Bisallylnickel, *see* Ni-00032
Bisallylpalladium, *see* Pd-00023
Bis(allyl)platinum, *see* Pt-00040
Bis(π-allyl)tetra-μ-bromotripalladium, *see* Pd-00020
Bis(ammine)iodotrimethylplatinum, *see* Pt-00021
Bis-*o*-*C,N*-(azobenzene)palladium, *see* Pd-00197
Bis(azobenzeneyl)di-μ-chlorodipalladium, *see* Pd-00196
Bis(benzene)di-μ-chlorobis(μ-chloropentachlorodialuminum)dipalladium, Pd-00071
Bis(μ-benzene)tetra-μ-chlorodecachlorotetraaluminumdipalladium, *see* Pd-00071
Bis(μ-benzenethiolato)di-π-cyclopentadienyldinickel, *see* Ni-00204
Bis[μ-(benzoato-*O,O′*)]bis[1,1′-(η^2-1,2-ethynediyl)-bis[benzene]]dicopper, *in* Cu-00054
▷Bis(benzonitrile)dichloropalladium, Pd-00094
▷Bis(benzonitrile)dichloroplatinum, Pt-00151
▷Bis(benzonitrile)palladium dichloride, *see* Pd-00094
Bis(bicyclo[2.2.1]hept-2-ene)(trimethylphosphine)nickel, Ni-00158
Bis(2,2′-bipyridine-*N,N′*)nickel, Ni-00181
Bis(bipyridyl)nickel, *see* Ni-00181
Bis[bis(di-*tert*-butylphosphino)propane]diplatinum, Pt-00390
Bis[1,2-bis(diethylphosphino)benzene]palladium, Pd-00232
Bis[2-[bis(1,1-dimethylethyl)arsino]-2-methylpropyl-*As,C*]-di-μ-hydrodipalladium, *see* Pd-00210
Bis[bis-(1,1-dimethylethyl)phenylphosphine]palladium, *see* Pd-00231
Bis[bis-(1,1-dimethylethyl)phenylphosphine]platinum, *see* Pt-00337
Bis[2-[bis(1,1-dimethylethyl)phosphine]-2,2-dimethylethyl-*C,P*]di-μ-chlorodiplatinum, *see* Pt-00298
Bis[3-[bis(1,1-dimethylethyl)phosphino]-2,2-dimethylpropyl-*C,P*]di-μ-chlorodiplatinum, *see* Pt-00320
Bis[2-[bis(1,1-dimethylethyl)phosphino]-2-methylpropyl-*C,P*]di-μ-chlorodiplatinum, *see* Pt-00298
Bis[1,2-bis(dimethylphosphino)ethane]nickel, Ni-00097
Bis[1,2-bis(diphenylphosphino)ethane]hydridonickel(1+), *see* Ni-00357
Bis[1,2-bis(diphenylphosphino)ethane]nickel, Ni-00356
Bis-μ-[bis(diphenylphosphino)methane]bis[di(methylethynyl)platinum], *see* Pt-00466
Bis-μ-bis(diphenylphosphino)methane-μ-hydridobis[hydridoplatinum](1+), *see* Pt-00439
Bis[bis[(4-methylphenyl)amino]methylene]diiodogold(1+), Au-00087
Bis[μ-[bis(trilfluoromethyl)phosphino]]di-π-cyclopentadienyldinickel, Ni-00111
Bis[(2,3-η)-2-butene]tetrachlorodipalladium, Pd-00042
Bis[(1,2,3-η)-2-butenyl]bis[μ-trifluoroacetato-*O:O′*]dinickel, Ni-00088
Bis[(1,2,3-η)-2-butenyl]bis(μ-trifluoroethanoato)dinickel, *see* Ni-00088
Bis[(1,2,3-η)-2-butenyl]di-μ-chlorodipalladium, Pd-00040
Bis[(1,2,3-η)-2-buten-1-yl]nickel, *see* Ni-00054
Bis(*tert*-butylisocyanide)-π-cyclopentadienylnickel(1+), *see* Ni-00132
Bis(*tert*-butylisocyanide)diiodopalladium, *see* Pd-00059
Bis(*tert*-butylisocyanide)(fumaronitrile)nickel, *see* Ni-00120
Bis((*tert*-butyl isocyanide)iodomethylpalladium, *see* Pd-00069
Bis(*tert*-butylisocyanide)palladium, *see* Pd-00061
Bis(*tert*-butylisocyanide)peroxypalladium, *see* Pd-00060
Bis(*tert*-butylisocyanide)(tetracyanoethylene)nickel, Ni-00144
Bis(*tert*-butylisonitrile)(azobenzene)nickel, *see* Ni-00210
Bis(*tert*-butylisonitrile)diiodopalladium, *see* Pd-00059
Bis(*tert*-butylisonitrile)(dioxygen)palladium, *see* Pd-00060
Bis(*tert*-butylisonitrile)iodomethylpalladium, *see* Pd-00069
Bis(*tert*-butylisonitrile)palladium, *see* Pd-00061
[1,2-Bis(carbomethoxy)ethyne]bis(triphenylphosphine)palladium, *see* Pd-00303
Bis(carbonylcyclopentadienylnickel), *see* Ni-00084
Bis[chloro(16,17,20-η)-3β-acetoxy-17-ethylidene-5-androstene)palladium], *see* Pd-00316
Bis(μ-chloro)bis[(1,4,5-η)-8-(α-chloroethyl)cyclooctenyl]dipalladium, *see* Pd-00175
Bis[chloro(η^3-5-*tert*-butyl-2-methylenecyclohexyl)palladium], *see* Pd-00190
Bis(1-chloroethenyl)bis(dimethylphenylphosphine)platinum, Pt-00248
Bis[chloro-(16,17,20-η)-3-methoxy-19-nor-1,3,5(10),17(20)-pregnatetraene)palladium], *see* Pd-00305
Bis[chloro(η^3-12-methoxy-2,6,10-trimethyl-12-oxo-2,6,10-dodecatrienyl)palladium], *see* Pd-00249
Bis[chloro(η^3-2-(4-methyl-5-oxo-3-cyclohexen-1-yl)-2-propenyl)palladium], *see* Pd-00173
Bis[chloro(9,10,11-η)methyl-10-undecenoate)palladium], Pd-00208
Bis[μ-chloro-η^3-(2-phenylpropenyl)palladium], *see* Pd-00143
Bis[chloro-(7,1,2-η^3-pinene)palladium], *see* Pd-00174
Bis(1-chlorovinyl)bis(dimethylphenylphosphine)platinum, *see* Pt-00248
Bis(π-crotylpalladium chloride), *see* Pd-00040
Bis(cyano-*C*)argentate(1−), Ag-00004
Bis(cyano-*C*)aurate(1−), Au-00003
Bis(cyano-*C*)bis(pentafluorophenyl)palladate(2−), *see* Pd-00091
▷Bis(cyano-*C*)cuprate(1−), Cu-00004
▷Bis(cyanoethylene)triphenylphosphinenickel, *see* Ni-00229
Bis(cyanomethyl)[1,2-ethanediylbis[diphenylphosphine]-*P,P′*]palladium, Pd-00239

Bis(dimethylphenylphosphine)(η^3-2-propenyl)palladium(1+), Pd-00164
Bis(dimethylphenylphosphine)(η^3-2-propenyl)platinum(1+), Pt-00230
Bis(dimethylphenylphosphine)(η^2-tetrafluoroethene)platinum, Pt-00200
Bis(dimethylphenylphosphine)(tetrafluoroethylene)platinum, *see* Pt-00200
Bis(dimethylphenylphosphine)tetramethylplatinum, Pt-00256
Bis[μ-[(dimethylphosphinidenio)bis(methylene)]]digold, Au-00059
Bis[μ-(dimethylphosphinidenio)bis[methylene]iodomethyldigold, Au-00062
Bis(dimethylsulfonium-η-methylide)di-μ-iododiiododipalladium, Pd-00026
Bis(diphenylacetylene)bis(trimethylphosphine)diplatinum, Pt-00354
Bis(diphenylacetylene)platinum, Pt-00328
Bis(μ-diphenylacetylene)tetrakis(triethylphosphine)triplatinum, Pt-00450
Bis(diphenylethyne)platinum, *see* Pt-00328
Bis(diphenylmethylphosphine)(σ-pentafluorophenyl)chloropalladium, *see* Pd-00246
Bis[η^2-1,5-diphenyl-1,4-pentadien-3-one]palladium, Pd-00253
Bis[(C^3,O^3-η)-1,5-diphenyl-1,4-pentadien-3-one]platinum, Pt-00353
Bis-μ-(diphenylphosphido)diphenylbis(tripropylphosphine)diplatinum, Pt-00454
(1,2-Bis(diphenylphosphino)ethane)bis(methylethynyl)palladium, *see* Pd-00247
[1,2-Bis(diphenylphosphino)ethane]bis(pentachlorophenyl)palladium, *see* Pd-00270
[1,2-Bis(diphenylphosphino)ethane]bis(phenylethynyl)palladium, *see* Pd-00300
[1,2-Bis(diphenylphosphino)ethane]diethynylpalladium, *see* Pd-00238
1,2-Bis(diphenylphosphino)ethane(dimethyl)palladium, *see* Pd-00228
(Bisdiphenylphosphinoethane)iodopentafluoroethylnickel, *see* Ni-00259
[1,2-bis(diphenylphosphino)ethane]nickel dichloride, *see* Ni-00246
1,2-Bis(diphenylphosphino)ethaneperfluoromethyliodopalladium, *see* Pd-00223
[1,2-Bis(diphenylphosphino)ethane](tetracyanoethylene)palladium, *see* Pd-00245
[1,2-Bis(diphenylphosphino)ethane]tetraphenylcyclobutadienenickel, *see* Ni-00360
[1,1′-Bis(diphenylphosphino)ferrocene-*P*,*P*′]dichloropalladium, Pd-00252
Bis(diphenylphosphino)hexacarbonyldinickel, *see* Ni-00275
[Bis(diphenylphosphino)methane]dimethylplatinum, Pt-00325
[Bis(diphenylphosphino)methanid]gold, *see* Au-00097
Bis[1,2-ethanediylbis(dimethylphosphine)-*P*,*P*′]nickel, *see* Ni-00097
Bis[1,2-ethanediylbis[diphenylphosphine]-*P*,*P*′]hydronickel(1+), Ni-00357
Bis[1,2-ethanediylbis(diphenylphosphine)-*P*,*P*′]nickel, *see* Ni-00356
▷Bis[(1,2-η)-ethenecarbonitrile]triphenylphosphinenickel, *see* Ni-00229
Bis(ethenediphenylnickelate)(4−), *see* Ni-00112
Bis[(η^2-ethene)diphenylnickel]pentakis(tetrahydrofuran)tetrasodium, *in* Ni-00112
Bis(η^2-ethene)ethylnickelate(1−), *see* Ni-00034
Bis(η^2-ethene)methylnickelate(1−), *see* Ni-00019
Bis(η^2-ethene)tricyclohexylphosphinenickel, *see* Ni-00214
Bis(η^2-ethene)(tricyclohexylphosphine)platinum, *see* Pt-00277
Bis(ethene)(trimethylphosphine)platinum, *see* Pt-00055
Bis(η^2-ethene)(triphenylarsine)platinum, *see* Pt-00271
Bisethene(triphenylphosphine)nickel, *see* Ni-00212
Bis(η^2-ethene)(triphenylphosphine)platinum, *see* Pt-00272
Bis(3-ethenylcyclohexene)(tricyclohexylphosphine)nickel, *see* Ni-00297
Bis(ethyldiphenylphosphine)dicarbonylplatinum, *see* Pt-00339
Bisethylenebis-μ-dicyclohexylphosphinedinickel, *see* Ni-00269
Bis[ethylenebis(dimethylphosphine)]nickel, *see* Ni-00097
Bis[ethylenebis(diphenylphosphine)]nickel, *see* Ni-00356
Bis(ethylene)dichloro-μ-dichloropalladium, *see* Pd-00011
Bis(ethylenedichloroplatinum), *see* Pt-00027
Bis(ethylene)methylnickelate(1−), Ni-00019
Bis(ethylene)tricyclohexylphosphinenickel, Ni-00214
Bis(ethylene)(tricyclohexylphosphine)platinum, Pt-00277
Bis(ethylene)(trimethylphosphine)platinum, Pt-00055
Bis(ethylene)(triphenylarsine)platinum, Pt-00271
Bisethylene(triphenylphosphine)nickel, Ni-00212
Bis(ethylene)(triphenylphosphine)platinum, Pt-00272
Bis(ethyl isocyanide)gold(1+), *see* Au-00036
[1,2-Bis(ethylthio)ethane-*S*,*S*′]dimethylplatinum, Pt-00075
[1,2-Bis(ethylthio)ethane-*S*,*S*′]diphenylplatinum, Pt-00201
Bis[1,1′-(η^2-1,2-ethynediyl)bis[benzene]]platinum, *see* Pt-00328
Bis[μ-[1,1′-(η^2:η^2-1,2-ethynediyl)bis[benzene]]]-tetrakis(triethylphosphine)triplatinum, *see* Pt-00450
Bis(fulvalene)dinickel, *see* Ni-00182
Bis(heptafluoropropyl)(2,2′-bipyridine)palladium, *see* Pd-00118
Bis[hexacarbonyltriplatinate](2−), *see* Pt-00136
Bis[(1,2,3,4,5,6-η)hexamethylbenzene]nickel(2+), Ni-00235
▷Bis(*N*-hydroxy-*N*-methylmethanethioamidato-*O*,*S*)copper, *see* Cu-00012
Bis[(1,2,3-η)-1*H*-inden-1-yl]nickel, Ni-00160
Bis(isocyanobenzene)palladium, Pd-00096
Bis(isocyanoethane)gold(1+), Au-00036
Bis(isocyanomethane)bis(pentafluorophenyl)palladium, Pd-00115
Bis(2-isocyano-2-methylpropane)(dioxygen)palladium, *see* Pd-00060
Bis[2-isocyano-2-methylpropane]palladium, Pd-00061
Bis(2-isocyano-2-methylpropane)peroxypalladium, Pd-00060
Bis[(2-mercaptoethylamine)nickel]dichlorophenylthallium, Ni-00074
Bis(3-methoxy-1-propenyl)bis(dimethylphenylphosphine)platinum, *see* Pt-00292
Bis(methylacetylide)bis(triethylphosphine)platinum, *see* Pt-00217
Bis(μ-2-methylallyl)bis(tricyclohexylphosphine)dipalladium, *see* Pd-00315
Bis(1-methyl-π-allyl)bis(μ-trifluoroacetato)dinickel, *see* Ni-00088
Bis(μ-2-methyl-π-allyl)bis(triisopropylphosphine)dipalladium, *see* Pd-00222
Bis[(2-methylallyl)chloropalladium], *see* Pd-00041
Bis(1-methyl-π-allyl)nickel, *see* Ni-00054
Bis(2-methyl-π-allyl)nickel, *see* Ni-00055
Bis(2-methylallyl)platinum, *see* Pt-00070
Bis(π-methylcyclopentadienyl)di-μ-carbonyldinickel, *see* Ni-00113
Bis(η^5-1-methyl-2,4-cyclopentadien-1-yl)nickel, Ni-00090
Bis(methyldiphenylphosphine)bis(pentafluorophenyl)nickel, Ni-00311
Bis(methyldiphenylphosphine)dicarbonylnickel, *see* Ni-00261
Bis(methyldiphenylphosphine)dimethylplatinum, *see* Pt-00333
Bis(methyldiphenylphosphine)methyliodopalladium, *see* Pd-00224
Bis(methyldiphenylphosphine)methylplatinum chloride, *see* Pt-00326
Bis(methyldiphenylphosphine)(pentachlorophenyl)-(pentafluorophenyl)nickel, Ni-00310
Bis(methyldiphenylphosphine)(pentafluoroethyl)platinum chloride, *see* Pt-00329
Bis(methyldiphenylphosphine)(phenylethene)palladium, *see* Pd-00254
Bis(methyldiphenylphosphine)phenylplatinum(II) chloride, *see* Pt-00351
Bis(methyldiphenylphosphine)(styrene)palladium, Pd-00254
Bis(methyldiphenylphosphine)tetramethylplatinum, *see* Pt-00342
Bis(methyldiphenylphosphine)(trifluoromethyl)platinum chloride, *see* Pt-00322

(Chlorodimethylstannyl)methylbis(triphenylphosphine)platinum, Pt-00400
Chloro(dimethyl sulfide)gold, Au-00012
Chlorodimethyl[thiobis[methane]]gold, *see* Au-00022
Chloro(2,8-dimethyl-2,10-undecadienyl)palladium, *in* Pd-00221
Chloro(diphenylacetylene)gold, Au-00068
Chloro[1,2-ethanediylbis[diphenylphosphine]-*P*,*P′*]ethylplatinum, *see* Pt-00330
Chloro[1,2-ethanediylbis[diphenylphosphine]-*P*,*P′*]methylplatinum, *see* Pt-00323
Chloro[1,2-ethanediylbis[diphenylphosphine]-*P*,*P′*]phenylplatinum, *see* Pt-00350
Chloro[(1,2,3-η)-4-ethoxy-1,2,3,4-tetraphenyl-2-cyclobuten-1-yl]palladium, *in* Pd-00336
Chloro(ethyl)bis(dimethylphenylphosphine)platinum, *see* Pt-00203
Chloroethylbis(triethylphosphine)platinum, Pt-00167
Chloro(ethyl)bis(triphenylphosphine)nickel, Ni-00319
Chloro[ethylenebis[diphenylphosphine]]methylplatinum, Pt-00323
Chloro[ethylenebis(diphenylphosphine)]phenylplatinum, Pt-00350
Chloroethyl[ethylenebis[diphenylphosphine]]platinum, Pt-00330
Chloro(ethylidenecyclohexyl)palladium, *in* Pd-00128
Chloro(2-ethylidene-6,6-dimethylbicyclo[3.1.1]hept-3-yl)palladium, *in* Pd-00189
Chloro[1,1′-(η^2-1,2-ethynediyl)bis[benzene]]gold, *see* Au-00068
Chloro(1,1,1,3,3,3-hexafluoro-2-propyl)-bis(triethylphosphine)platinum, Pt-00175
Chloro[(2,3,5-η)-3*a*,4,5,6,7,7*a*-hexahydro-6-methoxy-4,7-methano-1*H*-inden-5-yl]palladium, *in* Pd-00187
Chlorohydridobis(tricyclohexylphosphine)palladium, *see* Pd-00264
Chlorohydridobis(triethylarsine)platinum, *see* Pt-00123
Chlorohydridobis(triethylphosphine)palladium, *see* Pd-00084
Chlorohydridobis(triphenylphosphine)palladium, *see* Pd-00262
Chlorohydridobis(triphenylphosphine)platinum, *see* Pt-00357
Chlorohydridobis[tris(phenylmethyl)phosphine]platinum, *see* Pt-00420
Chlorohydrobis(dimethylphenylphosphine)platinum, Pt-00180
Chlorohydrobis(ethyldiphenylphosphine)platinum, Pt-00332
Chlorohydrobis(tribenzylphosphine)platinum, Pt-00420
Chlorohydrobis(tri-*tert*-butylphosphine)palladium, Pd-00212
Chlorohydrobis(tricyclohexylphosphine)nickel, Ni-00305
Chlorohydrobis(tricyclohexylphosphine)palladium, Pd-00264
Chlorohydrobis(triethylarsine)platinum, Pt-00123
Chlorohydrobis(triethylphosphine)palladium, Pd-00084
Chlorohydrobis(triethylphosphine)platinum, Pt-00126
Chlorohydrobis(triisopropylphosphine)nickel, Ni-00171
Chlorohydrobis(triisopropylphosphine)palladium, Pd-00160
Chlorohydrobis(trimethylphosphine)platinum, Pt-00047
Chlorohydrobis(triphenylphosphine)palladium, Pd-00262
Chlorohydrobis(triphenylphosphine)platinum, Pt-00357
Chlorohydrobis[tris(1-methylethyl)phosphine]nickel, *see* Ni-00171
Chlorohydrobis[tris(1-methylethyl)phosphine]palladium, *see* Pd-00160
Chlorohydrobis[tris(2-methyl-2-propyl)phosphine]palladium, *see* Pd-00212
Chlorohydrobis[tris(phenylmethyl)phosphine]platinum, *see* Pt-00420
Chloro[(1,2,3-η)-4-hydroxy-1-methyl-1-pentenyl]palladium, *in* Pd-00079
Chloro(3-hydroxypropyl-*N*,*N*-dimethylaminocarbene)-bis(dimethylphenylphosphine)platinum(1+), *see* Pt-00275
Chloro(isocyanocyclohexane)silver, Ag-00017
Chloro(isocyanomethane)bis(triethylarsine)palladium(1+), Pd-00105
Chloro(isocyanomethane)bis(triethylphosphine)palladium(1+), Pd-00106
Chloro(isocyanomethane)gold, Au-00005
Chloro(isocyanomethane)(pentafluorophenyl)palladium, *in* Pd-00114
Chloro(1-isocyano-4-methylbenzene)silver, Ag-00019
Chloromesitylbis(triethylphosphine)platinum, *see* Pt-00268
Chloro(methoxocarbonyl)bis(triethylphosphine)platinum, Pt-00163
Chloro(methoxycarbonyl)bis(triethylphosphine)platinum, *see* Pt-00163
Chloro[(1,4,5-η)-8-methoxy-4-cycloocten-1-yl]palladium, *in* Pd-00153
Chloro(2-methoxydicyclopentadienyl)palladium, *in* Pd-00187
Chloro[(1,2,3-η)-8-methoxy-2,6-dimethyl-8-oxo-2,6-octadienyl]palladium, *in* Pd-00188
Chloro[methoxy(methylamino)methylene]gold, Au-00018
Chloro(16,17,20-η)-3-methoxy-19-nor-1,3,5(10),17(20)-pregnatetraenepalladium, *in* Pd-00305
Chloro(8-methoxytricyclo[5.2.1.0^{2,6}]dec-3-ene)platinum, *in* Pt-00273
Chloro(12-methoxy-2,6,10-trimethyl-12-oxo-2,6,10-dodecatrienyl)palladium, *in* Pd-00249
μ-Chloro-μ-(2-methylallyl)bis(tricyclohexylphosphine)dipalladium, *see* Pd-00289
Chloro(2-methylallyl)nickel, *in* Ni-00052
Chloro(1-methyl-π-allyl)palladium, *in* Pd-00040
Chloro(2-methylallyl)palladium, *in* Pd-00041
Chloro(2-methylallyl)pyridinepalladium, *see* Pd-00046
Chloro(2-methyl-π-allyl)(triphenylarsine)palladium, *see* Pd-00185
Chloro(1-methylallyl)(triphenylphosphine)nickel, *see* Ni-00206
Chloro(2-methyl-π-allyl)(triphenylphosphine)palladium, *see* Pd-00186
Chloromethylbis(dimethylphenylphosphine)platinum, *see* Pt-00192
Chloro(methyl)bis(methyldiphenylphosphine)platinum, Pt-00326
Chloromethylbis(triethylphosphine)platinum, Pt-00147
Chloro(methyl)bis(trimethylarsine)platinum, Pt-00056
Chloro(methyl)bis(trimethylphosphine)nickel, Ni-00042
Chloromethylbis(triphenylphosphine)platinum, Pt-00373
Chloro(2-methylcyclohexenyl)palladium, *in* Pd-00101
Chloro[methylenebis[diphenylphosphine]-*P*,*P′*](η^3-2-propenyl)palladium, *in* Pd-00226
Chloro(2-methylenecyclohexyl)palladium, *in* Pd-00102
Chloro(methylenecyclopentyl)palladium, *in* Pd-00077
Chloro(methyl isocyanide)bis(triethylarsine)palladium(1+), *see* Pd-00105
Chloro(methyl isocyanide)bis(triethylphosphine)palladium(1+), *see* Pd-00106
Chloro(methyl isocyanide)gold, *see* Au-00005
Chloro(methylisonitrile)bis(triethylarsine)palladium(1+), *see* Pd-00105
Chloro(methylisonitrile)bis(triethylphosphine)palladium(1+), *see* Pd-00106
Chloro[2-(methylnitrosoamino)phenyl](triphenylphosphine)palladium, Pd-00216
Chloro[2-(4-methyl-5-oxo-3-cyclohexen-1-yl)-2-propenyl]palladium, *in* Pd-00173
Chloro(2-methyl-2-penten-1-yl)palladium, *in* Pd-00080
Chloro(3-methyl-3-penten-2-yl)palladium, *in* Pd-00081
Chloro(2-methylphenyl)bis(triethylphosphine)platinum, Pt-00237
Chloro(3-methylphenyl)bis(triethylphosphine)platinum, Pt-00238
Chloro(4-methylphenyl)bis(triethylphosphine)platinum, Pt-00236
μ-Chloro[μ-[(1-η:2,3-η)-2-methyl-2-propenyl]]-bis(tricyclohexylphosphine)dipalladium, Pd-00289
Chloro(2-methyl-2-propenyl)nickel, *in* Ni-00052
Chloro(2-methyl-2-propenyl)palladium, *in* Pd-00041
Chloro[(1,2,3-η)-2-methyl-2-propenyl]platinum, *in* Pt-00069
Chloro[(1,2,3-η)-2-methyl-2-propenyl](pyridine)palladium, Pd-00046
Chloro[(1,2,3-η)-2-methyl-2-propenyl](triphenylarsine)palladium, Pd-00185
Chloro[(1,2,3-η)-2-methyl-2-propenyl)](triphenylphosphine)palladium, Pd-00186
Chloro[(methylthio)methyl]bis(triphenylphosphine)palladium, Pd-00277

Molecular Formula Index

$CAgN_3O_6$
(Trinitromethyl)silver, Ag-00001
CAuClO
Carbonylchlorogold, Au-00001
CAuN
Gold cyanide, Au-00002
CBr_3KOPd
Tribromocarbonylpalladate(1−); K salt, *in* Pd-00001
CBr_3KOPt
Tribromocarbonylplatinate(1−); K salt, *in* Pt-00001
$CBr_3OPd^{\ominus}$
Tribromocarbonylpalladate(1−), Pd-00001
$CBr_3OPt^{\ominus}$
Tribromocarbonylplatinate(1−), Pt-00001
$CCl_3OPd^{\ominus}$
Carbonyltrichloropalladate(1−), Pd-00002
$CCl_3OPt^{\ominus}$
Carbonyltrichloroplatinate(1−), Pt-00002
$CCl_5OPt^{\ominus}$
Carbonylpentachloroplatinate(1−), Pt-00003
$CCl_7OPdSn_2^{\ominus}$
Carbonylchlorobis(trichlorostannyl)palladate(1−), Pd-00003
$CCuF_3O_3S$
Trifluoromethanesulfonic acid copper(1+) salt, Cu-00001
CCuN
▷Copper cyanide, Cu-00002
CF_3IPd
Iodo(trifluoromethyl)palladium, Pd-00004
$CHCl_2OPd^{\ominus}$
(Carbonyl)dichlorohydropalladate(1−), Pd-00005
CH_3Ag
Methylsilver, Ag-00002
$CH_3Cl_5Pt^{\ominus\ominus}$
Pentachloro(methyl)platinate(2−), Pt-00004
CH_3Cu
▷Methylcopper, Cu-00003
CI_3KOPt
Carbonyltriiodoplatinate(1−); K salt, *in* Pt-00005
$CI_3OPt^{\ominus}$
Carbonyltriiodoplatinate(1−), Pt-00005
C_2AgClF_4
(1-Chloro-1,2,2,2-tetrafluoroethyl)silver, Ag-00003
C_2AgKN_2
Potassium silver cyanide, *in* Ag-00004
$C_2AgN_2^{\ominus}$
Bis(cyano-*C*)argentate(1−), Ag-00004
C_2Ag_2
▷Silver acetylide, Ag-00005
C_2AuKN_2
Gold potassium cyanide, *in* Au-00003
$C_2AuN_2^{\ominus}$
Bis(cyano-*C*)aurate(1−), Au-00003
C_2Au_2
▷Gold acetylide, Au-00004
$C_2Br_2O_2Pt$
Dibromodicarbonylplatinum, Pt-00006
$C_2Cl_2O_2Pd$
Dicarbonyldichloropalladium, Pd-00006
$C_2Cl_2O_2Pt$
Dicarbonyldichloroplatinum, Pt-00007
$C_2Cl_4O_2Pt_2^{\ominus\ominus}$
Dicarbonyltetrachlorodiplatinate(2−), Pt-00008
C_2CuKN_2
Gold potassium cyanide, *in* Cu-00004
$C_2CuN_2^{\ominus}$
▷Bis(cyano-*C*)cuprate(1−), Cu-00004
C_2HCu
▷Ethynylcopper, Cu-00005
$C_2H_3AgO_2$
(Acetato)silver, Ag-00006
C_2H_3AuClN
Chloro(isocyanomethane)gold, Au-00005
$C_2H_3AuCl_3N$
Acetonitriletrichlorogold, Au-00006
$C_2H_3CuO_2$
(Acetato-*O,O'*)copper, Cu-00006
$C_2H_4Br_3KPt$
Tribromo(ethylene)platinate(1−); K salt, *in* Pt-00009
$C_2H_4Br_3Pt^{\ominus}$
Tribromo(ethylene)platinate(1−), Pt-00009
$C_2H_4Cl_2Pt$
Dichloro(η^2-ethene)platinum, *in* Pt-00027
$C_2H_4Cl_3KPt$
Zeise's salt, *in* Pt-00010
$C_2H_4Cl_3Pd^{\ominus}$
Trichloro(ethylene)palladate(1−), Pd-00007
$C_2H_4Cl_3Pt^{\ominus}$
Trichloro(η^2-ethene)platinate(1−), Pt-00010
$C_2H_6AgNO_3S$
Dimethylsulfide(nitrato)silver, Ag-00007
$C_2H_6Au^{\ominus}$
Dimethylaurate(1−), Au-00007
C_2H_6AuBr
Bromodimethylgold, Au-00008
C_2H_6AuBrS
Bromo(dimethyl sulfide)gold, Au-00009
$C_2H_6AuBr_3S$
Tribromo(dimethyl sulfide)gold, Au-00010
C_2H_6AuCl
Chlorodimethylgold, Au-00011
C_2H_6AuClS
Chloro(dimethyl sulfide)gold, Au-00012
$C_2H_6AuClSe$
Chloro[selenobis(methane)]gold, Au-00013
$C_2H_6AuCl_3S$
Trichloro(dimethylsulfide)gold, Au-00014
C_2H_6AuI
Iododimethylgold, Au-00015
C_2H_6AuLi
Dimethylaurate(1−); Li salt, *in* Au-00007
C_2H_6BrCuS
Bromo[thiobis(methane)]copper, Cu-00007
$C_2H_6Br_2Pt$
Dibromodimethylplatinum, Pt-00011
C_2H_6CuIS
Iodo(dimethylsulfide)copper, Cu-00008

C_2H_6CuLi
Lithium dimethylcuprate(1−), Cu-00009
C_2H_7AuO
▷Hydroxydimethylgold, Au-00016
$C_2H_8O_2Pt$
▷Dihydroxydimethylplatinum, Pt-00012
$C_2I_2O_2Pt$
Dicarbonyldiiodoplatinum, Pt-00013
$C_3ClNiO_3^{\ominus}$
Tricarbonylchloronickelate(1−), Ni-00001
$C_3Cl_3GeNiO_3^{\ominus}$
Tricarbonyl(trichlorogermyl)nickelate(1−), Ni-00002
$C_3Cl_3NiO_3P$
Tricarbonyl(phosphorus trichloride)nickel, Ni-00003
$C_3F_3NiO_3P$
Tricarbonyl(phosphorus trifluoride)nickel, Ni-00004
C_3H_3Cu
1-Propynylcopper, Cu-00010
$C_3H_4Cl_2Pd$
Chloro(2-chloro-2-propenyl)palladium, *in* Pd-00018
C_3H_5BrNi
Bromo(2-propenyl)nickel, *in* Ni-00029
C_3H_5BrPd
Bromo(2-propenyl)palladium, *in* Pd-00019
C_3H_5ClNi
Chloro(2-propenylnickel), *in* Ni-00030
C_3H_5ClPd
Chloro(η^3-2-propenyl)palladium, *in* Pd-00022
C_3H_5ClPt
Chloro(η^3-2-propenyl)platinum, Pt-00014
$C_3H_5Cl_2Pd^{\ominus}$
Dichloro(η^3-2-propenyl)palladate(1−), Pd-00008
C_3H_5INi
Iodo(η^3-2-propenylnickel), *in* Ni-00031
C_3H_5IPt
Iodo(η^3-2-propenyl)platinum, *in* Pt-00039
$C_3H_6AuNO_2S$
(Cysteinato-*O,S*)gold, Au-00017
$C_3H_6Cl_2Pt$
Dichloro-1,3-propanediylplatinum, Pt-00015
$C_3H_6Cl_3KOPt$
Trichloro[(2,3-η)-2-propen-1-ol]platinate(1−); K salt, *in* Pt-00016
$C_3H_6Cl_3KPt$
Trichloro[(1,2-η)-1-propene]platinate(1−); K salt, *in* Pt-00017
$C_3H_6Cl_3OPt^{\ominus}$
Trichloro[(2,3-η)-2-propen-1-ol]platinate(1−), Pt-00016
$C_3H_6Cl_3Pt^{\ominus}$
Trichloro[(1,2-η)-1-propene]platinate(1−), Pt-00017
$C_3H_6F_3NiP$
η^3-(1-Propenyl)hydrido(trifluorophosphine)nickel, Ni-00005
$C_3H_7AuClNO$
Chloro[methoxy(methylamino)methylene]gold, Au-00018
C_3H_9AgClP
Chloro(trimethylphosphine)silver, Ag-00008
C_3H_9AgIP
Iodo(trimethylphosphine)silver, Ag-00009
C_3H_9ClPt
Chlorotrimethylplatinum, Pt-00018
C_3H_9IPt
Iodotrimethylplatinum, Pt-00019
$C_3H_{10}OPt$
Trimethylplatinum hydroxide, Pt-00020
$C_3H_{15}FO_3Pt$
Tri(aqua)trimethylplatinum(1+); Fluoride, *in* Pt-00022
$C_3H_{15}IN_2Pt$
Diammineiodotrimethylplatinum, Pt-00021
$C_3H_{15}O_3Pt^{\oplus}$
Tri(aqua)trimethylplatinum(1+), Pt-00022
$C_3INaNiO_3$
Tricarbonyliodonickelate(1−); Na salt, *in* Ni-00006
$C_3INiO_3^{\ominus}$
Tricarbonyliodonickelate(1−), Ni-00006
$C_4H_3AuNa_2O_4S$
▷Gold sodium thiomalate, *in* Au-00019
$C_4H_5AuO_4S$
▷Mercaptobutanediato(1−)gold, Au-00019
$C_4H_6AgN_2^{\oplus}$
Bis(acetonitrile)silver(1+), Ag-00010
$C_4H_6Ag_2O_4$
Bis[μ-(acetato-*O:O'*)]disilver, *in* Ag-00006
C_4H_6AuCl
[(2,3-η)-2-Butyne]chlorogold, Au-00020
$C_4H_6AuN_2^{\oplus}$
Bis(acetonitrile)gold(1+), Au-00021
$C_4H_6ClAuN_2O_4$
Bis(acetonitrile)gold(1+); Perchlorate, *in* Au-00021
$C_4H_6Cl_2Cu_2$
Dichloro-μ-1,4-butadienedicopper, Cu-00011
$C_4H_6Cl_2N_2Pt$
Bis(acetonitrile)dichloroplatinum, Pt-00023
$C_4H_6Cl_6K_2Pt_2$
μ-[(1,2:3,4-η)-Butadiene]hexachlorodiplatinate(2−); Dipotassium salt, *in* Pt-00024
$C_4H_6Cl_6Pt_2^{\ominus\ominus}$
μ-[(1,2:3,4-η)-Butadiene]hexachlorodiplatinate(2−), Pt-00024
$C_4H_6O_2Pt$
Dicarbonyldimethylplatinum, Pt-00025
C_4H_7BrNi
Bromo(1,2,3-η-2-butenyl)nickel, *in* Ni-00048
Bromo(2-methyl-2-propenyl)nickel, *in* Ni-00049
C_4H_7ClNi
Chloro(2-methyl-2-propenyl)nickel, *in* Ni-00052
Di-μ-chlorobis[(1,2,3-η)-2-butenyl]dinickel; Monomer, *in* Ni-00051
C_4H_7ClPd
(2-Butenyl)chloropalladium, *in* Pd-00040
Chloro(2-methyl-2-propenyl)palladium, *in* Pd-00041
C_4H_7ClPt
Chloro[(1,2,3-η)-2-methyl-2-propenyl]platinum, *in* Pt-00069
$C_4H_7Cl_2Pd^{\ominus}$
Dichloro(η^3-2-butenyl)palladate(1−), Pd-00009
$C_4H_8Cl_2Pd$
Dichlorobis(ethylene)palladium, Pd-00010
Dichloro(2-methylpropene)palladium, *in* Pd-00043
$C_4H_8Cl_2Pt$
Dichlorobis(ethylene)platinum, Pt-00026
$C_4H_8Cl_4Pd_2$
Di-μ-chlorodichlorobis(ethylene)dipalladium, Pd-00011
$C_4H_8Cl_4Pt_2$
Di-μ-chlorodichlorobis(η^2-ethene)diplatinum, Pt-00027
$C_4H_8CuN_2O_2S_2$
▷Fluopsin *C*, Cu-00012
C_4H_8Ni
Methyl[(1,2,3-η)-2-propen-1-yl]nickel, Ni-00007

$C_4H_9Cl_2OPPt$
Carbonyldichloro(trimethylphosphine)platinum, Pt-00028
$C_4H_{11}Cl_2NPt$
Dichloro(ethylene)(dimethylamine)platinum, Pt-00029
$C_4H_{11}CuSi$
μ-[(Trimethylsilyl)methyl]copper, Cu-00013
$C_4H_{12}AuClS$
Chlorodimethyl(dimethyl sulfide)gold, Au-00022
$C_4H_{12}AuO_3P$
Methyl(trimethyl phosphite-*P*)gold, Au-00023
$C_4H_{12}AuP$
Methyl(trimethylphosphine)gold, Au-00024
$C_4H_{12}Au_2Br_2$
Di-μ-bromotetramethyldigold, *in* Au-00008
$C_4H_{12}Au_2Cl_2$
Di-μ-chlorotetramethyldigold, *in* Au-00011
$C_4H_{12}Au_2I_2$
▷Di-μ-iodotetramethyldigold, *in* Au-00015
$C_4H_{12}Li_2Ni$
Tetramethylnickelate(2−); Di-Li salt, *in* Ni-00008
$C_4H_{12}Li_2Pt$
Tetramethylplatinate(2−); Di-Li salt, *in* Pt-00030
$C_4H_{12}Ni^{\ominus\ominus}$
Tetramethylnickelate(2−), Ni-00008
$C_4H_{12}Pt^{\ominus\ominus}$
Tetramethylplatinate(2−), Pt-00030
$C_4H_{12}PtS$
Trimethyl(methylthio)platinum, Pt-00031
$C_4H_{13}NiOP$
Hydroxy(methyl)trimethylphosphinenickel, *in* Ni-00061
$C_4H_{22}AuB_{18}^{\ominus}$
Bis[undecahydro-1,2-dicarbaundecaborato(2−)]aurate(1−), Au-00025
Bis[undecahydro-1,2-dicarbaundecaborato(2−)]aurate(2−), Au-00026
$C_4H_{22}B_{18}Cu^{\ominus}$
Bis[(7,8,9,10,11-η)-undecahydro-7,8-dicarbaundecaborato(2−)]cuprate(1−), Cu-00014
Bis[(7,8,9,10,11-η)-undecahydro-7,8-dicarbaundecaborato(2−)]cuprate(2−), Cu-00015
$C_4H_{22}B_{18}CuK_2$
Bis[(7,8,9,10,11-η)-undecahydro-7,8-dicarbaundecaborato(2−)]cuprate(2−); Di-K salt, *in* Cu-00015
$C_4H_{22}B_{18}Ni$
Bis[(7,8,9,10,11-η)-undecahydro-7,8-dicarbaundecaborato(2−)]nickel, Ni-00009
Bis[(7,8,9,10,11-η)-undecahydro-7,8-dicarbaundecaborato(2−)]nickelate(1−), Ni-00010
Bis[(7,8,9,10,11-η)-undecahydro-7,8-dicarbaundecaborato(2−)]nickelate(2−), Ni-00011
Bis[(7,8,9,10,11-η)-undecahydro-7,9-dicarbaundecaborato(2−)]nickelate(1−), Ni-00012
$C_4H_{22}B_{18}NiRb$
Bis[(7,8,9,10,11-η)-undecahydro-7,8-dicarbaundecaborato(2−)]nickelate(1−); Rb salt, *in* Ni-00010
Bis[(7,8,9,10,11-η)-undecahydro-7,9-dicarbaundecaborato(2−)]nickelate(1−); Rb salt, *in* Ni-00012
$C_4K_2N_4Ni$
▷Tetrakis(cyano-*C*)nickelate(2−); Di-K salt, *in* Ni-00013
$C_4K_4N_4Pd$
Tetracyanopalladate(4−); Tetra-K salt, *in* Pd-00012
$C_4N_4Na_2Ni$
Tetrakis(cyano-*C*)nickelate(2−); Di-Na salt, *in* Ni-00013
$C_4N_4Ni^{\ominus\ominus}$
Tetrakis(cyano-*C*)nickelate(2−), Ni-00013
$C_4N_4Pd^{\ominus\ominus\ominus\ominus}$
Tetracyanopalladate(4−), Pd-00012
C_4NiO_4
▷Nickel carbonyl, Ni-00014
C_4NiS_4
Tetrakis(thiocarbonyl)nickel, Ni-00015
C_4O_4Pd
Tetracarbonylpalladium, Pd-00013
C_4O_4Pt
Tetracarbonylplatinum, Pt-00032
$C_5H_3NNiO_3$
Tricarbonyl(isocyanomethane)nickel, Ni-00016
C_5H_5Au
▷η-Cyclopentadienylgold, Au-00027
$C_5H_5BF_4Ni$
(η^5-2,4-Cyclopentadien-1-yl)nickel(1+); Tetrafluoroborate, *in* Ni-00018
C_5H_5Cu
3-Methyl-3-buten-1-ynylcopper, Cu-00016
$C_5H_5F_3NiO_2$
(η^3-Propenyl)(trifluoroacetato)nickel, *in* Ni-00067
C_5H_5NNiO
(η^5-2,4-Cyclopentadien-1-yl)nitrosylnickel, Ni-00017
C_5H_5NOPd
(η^5-2,4-Cyclopentadien-1-yl)nitrosylpalladium, Pd-00014
C_5H_5NOPt
(η^5-2,4-Cyclopentadien-1-yl)nitrosylplatinum, Pt-00033
$C_5H_5Ni^{\oplus}$
(η^5-2,4-Cyclopentadien-1-yl)nickel(1+), Ni-00018
C_5H_7Cu
1-Pentynylcopper, Cu-00017
C_5H_8AuCl
Chloro(cyclopentene)gold, Au-00028
$C_5H_8Cl_2N_2Pt$
Dichloro(ethylene)(pyrazole)platinum, Pt-00034
C_5H_9ClPd
Chloro[(2,3,4-η)-3-penten-2-yl]palladium, *in* Pd-00058
Di-μ-chlorobis[(1,2,3-η)-2-methyl-2-buten-1-yl]-dipalladium; Monomer, *in* Pd-00057
$C_5H_{11}Ni^{\ominus}$
Bis(ethylene)methylnickelate(1−), Ni-00019
$C_5H_{12}Cl_3NOPd$
Carbonyltrichloropalladate(1−); Diethylammonium salt, *in* Pd-00002
$C_5H_{13}BrN_4NiS_2$
(η^3-2-Propenyl)bis(thiourea-*S*)nickel(1+); Bromide, *in* Ni-00020
$C_5H_{13}CuN_3O^{\oplus}$
[*N*-(2-Aminoethyl)-1,2-ethanediamine-*N*,*N*′,*N*″]-carbonylcopper)(1+), Cu-00018
$C_5H_{13}N_4NiS_2^{\oplus}$
(η^3-2-Propenyl)bis(thiourea-*S*)nickel(1+), Ni-00020
$C_5H_{14}AuP$
Methyl(trimethylphosphonium η-methylide)gold, Au-00029
$C_5H_{49}F_6P_4Pt_2Sb$
μ-Hydrohydromethylbis[μ-[methylenebis(diphenylphosphine)-*P*:*P*′]]-diplatinum(1+); Hexafluoroantimonate, *in* Pt-00442
C_6AgF_5
(Pentafluorophenyl)silver, Ag-00011
C_6BrF_5Ni
Bromo(pentafluorophenyl)nickel, Ni-00021
C_6BrF_5Pd
Bromo(pentafluorophenyl)palladium, Pd-00015

C_6ClF_5Pd
Chloro(pentafluorophenyl)palladium, Pd-00016

C_6CuF_5
(Pentafluorophenyl)copper, Cu-00019

$C_6F_6NiO_2$
Dicarbonyl[(2,3-η)-1,1,1,4,4,4-hexafluoro-2-butyne]-nickel, Ni-00022

$C_6F_6O_2Pd$
Dicarbonyl(hexafluoro-2-butyne)palladium, Pd-00017

C_6H_5Ag
▷Phenylsilver, Ag-00012

$C_6H_5AuCl_2$
Dichlorophenylgold, Au-00030

$C_6H_5AuCl_3^{\ominus}$
Trichlorophenylgold(1−), Au-00031

C_6H_5Cu
Phenylcopper, Cu-00020

C_6H_5INiO
Carbonyl(η^5-2,4-cyclopentadien-1-yl)iodonickel, Ni-00023

C_6H_5IOPt
Carbonyl(η^5-2,4-cyclopentadien-1-yl)iodoplatinum, Pt-00035

$C_6H_5NiO^{\ominus}$
Carbonyl(η^5-2,4-cyclopentadien-1-yl)nickelate(1−), Ni-00024

$C_6H_6Ag^{\oplus}$
[(1,2-η)-Benzene]silver(1+), Ag-00013

$C_6H_6AgClO_4$
[(1,2-η)-Benzene]silver(1+); Perchlorate, *in* Ag-00013

$C_6H_6N_2Ni$
▷Bis[(2,3-η)-2-propenenitrile]nickel, Ni-00025

$C_6H_6N_2NiO_2$
Dicarbonylbis(isocyanomethane)nickel, Ni-00026

$C_6H_7Cl_2NOPd$
(Carbonyl)dichlorohydropalladate(1−); Pyridinium salt, *in* Pd-00005

$C_6H_7F_3NiO_2$
(2-Butenyl)(trifluoroacetato)nickel, *in* Ni-00088

C_6H_7NNiO
(η^5-1-Methyl-2,4-cyclopentadien-1-yl)nitrosylnickel, Ni-00027

$C_6H_8Cl_4Pd_2$
Di-μ-chlorobis(η^3-2-chloro-2-propenyl]dipalladium, Pd-00018

C_6H_9Ag
1-Hexynylsilver, Ag-00014

C_6H_9Au
(3,3-Dimethyl-1-butyne)gold, Au-00032

$C_6H_9AuFeNO_4P$
Tricarbonylnitrosyl[(trimethylphosphine)aurio]iron, Au-00033

$C_6H_9AuFeNO_7P$
Tricarbonylnitrosyl[(trimethyl phosphite-*P*)aurio]iron, Au-00034

$C_6H_9BrF_6N_3PPt$
Bromotris(isocyanomethane)platinum(1+); Hexafluorophosphate, *in* Pt-00036

$C_6H_9BrN_3Pt^{\oplus}$
Bromotris(isocyanomethane)platinum(1+), Pt-00036

$C_6H_9BrNiO_2$
Bromo(2-ethoxycarbonyl-2-propenyl)nickel, *in* Ni-00091

C_6H_9ClPd
Chloro(η^3-2-cyclohexenyl)palladium, *in* Pd-00076
Chloro(methylenecyclopentyl)palladium, *in* Pd-00077

C_6H_9Cu
(3,3-Dimethyl-1-butynyl)copper, Cu-00021

$C_6H_9N_3Pt^{\ominus\ominus}$
Tricyanotrimethylplatinate(2−), Pt-00037

$C_6H_9NiO_6P$
Tricarbonyl(trimethyl phosphite-*P*)nickel, Ni-00028

$C_6H_{10}Ag^{\oplus}$
[(1,2-η)-Cyclohexene]silver(1+), Ag-00015

$C_6H_{10}AgClO_4$
[(1,2-η)-Cyclohexene]silver(1+); Perchlorate, *in* Ag-00015

$C_6H_{10}AgNO_3$
[(1,2-η)-Cyclohexene]silver(1+); Nitrate, *in* Ag-00015

$C_6H_{10}AuCl$
Chloro(cyclohexene)gold, Au-00035

$C_6H_{10}AuClN_2O_4$
Bis(isocyanoethane)gold(1+); Perchlorate, *in* Au-00036

$C_6H_{10}AuN_2^{\oplus}$
Bis(isocyanoethane)gold(1+), Au-00036

$C_6H_{10}Br_2Ni_2$
Di-μ-bromobis(η^3-2-propenyl)dinickel, Ni-00029

$C_6H_{10}Br_2Pd_2$
Di-μ-bromobis(η^3-2-propenyl)dipalladium, Pd-00019

$C_6H_{10}Br_4Pd_3$
Tetra-μ-bromobis(η^3-2-propenyl)tripalladium, Pd-00020

$C_6H_{10}Cl_2Ni_2$
Di-μ-chlorobis(η^3-2-propenyl)dinickel, Ni-00030

$C_6H_{10}Cl_2Pd$
Dichloro[(1,2,5,6-η)-1,5-hexadiene]palladium, Pd-00021

$C_6H_{10}Cl_2Pd_2$
▷Di-μ-chlorobis(η^3-2-propenyl)dipalladium, Pd-00022

$C_6H_{10}Cl_2Pt$
Dichloro(1,2-η-cyclohexene)platinum, *in* Pt-00114
Dichloro[(1,2,5,6-η)-1,5-hexadiene]platinum, Pt-00038

$C_6H_{10}CuLi$
Di-1-propenylcopperlithium, Cu-00022

$C_6H_{10}I_2Ni_2$
Di-μ-iodobis(η^3-2-propenyl)dinickel, Ni-00031

$C_6H_{10}I_2Pt_2$
Di-μ-iodobis(η^3-2-propenyl)diplatinum, Pt-00039

$C_6H_{10}Ni$
Bis(η^3-2-propenyl)nickel, Ni-00032

$C_6H_{10}Pd$
Bis(η^3-2-propenyl)palladium, Pd-00023

$C_6H_{10}Pt$
Bis(η^3-2-propenyl)platinum, Pt-00040

$C_6H_{11}AuO_5S$
(1-Thioglucopyranosato)gold, Au-00037

$C_6H_{11}ClOPd$
Chloro[(1,2,3-η)-4-hydroxy-1-methyl-1-pentenyl]-palladium, *in* Pd-00079

$C_6H_{11}ClPd$
Chloro(2-methyl-2-penten-1-yl)palladium, *in* Pd-00080
Chloro(3-methyl-3-penten-2-yl)palladium, *in* Pd-00081

$C_6H_{11}CuSi$
[3-(Trimethylsilyl)-2-propynyl]copper, Cu-00023

$C_6H_{12}Ni$
Tris(η^2-ethene)nickel, Ni-00033

$C_6H_{12}Pd$
Tris(ethylene)palladium, Pd-00024

$C_6H_{12}Pt$
Tris(ethylene)platinum, Pt-00041

$C_6H_{13}LiNi$
Ethylbis(ethylene)nickelate(1−); Li salt, *in* Ni-00034

$C_6H_{13}Ni^{\ominus}$
Ethylbis(ethylene)nickelate(1−), Ni-00034

$C_6H_{14}ClNiP$
Chloro(η^3-2-propenyl)(trimethylphosphine)nickel, Ni-00035
$C_6H_{14}ClPPt$
Chloro(η^3-2-propenyl)(trimethylphosphine)platinum, Pt-00042
$C_6H_{14}I_2O_2Pd_2S_2$
Di-μ-iodobis[(methylsulfoxoniumylidene)bis(methylene)]-dipalladium, Pd-00025
$C_6H_{15}AuBrP$
Bromo(triethylphosphine)gold, Au-00038
$C_6H_{15}AuBr_3P$
Tribromo(triethylphosphine)gold, Au-00039
$C_6H_{15}AuClO_3P$
Chloro(triethyl phosphite-*P*)gold, Au-00040
$C_6H_{15}AuClP$
▷Chloro(triethylphosphine)gold, Au-00041
$C_6H_{15}AuCl_3P$
Trichloro(triethylphosphine)gold, Au-00042
$C_6H_{15}AuF_3P$
Dimethyl(trifluoromethyl)trimethylphosphinegold, Au-00043
$C_6H_{15}ClPt$
Chlorotriethylplatinum, Pt-00043
$C_6H_{15}CuIO_3P$
Iodo(triethyl phosphite-*P*)copper, Cu-00024
$C_6H_{15}CuIP$
Iodo(triethylphosphine)copper, Cu-00025
$C_6H_{16}I_4Pd_2S_2$
Bis(dimethylsulfonium-η-methylide)di-μ-iododiiododipalladium, Pd-00026
$C_6H_{17}AuOS$
(Dimethylsulfoxonium η-methylide)trimethylgold, Au-00044
$C_6H_{18}AgClP_2$
Chlorobis(trimethylphosphine)silver, Ag-00016
$C_6H_{18}As_2Cl_9PtSn_3^{\ominus}$
Tris(trichlorostannyl)bis(trimethylarsine)platinate(1−), Pt-00044
$C_6H_{18}AuClO_{10}P_2$
Bis(trimethyl phosphite)gold(1+); Perchlorate, *in* Au-00045
$C_6H_{18}AuO_6P_2^{\oplus}$
Bis(trimethyl phosphite)gold(1+), Au-00045
$C_6H_{18}Li_2Pt$
Hexamethylplatinate(2−); Di-Li salt, *in* Pt-00046
$C_6H_{18}O_2PtS_2$
Dimethylbis(dimethylsulfoxide)platinum, Pt-00045
$C_6H_{18}Pt^{\ominus\ominus}$
Hexamethylplatinate(2−), Pt-00046
$C_6H_{19}ClP_2Pt$
Chlorohydrobis(trimethylphosphine)platinum, Pt-00047
$C_6H_{30}F_6O_6Pt_2Si$
Tri(aqua)trimethylplatinum(1+); Hexafluorosilicate(2−), *in* Pt-00022
$C_6H_{30}F_6O_6Pt_3$
Tri(aqua)trimethylplatinum(1+); Hexafluoroplatinate(2−), *in* Pt-00022
$C_6K_2O_6Pt_3$
Tri-μ-carbonyltricarbonyltriplatinate(2−); Di-K salt, *in* Pt-00048
$C_6K_4N_6Ni_2$
Hexakiscyanodinickelate(4−); Tetrapotassium salt, *in* Ni-00036
$C_6N_6Ni_2^{\ominus\ominus\ominus\ominus}$
Hexakiscyanodinickelate(4−), Ni-00036
$C_6Na_2Ni_2O_6$
Hexacarbonyldinickelate(2−); Na salt, *in* Ni-00037
$C_6Ni_2O_6^{\ominus\ominus}$
Hexacarbonyldinickelate(2−), Ni-00037
$C_6O_6Pt_3^{\ominus\ominus}$
Tri-μ-carbonyltricarbonyltriplatinate(2−), Pt-00048
$C_7H_5F_3NiOS$
Carbonyl(η^5-2,4-cyclopentadien-1-yl)-(trifluoromethanethiolato)nickel, Ni-00038
$C_7H_5F_6NiP$
[Bis(trifluoromethyl)phosphino](cyclopentadienyl)-nickel, *in* Ni-00111
C_7H_7CuO
2-Methoxyphenylcopper, Cu-00026
$C_7H_8Br_2Pd$
[(2,3,5,6-η)-Bicyclo[2.2.1]hepta-2,5-diene]-dibromopalladium, Pd-00027
$C_7H_8Br_2Pt$
[(2,3,5,6-η)-Bicyclo[2.2.1]hepta-2,5-diene]-dibromoplatinum, Pt-00049
$C_7H_8Cl_2Pd$
[(2,3,5,6-η)-Bicyclo[2.2.1]hepta-2,5-diene]-dichloropalladium, Pd-00028
$C_7H_8Cl_2Pt$
[(2,3,5,6-η)-Bicyclo[2.2.1]hepta-2,5-diene]-dichloroplatinum, Pt-00050
C_7H_8CuN
(η^5-2,4-Cyclopentadien-1-yl)(isocyanomethane)copper, Cu-00027
$C_7H_8I_2Pt$
[(2,3,5,6-η)-Bicyclo[2.2.1]hepta-2,5-diene]-diiodoplatinum, Pt-00051
$C_7H_9Cl_2NPt$
Dichloro(ethylene)(pyridine)platinum, Pt-00052
$C_7H_9Cl_4N_2O_2Pt^{\ominus}$
Amminetetrachloro(4-methyl-3-nitrophenyl)platinate(1−), Pt-00053
$C_7H_9N_3NiO$
Carbonyltris(isocyanomethane)nickel, Ni-00039
$C_7H_{10}NiO_3S$
Tricarbonyl(diethylsulfide)nickel, Ni-00040
$C_7H_{11}AgClN$
Chloro(isocyanocyclohexane)silver, Ag-00017
$C_7H_{11}BrPd$
Bromo(2-cyclohepten-1-yl)palladium, *in* Pd-00098
$C_7H_{11}ClPd$
Chloro(2-methylcyclohexenyl)palladium, *in* Pd-00101
Chloro(2-methylenecyclohexyl)palladium, *in* Pd-00102
$C_7H_{13}Cl_4N_3O_2Pt$
Amminetetrachloro(4-methyl-3-nitrophenyl)platinate(1−); NH_4 salt, *in* Pt-00053
$C_7H_{14}ClNOPt$
Carbonylpentachloroplatinate(1−); Diisopropylammonium salt, *in* Pt-00003
$C_7H_{15}AuNPS$
(Thiocyanato-*S*)(triethylphosphine)gold, Au-00046
$C_7H_{15}Cl_2OPPt$
Carbonyldichloro(triethylphosphine)platinum, Pt-00054
$C_7H_{17}PPt$
Bis(ethylene)(trimethylphosphine)platinum, Pt-00055
$C_7H_{18}AuP$
Methyl(triethylphosphine)gold, Au-00047
$C_7H_{18}I_2NiOP_2$
Carbonyldiiodobis(trimethylphosphine)nickel, Ni-00041
$C_7H_{20}AuClP_2$
(Trimethylphosphine)(trimethylphosphonium η-methylide)gold(1+); Chloride, *in* Au-00050

$C_8H_{12}CuF_6N_4P$
Tetrakis(acetonitrile)copper(1+); Hexafluorophosphate, *in* Cu-00030

$C_8H_{12}CuN_4^{\oplus}$
Tetrakis(acetonitrile)copper(1+), Cu-00030

$C_8H_{12}F_{12}N_4P_2Pd$
Tetrakis(isocyanomethane)palladium(2+); Bis(hexafluorophosphate), *in* Pd-00038

$C_8H_{12}F_{12}N_4P_2Pt$
Tetrakis(isocyanomethane)platinum(2+); Bis(hexafluorophosphate), *in* Pt-00068

$C_8H_{12}I_2Pt$
[(1,2,5,6-η)-1,5-Cyclooctadiene]diiodoplatinum, Pt-00066

$C_8H_{12}N_4Ni$
Tetrakis(isocyanomethane)nickel, Ni-00047

$C_8H_{12}N_4Pd^{\oplus\oplus}$
Tetrakis(acetonitrile)palladium(2+), Pd-00037
Tetrakis(isocyanomethane)palladium(2+), Pd-00038

$C_8H_{12}N_4Pt^{\oplus\oplus}$
Tetrakis(acetonitrile)platinum(2+), Pt-00067
Tetrakis(isocyanomethane)platinum(2+), Pt-00068

$C_8H_{12}O_2Pd$
(2,4-Pentanedionato-*O,O'*)(η^3-2-propenyl)palladium, Pd-00039

$C_8H_{13}ClPd$
Chloro(ethylidenecyclohexyl)palladium, *in* Pd-00128

$C_8H_{14}AuCl$
Chloro[(1,2-η)-cyclooctene]gold, Au-00056

$C_8H_{14}Br_2Ni_2$
Di-μ-bromobis[(1,2,3-η)-2-butenyl]dinickel, Ni-00048
Di-μ-bromobis[(1,2,3-η)-2-methyl-2-propenyl]dinickel, Ni-00049

$C_8H_{14}Br_2Ni_2O_2$
Di-μ-bromobis[(1,2,3-η)-2-methoxy-2-propenyl]dinickel, Ni-00050

$C_8H_{14}Cl_2Ni_2$
Di-μ-chlorobis[(1,2,3-η)-2-butenyl]dinickel, Ni-00051
Di-μ-chlorobis[(1,2,3,-η)-2-methyl-2-propenyl]dinickel, Ni-00052

$C_8H_{14}Cl_2Pd_2$
Bis[(1,2,3-η)-2-butenyl]di-μ-chlorodipalladium, Pd-00040
Di-μ-chlorobis[(1,2,3-η)-2-methyl-2-propenyl]-dipalladium, Pd-00041

$C_8H_{14}Cl_2Pt_2$
Di-μ-chlorobis[(1,2,3,-η)-2-methyl-2-propenyl]-diplatinum, Pt-00069

$C_8H_{14}INiP$
(η^5-2,4-Cyclopentadien-1-yl)iodo(trimethylphosphine)-nickel, Ni-00053

$C_8H_{14}Ni$
Bis[(1,2,3-η)-(1-methyl-2-propenyl)]nickel, Ni-00054
Bis[(1,2,3-η)-2-methyl-2-propenyl]nickel, Ni-00055

$C_8H_{14}Pt$
Bis[(1,2,3-η)-2-methyl-2-propenyl]platinum, Pt-00070
(η^5-2,4-Cyclopentadien-1-yl)trimethylplatinum, Pt-00071

$C_8H_{16}As_2NiO_2$
Dicarbonyl[1,2-ethanediylbis[dimethylarsine]]nickel, Ni-00056

$C_8H_{16}Cl_4Pd_2$
Bis[(2,3-η)-2-butene]tetrachlorodipalladium, Pd-00042
Di-μ-chlorodichlorobis(2-methylpropene)dipalladium, Pd-00043

$C_8H_{16}Ni_2$
Dimethylbis[(1,2,3-η)-2-propen-1-yl]dinickel, *in* Ni-00007

$C_8H_{16}O_2Pt$
(Acetylacetonato)trimethylplatinum, Pt-00072

$C_8H_{17}Ni_2^{\ominus}$
Tetrakis(ethylene)(μ-hydrido)dinickelate(1−), Ni-00057

$C_8H_{18}Cl_2NPPt$
Dichloro(isocyanomethane)(triethylphosphine)platinuum, Pt-00073

$C_8H_{18}NiO_2P_2$
Dicarbonylbis(trimethylphosphine)nickel, Ni-00058

$C_8H_{20}Ag_2As_2$
Bis[μ-(dimethylarsinidenio)bis[methylene]]disilver, Ag-00021

$C_8H_{20}Ag_2P_2$
Bis[μ-[dimethyl(methylene)phosphoranyl]methyl]disilver, Ag-00022

$C_8H_{20}As_2Cu_2$
Bis[μ-[(dimethylarsinidenio)bis[methylene]]]dicopper, Cu-00031

$C_8H_{20}Au_2Cl_2P_2$
Dichlorobis[μ-[(dimethylphosphinidenio)bis(methylene)]]-digold, Au-00057

$C_8H_{20}Au_2Cl_4P_2$
Tetrachlorobis[μ-[(dimethylphosphinidenio)-bis[methylene]]]digold, Au-00058

$C_8H_{20}Au_2P_2$
Bis[μ-[(dimethylphosphinidenio)bis(methylene)]]digold, Au-00059

$C_8H_{20}Cl_2PtS_2$
Dichlorobis(diethyl sulfide)platinum, Pt-00074

$C_8H_{20}PtS_2$
[1,2-Bis(ethylthio)ethane-*S,S'*]dimethylplatinum, Pt-00075

$C_8H_{21}As_2F_6OPPt$
Carbonylmethylbis(trimethylarsine)platinum(1+); Hexafluorophosphate, *in* Pt-00076

$C_8H_{21}As_2OPt^{\oplus}$
Carbonylmethylbis(trimethylarsine)platinum(1+), Pt-00076

$C_8H_{21}ClNiOP_2$
Acetylchlorobis(trimethylphosphine)nickel, Ni-00059

$C_8H_{21}IOP_2Pd$
Acetyliodobis(trimethylphosphine)palladium, Pd-00044

$C_8H_{22}AuClP_2$
Bis(trimethylphosphonium η-methylide)gold(1+); Chloride, *in* Au-00060

$C_8H_{22}AuP_2^{\oplus}$
Bis(trimethylphosphonium η-methylide)gold(1+), Au-00060

$C_8H_{22}CuLiSi_2$
Bis[(trimethylsilylmethyl)]cuprate(1−); Li salt, *in* Cu-00032

$C_8H_{22}CuSi_2^{\ominus}$
Bis[(trimethylsilylmethyl)]cuprate(1−), Cu-00032

$C_8H_{22}P_2Pt$
Ethylenebis(trimethylphosphine)platinum, Pt-00077

$C_8H_{24}As_2Pt$
Dimethylbis(trimethylarsine)platinum, Pt-00078

$C_8H_{24}Cl_2Ni_2P_2$
Di-μ-chlorodimethylbis(trimethylphosphine)dinickel, Ni-00060

$C_8H_{24}Cu_2N_6O_2^{\oplus\oplus}$
Dicarbonyl[μ-(1,2-ethanediamine-*N,N'*)]bis(1,2-ethanediamine-*N,N'*)dicopper(2+), Cu-00033

$C_8H_{24}I_2Pt_2Se_2$
Di-μ-iodohexamethyl[μ-(dimethyldiselenide)-*Se,Se*]-diplatinum, Pt-00079

$C_8H_{26}Ni_2O_2P_2$
Di-μ-hydroxydimethylbis(trimethylphosphine)dinickel, Ni-00061

$C_8H_{34}B_{18}NNi$
Bis[(7,8,9,10,11-η)-undecahydro-7,8-dicarbaundecaborato(2−)]nickelate(1−); Tetramethylammonium salt, *in* Ni-00010

Bis[(7,8,9,10,11-η)-undecahydro-7,9-dicarbaundecaborato(2−)]nickelate(1−); Tetramethylammonium salt, *in* Ni-00012

$C_8Ni_3O_8^{\ominus\ominus}$
Tetra-μ-carbonyltetracarbonyltrinickelate(2−), Ni-00062

$C_9F_5N_3Pd^{\ominus\ominus}$
Tricyano(pentafluorophenyl)palladate(2−), Pd-00045

C_9H_9ClPd
Chloro(2-phenyl-2-propenyl)palladium, *in* Pd-00143
π-Phenylallylpalladium chloride, *in* Pd-00142

$C_9H_{10}Cl_2Pt$
Dichloro(2-phenyl-1,3-propanediyl)platinum, Pt-00080

$C_9H_{10}CuLiS$
Lithium phenylthio(cyclopropyl)cuprate, Cu-00034

$C_9H_{11}Ag$
(1,3,5-Trimethylbenzene)silver, Ag-00023

$C_9H_{11}Au$
(1,3,5-Trimethylbenzene)gold, Au-00061

$C_9H_{11}Cl_2OPPt$
Carbonyldichloro(dimethylphenylphosphine)platinum, Pt-00081

$C_9H_{11}Cu$
(1,3,5-Trimethylbenzene)copper, Cu-00035

$C_9H_{12}AgN$
[2-[(Dimethylamino)methyl]phenyl]silver, Ag-00024

$C_9H_{12}Ag_2BrN$
Bromo[2-[(dimethylamino)methyl]phenyl]disilver, Ag-00025

$C_9H_{12}ClNPd$
Chloro[2-[(dimethylamino)methyl]phenyl-*C*,*N*]palladium, *in* Pd-00148
Chloro[(1,2,3-η)-2-methyl-2-propenyl](pyridine)-palladium, Pd-00046

$C_9H_{12}Ni$
[(1,2,3-η)-2-Butenyl]($η^5$-2,4-cyclopentadien-1-yl)-nickel, Ni-00063
($η^5$-2,4-Cyclopentadien-1-yl)[(1,2,3-η)-2-methyl-2-propenyl]nickel, Ni-00064

$C_9H_{12}Pd$
($η^5$-2,4-Cyclopentadien-1-yl)($η^3$-2-methyl-2-propenyl)-palladium, Pd-00047

$C_9H_{12}Pt$
($η^5$-2,4-Cyclopentadien-1-yl)[(1,2,3-η)-2-methyl-2-propenyl]platinum, Pt-00082

$C_9H_{14}ClNOPd$
(1-Acetyl-4-ethylidenepiperidinyl)chloropalladium, *in* Pd-00151

$C_9H_{14}NiOSn$
Carbonyl($η^5$-2,4-cyclopentadien-1-yl)(trimethylstannyl)-nickel, Ni-00065

$C_9H_{14}Pt$
[(2,3,5,6-η)-Bicyclo[2.2.1]hepta-2,5-diene]-dimethylplatinum, Pt-00083

$C_9H_{14}PtS$
Trimethyl(phenylthio)platinum, Pt-00084

$C_9H_{15}ClOPd$
Chloro[(1,4,5-η)-8-methoxy-4-cycloocten-1-yl]palladium, *in* Pd-00153

$C_9H_{15}ClO_2Pt$
[(2,3-η)-2-Butene]chloro(2,4-pentanedionato-*O*,*O′*)-platinum, Pt-00085

$C_9H_{15}ClPd$
Chloro[(1,2,5,6-η)-1,5-cyclooctadiene]methylpalladium, Pd-00048

$C_9H_{15}ClPt$
Chloro[(1,2,5,6-η)-1,5-cyclooctadiene]methylplatinum, Pt-00086

$C_9H_{18}Cl_2OPt$
Dichloro[3,3-dimethyl-1-(1-methylethoxy)butylidene]-platinum, *in* Pt-00216

$C_9H_{19}NiO_2P$
Methyl(2,4-pentanedionato-*O*,*O′*)(trimethylphosphine)-nickel, Ni-00066

$C_9H_{20}BrPPd$
Bromo($η^3$-2-propenyl)(triethylphosphine)palladium, Pd-00049

$C_9H_{20}Cl_7NOPdSn_2$
Carbonylchlorobis(trichlorostannyl)palladate(1−); Tetraethylammonium salt, *in* Pd-00003

$C_9H_{23}Au_2IP_2$
Bis[μ-(dimethylphosphinidenio)bis[methylene]-iodomethyldigold, Au-00062

$C_9H_{28}P_3Pd^{\oplus}$
Hydrotris(trimethylphosphine)palladium(1+), Pd-00050

$C_{10}H_8Cl_2N_2Pt$
(2,2′-Bipyridine-*N*,*N′*)dichloroplatinum, Pt-00087

$C_{10}H_8Cu_2Fe$
1,1′-Ferrocenylenedicopper, Cu-00036

$C_{10}H_9Cl_2NOPd$
(Carbonyl)dichlorohydropalladate(1−); Quinolinium salt, *in* Pd-00005

$C_{10}H_{10}AgF_7O_2$
(6,6,7,7,8,8,8-Heptafluoro-2,2-dimethyl-3,5-octanedionato-*O*,*O′*)silver, Ag-00026

$C_{10}H_{10}BCuN_6O$
Carbonyl[hydrotris(1*H*-pyrazolato-N^1)borato(1−)-N^2,$N^{2′}$,$N^{2″}$]copper, Cu-00037

$C_{10}H_{10}ClNPd$
Benzonitrile(chloro)-2-propenylpalladium, Pd-00051

$C_{10}H_{10}Cl_4NPt^{\ominus}$
Amminetetrachloro-2-naphthalenylplatinate(1−), Pt-00088

$C_{10}H_{10}F_6Ni_2O_4$
Bis($η^3$-2-propenyl)bis[μ-(trifluoroacetato-*O*:*O′*)]-dinickel, Ni-00067

$C_{10}H_{10}Ni$
▷Nickelocene, Ni-00068

$C_{10}H_{11}Ni^{\oplus}$
($η^4$-Cyclopentadiene)($η^5$-2,4-cyclopentadien-1-yl)-nickel(1+), Ni-00069

$C_{10}H_{12}Br_2Pt$
Dibromo(dicyclopentadiene)platinum, Pt-00089

$C_{10}H_{12}Cl_2Pd$
Dichloro(dicyclopentadiene)palladium, Pd-00052

$C_{10}H_{12}Cl_2Pt$
Dichloro(dicyclopentadiene)platinum, Pt-00090

$C_{10}H_{12}F_6N_4O_6PdS_2$
Tetrakis(acetonitrile)palladium(2+); Bistrifluoromethanesulfonate, *in* Pd-00037

$C_{10}H_{12}Ni$
($η^5$-2,4-Cyclopentadien-1-yl)[(1,2,3-η)-2-cyclopenten-1-yl]nickel, Ni-00070

$C_{10}H_{12}NiO_2$
▷(2,3,5,6-Tetramethyl-2,5-cyclohexadiene-1,4-dione)-nickel, Ni-00071

$C_{10}H_{13}ClOPd$
Chloro[2-(4-methyl-5-oxo-3-cyclohexen-1-yl)-2-propenyl]-palladium, *in* Pd-00173

$C_{10}H_{14}ClKO_4Pt$
(1-Acetyl-2-oxopropyl)chloro(2,4-pentanedionato-*O*,*O′*)-platinate(1−); K salt, *in* Pt-00091

$C_{10}H_{14}ClO_4Pt^{\ominus}$
(1-Acetyl-2-oxopropyl)chloro(2,4-pentanedionato-*O*,*O′*)-platinate(1−), Pt-00091

$C_{10}H_{14}Cl_4N_2Pt$
Amminetetrachloro-2-naphthalenylplatinate(1−); NH_4 salt, *in* Pt-00088

$C_{10}H_{14}CuLiS$
Lithium phenylthio(*tert*-butyl)cuprate, Cu-00038

$C_{10}H_{14}CuN$
(η^5-2,4-Cyclopentadien-1-yl)(2-isocyano-2-methylpropane)copper, Cu-00039

$C_{10}H_{14}NiO_4$
▷Bis(2,4-pentanedionato-*O*,*O*′)nickel, Ni-00072

$C_{10}H_{14}Ni_2$
Bis[μ-(π-1-vinylallyl)dinickel, Ni-00073

$C_{10}H_{14}O_4Pd$
Bis(2,4-pentanedionato-*O*,*O*′)palladium, Pd-00053

$C_{10}H_{14}O_4Pt$
Bis(2,4-pentanedionato-*O*,*O*′)platinum, Pt-00092

$C_{10}H_{15}ClO_4Pt$
(1-Acetyl-2-oxopropyl)chloro(2,4-pentanedionato-*O*,*O*′)-platinate(1−); H deriv., *in* Pt-00091

$C_{10}H_{15}ClPd$
Chloro(η^3-6,6-dimethyl-4-methylenebicyclo[3.1.1]hept-3-yl)palladium, *in* Pd-00174

$C_{10}H_{15}Cl_2N_2NiS_2Tl$
Bis[(2-mercaptoethylamine)nickel]-dichlorophenylthallium, Ni-00074

$C_{10}H_{16}Cl_2Pd$
Chloro[(1,4,5-η)-8-(1-chloroethyl)-4-cycloocten-1-yl]-palladium, *in* Pd-00175
Dichloro[(1,2,3,4-η)-1,2,3,4,5-pentamethylcyclopentadiene]palladium, Pd-00054

$C_{10}H_{16}Cl_2Pt$
Dichloro[(1,2,3,4-η)-1,2,3,4,5-pentamethyl-1,3-cyclopentadiene]platinum, Pt-00093

$C_{10}H_{16}Ni_2$
Bis[μ-(η^3,η^3-1,3,5,7-cyclooctatetraene)]dinickel, Ni-00075

$C_{10}H_{16}OPt$
Acetyl(η^5-2,4-cyclopentadien-1-yl)ethylmethylplatinum, Pt-00094

$C_{10}H_{16}O_4Pd_2$
Bis[μ-(acetato-*O*:*O*′)]bis(η^3-2-propenyl)dipalladium, Pd-00055

$C_{10}H_{18}ClN_2Pd$
Chlorobis(2-isocyano-2-methylpropane)palladium, *in* Pd-00178

$C_{10}H_{18}Cl_2O_2Pd_2$
Di-μ-chlorobis[(1,2,3-η)-4-methoxy-2-buten-1-yl]-dipalladium, Pd-00056

$C_{10}H_{18}Cl_2Pd_2$
Di-μ-chlorobis[(1,2,3-η)-2-methyl-2-buten-1-yl]-dipalladium, Pd-00057
Di-μ-chlorobis[(2,3,4-η)-3-penten-2-yl]dipalladium, Pd-00058

$C_{10}H_{18}Cl_2Pt$
Dichloro(2,2,5,5-tetramethyl-3-hexyne)platinum, *in* Pt-00257

$C_{10}H_{18}Cl_3KPt$
Trichloro(2,2,5,5-tetramethyl-3-hexyne)platinate(1−); K salt, *in* Pt-00095

$C_{10}H_{18}Cl_3NaPt$
Trichloro(2,2,5,5-tetramethyl-3-hexyne)platinate(1−); Na salt, *in* Pt-00095

$C_{10}H_{18}Cl_3Pt^{\ominus}$
Trichloro(2,2,5,5-tetramethyl-3-hexyne)platinate(1−), Pt-00095

$C_{10}H_{18}Cl_4PtSn$
Chloro(2,2,5,5-tetramethyl-3-hexyne)(trichlorostannyl)-platinum, *in* Pt-00258

$C_{10}H_{18}I_2N_2Pd$
Diiodobis(2-isocyano-2-methylpropane)palladium, Pd-00059

$C_{10}H_{18}N_2O_2Pd$
Bis(2-isocyano-2-methylpropane)peroxypalladium, Pd-00060

$C_{10}H_{18}N_2Pd$
Bis[2-isocyano-2-methylpropane]palladium, Pd-00061

$C_{10}H_{18}Pd$
[(1,2,5,6-η)-1,5-Cyclooctadiene]dimethylpalladium, Pd-00062

$C_{10}H_{18}Pt$
[(1,2,5,6-η)-1,5-Cyclooctadiene]dimethylplatinum, Pt-00096

$C_{10}H_{19}NiO_3P$
Acetyl(2,4-pentanedionato-*O*,*O*′)(trimethylphosphine)-nickel, Ni-00076

$C_{10}H_{20}AuBF_4N_4$
Bis(1,3-dimethyl-2-imidazolidinylidene)gold(1+); Tetrafluoroborate, *in* Au-00063

$C_{10}H_{20}AuN_4^{\oplus}$
Bis(1,3-dimethyl-2-imidazolidinylidene)gold(1+), Au-00063

$C_{10}H_{20}AuO_4PS$
[Mercaptobutanedioato(1−)]triethylphosphinegold, Au-00064

$C_{10}H_{24}BF_4N_2Pd$
(η^3-2-Butenyl)[1,2-bis(dimethylamino)ethane]-palladium(1+); Tetrafluoroborate, *in* Pd-00063

$C_{10}H_{24}N_2Pd^{\oplus}$
(η^3-2-Butenyl)[1,2-bis(dimethylamino)ethane]-palladium(1+), Pd-00063

$C_{10}H_{27}NiOP_3$
Carbonyltris(trimethylphosphine)nickel, Ni-00077

$C_{10}H_{28}P_2Pt$
Dimethylbis(trimethylphosphonium-η-methylide)platinum, Pt-00097

$C_{10}H_{30}P_3Pd^{\oplus}$
Methyltris(trimethylphosphine)palladium(1+), Pd-00064

$C_{10}H_{33}Cl_2N_2Pd_2$
Dichloro(η^3-2-butenyl)palladate(1−); (η^3-2-Butenyl)(*N*,*N*,*N*′-,*N*′-tetramethylethylenediamine)palladium(1+) salt, *in* Pd-00009

$C_{11}H_8ClN_2OPt^{\oplus}$
(2,2′-Bipyridine-*N*,*N*′)carbonylchloroplatinum(1+), Pt-00098

$C_{11}H_{10}NiS$
(Cyclopentadienyl)(phenylthiolato)nickel, *in* Ni-00204

$C_{11}H_{11}ClN_2Pt$
(2,2′-Bipyridine-*N*,*N*′)chloromethylplatinum, Pt-00099

$C_{11}H_{12}F_6Ni$
[(1,2,5,6-η)-1,5-Cyclooctadiene][(1,2-η)-hexafluoropropene]nickel, Ni-00078

$C_{11}H_{14}AgP$
(Phenylethynyl)(trimethylphosphine)silver, Ag-00027

$C_{11}H_{15}ClOPd$
Chloro[(2,3,5-η)-3*a*,4,5,6,7,7*a*-hexahydro-6-methoxy-4,7-methano-1*H*-inden-5-yl]palladium, *in* Pd-00187

$C_{11}H_{15}ClOPt$
Chloro(8-methoxytricyclo[5.2.1.0^{2,6}]dec-3-ene)platinum, *in* Pt-00273

$C_{11}H_{15}Cl_2PPt$
Dichloro(dimethylphenylphosphine)[(1,2-η)-1,2-propadiene]platinum, Pt-00100

$C_{11}H_{15}CuO$
Carbonyl(η^5-pentamethylcyclopentadienyl)copper, Cu-00040

$C_{11}H_{15}INiO$
Carbonyl(iodo)(pentamethylcyclopentadienyl)nickel, Ni-00079

$C_{11}H_{17}BF_4Pd$
[(1,2,5,6-η)-1,5-Cyclooctadiene](η^3-2-propenyl)-palladium(1+); Tetrafluoroborate, *in* Pd-00065

$C_{11}H_{17}BF_4Pt$
[(1,2,5,6-η)-1,5-Cyclooctadiene](η^3-2-propenyl)-platinum(1+); Tetrafluoroborate, *in* Pt-00102

$C_{11}H_{17}ClNi$
[(2,3-η)-Bicyclo[2.2.1]hept-2-ene]chloro[(1,2,3-η)-2-methyl-2-propenyl]nickel, Ni-00080

$C_{11}H_{17}ClO_2Pd$
Chloro[(1,2,3-η)-8-methoxy-2,6-dimethyl-8-oxo-2,6-octadienyl]palladium, *in* Pd-00188

$C_{11}H_{17}ClPd$
Chloro(2-ethylidene-6,6-dimethylbicyclo[3.1.1]hept-3-yl)palladium, *in* Pd-00189

$C_{11}H_{17}Cl_2NPt$
Dichloro(ethylene)(*N*-methyl-α-methylbenzylamine)-platinum, Pt-00101

$C_{11}H_{17}Pd^{\oplus}$
[(1,2,5,6-η)-1,5-Cyclooctadiene](η^3-2-propenyl)-palladium(1+), Pd-00065

$C_{11}H_{17}Pt^{\oplus}$
[(1,2,5,6-η)-1,5-Cyclooctadiene](η^3-2-propenyl)-platinum(1+), Pt-00102

$C_{11}H_{19}ClPd$
Di-μ-chlorobis(η^3-5-*tert*-butyl-2-methylenecyclohexyl)-dipalladium; Monomer, *in* Pd-00190

$C_{11}H_{20}BrPPd$
Bromo(η^5-2,4-cyclopentadien-1-yl)(triethylphosphine)-palladium, Pd-00066

$C_{11}H_{20}ClPPd$
Chloro(η^5-2,4-cyclopentadien-1-yl)(triethylphosphine)-palladium, Pd-00067

$C_{11}H_{20}Cl_3GeNNiO_3$
Tricarbonyl(trichlorogermyl)nickelate(1−); Tetraethylammonium salt, *in* Ni-00002

$C_{11}H_{20}CuP$
(η^5-2,4-Cyclopentadien-1-yl)(triethylphosphine)copper, Cu-00041

$C_{11}H_{20}IPPd$
(η^5-2,4-Cyclopentadien-1-yl)iodo(triethylphosphine)-palladium, Pd-00068

$C_{11}H_{20}IPPt$
(η^5-2,4-Cyclopentadien-1-yl)iodo(triethylphosphine)-platinum, Pt-00103

$C_{11}H_{21}ClPd$
Chloro(1,1,5-trimethyl-2-octenyl)palladium, *in* Pd-00191

$C_{11}H_{21}IN_2Pd$
Iodobis(2-isocyano-2-methylpropane)methylpalladium, Pd-00069

$C_{11}H_{29}AuLiN_3$
[*N*-[2-(dimethylimino)ethyl]-*N*,*N'*,*N'*-trimethyl-1,2-ethanediamine-*N*,*N'*,*N''*]lithium(1+) salt, *in* Au-00007

$C_{11}H_{30}OP_3Pd^{\oplus}$
Acetyltris(trimethylphosphine)palladium(1+), Pd-00070

$C_{12}AuF_{10}^{\ominus}$
Bis(pentafluorophenyl)aurate(1−), Au-00065

$C_{12}ClF_{10}Pd^{\ominus}$
Chlorobis(pentafluorophenyl)palladate(1−), *in* Pd-00194

$C_{12}F_{10}Ni$
Bis(pentafluorophenyl)nickel, Ni-00081

$C_{12}H_8Cl_4N_2O_2Pt_2$
Carbonyltrichloroplatinate(1−); (2,2'-Bipyridine-*N*,*N'*)carbonylchloroplatinum(1+) salt, *in* Pt-00002

$C_{12}H_8F_4N_2Pt$
(2,2'-Bipyridine)(tetrafluoroethylene)platinum, Pt-00104

$C_{12}H_8N_2NiO_2$
(2,2'-Bipyridine)dicarbonylnickel, Ni-00082

$C_{12}H_9ClN_2Pd$
Chloro[2-(phenylazo)phenyl]palladium, *in* Pd-00196

$C_{12}H_{10}Au_2Cl_4$
Bis[dichlorophenylgold], *in* Au-00030

$C_{12}H_{10}Br_2Ni_2O_2Sn$
Dicarbonylbis(η^5-2,4-cyclopentadien-1-yl)[μ-(dibromostannylene)]dinickel, Ni-00083

$C_{12}H_{10}CuLi$
Lithium diphenylcuprate(1−), Cu-00042

$C_{12}H_{10}Ni_2O_2$
Di-μ-carbonylbis(η^5-2,4-cyclopentadien-1-yl)dinickel, Ni-00084

$C_{12}H_{10}O_2Pt_2$
Dicarbonylbis(η^5-2,4-cyclopentadien-1-yl)diplatinum, Pt-00105

$C_{12}H_{12}Al_4Cl_{14}Pd_2$
Bis(benzene)di-μ-chlorobis(μ-chloropentachlorodialuminum)dipalladium, Pd-00071

$C_{12}H_{12}F_6Pt$
[(1,2,5,6-η)-1,5-cyclooctadiene][(2,3-η)-1,1,1,4,4,4-hexafluoro-2-butyne]platinum, Pt-00106

$C_{12}H_{12}N_8Pt_2$
Tetrakis(isocyanomethane)platinum(2+); Tetrakis(cyano-*C*)-platinate(2−), *in* Pt-00068

$C_{12}H_{12}Ni_2$
Bis(η^5-2,4-cyclopentadien-1-yl)[μ-(η^2:η^2-ethyne)-dinickel], Ni-00085

$C_{12}H_{13}BF_4Ni$
[(2,3,5,6-η)-Bicyclo[2.2.1]hepta-2,5-diene](η^5-2,4-cyclopentadien-1-yl)nickel(1+); Tetrafluoroborate, *in* Ni-00087

$C_{12}H_{13}BrN_2Ni$
(2,2'-Bipyridine)bromo(ethyl)nickel, Ni-00086

$C_{12}H_{13}Ni^{\oplus}$
[(2,3,5,6-η)-Bicyclo[2.2.1]hepta-2,5-diene](η^5-2,4-cyclopentadien-1-yl)nickel(1+), Ni-00087

$C_{12}H_{14}F_6Ni_2O_4$
Bis[(1,2,3-η)-2-butenyl]bis[μ-trifluoroacetato-*O*:*O'*]-dinickel, Ni-00088

$C_{12}H_{14}N_2Ni$
(2,2'-Bipyridine-*N*,*N'*)dimethylnickel, Ni-00089

$C_{12}H_{14}N_2Pd$
(2,2'-Bipyridine-*N*,*N'*)dimethylpalladium, Pd-00072

$C_{12}H_{14}N_2Pt$
(2,2'-Bipyridine-*N*,*N'*)dimethylplatinum, Pt-00107

$C_{12}H_{14}Ni$
Bis(η^5-1-methyl-2,4-cyclopentadien-1-yl)nickel, Ni-00090

$C_{12}H_{15}BF_4O_2Pd$
[(2,3,5,6-η)-Bicyclo[2.2.1]hepta-2,5-diene][2,4-pentanedionato-*O*,*O'*]palladium(1+); Tetrafluoroborate, *in* Pd-00073

$C_{12}H_{15}F_3O_2Pd$
(η^3-6,6-Dimethyl-4-methylenebicyclo[3.3.1]hept-3-yl)-palladium trifluoroacetate, *in* Pd-00202

$C_{12}H_{15}O_2Pd^{\oplus}$
[(2,3,5,6-η)-Bicyclo[2.2.1]hepta-2,5-diene][2,4-pentanedionato-*O*,*O'*]palladium(1+), Pd-00073

$C_{12}H_{16}Br_2N_2Pt$
Dibromodimethylbis(pyridine)platinum, Pt-00108

$C_{12}H_{16}Cl_4Pd_2$
Di-μ-chlorobis[η^3-3-(chloromethyl)-2-methylene-3-butenyl]dipalladium, Pd-00074

$C_{12}H_{16}N_2Pt$
Dimethylbispyridineplatinum, Pt-00109

$C_{12}H_{17}BrPt$
Bromo(1,2,4,5,6-pentamethyl-3-methylenebicyclo[2.2.0]-hex-5-en-2-yl)platinum, *in* Pt-00288

$C_{12}H_{17}ClPd$
Chloro(1,2,4,5,6-pentamethyl-3-methylenebicyclo[2.2.0]-hex-5-en-2-yl)palladium, *in* Pd-00204

$C_{12}H_{17}ClPt$
Chloro(1,2,4,5,6-pentamethyl-3-methylenebicyclo[2.2.0]-hex-5-en-1-yl)platinum, *in* Pt-00290

$C_{12}H_{18}B_2F_8N_6Pt_2$
Hexakis(isocyanomethane)diplatinum(2+); Bis(tetrafluoroborate), *in* Pt-00113

$C_{12}H_{18}Br_2N_6Pd_2$
Hexakis(isocyanomethane)dipalladium(2+); Dibromide, *in* Pd-00078

$C_{12}H_{18}Br_2Ni_2O_4$
Di-μ-bromobis[(1,2,3-η)-2(ethoxycarbonyl)-2-propenyl]-dinickel, Ni-00091

$C_{12}H_{18}Br_2Pt$
Dibromo[(2,3,5,6-η)-1,2,3,4,5,6-hexamethylbicyclo[2.2.0]hexa-2,5-diene]platinum, Pt-00110

$C_{12}H_{18}Cl_2N_6Pd_2$
Hexakis(isocyanomethane)dipalladium(2+); Dichloride, *in* Pd-00078

$C_{12}H_{18}Cl_2Pd$
Dichloro[(2,3,5,6-η)-1,2,3,4,5,6-hexamethylbicyclo[2.2.0]hexa-2,5-diene]palladium, Pd-00075

$C_{12}H_{18}Cl_2Pd_2$
Di-μ-chlorobis[(1,2,3-η)-2-cyclohexen-1-yl]dipalladium, Pd-00076
Di-μ-chlorobis(η^3-2-methylenecyclopentyl)dipalladium, Pd-00077

$C_{12}H_{18}Cl_2Pt$
Dichloro[(2,3,5,6-η)-1,2,3,4,5,6-hexamethylbicyclo[2.2.0]hexa-2,5-diene]platinum, Pt-00111

$C_{12}H_{18}F_{12}N_6P_2Pd_2$
Hexakis(isocyanomethane)dipalladium(2+); Bis(hexafluorophosphate), *in* Pd-00078

$C_{12}H_{18}F_{12}N_6P_2Pt_2$
Hexakis(isocyanomethane)diplatinum(2+); Bis(hexafluorophosphate), *in* Pt-00113

$C_{12}H_{18}I_2Pt$
[(2,3,5,6-η)-1,2,3,4,5,6-Hexamethylbicyclo[2.2.0]hexa-2,5-diene]diiodoplatinum, Pt-00112

$C_{12}H_{18}N_6Pd_2^{\oplus\oplus}$
Hexakis(isocyanomethane)dipalladium(2+), Pd-00078

$C_{12}H_{18}N_6Pt_2^{\oplus\oplus}$
Hexakis(isocyanomethane)diplatinum(2+), Pt-00113

$C_{12}H_{18}Ni$
Bis[(1,2,3-η)-2-cyclohexen-1-yl]nickel, Ni-00092
[(1,2,5,6,9,10-η)-1,5,9-Cyclododecatriene]nickel, Ni-00093
[(1,2,3,10,11,12-η)-2,6,10-Dodecatriene-1,12-diyl]-nickel, Ni-00094

$C_{12}H_{18}O_2Pd$
(Acetato)(6,6-dimethyl-2-methylenebicyclo[3.3.1]hept-3-yl)palladium, *in* Pd-00205

$C_{12}H_{19}ClO_2Pd$
[η^3-2-[2-(Acetyloxy)ethylidene]-6-methyl-5-heptenyl]-chloropalladium, *in* Pd-00206

$C_{12}H_{20}Cl_4Pt_2$
Di-μ-chlorodichlorobis[(1,2-η)-cyclohexene]diplatinum, Pt-00114

$C_{12}H_{20}Cl_4Pt_4$
Tetra-μ-chlorotetrakis[(1-η:2,3-η)-2-propenyl]-tetraplatinum, *in* Pt-00014

$C_{12}H_{20}GeNiO$
Carbonyl(η^5-2,4-cyclopentadien-1-yl)(triethylgermyl)-nickel, Ni-00095

$C_{12}H_{20}Pt$
1,4-Butanediyl[(1,2,5,6-η)-1,5-cyclooctadiene]platinum, Pt-00115

$C_{12}H_{20}Pt_2$
[μ-(1,2,5,6:3,4,7,8-η)-Cyclooctatetraene]-tetramethyldiplatinum, Pt-00116

$C_{12}H_{21}ClOPd$
Chloro(methyl 10-undecenoate)palladium, *in* Pd-00208

$C_{12}H_{21}Cl_4NPtSn$
Acetonitrilechloro[(3,4-η)-2,2,5,5-tetramethyl-3-hexyne](trichlorostannyl)platinum, Pt-00117

$C_{12}H_{22}Cl_2O_2Pd_2$
Di-μ-chlorobis[(1,2,3-η)-4-hydroxy-1-methyl-1-pentenyl]-dipalladium, Pd-00079

$C_{12}H_{22}Cl_2Pd_2$
Di-μ-chlorobis[(1,2,3-η)-2-methyl-2-penten-1-yl]-dipalladium, Pd-00080
Di-μ-chlorobis[(2,3,4-η)-3-methyl-3-penten-2-yl]-dipalladium, Pd-00081

$C_{12}H_{23}IP_2Pd$
Iodo(phenyl)bis(trimethylphosphine)palladium, Pd-00082

$C_{12}H_{24}As_2Pt$
Di-1-propynylbis(trimethylarsine)platinum, Pt-00118

$C_{12}H_{24}Cl_2Pt$
Dichloro-1-dodeceneplatinum, *in* Pt-00297

$C_{12}H_{25}Cl_2PPt$
Dichloro[(1,2-η)-1,2-propadiene](tripropylphosphine)-platinum, Pt-00119

$C_{12}H_{26}AuO_5PS$
(1-Thioglucopyranosato-*S*)(triethylphosphine)gold, Au-00066

$C_{12}H_{27}AsPd$
Bis[(2,2-di-*tert*-butylarsino)-2-methylpropyl]di-μ-hydridodipalladium; Monomer, *in* Pd-00210

$C_{12}H_{27}Cl_2PPt$
Dichloro(tributylphosphine)platinum, *in* Pt-00300

$C_{12}H_{27}CuIP$
Iodo(tributylphosphine)copper, Cu-00043

$C_{12}H_{28}Au_2P_2S_2$
Bis[μ-[2-(diethylphosphino)ethanethiolato-*P*,*S*]digold, Au-00067

$C_{12}H_{28}Cl_2N_2O_2Pd_2$
Di-μ-chlorobis[3-(dimethylamino)-2-methoxypropyl]-dipalladium, Pd-00083

$C_{12}H_{30}Cl_2NiP_2$
Dichlorobis(triethylphosphine)nickel, Ni-00096

$C_{12}H_{30}Cl_4P_2PtSn$
Chloro(trichlorostannyl)bis(triethylphosphine)platinum, Pt-00120

$C_{12}H_{30}Cl_6P_2PtSn_2$
Bis(trichlorostannyl)bis(triethylphosphine)platinum, Pt-00121

$C_{12}H_{31}As_2BrPt$
Bromohydrobis(triethylarsine)platinum, Pt-00122

$C_{12}H_{31}As_2ClPt$
Chlorohydrobis(triethylarsine)platinum, Pt-00123

$C_{12}H_{31}As_2IPt$
Hydroiodobis(triethylarsine)platinum, Pt-00124

$C_{12}H_{31}BrP_2Pt$
Bromohydrobis(triethylphosphine)platinum, Pt-00125

$C_{12}H_{31}ClP_2Pd$
Chlorohydrobis(triethylphosphine)palladium, Pd-00084

$C_{12}H_{31}ClP_2Pt$
Chlorohydrobis(triethylphosphine)platinum, Pt-00126

$C_{12}H_{31}Cl_3P_2PtSn$
Hydro(trichlorostannyl)bis(triethylphosphine)platinum, Pt-00127

$C_{12}H_{31}IP_2Pt$
Hydroiodobis(triethylphosphine)platinum, Pt-00128

$C_{12}H_{31}NO_2P_2Pt$
Hydronitrobis(triethylphosphine)platinum, Pt-00129

$C_{12}H_{31}NO_3P_2Pt$
Hydro(nitrato-*O*)bis(triethylphosphine)platinum, Pt-00130

$C_{12}H_{32}Cl_2P_2Pt$
Dichlorodihydrobis(triethylphosphine)platinum, Pt-00131

$C_{12}H_{32}NiP_4$
Bis[1,2-bis(dimethylphosphino)ethane]nickel, Ni-00097

$C_{12}H_{32}P_2Pt$
Dihydrobis(triethylphosphine)platinum, Pt-00132

$C_{12}H_{36}AgOP_3Si$
Tris(trimethylphosphine)(trimethylsilanolato)silver, Ag-00028

$C_{12}H_{36}Ag_2Cl_2P_4$
Di-μ-chlorotetrakis(trimethylphosphine)disilver, *in* Ag-00016

$C_{12}H_{36}Ag_4Cl_4P_4$
Tetra-μ_3-chlorotetrakis(trimethylphosphine)tetrasilver, *in* Ag-00008

$C_{12}H_{36}Ag_4I_4P_4$
Tetra-μ_3-iodotetrakis(trimethylphosphine)tetrasilver, *in* Ag-00009

$C_{12}H_{36}Cl_4Pt_4$
Tetra-μ_3-chlorododecamethyltetraplatinum, *in* Pt-00018

$C_{12}H_{36}Cl_{15}N_3PtSn_5$
Pentakis(trichlorostannyl)platinate(3−); Tris(tetramethylammonium) salt, *in* Pt-00476

$C_{12}H_{36}CuOP_3Si$
Tris(trimethylphosphine)(trimethylsilanolato)copper, Cu-00044

$C_{12}H_{36}I_4Pt_4$
Tetra-μ_3-iodododecamethyltetraplatinum, *in* Pt-00019

$C_{12}H_{36}NiO_{12}P_4$
Tetrakis(trimethylphosphite-*P*)nickel, Ni-00098

$C_{12}H_{36}NiP_4$
Tetrakis(trimethylphosphine)nickel, Ni-00099

$C_{12}H_{37}Cl_{12}N_3PtSn_4$
Hydrotetrakis(trichlorostannyl)platinate(3−); Tris(tetramethylammonium) salt, *in* Pt-00475

$C_{12}H_{40}O_4Pt_4$
Tetra-μ_3-hydroxydodecamethyltetraplatinum, *in* Pt-00020

$C_{12}H_{42}AuB_{18}N$
Bis[undecahydro-1,2-dicarbaundecaborato(2−)]aurate(1−); Tetraethylammonium salt, *in* Au-00025

$C_{12}H_{42}B_8P_2Pt$
[η^3-Dodecahydrooctaborato(2−)]bis(triethylphosphine)-platinum, Pt-00133

$C_{12}H_{42}B_{10}P_2Pt$
[(5,6,7,8,9,10-η)Dodecahydrodecaborato(2−)]-bis(triethylphosphine)platinum, Pt-00134

$C_{12}H_{46}B_{18}N_2Ni$
Bis[(7,8,9,10,11-η)-undecahydro-7,8-dicarbaundecaborato(2−)]nickelate(2−); Bis(tetramethylammonium) salt, *in* Ni-00011

$C_{12}K_2Ni_6O_{12}$
Dodecacarbonylhexanickelate(2−); Di-K salt, *in* Ni-00102

$C_{12}Ni_3O_{12}Pt_3^{\ominus\ominus}$
Dodecacarbonyltrinickelatetriplatinate(2−), Pt-00135

$C_{12}Ni_5O_{12}^{\ominus\ominus}$
Dodecacarbonylpentanickelate(2−), Ni-00101

$C_{12}Ni_6O_{12}^{\ominus\ominus}$
Dodecacarbonylhexanickelate(2−), Ni-00102

$C_{12}O_{12}Pt_6^{\ominus\ominus}$
Hexa-μ-carbonylhexacarbonylhexaplatinate(2−), Pt-00136

$C_{13}H_{13}AgF_6O_2$
[(1,2-η)-1,5-Cyclooctadiene](1,1,1,5,5,5-hexafluoro-2,4-pentanedionato-*O,O'*)silver, Ag-00029

$C_{13}H_{14}Ni_2$
Bis(η^5-2,4-cyclopentadien-1-yl)[μ-[(1,2-η:1,2-η)-1-propyne]]dinickel, Ni-00103

$C_{13}H_{16}AgFeN$
[2-[(Dimethylamino)methyl]ferrocenyl-*C,N*]silver, Ag-00030

$C_{13}H_{16}ClNNiO_3$
Tricarbonylchloronickelate(1−); Benzyltrimethylammonium salt, *in* Ni-00001

$C_{13}H_{16}Cl_2N_2Pt$
Dichloro-1,3-propanediylbis(pyridine)platinum, Pt-00137

$C_{13}H_{16}CuFeN$
[2-[(Dimethylamino)methyl]ferrocenyl-*C,N*]copper, Cu-00045

$C_{13}H_{17}BF_4Ni$
[(1,2,5,6-η)-1,5-Cyclooctadiene](η^5-2,4-cyclopentadien-1-yl)nickel(1+); Tetrafluoroborate, *in* Ni-00104

$C_{13}H_{17}BF_4Pd$
[(1,2,5,6-η)-1,5-Cyclooctadiene](η^5-2,4-cyclopentadien-1-yl)palladium(1+); Tetrafluoroborate, *in* Pd-00085

$C_{13}H_{17}BF_4Pt$
[(1,2,5,6-η)-1,5-Cyclooctadiene](η^5-2,4-cyclopentadien-1-yl)platinum(1+); Tetrafluoroborate, *in* Pt-00139

$C_{13}H_{17}ClPt$
[(1,2,5,6-η)-1,5-Cyclooctadiene](η^5-2,4-cyclopentadien-1-yl)platinum(1+); Chloride, *in* Pt-00139

$C_{13}H_{17}F_6PPt$
[(1,2,5,6-η)-1,5-Cyclooctadiene](η^5-2,4-cyclopentadien-1-yl)platinum(1+); Hexafluorophosphate, *in* Pt-00139

$C_{13}H_{17}IN_2Pt$
(2,2'-Bipyridine-*N,N'*)iodotrimethylplatinum, Pt-00138

$C_{13}H_{17}Ni^{\oplus}$
[(1,2,5,6-η)-1,5-Cyclooctadiene](η^5-2,4-cyclopentadien-1-yl)nickel(1+), Ni-00104

$C_{13}H_{17}Pd^{\oplus}$
[(1,2,5,6-η)-1,5-Cyclooctadiene](η^5-2,4-cyclopentadien-1-yl)palladium(1+), Pd-00085

$C_{13}H_{17}Pt^{\oplus}$
[(1,2,5,6-η)-1,5-Cyclooctadiene](η^5-2,4-cyclopentadien-1-yl)platinum(1+), Pt-00139

$C_{13}H_{18}O_2Pd$
[(1,2,3-η)-2,4-Cyclooctadien-1-yl](2,4-pentanedionato-*O,O'*)palladium, Pd-00086

$C_{13}H_{19}BF_4O_2Pd$
[(1,2,5,6-η)-1,5-Cyclooctadiene](2,4-pentadionato-*O,O'*)-palladium(1+); Tetrafluoroborate, *in* Pd-00087

$C_{13}H_{19}BF_4O_2Pt$
[(1,2,5,6-η)-1,5-Cyclooctadiene](2,4-pentanedionato-*O,O'*)platinum(1+); Tetrafluoroborate, *in* Pt-00141

$C_{13}H_{19}IN_2Pt$
Iodotrimethylbis(pyridine)platinum, Pt-00140

$C_{13}H_{19}O_2Pd^{\oplus}$
[(1,2,5,6-η)-1,5-Cyclooctadiene](2,4-pentadionato-*O,O'*)-palladium(1+), Pd-00087

$C_{13}H_{19}O_2Pt^{\oplus}$
[(1,2,5,6-η)-1,5-Cyclooctadiene](2,4-pentanedionato-*O,O'*)platinum(1+), Pt-00141

$C_{13}H_{20}Cl_2NPPt$
Dichloro(isocyanobenzene)(triethylphosphine)platinum, Pt-00142

$C_{13}H_{20}NiO_2$
(1,4,5-η)-4-Cycloocten-1-yl(2,4-pentanedionato-*O,O'*)-nickel, Ni-00105

$C_{13}H_{23}ClPd$
Chloro(2,8-dimethyl-2,10-undecadienyl)palladium, *in* Pd-00221

$C_{13}H_{23}CuSi_2$
[η-Bis(trimethylsilyl)acetylene](η^5-cyclopentadienyl)-copper, Cu-00046

$C_{15}H_{26}BrPPt$
Bromophenyl(tripropylphosphine)platinum, *in* Pt-00343

$C_{15}H_{26}Cl_2NOPPt$
Dichloro[ethoxy(phenylamino)methylene]-(triethylphosphine)platinum, Pt-00174

$C_{15}H_{26}IPPt$
Iodophenyl(tripropylphosphine)platinum, *in* Pt-00344

$C_{15}H_{27}NiO_3P$
Tricarbonyl(tributylphosphine)nickel, Ni-00134
Tricarbonyl(tri-*tert*-butylphosphine)nickel, Ni-00135

$C_{15}H_{27}NiP$
[(1,2,5,6,9,10-η)-1,5,9-Cyclododecatriene]-(trimethylphosphine)nickel, Ni-00136

$C_{15}H_{31}ClF_6P_2Pt$
Chloro(1,1,1,3,3,3-hexafluoro-2-propyl)-bis(triethylphosphine)platinum, Pt-00175

$C_{15}H_{35}BrP_2Pd$
Bromo(2-propenyl)bis(triethylphosphine)palladium, Pd-00111

$C_{15}H_{35}BrP_2Pt$
Bromo(2-propenyl)bis(triethylphosphine)platinum, Pt-00176

$C_{15}H_{35}ClP_2Pd$
π-Allylchlorobis(triethylphosphine)palladium, *in* Pd-00112

$C_{15}H_{35}N_4Ni^{\oplus}$
Methyl(1,4,8,11-tetramethyl-1,4,8,11-tetraazacyclotetradecane-N^1,N^4,N^8,N^{11})nickel(1+), Ni-00137

$C_{15}H_{35}P_2Pd^{\oplus}$
(η^3-2-Propenyl)bis(triethylphosphine)palladium(1+), Pd-00112

$C_{15}H_{39}ClP_2PtSi$
Chlorobis(triethylphosphine)(trimethylsilyl)platinum, Pt-00177

$C_{15}H_{45}B_2F_8NiO_{15}P_5$
Pentakis(trimethylphosphite)nickel(2+); Bis(tetrafluoroborate), *in* Ni-00138

$C_{15}H_{45}Cl_2NiO_{23}P_5$
Pentakis(trimethylphosphite)nickel(2+); Diperchlorate, *in* Ni-00138

$C_{15}H_{45}F_6NiO_{15}P_5Si$
Pentakis(trimethylphosphite)nickel(2+); Hexafluorosilicate, *in* Ni-00138

$C_{15}H_{45}NiO_{15}P_5^{\oplus\oplus}$
Pentakis(trimethylphosphite)nickel(2+), Ni-00138

$C_{16}F_{18}Ni_4O_4$
Tetracarbonyltris[μ_3-[(1-η:1,2-η:1,2-η)-1,1,1,4,4,4-hexafluoro-2-butyne]]tetranickel, Ni-00139

$C_{16}F_{18}O_4Pd_4$
Tetracarbonyltris(hexafluoro-2-butyne)tetrapalladium, Pd-00113

$C_{16}H_6Cl_2F_{10}N_2Pd_2$
Di-μ-chlorobis(isocyanomethane)bis(pentafluorophenyl)-dipalladium, Pd-00114

$C_{16}H_6F_{10}N_2Pd$
Bis(isocyanomethane)bis(pentafluorophenyl)palladium, Pd-00115

$C_{16}H_8ClF_5N_2Pd$
(2,2′-Bipyridine-*N*,*N*′)chloro(pentafluorophenyl)-palladium, Pd-00116

$C_{16}H_8Cl_3F_5N_2Pd$
(2,2′-Bipyridine-*N*,*N*′)trichloro(pentafluorophenyl)-palladium, Pd-00117

$C_{16}H_8F_{14}N_2Pd$
(2,2′-Bipyridine)bis(heptafluoropropyl)palladium, Pd-00118

$C_{16}H_{12}Ni_2$
Bis[(1,2,3,3*a*,6*a*-η:3*a*,4,5,6,6*a*-η)pentalene]dinickel, Ni-00140

$C_{16}H_{13}ClN_2Ni$
(2,2′-Bipyridine-*N*,*N*′)chlorophenylnickel, Ni-00141

$C_{16}H_{14}Cl_4N_2Pd_2$
Di-μ-chlorodichlorobis(1-isocyano-4-methylbenzene)-dipalladium, Pd-00119

$C_{16}H_{14}N_4Ni$
(2,2′-Bipyridine-*N*,*N*′)bis(2-propenenitrile)nickel, Ni-00142

$C_{16}H_{16}Cl_4Pd_2$
Di-μ-chlorodichlorobis(styrene)dipalladium, Pd-00120

$C_{16}H_{16}Cl_4Pt_2$
Di-μ-chlorodichlorobis(styrene)diplatinum, Pt-00178

$C_{16}H_{16}Ni$
Bis[(1,2,3,4-η)-1,3,5,7-cyclooctatetraene]nickel, Ni-00143

$C_{16}H_{18}Cl_2N_2Pd_2$
Dichloro(η^3-2-propenyl)palladate(1−); π-Allylbipyridylpalladium salt, *in* Pd-00008

$C_{16}H_{18}N_6Ni$
Bis(*tert*-butylisocyanide)(tetracyanoethylene)nickel, Ni-00144

$C_{16}H_{18}Ni$
Bis[(1,2,3-η)-2,4,7-cyclooctatrien-1-yl]nickel, Ni-00145

$C_{16}H_{18}Ni_2$
[μ-[η^3:η^3-2,3-Bis(methylene)-1,4-butanediyl]]-bis[(1,2,3-η)-2,4-cyclopentadien-1-yl]dinickel, Ni-00146

$C_{16}H_{18}Pd_2$
[μ-[η^3:η^3-2,3-Bismethylene-1,4-butanediyl]]bis(η^5-2,4-cyclopentadien-1-yl)dipalladium, Pd-00121

$C_{16}H_{20}AuIS$
Iododimethyl(dibenzylsulfide)gold, Au-00070

$C_{16}H_{22}Cl_2O_2Pd_2$
Di-μ-chlorobis[(2,5,6-η)-3-methoxybicyclo[2.2.1]hept-5-en-2-yl]dipalladium, Pd-00122

$C_{16}H_{22}Cl_2Pd_2$
Di-μ-chlorobis[(1,5,6-η)-2,5-cyclooctadien-1-yl]-dipalladium, Pd-00123

$C_{16}H_{22}N_2Ni$
(2,2′-Bipyridine-*N*,*N*′)dipropylnickel, Ni-00147

$C_{16}H_{22}O_2PtS_2$
Diphenylbis(dimethylsulfoxide)platinum, Pt-00179

$C_{16}H_{22}O_4Pd_2$
[μ-[η^3:η^3-2,3-Bismethylene-1,4-butanediyl]]bis(2,4-pentanedionato-*O*,*O*′)dipalladium, Pd-00124

$C_{16}H_{23}ClP_2Pt$
Chlorohydrobis(dimethylphenylphosphine)platinum, Pt-00180

$C_{16}H_{24}B_2Cl_2F_8Pd_2$
Di-μ-chlorobis[(1,2,5,6-η)-1,5-cyclooctadiene]-dipalladium(2+); Bis(tetrafluoroborate), *in* Pd-00125

$C_{16}H_{24}Br_2Ni$
Dibromo(1,2,3,4,5,6,7,8,9,10,11,12-dodecahydrocyclobuta[1,2:3,4]dicyclooctenenickel, Ni-00148

$C_{16}H_{24}Br_4Ni_2$
Di-μ-bromodibromobis[(1,2,3,4-η)-1,2,3,4-tetramethyl-1,3-cyclobutadiene]dinickel, Ni-00149

$C_{16}H_{24}Cl_2Cu_2$
Di-μ-chlorobis[(1,2,5,6-η)-1,5-cyclooctadiene]dicopper, *in* Cu-00029

$C_{16}H_{24}Cl_2Pd_2^{\oplus\oplus}$
Di-μ-chlorobis[(1,2,5,6-η)-1,5-cyclooctadiene]-dipalladium(2+), Pd-00125

$C_{16}H_{24}Cl_4Ni_2$
Di-μ-chlorodichlorobis[(1,2,3,4-η)-1,2,3,4-tetramethyl-1,3-cyclobutadiene]dinickel, Ni-00150

$C_{16}H_{24}Cl_4Pt_2$
Di-μ-chlorodichlorobis[(1,2,3,4-η)-1,2,3,4-tetramethyl-1,3-cyclobutadiene]diplatinum, Pt-00181

$C_{16}H_{24}F_{12}N_8P_2Pd_3$
Octakis(isocyanomethane)tripalladium(2+); Bis(hexafluorophosphate), *in* Pd-00126

$C_{16}H_{24}N_8Pd_3^{\oplus\oplus}$
Octakis(isocyanomethane)tripalladium(2+), Pd-00126

$C_{16}H_{24}Ni$
Bis[(1,2,5,6-η)-1,5-cyclooctadiene]nickel, Ni-00151

$C_{16}H_{24}O_4Pt_2$
Bis(2,4-pentanedionato-*O,O'*)bis[μ-[(1-η:2,3-η)-propenyl]]diplatinum, Pt-00182

$C_{16}H_{24}Pd$
Bis[(1,2,5,6-η)-1,5-cyclooctadiene]palladium, Pd-00127

$C_{16}H_{24}Pt$
Bis[(1,2,5,6-η)-1,5-cyclooctadiene]platinum, Pt-00183

$C_{16}H_{25}ClO_2Pd$
Chloro(12-methoxy-2,6,10-trimethyl-12-oxo-2,6,10-dodecatrienyl)palladium, *in* Pd-00249

$C_{16}H_{26}Cl_2Pd_2$
Di-μ-chlorobis(η^3-2-ethylidenecyclohexyl)dipalladium, Pd-00128

$C_{16}H_{26}Ni$
Bis[(1,2,3-η)-2-cycloocten-1-yl]nickel, Ni-00152

$C_{16}H_{26}NiSi_2$
1,1'-Bis(trimethylsilyl)nickelocene, Ni-00153

$C_{16}H_{28}Cl_6N_4Pt_3$
Trichloro(styrene)platinate(1−); Tetraammineplatinum(2+) salt, *in* Pt-00059

$C_{16}H_{29}INNiP$
(η^5-2,4-Cyclopentadien-1-yl)(2-isocyano-2-methylpropane)(triethylphosphine)nickel(1+); Iodide, *in* Ni-00154

$C_{16}H_{29}NNiP^{\oplus}$
(η^5-2,4-Cyclopentadien-1-yl)(2-isocyano-2-methylpropane)(triethylphosphine)nickel(1+), Ni-00154

$C_{16}H_{29}O_2PPd$
Acetato(cyclopentadienyl)-triisopropylphosphinepalladium, Pd-00129

$C_{16}H_{30}CuP$
(η^5-Pentamethylcyclopentadienyl)(triethylphosphine)-copper, Cu-00047

$C_{16}H_{30}F_6P_2Pt$
[(2,3-η)-1,1,1,4,4,4-Hexafluoro-2-butyne]-bis(triethylphosphine)platinum, Pt-00184

$C_{16}H_{31}ClF_6P_2Pt$
Chloro[1,2-bis(trifluoromethyl)vinyl]-bis(triethylphosphine)platinum, Pt-00185

$C_{16}H_{32}OP_3Pd^{\oplus}$
Benzoyltris(trimethylphosphine)palladium(1+), Pd-00130

$C_{16}H_{32}O_4Pt_2$
Hexamethylbis(μ-(2,4-pentanedionato-C^3:O^2,O^4))]-diplatinum, *in* Pt-00072

$C_{16}H_{32}P_2Pt$
Diethynylbis(triethylphosphine)platinum, Pt-00186

$C_{16}H_{35}F_3N_4NiO_3S$
Methyl(1,4,8,11-tetramethyl-1,4,8,11-tetraazacyclotetradecane-N^1,N^4,N^8,N^{11})nickel(1+); Trifluoromethanesulphonate, *in* Ni-00137

$C_{16}H_{36}AgP$
Butyl(tributylphosphine)silver, Ag-00031

$C_{16}H_{36}CuP$
Butyl(tributylphosphine)copper, Cu-00048

$C_{16}H_{37}BF_4P_2Pd$
[(1,2,3-η)-2-Methyl-2-propenyl]bis(triethylphosphine)-palladium(1+); Tetrafluoroborate, *in* Pd-00132

$C_{16}H_{37}F_6NiO_6P_3$
[(1,2,3-η)-2-Buten-1-yl]bis[(triethyl phosphite)-*P*]nickel(1+); Hexafluorophosphate, *in* Ni-00155

$C_{16}H_{37}F_6P_3Pt$
[(1,2,3-η)-2-Butenyl]bis(triethylphosphine)platinum(1+); Hexafluorophosphate, *in* Pt-00187

$C_{16}H_{37}NiO_6P_2^{\oplus}$
[(1,2,3-η)-2-Buten-1-yl]bis[(triethyl phosphite)-*P*]nickel(1+), Ni-00155

$C_{16}H_{37}P_2Pd^{\oplus}$
[(1,2,3-η)-2-Butenyl]bis(triethylphosphine)-palladium(1+), Pd-00131
[(1,2,3-η)-2-Methyl-2-propenyl]bis(triethylphosphine)-palladium(1+), Pd-00132

$C_{16}H_{37}P_2Pt^{\oplus}$
[(1,2,3-η)-2-Butenyl]bis(triethylphosphine)platinum(1+), Pt-00187

$C_{16}H_{40}P_2Pt$
Diethylbis(triethylphosphine)platinum, Pt-00188

$C_{16}H_{42}P_2Pt$
Tetramethylbis(triethylphosphine)platinum, Pt-00189

$C_{16}H_{44}Cu_4Si_4$
Tetrakis(μ-[(trimethylsilyl)methyl]tetracopper, *in* Cu-00013

$C_{16}H_{48}Pt_4S_4$
Tetrakis[μ_3-(methanethiolato)]-dodecamethyltetraplatinum, *in* Pt-00031

$C_{17}H_8ClF_5N_2O_5Pd$
(2,2'-Bipyridine)carbonyl(pentafluorophenyl)-palladium(1+); Perchlorate, *in* Pd-00133

$C_{17}H_8F_5N_2OPd^{\oplus}$
(2,2'-Bipyridine)carbonyl(pentafluorophenyl)-palladium(1+), Pd-00133

$C_{17}H_{14}N_2Ni$
η^5-2,4-Cyclopentadien-1-yl[2-(phenylazo)phenyl]nickel, Ni-00156

$C_{17}H_{15}Ni_3O_2$
Tricyclopentadienyltrinickeldicarbonyl, Ni-00157

$C_{17}H_{22}BClF_4OP_2Pt$
Carbonylchlorobis(dimethylphenylphosphine)platinum(1+); Tetrafluoroborate, *in* Pt-00190

$C_{17}H_{22}ClOP_2Pt^{\oplus}$
Carbonylchlorobis(dimethylphenylphosphine)platinum(1+), Pt-00190

$C_{17}H_{22}Cl_2O_5P_2Pt$
Carbonylchlorobis(dimethylphenylphosphine)platinum(1+); Perchlorate, *in* Pt-00190

$C_{17}H_{24}O_2Pd$
η^3-(1,2,4,5,6-Pentamethyl-3-methylenebicyclo[2.2.0]hex-5-en-2-yl)(2,4-pentanedionato-*O,O'*)palladium, Pd-00134

$C_{17}H_{25}BrP_2Pt$
Bromobis(dimethylphenylphosphine)methylplatinum, Pt-00191

$C_{17}H_{25}ClP_2Pd$
Chlorobis(dimethylphenylphosphine)methylpalladium, Pd-00135

$C_{17}H_{25}ClP_2Pt$
Chlorobis(dimethylphenylphosphine)methylplatinum, Pt-00192

$C_{17}H_{25}IP_2Pd$
Bis(dimethylphenylphosphine)iodo(methyl)palladium, Pd-00136

$C_{17}H_{25}IP_2Pt$
Bis(dimethylphenylphosphine)iodomethylplatinum, Pt-00193

$C_{17}H_{25}PPd$
(η^5-2,4-Cyclopentadien-1-yl)phenyl(triethylphosphine)-palladium, Pd-00137

$C_{17}H_{25}PPt$
(η^5-2,4-Cyclopentadien-1-yl)phenyl(triethylphosphine)-platinum, Pt-00194

$C_{17}H_{27}Cl_2NPt$
Dichloro(4-methylaniline)[(3,4-η)-2,2,5,5-tetramethyl-3-hexyne]platinum, Pt-00195

$C_{17}H_{29}NiP$
Bis(bicyclo[2.2.1]hept-2-ene)(trimethylphosphine)-nickel, Ni-00158

$C_{17}H_{32}ClNiP$
Chloro(η^5-2,4-cyclopentadien-1-yl)(tributylphosphine)-nickel, Ni-00159

$C_{17}H_{34}BrNP_2Pd$
Bromo(2-pyridinyl)bis(triethylphosphine)palladium, Pd-00138
Bromo(3-pyridinyl)bis(triethylphosphine)palladium, Pd-00139
Bromo(4-pyridinyl)bis(triethylphosphine)palladium, Pd-00140

$C_{17}H_{35}ClO_4P_2Pt$
(η^5-2,4-Cyclopentadien-1-yl)bis(triethylphosphine)-platinum(1+); Perchlorate, *in* Pt-00196

$C_{17}H_{35}ClP_2Pt$
(η^5-2,4-Cyclopentadien-1-yl)bis(triethylphosphine)-platinum(1+); Chloride, *in* Pt-00196

$C_{17}H_{35}P_2Pd^{\oplus}$
(η^5-2,4-Cyclopentadien-1-yl)bis(triethylphosphine)-palladium(1+), Pd-00141

$C_{17}H_{35}P_2Pt^{\oplus}$
(η^5-2,4-Cyclopentadien-1-yl)bis(triethylphosphine)-platinum(1+), Pt-00196

$C_{17}H_{36}Br_3NOPd$
Tribromocarbonylpalladate(1−); Tetrabutylammonium salt, *in* Pd-00001

$C_{17}H_{36}Cl_3NOPd$
Carbonyltrichloropalladate(1−); Tetrabutylammonium salt, *in* Pd-00002

$C_{17}H_{36}Cl_3NOPt$
Carbonyltrichloroplatinate(1−); Tetrabutylammonium salt, *in* Pt-00002

$C_{17}H_{36}I_3NOPt$
Carbonyltriiodoplatinate(1−); Tetrabutylammonium salt, *in* Pt-00005

$C_{17}H_{38}O_2P_2Pd$
(η^3-2-Propenyl)bis(triethylphosphine)palladium(1+); Acetate, *in* Pd-00112

$C_{17}H_{40}P_2Pt$
(2,2-Dimethyl-1,3-propanediyl)bis(triethylphosphine)-platinium, Pt-00197

$C_{17}H_{43}LiN_4Ni$
Bis(ethylene)methylnickelate(1−); Bis(tetramethylethylenediamine)lithium(1+) salt, *in* Ni-00019

$C_{18}H_{12}CuN_2O_2$
▷Bis(8-quinolinolato-N^1,O^8)copper, Cu-00049

$C_{18}H_{14}Ni$
Bis[(1,2,3-η)-1*H*-inden-1-yl]nickel, Ni-00160

$C_{18}H_{15}AuClP$
Chloro(triphenylphosphine)gold, Au-00071

$C_{18}H_{15}Li_3Ni$
Triphenylnickelate(3−); Tri-Li salt, *in* Ni-00161

$C_{18}H_{15}Ni^{\ominus\ominus\ominus}$
Triphenylnickelate(3−), Ni-00161

$C_{18}H_{16}CuP$
Hydrido(triphenylphosphine)copper, Cu-00050

$C_{18}H_{18}Cl_2Pd_2$
Di-μ-chlorobis[(1,2,3-η)-1-phenyl-2-propenyl]-dipalladium, Pd-00142
Di-μ-chlorobis[(1,2,3-η)-2-phenyl-2-propenyl]-dipalladium, Pd-00143

$C_{18}H_{18}Cl_2Pt_2$
Di-μ-chlorobis(η^3-1-phenyl-2-propenyl)diplatinum, Pt-00198

$C_{18}H_{18}F_{18}P_2Pt$
[1,2,3,4,5,6-Hexakis(trifluoromethyl)-1,3,5-hexatriene-1,6-diyl]bis(trimethylphosphine)platinum, Pt-00199

$C_{18}H_{20}Cl_2N_2O_8Pd$
(2,2′-Bipyridine-*N*,*N*′)[(1,2,5,6-η)-1,5-cyclooctadiene]-palladium(2+); Diperchlorate, *in* Pd-00144

$C_{18}H_{20}N_2Ni$
(2,2′-Bipyridine-*N*,*N*′)[(1,2,5,6-η)-1,5-cyclooctadiene]-nickel, Ni-00162
(2,2′-Bipyridine-*N*,*N*′)[(1,2,3,4-η)-1,2,3,4-tetramethyl-1,3-cyclobutadiene]nickel, Ni-00163

$C_{18}H_{20}N_2Pd^{\oplus\oplus}$
(2,2′-Bipyridine-*N*,*N*′)[(1,2,5,6-η)-1,5-cyclooctadiene]-palladium(2+), Pd-00144

$C_{18}H_{20}Pd_2$
Bis[η^5-2,4-cyclopentadien-1-yl][μ-[(1,2,3-η:6,7,8-η)-2,6-octadien-1,8-diyl]]dipalladium, Pd-00145

$C_{18}H_{21}ClN_2OPd$
[(2,5,6-η)-3-Methoxybicyclo[2.2.1]hept-5-en-2-yl]-bis(pyridine)palladium(1+); Chloride, *in* Pd-00146

$C_{18}H_{21}N_2OPd^{\oplus}$
[(2,5,6-η)-3-Methoxybicyclo[2.2.1]hept-5-en-2-yl]-bis(pyridine)palladium(1+), Pd-00146

$C_{18}H_{22}F_4P_2Pt$
Bis(dimethylphenylphosphine)(η^2-tetrafluoroethene)-platinum, Pt-00200

$C_{18}H_{22}Ni$
Bis[(1,2,3,3*a*,7*a*-η)-4,5,6,7-tetrahydro-1*H*-inden-1-yl]-nickel, Ni-00164
Bis(2,4,6-trimethylphenyl)nickel, Ni-00165

$C_{18}H_{23}FeNO_2Pd$
[2-[(Dimethylamino)methyl]ferrocenyl-*C*,*N*]-(2,4-pentanedionato-*O*,*O*′)palladium, Pd-00147

$C_{18}H_{24}Cl_2N_2Pd_2$
Di-μ-chlorobis[2-[(dimethylamino)methyl]phenyl-*C*,*N*]-dipalladium, Pd-00148

$C_{18}H_{24}N_2Pd$
Bis[2-[(dimethylamino)methyl]phenyl-*C*,*N*]palladium, Pd-00149

$C_{18}H_{24}NiO_2$
(1,5-Cyclooctadiene)(2,3,5,6-tetramethyl-*p*-benzoquinone)nickel, Ni-00166

$C_{18}H_{24}PtS_2$
[1,2-Bis(ethylthio)ethane-*S*,*S*′]diphenylplatinum, Pt-00201

$C_{18}H_{25}ClOP_2Pt$
Acetylchlorobis(dimethylphenylphosphine)platinum, Pt-00202

$C_{18}H_{26}O_4Pd$
[8-(1-Acetylacetonyl)-π-4-cycloocten-1-yl](2,4-pentanedionato)palladium, Pd-00150

$C_{18}H_{27}ClP_2Pt$
Chlorobis(dimethylphenylphosphine)ethylplatinum, Pt-00203

$C_{18}H_{28}Br_2P_2Pt$
Dibromobis(dimethylphenylphosphine)dimethylplatinum, Pt-00204

$C_{18}H_{28}Cl_2N_2O_2Pd_2$
Bis(η^3-1-acetyl-4-ethylidenepiperidinyl)di-μ-chlorodipalladium, Pd-00151

$C_{18}H_{28}Cl_2P_2Pt$
Dichlorobis(dimethylphenylphosphine)dimethylplatinum, Pt-00205

$C_{18}H_{28}I_2P_2Pt$
Bis(dimethylphenylphosphine)diiododimethylplatinum, Pt-00206

$C_{18}H_{28}LiPPt$
(Methyldiphenylphosphine)pentamethylplatinate(1−); Li salt, *in* Pt-00207

$C_{18}H_{28}PPt^{\ominus}$
(Methyldiphenylphosphine)pentamethylplatinate(1−), Pt-00207

$C_{18}H_{28}P_2Pt$
Bis(dimethylphenylphosphine)dimethylplatinum, Pt-00208

$C_{18}H_{30}BrF_5NiP_2$
Bromo(pentafluorophenyl)bis(triethylphosphine)nickel, Ni-00167

$C_{18}H_{30}BrF_5P_2Pd$
Bromo(pentafluorophenyl)bis(triethylphosphine)-palladium, Pd-00152

$C_{18}H_{30}ClF_5P_2Pt$
Chloro(pentafluorophenyl)bis(triethylphosphine)-platinum, Pt-00209

$C_{18}H_{30}Cl_2O_2Pd_2$
Di-μ-chlorobis[(1,4,5-η)-8-methoxy-4-cycloocten-1-yl]-dipalladium, Pd-00153

$C_{18}H_{30}Cl_3F_5P_2Pt$
Trichloro(pentafluorophenyl)bis(triethylphosphine)-platinum, Pt-00210

$C_{18}H_{30}Cl_6P_2Pd$
Chloro(pentachlorophenyl)bis(triethylphosphine)-palladium, Pd-00154

$C_{18}H_{30}F_6P_2Pd$
Bis(triethylphosphine)bis(3,3,3-trifluoro-1-propynyl)-palladium, Pd-00155

$C_{18}H_{32}Cl_2NOPPt$
Dichloro[ethoxy(phenylamino)methylene]-(tripropylphosphine)platinum, Pt-00211

$C_{18}H_{33}NiP$
(1,5,9-Cyclododecatriene)(triethylphosphine)nickel, Ni-00168

$C_{18}H_{33}PPd$
(π-Cyclopentadienyl)(2-methyl-2-propenyl)-(triisopropylphosphine)palladium, Pd-00156
(η^1-2,4-Cyclopentadien-1-yl)[(1,2,3-η)-2-methyl-2-propenyl][tris(1-methylethyl)phosphine]palladium, Pd-00157

$C_{18}H_{35}BrNiP_2$
Bromo(phenyl)bis(triethylphosphine)nickel, Ni-00169

$C_{18}H_{35}BrP_2Pd$
Bromo(phenyl)bis(triethylphosphine)palladium, Pd-00158

$C_{18}H_{35}ClP_2Pd$
Chloro(phenyl)bis(triethylphosphine)palladium, Pd-00159

$C_{18}H_{35}ClP_2Pt$
Chlorophenylbis(triethylphosphine)platinum, Pt-00212

$C_{18}H_{35}Cl_3P_2Pt$
Trichlorophenylbis(triethylphosphine)platinum, Pt-00213

$C_{18}H_{35}Cl_3P_2PtSn$
Phenyl(trichlorostannyl)bis(triethylphosphine)platinum, Pt-00214

$C_{18}H_{35}IP_2Pt$
Iodo(phenyl)bis(triethylphosphine)platinum, Pt-00215

$C_{18}H_{35}NiP$
η^5-Cyclopentadienyl(methyl)(tributylphosphine)nickel, Ni-00170

$C_{18}H_{36}Cl_4O_2Pt_2$
Di-μ-chlorodichlorobis[3,3-dimethyl-1-(1-methylethoxy)-butylidene]diplatinum, Pt-00216

$C_{18}H_{36}P_2Pt$
Di(1-propynyl)bis(triethylphosphine)platinum, Pt-00217

$C_{18}H_{40}Cl_3NPd$
Trichloro(ethylene)palladate(1−); Tetrabutylammonium salt, *in* Pd-00007

$C_{18}H_{40}N_2O_4Pt_2$
(μ-Ethylenediamine)hexamethylbis(2,4-pentanedionato)-diplatinum, Pt-00218

$C_{18}H_{43}ClNiP_2$
Chlorohydrobis(triisopropylphosphine)nickel, Ni-00171

$C_{18}H_{43}ClP_2Pd$
Chlorohydrobis(triisopropylphosphine)palladium, Pd-00160

$C_{18}H_{45}P_3Pt$
Tris(triethylphosphine)platinum, Pt-00219

$C_{18}H_{46}ClO_4P_3Pt$
Hydrotris(triethylphosphine)platinum(1+); Perchlorate, *in* Pt-00220

$C_{18}H_{46}P_3Pt^{\oplus}$
Hydrotris(triethylphosphine)platinum(1+), Pt-00220

$C_{18}Ni_9O_{18}^{\ominus\ominus}$
Octadecacarbonylnonanickelate(2−), Ni-00172

$C_{18}O_{18}Pt_9^{\ominus\ominus}$
Nona-μ-carbonylnonacarbonylnonaplatinate(2−), Pt-00221

$C_{19}F_{15}NPd^{\ominus\ominus}$
(Cyano-*C*)tris(pentafluorophenyl)palladate(2−), Pd-00161

$C_{19}H_8F_{10}Ni$
[(1,2,3,4,5,6-η)-Methylbenzene]bis(pentafluorophenyl)-nickel, Ni-00173

$C_{19}H_{15}AsCl_2OPt$
Carbonyldichloro(triphenylarsine)platinum, Pt-00222

$C_{19}H_{15}Cl_2OPPt$
Carbonyldichloro(triphenylphosphine)platinum, Pt-00223

$C_{19}H_{16}Pt$
[(2,3,5,6-η)-Bicyclo[2.2.1]hepta-2,5-diene](1,1′-biphenyl-2,2′-diyl)platinum, Pt-00224

$C_{19}H_{18}AuP$
Methyl(triphenylphosphine)gold, Au-00072

$C_{19}H_{18}N_2Ni$
(η^5-2,4-Cyclopentadien-1-yl)[5-methyl-2-[(4-methylphenyl)azo]phenyl]nickel, Ni-00174

$C_{19}H_{18}Pt$
[(2,3,5,6-η)-Bicyclo[2.2.1]hepta-2,5-diene]-diphenylplatinum, Pt-00225

$C_{19}H_{20}Cl_2N_2Pt$
Dichloro(2-phenyl-1,3-propanediyl)bis(pyridine)-platinum, Pt-00226

$C_{19}H_{24}F_6OPt_2$
Bis[(1,2,5,6-η)-1,5-cyclooctadiene][μ-[(1,1,1,3,3,3-hexafluoro-2-propanolato(2−)-C^2,*O*]diplatinum, Pt-00227

$C_{19}H_{24}NNi_3$
Tris(π-cyclopentadienyl)(μ_3-*tert*-butylaminato)-trinickel, Ni-00175

$C_{19}H_{25}FeNO_2Pd$
[2-[1-(Dimethylamino)ethyl]ferrocenyl-*C*,*N*](2,4-pentanedionato-*O*,*O′*)palladium, Pd-00162

$C_{19}H_{27}ClP_2Pt$
Chloro(cyclopropyl)bis(dimethylphenylphosphine)-platinum, Pt-00228

$C_{19}H_{27}Cl_2N_2PPt$
Dichloro[bis(phenylamino)methylene](triethylphosphine)-platinum, Pt-00229

$C_{19}H_{27}F_6P_3Pt$
Bis(dimethylphenylphosphine)(η^3-2-propenyl)platinum(1+); Hexafluorophosphate, *in* Pt-00230

$C_{19}H_{27}PPd$
[2-(*tert*-Butylphenylphosphino)-2-methylpropyl]-cyclopentadienylpalladium, Pd-00163

$C_{19}H_{27}P_2Pd^{\oplus}$
Bis(dimethylphenylphosphine)(η^3-2-propenyl)-palladium(1+), Pd-00164

$C_{19}H_{27}P_2Pt^{\oplus}$
Bis(dimethylphenylphosphine)(η^3-2-propenyl)platinum(1+), Pt-00230

$C_{19}H_{28}ClO_4PPd$
Cyclopentadienyl(styrene)(triethylphosphine)-palladium(1+); Perchlorate, *in* Pd-00165

$C_{19}H_{28}PPd^{\oplus}$
Cyclopentadienyl(styrene)(triethylphosphine)-palladium(1+), Pd-00165

$C_{19}H_{29}As_2IPt$
[1,2-Ethanediylbis(methylphenylarsine)-*As*,*As'*]-iodotrimethylplatinum, Pt-00231

$C_{19}H_{31}IP_2Pt$
Bis(dimethylphenylphosphine)iodotrimethylplatinum, Pt-00232

$C_{19}H_{31}PPd$
2,4-Cyclopentadien-1-yl(η^5-2,4-cyclopentadien-1-yl)-[tris(1-methylethyl)phosphine]palladium, Pd-00166

$C_{19}H_{33}Cl_2OPPt$
Carbonyldichloro(tricyclohexylphosphine)platinum, Pt-00233

$C_{19}H_{33}F_5P_2Pt$
Methyl(pentafluorophenyl)bis(triethylphosphine)-platinum, Pt-00234

$C_{19}H_{35}NNiP_2$
(Cyano-*C*)phenylbis(triethylphosphine)nickel, Ni-00176

$C_{19}H_{35}NP_2Pd$
Cyano(phenyl)bis(triethylphosphine)palladium, Pd-00167

$C_{19}H_{35}NP_2Pt$
(Cyano-*C*)phenylbis(triethylphosphine)platinum, Pt-00235

$C_{19}H_{36}ClNNiO_3$
Tricarbonylchloronickelate(1−); Tetrabutylammonium salt, *in* Ni-00001

$C_{19}H_{36}CuP$
Methyl(tricyclohexylphosphine)copper, Cu-00051

$C_{19}H_{36}INNiO_3$
Tricarbonyliodonickelate(1−); Tetrabutylammonium salt, *in* Ni-00006

$C_{19}H_{37}BF_4P_2Pd$
(η^3-6-Methylene-2,4-cyclohexadien-1-yl)-bis(triethylphosphine)palladium(1+); Tetrafluoroborate, *in* Pd-00168

$C_{19}H_{37}BrNiP_2$
Bromo(2-methylphenyl)bis(triethylphosphine)nickel, Ni-00177

$C_{19}H_{37}ClP_2Pt$
Chloro(2-methylphenyl)bis(triethylphosphine)platinum, Pt-00237
Chloro(3-methylphenyl)bis(triethylphosphine)platinum, Pt-00238
Chloro(4-methylphenyl)bis(triethylphosphine)platinum, Pt-00236

$C_{19}H_{37}P_2Pd^{\oplus}$
(η^3-6-Methylene-2,4-cyclohexadien-1-yl)-bis(triethylphosphine)palladium(1+), Pd-00168

$C_{19}H_{38}NiP_2$
Methylphenylbis(triethylphosphine)nickel, Ni-00178

$C_{19}H_{42}Cl_3NOPt$
Trichloro[(2,3-η)-2-propen-1-ol]platinate(1−); Tetrabutylammonium salt, *in* Pt-00016

$C_{19}H_{42}Cl_3NPt$
Trichloro[(1,2-η)-1-propene]platinate(1−); Tetrabutylammonium salt, *in* Pt-00017

$C_{19}H_{43}OP_2Pt^{\oplus}$
Carbonyl(hydrido)bis(triisopropylphosphine)platinum(1+), Pt-00239

$C_{19}H_{44}O_2P_2Pt$
Carbonyl(hydrido)bis(triisopropylphosphine)platinum(1+); Hydroxide, *in* Pt-00239

$C_{19}H_{45}BrNiP_2$
Bromo(methyl)bis(triisopropylphosphine)nickel, Ni-00179

$C_{19}H_{45}OP_3Pt$
Carbonyltris(triethylphosphine)platinum, Pt-00240

$C_{19}H_{46}P_2Pt$
Hydridomethylbis(triisopropylphosphine)platinum, Pt-00241

$C_{20}H_{12}F_{18}Ni$
[(1,2,5,6-η)-1,5-Cyclooctadiene]-[hexakis(trifluoromethyl)benzene]nickel, Ni-00180

$C_{20}H_{16}Cl_2N_2Pd_2$
Di-μ-chlorobis(8-quinolinylmethyl-*C*,*N*)dipalladium, Pd-00169

$C_{20}H_{16}N_4Ni$
Bis(2,2'-bipyridine-*N*,*N'*)nickel, Ni-00181

$C_{20}H_{16}Ni_2$
1,1'':1',1''-Binickelocene, Ni-00182

$C_{20}H_{17}AsCl_2Pt$
Dichloro[[2-(η^2-ethenyl)phenyl]diphenylarsine-*As*]-platinum, Pt-00242

$C_{20}H_{18}AuP$
(Triphenylphosphine)vinylgold, Au-00073

$C_{20}H_{18}Cl_2NPPt$
Dichloro(isocyanomethane)(triphenylphosphine)platinum, Pt-00243

$C_{20}H_{18}IOPPt$
Carbonyl(iodo)methyl(triphenylphosphine)platinum, Pt-00244

$C_{20}H_{19}AsCl_2Pt$
Dichloro(ethylene)(triphenylarsine)platinum, Pt-00245

$C_{20}H_{19}Cl_2PPt$
Dichloro(ethylene)(triphenylphosphine)platinum, Pt-00246

$C_{20}H_{20}ClPPdS$
Chloro[(methylthio)methyl-*C*,*S*](triphenylphosphine)-palladium, Pd-00170

$C_{20}H_{20}Cl_2N_2O_2Pd_2$
Di-μ-chlorobis[5,6,7,8-tetrahydro-8-(hydroxyimino)-1-naphthalenyl-*C*,*N*]dipalladium, Pd-00171

$C_{20}H_{20}Ni_5S_4$
Tetra-π-cyclopentadienyltetra-μ_3-thioxopentanickel, Ni-00183

$C_{20}H_{22}F_6P_2Pd$
[(2,3-η)-Hexafluoro-2-butyne]-bis(dimethylphenylphosphine)palladium, Pd-00172

$C_{20}H_{22}Li_2Ni$
[(1,2,5,6-η)-1,5-Cyclooctadiene]diphenylnickelate(2−); Di-Li salt, *in* Ni-00185

$C_{20}H_{22}N_2Ni$
Azobenzene(1,5-cyclooctadiene)nickel, Ni-00184

$C_{20}H_{22}Ni^{\ominus\ominus}$
[(1,2,5,6-η)-1,5-Cyclooctadiene]diphenylnickelate(2−), Ni-00185

$C_{20}H_{22}Pt$
[(1,2,5,6-η)-1,5-Cyclooctadiene]diphenylplatinum, Pt-00247

$C_{20}H_{23}Ni_4$
Tetrakis(η^5-2,4-cyclopentadien-1-yl)tri-μ_3-hydrotetranickel, Ni-00186

$C_{20}H_{24}N_2Ni_5O_{12}$
Dodecacarbonylpentanickelate(2−); Bis(tetramethylammonium) salt, *in* Ni-00101

$C_{20}H_{24}N_2Ni_6O_{12}$
Dodecacarbonylhexanickelate(2−); Bis(tetramethylammonium) salt, *in* Ni-00102

$C_{20}H_{24}Ni_3$
Tris(η^5-2,4-cyclopentadien-1-yl)[μ_3-(2,2-dimethylpropylidyne)]trinickel, Ni-00187

$C_{20}H_{26}AgB_8P$
Triphenylphosphine[(7,8,9-η)undecahydro-5,6-dicarbadecaborato(1−)]silver, Ag-00032

$C_{20}H_{26}B_8CuP$
(Triphenylphosphine)[(7,8,9-η)-undecahydro-5,6-dicarbadecaborato(1−)]copper, Cu-00052

$C_{20}H_{26}Cl_2O_2Pd_2$
Di-μ-chlorobis[μ-[(1,2,3-η)-2-(4-methyl-5-oxo-3-cyclohexen-1-yl)-2-propenyl]]dipalladium, Pd-00173

$C_{20}H_{26}Cl_2P_2Pt$
Bis(1-chloroethenyl)bis(dimethylphenylphosphine)-platinum, Pt-00248

$C_{20}H_{26}Cl_3Pt$
Trichloro(diphenylacetylene)platinate(1−); Triethylammonium salt, *in* Pt-00152

$C_{20}H_{26}F_6N_2O_4Pt_2$
Tetramethylbis(4-methylpyridine)bis[μ-(trifluoroacetate-*O*,*O'*)]diplatinum, Pt-00249

$C_{20}H_{28}Cl_4P_2Pt_2$
μ-[(1,2:3,4-η)Butadiene]-tetrachlorobis(dimethylphenylphosphine)-diplatinum, Pt-00250

$C_{20}H_{28}P_2Pt$
(Diphenylacetylene)bis(trimethylphosphine)platinum, Pt-00251

$C_{20}H_{30}Cl_2Pd_2$
Di-μ-chlorobis(η^3-6,6-dimethyl-4-methylenebicyclo[3.1.1]hept-3-yl)dipalladium, Pd-00174

$C_{20}H_{30}I_2P_2Pt$
1,4-Butanediylbis(dimethylphenylphosphine)-diiodoplatinum, Pt-00252

$C_{20}H_{30}Ni$
Bis(η^5-pentamethylcyclopentadienyl)nickel, Ni-00188

$C_{20}H_{31}F_6OP_3Pt$
Bis(dimethylphenylphosphine)methyl[methyl(methoxy)-methylene]platinum(1+); Hexafluorophosphate, *in* Pt-00253

$C_{20}H_{31}OP_2Pt^{\oplus}$
Bis(dimethylphenylphosphine)methyl[methyl(methoxy)-methylene]platinum(1+), Pt-00253

$C_{20}H_{32}As_4Ni$
Bis[1,2-phenylenebis[dimethylarsine]-*As*,*As'*]nickel, Ni-00189

$C_{20}H_{32}Cl_4Pd_2$
Di-μ-chlorobis[(1,4,5-η)-8-(1-chloroethyl)-4-cycloocten-1-yl]dipalladium, Pd-00175

$C_{20}H_{33}ClF_6P_2PdSi$
Chloro[(1,2,5,6-η)-1,5-cyclooctadiene]-[dimethylphenylphosphonium(1-η)-(trimethylsilyl)-methylide]palladium(1+); Hexafluorophosphate, *in* Pd-00176

$C_{20}H_{33}ClPPdSi^{\oplus}$
Chloro[(1,2,5,6-η)-1,5-cyclooctadiene]-[dimethylphenylphosphonium(1-η)-(trimethylsilyl)-methylide]palladium(1+), Pd-00176

$C_{20}H_{33}ClP_2PtSi$
Chlorobis(dimethylphenylphosphine)-(trimethylsilylmethyl)platinum, Pt-00254

$C_{20}H_{34}As_2Pt$
Bis(dimethylphenylarsine)tetramethylplatinum, Pt-00255

$C_{20}H_{34}AuO_9PS$
[1-Thioglucopyranose-2,3,4,6-tetrakis(methylcarbamato)-*S*]triethylphosphinegold, Au-00074

$C_{20}H_{34}P_2Pt$
Bis(dimethylphenylphosphine)tetramethylplatinum, Pt-00256

$C_{20}H_{35}ClP_2Pd$
Chloro(phenylethynyl)bis(triethylphosphine)palladium, Pd-00177

$C_{20}H_{36}Au_4$
Tetrakis(3,3-dimethyl-1-butyne)tetragold, *in* Au-00032

$C_{20}H_{36}Cl_2N_4Pd_2$
Di-μ-chlorotetrakis[2-isocyano-2-methylpropane]-dipalladium, Pd-00178

$C_{20}H_{36}Cl_4Pd_2$
Di-μ-chlorodichlorobis[(3,4-η)-2,2,5,5-tetramethyl-3-hexyne]dipalladium, Pd-00179

$C_{20}H_{36}Cl_4Pt_2$
Di-μ-chlorodichlorobis[(3,4-η)-2,2,5,5-tetramethyl-3-hexyne]diplatinum, Pt-00257

$C_{20}H_{36}Cl_8Pt_2Sn_2$
Di-μ-chlorobis[(3,4-η)-2,2,5,5-tetramethyl-3-hexyne]-bis(trichlorostannyl)diplatinum, Pt-00258

$C_{20}H_{36}N_4Ni$
Tetrakis(2-isocyano-2-methylpropane)nickel, Ni-00190

$C_{20}H_{36}O_4Pt_2$
Di-μ-methoxobis[(1,4,5-η)-8-methoxy-4-cycloocten-1-yl]-diplatinum, Pt-00259

$C_{20}H_{37}Cu_2N_4O_3^{\oplus}$
(μ-Carbonyl)(μ-benzoato-*O*,*O'*)bis(*N*,*N*,*N'*,*N'*-tetramethylethylenediamine)dicopper(1+), Cu-00053

$C_{20}H_{38}LiNi_2P$
(μ-Dicyclohexylphosphine)tetrakis(ethylene)-dinickelate(1−); Li salt, *in* Ni-00191

$C_{20}H_{38}Ni_2P^{\ominus}$
(μ-Dicyclohexylphosphine)tetrakis(ethylene)-dinickelate(1−), Ni-00191

$C_{20}H_{39}NiP$
Dimethyl(tricyclohexylphosphine)nickel, Ni-00192

$C_{20}H_{39}NiPS$
(η^5-2,4-Cyclopentadien-1-yl)(1-propanethiolato)-(tributylphosphine)nickel, Ni-00193

$C_{20}H_{62}AuB_{18}N_2$
Bis[undecahydro-1,2-dicarbaundecaborato(2−)]aurate(2−); Bis(tetraethylammonium) salt, *in* Au-00026

$C_{21}H_{12}F_{10}Ni$
Bis(pentafluorophenyl)[(1,2,3,4,5,6-η)-1,3,5-trimethylbenzene]nickel, Ni-00194

$C_{21}H_{15}AuFeNO_4P$
Tricarbonylnitrosyl[(triphenylphosphine)aurio]iron, Au-00075

$C_{21}H_{15}BrNi$
Bromo(η^3-triphenyl-2-cyclopropen-1-yl)nickel, *in* Ni-00332

$C_{21}H_{15}ClF_5N_3O_4Pd$
(Pentafluorophenyl)tris(pyridine)palladium(1+); Perchlorate, *in* Pd-00180

$C_{21}H_{15}Cl_5N_3Ni^{\oplus}$
Pentachlorophenyltris(pyridine)nickel(1+), Ni-00195

$C_{21}H_{15}Cl_6N_3NiO_4$
Pentachlorophenyltris(pyridine)nickel(1+); Perchlorate, *in* Ni-00195

$C_{21}H_{15}CuO_2$
(Benzoato)(diphenylacetylene)copper, Cu-00054

$C_{21}H_{15}F_5N_3Pd^{\oplus}$
(Pentafluorophenyl)tris(pyridine)palladium(1+), Pd-00180

$C_{21}H_{15}NiO_3P$
Tricarbonyl(triphenylphosphine)nickel, Ni-00196

$C_{21}H_{15}O_3PPt$
Tricarbonyl(triphenylphosphine)platinum, Pt-00260

$C_{21}H_{20}AsClOPt$
Carbonylchloro(ethyl)(triphenylarsine)platinum, Pt-00261

$C_{21}H_{20}BrNiP$
Bromo(η^3-2-propenyl)(triphenylphosphine)nickel, Ni-00197

$C_{21}H_{20}ClNiP$
Chloro(η^3-2-propenyl)triphenylphosphinenickel, Ni-00198

$C_{21}H_{20}ClPPt$
Chloro(η^3-2-propenyl)(triphenylphosphine)platinum, Pt-00262

$C_{21}H_{20}Cl_3PPdSn$
(η^3-2-Propenyl)(trichlorostannyl)(triphenylphosphine)-palladium, Pd-00181

$C_{21}H_{21}NiP$
Hydro-η^3-propenyl(triphenylphosphine)nickel, Ni-00199

$C_{21}H_{24}AuP$
Trimethyl(triphenylphosphine)gold, Au-00076

$C_{21}H_{27}ClOPd$
Chloro(16,17,20-η)-3-methoxy-19-nor-1,3,5(10),17(20)-pregnatetraenepalladium, *in* Pd-00305

$C_{21}H_{30}Ni$
Tris[(2,3-η)-bicyclo[2.2.1]hept-2-ene]nickel, Ni-00200

$C_{21}H_{31}F_6OP_3Pt$
[Dihydro-2(3*H*)-furanylidene]-bis(dimethylphenylphosphine)methylplatinum(1+); Hexafluorophosphate, *in* Pt-00263

$C_{21}H_{31}F_6P_3Pt$
[(2,3-η)-2-Butyne]bis(dimethylphenylphosphine)-methylplatinum(1+); Hexafluorophosphate, *in* Pt-00264

$C_{21}H_{31}OP_2Pt^{\oplus}$
[Dihydro-2(3*H*)-furanylidene]-bis(dimethylphenylphosphine)methylplatinum(1+), Pt-00263

$C_{21}H_{31}PPtS$
Phenyl(phenylthio)(tripropylphosphine)platinum, *in* Pt-00422

$C_{21}H_{31}P_2Pt^{\oplus}$
[(2,3-η)-2-Butyne]bis(dimethylphenylphosphine)-methylplatinum(1+), Pt-00264

$C_{21}H_{34}F_6NP_3Pt$
[(Dimethylamino)ethylidene]bis(dimethylphenylphosphine)-methylplatinum(1+); Hexafluorophosphate, *in* Pt-00265

$C_{21}H_{34}NP_2Pt^{\oplus}$
[(Dimethylamino)ethylidene]bis(dimethylphenylphosphine)-methylplatinum(1+), Pt-00265

$C_{21}H_{38}BrNiP$
Bromo(η^3-2-propenyl)(tricyclohexylphosphine)nickel, Ni-00201

$C_{21}H_{38}ClPPt$
Chloro(η^3-2-propenyl)(tricyclohexylphosphine)platinum, Pt-00266

$C_{21}H_{41}BrP_2Pt$
Bromobis(triethylphosphine)(2,4,6-trimethylphenyl)-platinum, Pt-00267

$C_{21}H_{41}ClP_2Pt$
Chlorobis(triethylphosphine)(2,4,6-trimethylphenyl)-platinum, Pt-00268

$C_{22}H_8Cl_2F_{10}N_2Pd$
Dichloro(2,2′-bipyridine)bis(pentafluorophenyl)-palladium, Pd-00182

$C_{22}H_8F_{10}N_2Pd$
(2,2′-Bipyridine)bis(pentafluorophenyl)palladium, Pd-00183

$C_{22}H_{15}BrNiO$
Bromo(carbonyl)(η^3-1,2,3-triphenyl-2-cyclopropen-1-yl)-nickel, Ni-00202

$C_{22}H_{15}ClNiO$
Carbonylchloro(η^3-1,2,3-triphenyl-2-cyclopropen-1-yl)-nickel, Ni-00203

$C_{22}H_{16}Cl_2N_2Pd_2$
Di-μ-chlorobis[2-(2-pyridinyl)phenyl-*C*,*N*]dipalladium, Pd-00184

$C_{22}H_{18}N_2Pt$
(2,2′-Bipyridine-*N*,*N*′)diphenylplatinum, Pt-00269

$C_{22}H_{20}N_2Pt$
Diphenylbis(pyridine)platinum, Pt-00270

$C_{22}H_{20}Ni_2S_2$
Bis(η^5-2,4-cyclopentadien-1-yl)bis(μ-phenylthiolato)-dinickel, Ni-00204

$C_{22}H_{20}Ni_3$
Tris(η^5-2,4-cyclopentadien-1-yl)[μ_3-(phenylmethylidyne)]-trinickel, Ni-00205

$C_{22}H_{22}AsClPd$
Chloro[(1,2,3-η)-2-methyl-2-propenyl](triphenylarsine)-palladium, Pd-00185

$C_{22}H_{22}ClNiP$
[(1,2,3-η)-2-Butenyl]chloro(triphenylphosphine)nickel, Ni-00206

$C_{22}H_{22}ClPPd$
Chloro[(1,2,3-η)-2-methyl-2-propenyl)]-(triphenylphosphine)palladium, Pd-00186

$C_{22}H_{22}Ni$
(1,5-Cyclooctadiene)(diphenylacetylene)nickel, Ni-00207

$C_{22}H_{23}AsPt$
Bis(ethylene)(triphenylarsine)platinum, Pt-00271

$C_{22}H_{23}NiP$
Methyl(η^3-2-propenyl)(triphenylphosphine)nickel, Ni-00208

$C_{22}H_{23}PPt$
Bis(ethylene)(triphenylphosphine)platinum, Pt-00272

$C_{22}H_{25}NiO_2P$
Cyclooctenyl[(diphenylphosphino)acetato-*O*,*P*]nickel, Ni-00209

$C_{22}H_{26}AuP$
Trimethyl(triphenylmethylenephosphorane)gold, Au-00077

$C_{22}H_{28}N_4Ni$
(Azobenzene)bis(*tert*-butylisocyanide)nickel, Ni-00210

$C_{22}H_{30}Cl_2O_2Pd_2$
Di-μ-chlorobis[(2,3,5-η)-3*a*,4,5,6,7,7*a*-hexahydro-6-methoxy-4,7-methano-1*H*-inden-5-yl]dipalladium, Pd-00187

$C_{22}H_{30}Cl_2O_2Pt_2$
Di-μ-chlorobis[(2,3,5-η)-3*a*,4,5,6,7,7*a*-hexahydro-6-methoxy-4,7-methano-1*H*-inden-5-yl]diplatinum, Pt-00273

$C_{22}H_{30}Ni_2O_2$
Di-μ-carbonylbis[(1,2,3,4,5-η)-1,2,3,4,5-pentamethyl-2,4-cyclopentadien-1-yl]dinickel, Ni-00211

$C_{22}H_{33}ClP_2Pt$
Chlorobis(diethylphenylphosphine)ethenylplatinum, Pt-00274

$C_{22}H_{33}NiP$
Bisethylene(triphenylphosphine)nickel, Ni-00212

$C_{22}H_{34}Cl_2O_4Pd_2$
Di-μ-chlorobis[(1,2,3-η)-8-methoxy-2,6-dimethyl-8-oxo-2,6-octadienyl]dipalladium, Pd-00188

$C_{22}H_{34}Cl_2Pd_2$
Di-μ-chlorobis(η^3-2-ethylidene-6,6-dimethylbicyclo[3.1.1]hept-3-yl)dipalladium, Pd-00189

$C_{22}H_{35}ClF_6NOP_3Pt$
Chloro[dimethylamino(3-hydroxypropyl)methylene]-bis(dimethylphenylphosphine)platinum(1+); Hexafluorophosphate, *in* Pt-00275

$C_{22}H_{35}ClNOP_2Pt^{\oplus}$
Chloro[dimethylamino(3-hydroxypropyl)methylene]-bis(dimethylphenylphosphine)platinum(1+), Pt-00275

$C_{22}H_{36}NiP_2$
(3-Methylphenyl)(2,4,6-trimethylphenyl)-bis(trimethylphosphine)nickel, Ni-00213

$C_{22}H_{36}P_2Pt$
Biscyclopropylbis(dimethylphenylphosphine)platinum, Pt-00276

$C_{22}H_{38}Cl_2Pd_2$
Di-μ-chlorobis(η^3-5-*tert*-butyl-2-methylenecyclohexyl)-dipalladium, Pd-00190

$C_{22}H_{41}AuCl_3N$
N,*N*,*N*-Tributyl-1-butanaminium trichlorophenylaurate, *in* Au-00031

$C_{22}H_{41}NiP$
Bis(ethylene)tricyclohexylphosphinenickel, Ni-00214

$C_{22}H_{41}PPt$
Bis(ethylene)(tricyclohexylphosphine)platinum, Pt-00277

$C_{22}H_{42}Cl_2Pd_2$
Di-μ-chlorobis[(1,2,3-η)-1,1,5-trimethyl-2-octenyl]-dipalladium, Pd-00191

$C_{22}H_{47}Cl_2NPd$
Dichloro(η3-2-propenyl)palladate(1−); Hexadecyltrimethylammonium salt, *in* Pd-00008

$C_{22}O_{22}Pt_{19}^{\ominus\ominus\ominus\ominus}$
Deca-μ-carbonyldodecacarbonylnonadecaplatinate(4−), Pt-00278

$C_{23}H_{20}AgP$
(η5-2,4-Cyclopentadien-1-yl)triphenylphosphinesilver, Ag-00033

$C_{23}H_{20}AuP$
2,4-Cyclopentadien-1-yl(triphenylphosphine)gold, Au-00078

$C_{23}H_{20}BrNiP$
Bromo(η5-2,4-cyclopentadien-1-yl)(triphenylphosphine)-nickel, Ni-00215

$C_{23}H_{20}BrPPd$
Bromo(η5-2,4-cyclopentadien-1-yl)(triphenylphosphine)-palladium, Pd-00192

$C_{23}H_{20}ClNiP$
Chloro(η5-2,4-cyclopentadien-1-yl)-triphenylphosphinenickel, Ni-00216

$C_{23}H_{20}Cl_3GeNiP$
(η5-2,4-Cyclopentadien-1-yl)(trichlorogermyl)-(triphenylphosphine)nickel, Ni-00217

$C_{23}H_{20}Cl_3NiPSn$
(η5-2,4-Cyclopentadien-1-yl)(trichlorostannyl)-(triphenylphosphine)nickel, Ni-00218

$C_{23}H_{20}CuP$
(η5-2,4-Cyclopentadien-1-yl)triphenylphosphinecopper, Cu-00055

$C_{23}H_{21}IN_2Pt$
(2,2′-Bipyridine-*N*,*N*′)iodomethyldiphenylplatinum, Pt-00279

$C_{23}H_{22}AuO_2P$
(1-Acetyl-2-oxopropyl)(triphenylphosphine)gold, Au-00079

$C_{23}H_{23}NiO_2P$
(Acetato-*O*)(η3-2-propenyl)(triphenylphosphine)nickel, Ni-00219

$C_{23}H_{28}B_9NiP$
[Decahydro-7-methyl-π-7-phospha-10-carbaundecaborato(1−)](triphenyl-π-cyclopropenyl)-nickel, Ni-00220

$C_{23}H_{33}ClO_2Pd$
Chloro(16,17,20-η)-3β-acetoxy-17-ethylidene-5-androstenepalladium, *in* Pd-00316

$C_{23}H_{37}NiO_3P$
Tricarbonyl[1-(tricyclohexylphosphonio)ethyl]nickel, Ni-00221

$C_{23}H_{39}NiP$
(η5-2,4-Cyclopentadien-1-yl)-hydro(tricyclohexylphosphine)nickel, Ni-00222

$C_{23}H_{40}AuB_{18}P$
Bis[undecahydro-1,2-dicarbaundecaborato(2−)]aurate(1−); Methyltriphenylphosphonium salt, *in* Au-00025

$C_{23}H_{40}B_{18}CuP$
Bis[(7,8,9,10,11-η)-undecahydro-7,8-dicarbaundecaborato(2−)]cuprate(1−); Methyltriphenylphosphonium salt, *in* Cu-00014

$C_{24}Br_2F_{20}Pd_2^{\ominus\ominus}$
Di-μ-bromotetrakis(pentafluorophenyl)dipalladate(2−), Pd-00193

$C_{24}Cl_2F_{20}Pd_2^{\ominus\ominus}$
Di-μ-chlorotetrakis(pentafluorophenyl)dipalladate(2−), Pd-00194

$C_{24}Cu_4F_{20}$
(Pentafluorophenyl)copper; Tetramer(?), *in* Cu-00019

$C_{24}F_{20}Ni^{\ominus\ominus}$
Tetrakis(pentafluorophenyl)nickelate(2−), Ni-00223

$C_{24}F_{20}Pd^{\ominus\ominus}$
Tetrakis(pentafluorophenyl)palladate(2−), Pd-00195

$C_{24}H_{15}ClF_5PPd$
Chloro(pentafluorophenyl)(triphenylphosphine)palladium, *in* Pd-00318

$C_{24}H_{15}Cl_6NiP$
Chloro(pentachlorophenyl)(triphenylphosphine)nickel, *in* Ni-00348

$C_{24}H_{16}N_4Ni$
Bis[1,10-phenanthroline-N^1,N^{10}]nickel, Ni-00224

$C_{24}H_{18}Cl_2N_4Pd_2$
Di-μ-chlorobis[2-(phenylazo)phenyl]dipalladium, Pd-00196

$C_{24}H_{18}N_2Ni$
(2,2′-Bipyridine)(diphenylacetylene)nickel, Ni-00225

$C_{24}H_{18}N_4Pd$
Bis[2-phenylazo(phenyl)-*C*,*N*]palladium, Pd-00197

$C_{24}H_{20}AgB$
Silver(1+) tetraphenylborate(1−), Ag-00034

$C_{24}H_{20}AuFeO_3P$
Tricarbonyl(η3-2-propenyl)[(triphenylphosphine)gold]-iron, Au-00080

$C_{24}H_{20}AuP$
Phenyl(triphenylphosphine)gold, Au-00081

$C_{24}H_{20}ClOPPt$
Carbonylchloro(η1-2,4-cyclopentadien-1-yl)-(triphenylphosphine)platinum, Pt-00280

$C_{24}H_{20}ClO_5PPd$
Carbonyl(η5-2,4-cyclopentadien-1-yl)-(triphenylphosphine)palladium(1+); Perchlorate, *in* Pd-00198

$C_{24}H_{20}ClO_5PPt$
▷Carbonyl(η5-2,4-cyclopentadien-1-yl)-(triphenylphosphine)platinum(1+); Perchlorate, *in* Pt-00281

$C_{24}H_{20}Li_2Ni$
Tetraphenylnickelate(2−); Di-Li salt, *in* Ni-00227

$C_{24}H_{20}N_2Ni_2$
Bis(η5-2,4-cyclopentadien-1-yl)bis[μ-phenylisonitrile]-dinickel, Ni-00226

$C_{24}H_{20}Ni^{\ominus\ominus}$
Tetraphenylnickelate(2−), Ni-00227

$C_{24}H_{20}Ni_2$
Di-π-cyclopentadienyl(μ-diphenylacetylene)dinickel, Ni-00228

$C_{24}H_{20}OPPd^{\oplus}$
Carbonyl(η5-2,4-cyclopentadien-1-yl)-(triphenylphosphine)palladium(1+), Pd-00198

$C_{24}H_{20}OPPt^{\oplus}$
Carbonyl(η5-2,4-cyclopentadien-1-yl)-(triphenylphosphine)platinum(1+), Pt-00281

$C_{24}H_{21}N_2NiP$
▷Bis[(1,2-η)-2-propenenitrile]triphenylphosphinenickel, Ni-00229

$C_{24}H_{22}O_2Pd$
[η3-6-(Diphenylmethylene)-2,4-cyclohexadien-1-yl](2,4-pentanedionato-*O*,*O*′)palladium, Pd-00199

$C_{24}H_{22}O_2Pt$
Acetylacetonato(η3-triphenylmethyl)platinum, Pt-00282

$C_{24}H_{23}NiP$
(η5-2,4-Cyclopentadien-1-yl)methyl(triphenylphosphine)-nickel, Ni-00230

$C_{24}H_{23}PPd$
(η^5-2,4-Cyclopentadien-1-yl)methyl(triphenylphosphine)-palladium, Pd-00200

$C_{24}H_{24}Ni$
Tris(η^2-phenylethylene)nickel, Ni-00231

$C_{24}H_{25}NiO_2P$
Methyl(2,4-pentanedionato-*O,O′*)(triphenylphosphine)-nickel, Ni-00232

$C_{24}H_{26}ClPPt$
Chloro(η^3-2-propenyl)[tris(4-methylphenyl)phosphine]-platinum, Pt-00283

$C_{24}H_{28}N_2Ni$
Di(*tert*-butylisocyanide)diphenylacetylenenickel, Ni-00233

$C_{24}H_{28}Ni^{\ominus\ominus}$
Cyclododecatrienediphenylnickelate(2−), Ni-00234

$C_{24}H_{29}PPtSn$
(η^3-2-Propenyl)(trimethylstannyl)(triphenylphosphine)-platinum, Pt-00284

$C_{24}H_{30}Cl_2F_{10}P_2Pt$
Dichlorobis(pentafluorophenyl)bis(triethylphosphine)-platinum, Pt-00285

$C_{24}H_{30}Cl_5F_5P_2Pd$
(Pentachlorophenyl)(pentafluorophenyl)-bis(triethylphosphine)palladium, Pd-00201

$C_{24}H_{30}F_6O_4Pd_2$
Bis(η^3-6,6-dimethyl-4-methylenebicyclo[3.1.1]hept-3-yl)-di-μ-(trifluoroacetato)dipalladium, Pd-00202

$C_{24}H_{30}F_{10}P_2Pt$
Bis(pentafluorophenyl)bis(triethylphosphine)platinum, Pt-00286

$C_{24}H_{30}F_{18}P_2Pt$
[(1,2-η)-Hexakis(trifluoromethyl)benzene]-bis(triethylphosphine)platinum, Pt-00287

$C_{24}H_{32}O_2Pd$
[η^3-2-(4-Methylphenyl)-2-(1,2,3,4,5-pentamethyl-2,4-cyclopentadien-1-yl)ethyl](2,4-pentanedionato-*O,O′*]palladium, Pd-00203

$C_{24}H_{34}Br_2Pt_2$
Di-μ-bromobis(η^3-1,2,4,5,6-pentamethyl-3-methylenebicyclo[2.2.0]hex-5-en-2-yl)diplatinum, Pt-00288

$C_{24}H_{34}Cl_2Pd_2$
Di-μ-chlorobis(η^3-1,2,4,5,6-pentamethyl-3-methylenebicyclo[2.2.0]hex-5-en-2-yl)dipalladium, Pd-00204

$C_{24}H_{34}Cl_2Pt_2$
Dichlorobis[μ-[η,η^4-(1,3,4,5,6-pentamethylbicyclo[2.2.0]hexa-2,5-dien-2-yl)-methyl]]diplatinum, Pt-00289
Di-μ-chlorobis(η^3-1,2,4,5,6-pentamethyl-3-methylenebicyclo[2.2.0]hex-5-en-1-yl)diplatinum, Pt-00290

$C_{24}H_{34}O_2P_2Pd$
Bis(dimethylphenylphosphine)(η^3-2-propenyl)-palladium(1+); 2,4-Pentanedionate, *in* Pd-00164

$C_{24}H_{36}Cl_6NiPt$
Bis[(1,2,3,4,5,6-η)hexamethylbenzene]nickel(2+); Hexachloro-platinate, *in* Ni-00235

$C_{24}H_{36}Cl_6Pt_3Sn_2$
Tris[(1,2,5,6-η)-1,5-cyclooctadiene]bis(μ_3-trichlorostannyl)triplatinum, Pt-00291

$C_{24}H_{36}Cl_{12}Pt_3Sn_3$
[(1,2,3,4-η)-1,2,3,4-Tetramethyl-1,3-cyclobutadiene]-tris(trichlorostannyl)platinate(1−); Trichlorobis(tetramethyl-cyclobutadiene)diplatinum salt, *in* Pt-00065

$C_{24}H_{36}Ni^{\oplus\oplus}$
Bis[(1,2,3,4,5,6-η)hexamethylbenzene]nickel(2+), Ni-00235

$C_{24}H_{36}O_2P_2Pt$
Bis(dimethylphenylphosphine)bis(3-methoxy-1-propenyl)-platinum, Pt-00292

$C_{24}H_{36}O_4Pd_2$
Bis[μ-(acetato-*O:O*)](η^3-6,6-dimethyl-2-methylenebicyclo[3.1.1]hept-3-yl)dipalladium, Pd-00205

$C_{24}H_{38}Cl_2O_4Pd_2$
Bis[η^3-2-[2-(acetyloxy)ethylidene]-6-methyl-5-heptenyl]-di-μ-chlorodipalladium, Pd-00206

$C_{24}H_{38}F_{12}N_2OP_4Pt$
Bis(dimethylphenylphosphine)[ethoxy(ethylamino)-methylene](isocyanoethane)platinum(2+); Bishexafluoro-phosphate, *in* Pt-00293

$C_{24}H_{38}N_2OP_2Pt^{\oplus\oplus}$
Bis(dimethylphenylphosphine)[ethoxy(ethylamino)-methylene](isocyanoethar e)platinum(2+), Pt-00293

$C_{24}H_{39}ClN_2P_2Pd$
Chloro[2-(phenylazo)phenyl]bis(triethylphosphine)-palladium, Pd-00207

$C_{24}H_{40}I_2P_2Pt$
Diiododiphenylbis(triethylphosphine)platinum, Pt-00294

$C_{24}H_{40}N_2NiP_2$
(Azobenzene)bis(triethylphosphine)nickel, Ni-00236

$C_{24}H_{40}NiP_2$
Diphenylbis(triethylphosphine)nickel, Ni-00237

$C_{24}H_{40}P_2Pt$
Diphenylbis(triethylphosphine)platinum, Pt-00295

$C_{24}H_{42}Cl_2O_2Pd_2$
Bis[chloro(9,10,11-η)methyl-10-undecenoate)palladium], Pd-00208

$C_{24}H_{43}NiO_2P$
Methyl(2,4-pentanedionato-*O,O′*)-tricyclohexylphosphinenickel, Ni-00238

$C_{24}H_{45}ClF_5O_4P_3Pd$
(Pentafluorophenyl)tris(triethylphosphine)palladium(1+) ; Perchlorate, *in* Pd-00209

$C_{24}H_{45}F_5P_3Pd^{\oplus}$
(Pentafluorophenyl)tris(triethylphosphine)palladium(1+) , Pd-00209

$C_{24}H_{46}P_2Pt$
Dihydro[[1,2-phenylenebis(methylene)]bis[bis(1,1-dimethylethyl)phosphine]-*P,P′*]platinum, Pt-00296

$C_{24}H_{48}Cl_4Pt_2$
Di-μ-chlorodichlorobis(1-dodecene)diplatinum, Pt-00297

$C_{24}H_{52}Cl_2P_2Pt_2$
Bis[2-(di-*tert*-butylphosphino)-2-methylpropyl-*C,P*]di-μ-chlorodiplatinum, Pt-00298

$C_{24}H_{54}As_2Pd_2$
Bis[(2,2-di-*tert*-butylarsino)-2-methylpropyl]di-μ-hydridodipalladium, Pd-00210

$C_{24}H_{54}Cl_2P_2Pt$
Dichlorobis(tributylphosphine)platinum, Pt-00299

$C_{24}H_{54}Cl_4P_2Pt_2$
Di-μ-chlorodichlorobis(tributylphosphine)diplatinum, Pt-00300

$C_{24}H_{54}P_2Pd$
Bis(tri-*tert*-butylphosphine)palladium, Pd-00211

$C_{24}H_{54}P_2Pt$
Bis(tri-*tert*-butylphosphine)platinum, Pt-00301

$C_{24}H_{55}ClP_2Pd$
Chlorohydrobis(tri-*tert*-butylphosphine)palladium, Pd-00212

$C_{24}H_{55}F_6P_3Pt$
Hydrobis(tri-*tert*-butylphosphine)platinum(1+); Hexafluoro-phosphate, *in* Pt-00302

$C_{24}H_{55}P_2Pt^{\oplus}$
Hydrobis(tri-*tert*-butylphosphine)platinum(1+), Pt-00302
$C_{24}H_{56}As_2Pt$
Dihydrobis(tri-*tert*-butylarsine)platinum, Pt-00303
$C_{24}H_{56}P_2Pt$
Dihydrobis(tri-*tert*-butylphosphine)platinum, Pt-00304
$C_{24}H_{60}Cl_4Pt_4$
Tetra-μ_3-chlorododecaethyltetraplatinum, *in* Pt-00043
$C_{24}H_{60}Cl_{15}N_3PtSn_5$
Pentakis(trichlorostannyl)platinate(3−); Tris(tetraethylammonium) salt, *in* Pt-00476
$C_{24}H_{60}Cu_4I_4O_{12}P_4$
Iodo(triethyl phosphite-*P*)copper; Tetramer(?), *in* Cu-00024
$C_{24}H_{60}Cu_4I_4P_4$
Tetra-μ_3-iodotetrakis(triethylphosphine)tetracopper, *in* Cu-00025
$C_{24}H_{60}NiO_{12}P_4$
Tetrakis(triethylphosphite-*P*)nickel, Ni-00239
$C_{24}H_{60}NiP_4$
▷Tetrakis(triethylphosphine)nickel, Ni-00240
$C_{24}H_{60}O_{12}P_4Pd$
Tetrakis(triethylphosphite-*P*)palladium, Pd-00213
$C_{24}H_{60}O_{12}P_4Pt$
Tetrakis(triethylphosphite-*P*)platinum, Pt-00305
$C_{24}H_{60}P_4Pt$
Tetrakis(triethylphosphine)platinum, Pt-00306
$C_{24}H_{61}Cl_{12}N_3PtSn_4$
Hydrotetrakis(trichlorostannyl)platinate(3−); Tris(tetraethylammonium) salt, *in* Pt-00475
$C_{24}H_{61}NiO_{12}P_4^{\oplus}$
Hydrotetrakis(triethylphosphite-*P*)nickel(1+), Ni-00241
$C_{24}H_{63}P_4Pt_2^{\oplus}$
Di-μ-hydrohydrotetrakis(triethylphosphine)diplatinum(1+), Pt-00307
$C_{24}H_{64}ClP_5Pt_2$
Dihydro-μ-phosphinotetrakis(triethylphosphine)diplatinum(1+); Chloride, *in* Pt-00308
$C_{24}H_{64}P_5Pt_2^{\oplus}$
Dihydro-μ-phosphinotetrakis(triethylphosphine)diplatinum(1+), Pt-00308
$C_{24}H_{65}Cl_2P_5Pt_2^{\oplus}$
Chlorotrihydro-μ-phosphinotetrakis(triethylphosphine)diplatinum(1+), Pt-00309
$C_{24}H_{66}Cl_2P_5Pt_2^{\oplus}$
Dichlorotetrahydro-μ-phosphinotetrakis(triethylphosphine)diplatinum(1+), Pt-00310
$C_{24}O_{24}Pt_{12}^{\ominus\ominus}$
Dodeca-μ-carbonyldodecacarbonyldodecaplatinate(2−), Pt-00311
$C_{25}H_{20}AsCl_2NPd$
Dichloro(isocyanobenzene)(triphenylarsine)palladium, Pd-00214
$C_{25}H_{20}Cl_2NPPd$
Dichloro(isocyanobenzene)(triphenylphosphine)palladium, Pd-00215
$C_{25}H_{20}Cl_2NPPt$
Dichloro(isocyanobenzene)(triphenylphosphine)platinum, Pt-00312
$C_{25}H_{21}AsCl_2OPd$
(Carbonyl)dichlorohydropalladate(1−); Tetraphenylarsonium salt, *in* Pd-00005
$C_{25}H_{21}NiP$
(η^5-2,4-Cyclopentadien-1-yl)ethynyl(triphenylphosphine)nickel, Ni-00242
$C_{25}H_{22}ClPPd$
Benzylchloro(triphenylphosphine)palladium, *in* Pd-00320
$C_{25}H_{22}Cl_2N_2OPPd$
Chloro[2-(methylnitrosoamino)phenyl](triphenylphosphine)palladium, Pd-00216
$C_{25}H_{24}AuGeO_4PRu$
Tetracarbonyl(trimethylgermyl)[(triphenylphosphine)aurio]ruthenium, Au-00082
$C_{25}H_{24}AuO_4PRuSi$
Tetracarbonyl(trimethylsilyl)[(triphenylphosphine)aurio]ruthenium, Au-00083
$C_{25}H_{24}ClO_4PPd$
▷(π-Cyclopentadienyl)ethylene(triphenylphosphine)palladium(1+); Perchlorate, *in* Pd-00217
$C_{25}H_{24}ClO_4PPt$
▷Cyclopentadienyl(ethylene)(triphenylphosphine)platinum(1+); Perchlorate, *in* Pt-00314
$C_{25}H_{24}Cl_2N_2Pt$
Dichloro(1,2-diphenyl-1,3-propanediyl)bis(pyridine)platinum, Pt-00313
$C_{25}H_{24}PPd^{\oplus}$
(π-Cyclopentadienyl)ethylene(triphenylphosphine)palladium(1+), Pd-00217
$C_{25}H_{24}PPt^{\oplus}$
Cyclopentadienyl(ethylene)(triphenylphosphine)platinum(1+), Pt-00314
$C_{25}H_{25}NiP$
(η^5-2,4-Cyclopentadien-1-yl)ethyl(triphenylphosphine)nickel, Ni-00243
$C_{25}H_{25}PPdS$
(η^5-2,4-Cyclopentadien-1-yl)[(methylthio)methyl](triphenylphosphine)palladium, Pd-00218
$C_{25}H_{28}NiO_2P$
Ethyl(2,4-pentanedionato-*O*,*O'*)triphenylphosphinenickel, Ni-00244
$C_{25}H_{31}NO_2P_2Pd$
Bis(dimethylphenylphosphine)(η^3-2-propenyl)palladium(1+); 2-Pyridinecarboxylate, *in* Pd-00164
$C_{25}H_{50}O_2P_2Pd_2$
(μ-π-Cyclopentadienyl)(μ-acetato)bis(triisopropylphosphine)dipalladium, Pd-00219
$C_{25}H_{62}F_6NP_5Pt_2$
[μ-(Cyano-*C*:*N*)]dihydrotetrakis(triethylphosphine)diplatinum(1+); Hexafluorophosphate, *in* Pt-00315
$C_{25}H_{62}NP_4Pt_2^{\oplus}$
[μ-(Cyano-*C*:*N*)]dihydrotetrakis(triethylphosphine)diplatinum(1+), Pt-00315
$C_{25}H_{64}O_2P_4Pt_2$
Di-μ-hydrohydrotetrakis(triethylphosphine)diplatinum(1+); Formate, *in* Pt-00307
$C_{26}H_{13}CuN_3O_6$
Matchamycin, Cu-00056
$C_{26}H_{20}Ni$
(η^5-2,4-Cyclopentadien-1-yl)[(1,2,3-η)-1,2,3-triphenyl-2-cyclopropen-1-yl]nickel, Ni-00245
$C_{26}H_{24}Cl_2NiP_2$
Dichloro[1,2-ethanediylbis(diphenylphosphine)-*P*,*P'*]nickel, Ni-00246
$C_{26}H_{27}AsBClF_4Pt$
Chloro[(1,2,5,6-η)-1,5-cyclooctadiene](triphenylarsine)platinum(1+); Tetrafluoroborate, *in* Pt-00316
$C_{26}H_{27}AsClPt^{\oplus}$
Chloro[(1,2,5,6-η)-1,5-cyclooctadiene](triphenylarsine)platinum(1+), Pt-00316
$C_{26}H_{27}NiP$
(π-Cyclopentadienyl)isopropyl(triphenylphosphine)nickel, Ni-00247
(η^5-2,4-Cyclopentadien-1-yl)propyl(triphenylphosphine)nickel, Ni-00248
[(1,2,3,6,7,8-η)-2,6-Octadiene-1,8-diyl](triphenylphosphine)nickel, Ni-00249

$C_{26}H_{32}Cl_2Fe_2N_2Pd_2$
Di-μ-chlorobis[2-[(dimethylamino)methyl]ferrocenyl-*C*,*N*]-dipalladium, Pd-00220

$C_{26}H_{35}F_6O_2P_3Pt$
Bis(dimethylphenylphosphine)-methyl[methoxy(phenylmethyl)methylene]-platinum(1+); Hexafluorophosphate, *in* Pt-00317

$C_{26}H_{35}OP_2Pt^{\oplus}$
Bis(dimethylphenylphosphine)-methyl[methoxy(phenylmethyl)methylene]-platinum(1+), Pt-00317

$C_{26}H_{39}NiP_3$
Tris(dimethylphenylphosphine)dimethylnickel, Ni-00250

$C_{26}H_{44}P_2Pt$
Bis(2-methylphenyl)bis(triethylphosphine)platinum, Pt-00318
Dibenzylbis(triethylphosphine)platinum, Pt-00319

$C_{26}H_{45}NiP$
[(1,2,3,8-η)-2,6-Octadiene-1,8-diyl]-(tricyclohexylphosphine)nickel, Ni-00251

$C_{26}H_{46}Cl_2Pd_2$
Di-μ-chlorobis[(1,2,3-η)-2,8-dimethyl-2,10-undecadienyl]dipalladium, Pd-00221

$C_{26}H_{54}Br_2Ni_2P_2$
Dibromo(2,6-octadiene-1,8-diyl)-bis(triisopropylphosphine)dinickel, Ni-00252

$C_{26}H_{56}Cl_2P_2Pt_2$
Bis[3-(di-*tert*-butylphosphino)-2,2-dimethylpropyl-*C*,*P*]-di-μ-chlorodiplatinum, Pt-00320

$C_{26}H_{56}Cl_4N_2O_2Pt_2$
Dicarbonyltetrachlorodiplatinate(2−); Bistetrapropylammonium salt, *in* Pt-00008

$C_{26}H_{56}P_2Pd_2$
Bis[μ-[(1-η:2,3-η)-2-methyl-2-propenyl]]bis[tris(1-methylethyl)phosphine]dipalladium, Pd-00222

$C_{27}H_{20}F_5PPt$
Pentafluorophenyl(η^3-2-propenyl)(triphenylphosphine)-platinum, Pt-00321

$C_{27}H_{24}F_3IP_2Pd$
[Ethylenebis[diphenylphosphine]]iodo(trifluoromethyl)-palladium, Pd-00223

$C_{27}H_{25}AuNOP$
[Methoxy[(4-methylphenyl)imino]methyl]-(triphenylphosphine)gold(I), Au-00084

$C_{27}H_{25}Cl_2PPd$
Dichloro(η^3-2-propenyl)palladate(1−); Tetraphenylphosphonium salt, *in* Pd-00008

$C_{27}H_{26}ClF_3P_2Pt$
Chlorobis(methyldiphenylphosphine)(trifluoromethyl)-platinum, Pt-00322

$C_{27}H_{27}ClP_2Pt$
Chloro[ethylenebis[diphenylphosphine]]methylplatinum, Pt-00323

$C_{27}H_{28}OP_2Pt$
[1,2-Ethanediylbis(diphenylphosphine)-*P*,*P′*]-hydroxy(methyl)platinum, Pt-00324

$C_{27}H_{28}P_2Pt$
[Bis(diphenylphosphino)methane]dimethylplatinum, Pt-00325

$C_{27}H_{29}ClP_2Pt$
Chloro(methyl)bis(methyldiphenylphosphine)platinum, Pt-00326

$C_{27}H_{29}IP_2Pd$
Iodo(methyl)bis(methyldiphenylphosphine)palladium, Pd-00224

$C_{27}H_{29}NiP$
Butyl(η^5-2,4-cyclopentadien-1-yl)(triphenylphosphine)-nickel, Ni-00253

$C_{27}H_{29}PPd$
Butyl(η^5-2,4-cyclopentadien-1-yl)(triphenylphosphine)-palladium, Pd-00225

$C_{27}H_{35}NiP_2$
Bis(dimethylphenylphosphine)ethynyl(2,4,6-trimethylphenyl)nickel, Ni-00254

$C_{27}H_{43}ClOPd$
Chloro[(4,5,6-η)-3-oxo-5-cholesten-4-yl]palladium, *in* Pd-00327

$C_{27}H_{45}NiP$
(Tricyclohexylphosphine)[(1,2,2′,5,5′,6-η)-2,3,5-tris(methylene)-1,6-hexanediyl]nickel, Ni-00255

$C_{27}H_{63}P_3Pt$
Tris(triisopropylphosphine)platinum, Pt-00327

$C_{28}H_{20}Br_2Ni$
(Tetraphenylcyclobutadienyl)dibromonickel, Ni-00256

$C_{28}H_{20}Br_2Pd$
Dibromo(tetraphenylcyclobutadiene)palladium, *in* Pd-00330

$C_{28}H_{20}Cl_2Pd$
Dichloro(tetraphenylcyclobutadiene)palladium, *in* Pd-00331

$C_{28}H_{20}Cl_2Pt$
Dichloro(tetraphenylcyclobutadiene)platinum, *in* Pt-00461

$C_{28}H_{20}Ni_2O_4P_2$
Tetracarbonylbis[μ-(diphenylphosphino)]dinickel, Ni-00257

$C_{28}H_{20}Pt$
Bis(diphenylacetylene)platinum, Pt-00328

$C_{28}H_{24}As_2NiO_2$
Dicarbonyl[1,2-ethanediylbis[diphenylarsine]]nickel, Ni-00258

$C_{28}H_{24}AuFeP$
1-[(Triphenylphosphine)aurio]ferrocene, Au-00085

$C_{28}H_{24}F_5INiP_2$
[1,2-Ethanediylbis(diphenylphosphine)-*P*,*P′*]-iodopentafluoroethylnickel, Ni-00259

$C_{28}H_{24}NiO_2P_2$
Dicarbonyl[ethylenebis[diphenylphosphine]]nickel, Ni-00260

$C_{28}H_{26}ClF_5P_2Pt$
Chlorobis(methyldiphenylphosphine)(pentafluoroethyl)-platinum, Pt-00329

$C_{28}H_{26}NiO_2P_2$
Dicarbonylbis(methyldiphenylphosphine)nickel, Ni-00261

$C_{28}H_{27}ClP_2Pd$
Chloro[methylenebis[diphenylphosphine]-*P*,*P′*](η^3-2-propenyl)palladium, *in* Pd-00226

$C_{28}H_{27}P_2Pd^{\oplus}$
[Methylenebis[diphenylphosphine]-*P*,*P′*](η^3-2-propenyl)-palladium(1+), Pd-00226

$C_{28}H_{29}ClP_2Pt$
Chloroethyl[ethylenebis[diphenylphosphine]]platinum, Pt-00330

$C_{28}H_{29}INNiP$
(η^5-2,4-Cyclopentadien-1-yl)(2-isocyano-2-methylpropane)(triphenylphosphine)nickel(1+); Iodide, *in* Ni-00262

$C_{28}H_{29}NNiP^{\oplus}$
(η^5-2,4-Cyclopentadien-1-yl)(2-isocyano-2-methylpropane)(triphenylphosphine)nickel(1+), Ni-00262

$C_{28}H_{29}O_4PPd$
(1-Acetyl-2-oxopropyl)(2,4-pentanedionato-*O*,*O′*)-(triphenylphosphine)palladium, Pd-00227

$C_{28}H_{30}AuClP_2$
[1,2-Ethanediylbis[diphenylphosphine]-*P*,*P′*]-dimethylgold(1+); Chloride, *in* Au-00086

$C_{28}H_{30}AuP_2^{\oplus}$
[1,2-Ethanediylbis[diphenylphosphine]-*P*,*P′*]-dimethylgold(1+), Au-00086

$C_{28}H_{30}BrNiP$
Bromo[(1,2,3,4,5-η)-1,2,3,4,5-pentamethyl-2,4-cyclopentadien-1-yl](triphenylphosphine)nickel, Ni-00263

$C_{28}H_{30}CuP$
(η^5-Pentamethylcyclopentadienyl)-triphenylphosphinecopper, Cu-00057

$C_{28}H_{30}INiP$
Iodo[(1,2,3,4,5-η)-1,2,3,4,5-pentamethyl-2,4-cyclopentadien-1-yl](triphenylphosphine)nickel, Ni-00264

$C_{28}H_{30}P_2Pd$
[Ethylenebis[diphenylphosphine]]dimethylpalladium, Pd-00228

$C_{28}H_{30}P_2Pt$
[Ethylenebis[diphenylphosphine]]dimethylplatinum, Pt-00331

$C_{28}H_{31}ClP_2Pt$
Chlorohydrobis(ethyldiphenylphosphine)platinum, Pt-00332

$C_{28}H_{32}P_2Pd$
Dimethylbis(methyldiphenylphosphine)palladium, Pd-00229

$C_{28}H_{32}P_2Pt$
Dimethylbis(methyldiphenylphosphine)platinum, Pt-00333

$C_{28}H_{35}ClP_2Pt$
Chlorobis(diethylphenylphosphine)(phenylethynyl)-platinum, Pt-00334

$C_{28}H_{36}AuF_{10}N$
Bis(pentafluorophenyl)aurate(1−); Tetrabutylammonium salt, *in* Au-00065

$C_{28}H_{39}ClNiO_5P_2$
Bis(dimethylphenylphosphine)(1-methoxyethylidene)-(2,4,6-trimethylphenyl)nickel(1+); Perchlorate, *in* Ni-00265

$C_{28}H_{39}NiOP_2^{\oplus}$
Bis(dimethylphenylphosphine)(1-methoxyethylidene)-(2,4,6-trimethylphenyl)nickel(1+), Ni-00265

$C_{28}H_{40}As_2Pt$
Bis(phenylethynyl)bis(triethylarsine)platinum, Pt-00335

$C_{28}H_{40}N_2O_{12}Pt_6$
Hexa-μ-carbonylhexacarbonylhexaplatinate(2−); Bis(tetraethylammonium) salt, *in* Pt-00136

$C_{28}H_{40}NiP_2$
Bis(phenylethynyl)bis(triethylphosphine)nickel, Ni-00266

$C_{28}H_{40}P_2Pd$
Bis(phenylethynyl)bis(triethylphosphine)palladium, Pd-00230

$C_{28}H_{40}P_2Pt$
Bis(phenylethynyl)bis(triethylphosphine)platinum, Pt-00336

$C_{28}H_{46}P_2Pd$
Bis(di-*tert*-butylphenylphosphine)palladium, Pd-00231

$C_{28}H_{46}P_2Pt$
Bis(di-*tert*-butylphenylphosphine)platinum, Pt-00337

$C_{28}H_{48}P_4Pd$
Bis[1,2-bis(diethylphosphino)benzene]palladium, Pd-00232

$C_{28}H_{49}NiP$
[(1,2,3,8-η)-2,6-dimethyl-2,6-octadiene-1,8-diyl]-tricyclohexylphosphinenickel, Ni-00267

$C_{28}H_{52}N_2Ni_5O_{12}$
Dodecacarbonylpentanickelate(2−); Bis(tetraethylammonium) salt, *in* Ni-00101

$C_{28}H_{52}N_4Ni$
Tetrakis(isocyanocyclohexane)nickel, Ni-00268

$C_{28}H_{52}Ni_2P_2$
Bis[μ-(dicyclohexylphosphino)]bis(η^2-ethene)dinickel, Ni-00269

$C_{28}H_{52}P_2Pd_2$
Di-μ-cyclopentadienylbis(triisopropylphosphine)-dipalladium, Pd-00233

$C_{28}H_{56}NiP_2$
Diethynylbis(tributylphosphine)nickel, Ni-00270

$C_{29}H_{20}F_5NiP$
(η^5-2,4-Cyclopentadien-1-yl)(pentafluorophenyl)-(triphenylphosphine)nickel, Ni-00271

$C_{29}H_{25}BrNPPd$
Bromo[1-(8-quinolinyl)ethyl-*C*,*N*](triphenylphosphine)-palladium, Pd-00234

$C_{29}H_{25}BrNPPt$
Bromo[1-(8-quinolinyl)ethyl-*C*,*N*]-triphenylphosphineplatinum, Pt-00338

$C_{29}H_{25}ClNPPd$
Chloro[1-(8-quinolinyl)ethyl-*C*,*N*](triphenylphosphine)-palladium, Pd-00235

$C_{29}H_{25}NiP$
(η^5-2,4-Cyclopentadien-1-yl)phenyl(triphenylphosphine)-nickel, Ni-00272

$C_{29}H_{25}PPd$
(η^5-2,4-Cyclopentadien-1-yl)phenyl(triphenylphosphine)-palladium, Pd-00236

$C_{29}H_{27}NiO_2P$
(2,4-Pentanedionato-*O*,*O′*)phenyl(triphenylphosphine)-nickel, Ni-00273

$C_{29}H_{33}BCuN_3O$
[*N*-(2-Aminoethyl)-1,2-ethanediamine-*N*,*N′*,*N″*]-carbonylcopper)(1+); Tetraphenylborate, *in* Cu-00018

$C_{29}H_{33}NiP$
Methyl[(1,2,3,4,5-η)-1,2,3,4,5-pentamethyl-2,4-cyclopentadien-1-yl](triphenylphosphine)nickel, Ni-00274

$C_{30}H_{20}Ni_2O_6P_2$
Hexacarbonylbis[μ-(diphenylphosphino)]dinickel, Ni-00275

$C_{30}H_{25}ClOPd$
Chloro[(1,2,3-η)-4-ethoxy-1,2,3,4-tetraphenyl-2-cyclobuten-1-yl]palladium, *in* Pd-00336

$C_{30}H_{26}O_3P_2Pd$
[1,2-Ethanediylbis(diphenylphosphine)-*P*,*P′*][(3,4-η)-2,5-furandione]palladium, Pd-00237

$C_{30}H_{26}P_2Pd$
[1,2-Ethanediylbis(diphenylphosphine)-*P*,*P′*]-diethynylpalladium, Pd-00238

$C_{30}H_{27}NiO_3P$
Benzoyl(2,4-pentanedionato-*O*,*O′*)(triphenylphosphine)-nickel, Ni-00277

$C_{30}H_{28}N_2P_2Pd$
Bis(cyanomethyl)[1,2-ethanediylbis[diphenylphosphine]-*P*,*P′*]palladium, Pd-00239

$C_{30}H_{30}F_6Ni_6P$
Hexakis(η^5-2,4-cyclopentadien-1-yl)hexanickel(1+); Hexafluorophosphate, *in* Ni-00279

$C_{30}H_{30}Ni_6$
Hexakis(η^5-2,4-cyclopentadien-1-yl)hexanickel, Ni-00278
Hexakis(η^5-2,4-cyclopentadien-1-yl)hexanickel(1+), Ni-00279

$C_{30}H_{30}O_2P_2Pt$
Dicarbonylbis(ethyldiphenylphosphine)platinum, Pt-00339

$C_{30}H_{31}BrNiP_2$
Bromo[ethane-1,2-diylbis[diphenylphosphine]](η^3-2-methyl-2-propenyl)nickel, Ni-00280

$C_{30}H_{31}Cl_3GeNNiP$
(η^5-2,4-Cyclopentadien-1-yl)(isocyanocyclohexane)-(triphenylphosphine)nickel(1+); Trichlorogermanate, *in* Ni-00281

$C_{30}H_{31}F_6P_3Pt$
[1,2-Ethanediylbis(diphenylphosphine)-*P*,*P'*](1,2,3-η)-2-methyl-2-propenyl]platinum(1+); Hexafluorophosphate, *in* Pt-00340

$C_{30}H_{31}INNiP$
(η^5-2,4-Cyclopentadien-1-yl)(isocyanocyclohexane)-(triphenylphosphine)nickel(1+); Iodide, *in* Ni-00281

$C_{30}H_{31}NNiP^{\oplus}$
(η^5-2,4-Cyclopentadien-1-yl)(isocyanocyclohexane)-(triphenylphosphine)nickel(1+), Ni-00281

$C_{30}H_{31}P_2Pt^{\oplus}$
[1,2-Ethanediylbis(diphenylphosphine)-*P*,*P'*](1,2,3-η)-2-methyl-2-propenyl]platinum(1+), Pt-00340

$C_{30}H_{32}AuClI_2N_4O_4$
Bis[bis[(4-methylphenyl)amino]methylene]diiodogold(1+); Perchlorate, *in* Au-00087

$C_{30}H_{32}AuI_2N_4^{\oplus}$
Bis[bis[(4-methylphenyl)amino]methylene]diiodogold(1+), Au-00087

$C_{30}H_{33}NiP$
[(1,2,5,6,9,10-η)-1,5,9-Cyclododecatriene]-(triphenylphosphine)nickel, Ni-00282

$C_{30}H_{34}NiP_2$
[1,2-Ethanediylbis[diphenylphosphine]-*P*,*P'*]-diethylnickel, Ni-00283

$C_{30}H_{34}Ni_2$
Bis(cyclooctadiene)(μ-diphenylacetylene)dinickel, Ni-00284

$C_{30}H_{34}P_2Pd$
Diethyl[ethylenebis[diphenylphosphine]]palladium, Pd-00240

$C_{30}H_{34}P_2Pt$
Diethyl[ethylenebis[diphenylphosphine]]platinum, Pt-00341

$C_{30}H_{36}NiP_2$
Bis(dimethylphenylphosphine)bis(2-methylphenyl)nickel, Ni-00285

$C_{30}H_{36}P_2Pd$
Diethylbis(methyldiphenylphosphine)palladium, Pd-00241

$C_{30}H_{38}P_2Pt$
Tetramethylbis(methyldiphenylphosphine)platinum, Pt-00342

$C_{30}H_{52}Br_2P_2Pt_2$
Di-μ-bromodiphenylbis(tripropylphosphine)diplatinum, Pt-00343

$C_{30}H_{52}I_2P_2Pt_2$
Di-μ-iododiphenylbis(tripropylphosphine)diplatinum, Pt-00344

$C_{30}H_{54}F_{12}N_6P_2Pd_2$
Hexakis(2-isocyano-2-methylpropane)dipalladium(2+); Bis(hexafluorophosphate), *in* Pd-00242

$C_{30}H_{54}N_6Pd_2^{\oplus\oplus}$
Hexakis(2-isocyano-2-methylpropane)dipalladium(2+), Pd-00242

$C_{30}H_{54}N_6Pt_3$
Tris-μ-(2-isocyano-2-methylpropane)tris(2-isocyano-2-methylpropane)triplatinum, Pt-00345

$C_{30}H_{67}F_6P_5Pt_2$
μ-Hydrohydrophenyltetrakis(triethylphosphine)-diplatinum(1+); Hexafluorophosphate, *in* Pt-00346

$C_{30}H_{67}P_4Pt_2^{\oplus}$
μ-Hydrohydrophenyltetrakis(triethylphosphine)-diplatinum(1+), Pt-00346

$C_{30}O_{30}Pt_{15}^{\ominus\ominus}$
Pentadeca-μ-carbonylpentadecacarbonylpentadecaplatinate(2−), Pt-00347

$C_{31}H_{25}ClN_2Ni$
Chlorobis(pyridine)[(1,2,3-η)-1,2,3-triphenyl-2-cyclopropen-1-yl]nickel, Ni-00286

$C_{31}H_{29}Br_4Ni_2P_2$
(π-Cyclopentadienyl)[ethylenebis[diphenylphosphine]]-nickel(1+); Tetrabromonickelate, *in* Ni-00287

$C_{31}H_{29}Cl_4Ni_2P_2$
(π-Cyclopentadienyl)[ethylenebis[diphenylphosphine]]-nickel(1+); Tetrachloronickelate, *in* Ni-00287

$C_{31}H_{29}F_6NiP_3$
(π-Cyclopentadienyl)[ethylenebis[diphenylphosphine]]-nickel(1+); Hexafluorophosphate, *in* Ni-00287

$C_{31}H_{29}INiP_2$
(π-Cyclopentadienyl)[ethylenebis[diphenylphosphine]]-nickel(1+); Iodide, *in* Ni-00287

$C_{31}H_{29}NiP_2^{\oplus}$
(π-Cyclopentadienyl)[ethylenebis[diphenylphosphine]]-nickel(1+), Ni-00287

$C_{31}H_{31}BF_4OP_2Pt$
Carbonylhydrobis(triethylphosphine)platinum(1+); Tetrafluoroborate, *in* Pt-00145

$C_{31}H_{34}AsClO_2Pt$
[8-(1-Acetyl-2-oxopropyl)-4-cycloocten-1-yl]-chloro(triphenylarsine)platinum, Pt-00348

$C_{31}H_{35}P_3Pd$
[(Diethylphosphinidenio)bis(methylene)]-[[methylenebis(diphenylphosphinato)](1−)-*P*,*P'*]-palladium, Pd-00243

$C_{32}H_{20}K_2Pd$
Tetrakis(phenylethynyl)palladate(2−); Di-K salt, *in* Pd-00244

$C_{32}H_{20}K_4Ni$
▷Tetrakis(phenylethynyl)nickelate(4−); Tetra-K salt, *in* Ni-00289

$C_{32}H_{20}Li_2Ni$
Tetrakis(phenylethynyl)nickelate(2−); Di-Li salt, *in* Ni-00288

$C_{32}H_{20}Ni^{\ominus\ominus}$
Tetrakis(phenylethynyl)nickelate(2−), Ni-00288
Tetrakis(phenylethynyl)nickelate(4−), Ni-00289

$C_{32}H_{20}Pd^{\ominus\ominus}$
Tetrakis(phenylethynyl)palladate(2−), Pd-00244

$C_{32}H_{24}N_4P_2Pd$
[Ethylenebis[diphenylphosphine]](tetracyanoethylene)-palladium, Pd-00245

$C_{32}H_{26}ClF_5P_2Pd$
Chlorobis(methyldiphenylphosphine)(pentafluorophenyl)-palladium, Pd-00246

$C_{32}H_{28}Cl_2Pd$
Dichloro[tetrakis(4-methylphenyl)cyclobutadiene]-palladium, *in* Pd-00338

$C_{32}H_{28}Pt_2$
[μ-[(1,2,5,6-η:3,4,7,8-η)-Cyclooctatetraene]]-tetraphenyldiplatinum, Pt-00349

$C_{32}H_{29}ClP_2Pt$
Chloro[ethylenebis(diphenylphosphine)]phenylplatinum, Pt-00350

$C_{32}H_{30}P_2Pd$
[Ethylenebis[diphenylphosphine]]bis(propynyl)palladium, Pd-00247

$C_{32}H_{31}ClP_2Pt$
Chlorobis(methyldiphenylphosphine)phenylplatinum, Pt-00351

$C_{32}H_{32}AsAuN_{16}$
Tetrakis(1-methyl-1*H*-tetrazol-5-yl)aurate(1−); Tetraphenylarsonium salt, *in* Au-00055

$C_{32}H_{32}P_2Pt$
Bis(dimethylphenylphosphine)bis(phenylethynyl)platinum, Pt-00352

$C_{32}H_{35}B_9Pd$
(1,2,3,4-Tetraphenyl-1,3-cyclobutadiene)[nonahydro-1,2-dimethyl-1,2-dicarbaundecaborato(2−)]palladium, Pd-00248

$C_{32}H_{40}Ag_6Br_2N_4$
Di-μ-bromotetrakis[μ_3-(2-dimethylamino)phenyl-*C*,*C*,*N*]-hexasilver, Ag-00035

$C_{32}H_{40}Br_2Cu_6N_4$
Di-μ-bromotetrakis[μ_3-(2-dimethylaminophenyl-*C*:*C*:*N*)]-hexacopper, Cu-00058

$C_{32}H_{40}NiP_2$
Bis(4-phenyl-1,3-butadiynyl)bis(triethylphosphine)-nickel, Ni-00290

$C_{32}H_{44}NiP_4$
Tetrakis(dimethylphenylphosphine)nickel, Ni-00291

$C_{32}H_{48}Br_4Ni_2$
Dibromo(1,2,3,4,5,6,7,8,9,10,11,12-dodecahydrocyclobuta[1,2:3,4]dicyclooctenenickel; Dimer, *in* Ni-00148

$C_{32}H_{50}Cl_2O_4Pd_2$
Di-μ-chlorobis[(1,2,3-η)-12-methoxy-2,6,10-trimethyl-12-oxo-2,6,10-dodecatrienyl]dipalladium, Pd-00249

$C_{32}H_{60}NiP_2$
[(2,3-η)-2,3-Dimethyl-2-butene][1,2-ethanediylbis(dicyclohexylphosphine)-*P*,*P*′]nickel, Ni-00292

$C_{32}H_{66}NiP_2$
▷[(1,2,5,6-η)-1,5-Cyclooctadiene]bis(tributylphosphine)-nickel, Ni-00293

$C_{33}H_{25}BrNi$
(η^5-2,4-Cyclopentadien-1-yl)(1,2,3,4-tetraphenyl-1,3-cyclobutadiene)nickel(1+); Bromide, *in* Ni-00294

$C_{33}H_{25}BrPd$
(η^5-2,4-Cyclopentadien-1-yl)(tetraphenyl-1,3-cyclobutadiene)palladium(1+); Bromide, *in* Pd-00250

$C_{33}H_{25}Br_4FePd$
(η^5-2,4-Cyclopentadien-1-yl)(tetraphenyl-1,3-cyclobutadiene)palladium(1+); Tetrabromoferrate, *in* Pd-00250

$C_{33}H_{25}Ni^{\oplus}$
(η^5-2,4-Cyclopentadien-1-yl)(1,2,3,4-tetraphenyl-1,3-cyclobutadiene)nickel(1+), Ni-00294

$C_{33}H_{25}Pd^{\oplus}$
(η^5-2,4-Cyclopentadien-1-yl)(tetraphenyl-1,3-cyclobutadiene)palladium(1+), Pd-00250

$C_{33}H_{35}BF_4P_2Pd$
[1,2-Ethanediylbis[diphenylphosphine]-*P*,*P*′](η^3-2-methylenecyclohexyl)palladium(1+); Tetrafluoroborate, *in* Pd-00251

$C_{33}H_{35}P_2Pd^{\oplus}$
[1,2-Ethanediylbis[diphenylphosphine]-*P*,*P*′](η^3-2-methylenecyclohexyl)palladium(1+), Pd-00251

$C_{33}H_{48}BP_3Pd$
Hydrotris(trimethylphosphine)palladium(1+); Tetraphenylborate, *in* Pd-00050

$C_{34}H_{28}Cl_2FeP_2Pd$
[1,1′-Bis(diphenylphosphino)ferrocene-*P*,*P*′]-dichloropalladium, Pd-00252

$C_{34}H_{28}O_2Pd$
Bis[η^2-1,5-diphenyl-1,4-pentadien-3-one]palladium, Pd-00253

$C_{34}H_{28}O_2Pt$
Bis[(C^3,O^3-η)-1,5-diphenyl-1,4-pentadien-3-one]-platinum, Pt-00353

$C_{34}H_{30}Ni_2P_2$
Bis(η^5-2,4-cyclopentadien-1-yl)bis[μ-(diphenylphosphino)]dinickel, Ni-00295

$C_{34}H_{34}P_2Pd$
Bis(methyldiphenylphosphine)(styrene)palladium, Pd-00254

$C_{34}H_{36}F_{12}P_4Pd$
[(1,2,5,6-η)-1,5-Cyclooctadiene][1,2-ethanediylbis[diphenylphosphine]-*P*,*P*′]-palladium(2+); Bis(hexafluorophosphate), *in* Pd-00255

$C_{34}H_{36}P_2Pd^{\oplus\oplus}$
[(1,2,5,6-η)-1,5-Cyclooctadiene][1,2-ethanediylbis[diphenylphosphine]-*P*,*P*′]-palladium(2+), Pd-00255

$C_{34}H_{38}P_2Pt_2$
Bis(diphenylacetylene)bis(trimethylphosphine)-diplatinum, Pt-00354

$C_{34}H_{39}NiP$
Bis[(1,2,5,6-η)-1,5-cyclooctadiene]-triphenylphosphinenickel, Ni-00296

$C_{34}H_{40}N_2O_{18}Pt_9$
Nona-μ-carbonylnonacarbonylnonaplatinate(2−); Bis(tetraethylammonium) salt, *in* Pt-00221

$C_{34}H_{50}BP_3Pd$
Methyltris(trimethylphosphine)palladium(1+); Tetraphenylborate, *in* Pd-00064

$C_{34}H_{57}NiP$
(Tricyclohexylphosphine)bis(3-vinylcyclohexene)nickel, Ni-00297

$C_{34}H_{64}Cl_2P_4Pd_2$
Dichloro[μ-(1,4-phenylenedi-1,2-ethynediyl)]-tetrakis(triethylphosphine)dipalladium, Pd-00256

$C_{34}H_{66}NiO_2P_2$
(2,3,5,6-Tetramethyl-2,5-cyclohexadiene-1,4-dione)-bis(tributylphosphine)nickel, Ni-00298

$C_{35}H_{25}NOPd$
Nitrosyl[(1,2,3,4,5-η)-1,2,3,4,5-pentaphenyl-2,4-cyclopentadien-1-yl]palladium, Pd-00257

$C_{35}H_{30}OPd$
(η^5-2,4-Cyclopentadien-1-yl)[(1,2,3-η)-4-ethoxy-1,2,3,4-tetraphenyl-2-cyclobuten-1-yl]palladium, Pd-00258

$C_{35}H_{50}BOP_3Pd$
Acetyltris(trimethylphosphine)palladium(1+); Tetraphenylborate, *in* Pd-00070

$C_{35}H_{63}N_7Ni_4$
Heptakis(2-isocyano-2-methylpropane)tetranickel, Ni-00299

$C_{36}H_{28}Cl_2N_2O_2P_2Pd_2$
Dicarbonyldichlorobis[2-(diphenylphosphino)pyridine-*P*]-dipalladium, Pd-00259

$C_{36}H_{28}Ni$
(Cyclooctatetraene)(η^4-1,2,3,4-tetraphenylcyclobutadiene)nickel, Ni-00300

$C_{36}H_{30}Au_2Zn_2$
Tetra-μ-phenylbis(phenylzinc)digold, Au-00088

$C_{36}H_{30}Br_2NiP_2$
Dibromobis(triphenylphosphine)nickel, Ni-00301

$C_{36}H_{30}Cl_2NiP_2$
▷Dichlorobis(triphenylphosphine)nickel, Ni-00302

$C_{36}H_{30}Cl_2P_2Pd$
▷Dichlorobis(triphenylphosphine)palladium, Pd-00260

$C_{36}H_{30}Cl_2P_2Pt$
▷Dichlorobis(triphenylphosphine)platinum, Pt-00355

$C_{36}H_{30}CuNO_3P_2$
Nitratobis(triphenylphosphine)copper, Cu-00059

$C_{36}H_{30}Cu_5^{\ominus}$
Hexa-μ-phenylpentacuprate(1−), Cu-00060

$C_{36}H_{30}NOP_2Pd$
Nitrosylbis(triphenylphosphine)palladium, Pd-00261

$C_{36}H_{30}O_2P_2Pt$
(Dioxygen)bis(triphenylphosphine)platinum, Pt-00356

$C_{36}H_{31}ClP_2Pd$
Chlorohydrobis(triphenylphosphine)palladium, Pd-00262

$C_{36}H_{31}ClP_2Pt$
Chlorohydrobis(triphenylphosphine)platinum, Pt-00357

$C_{36}H_{31}Cl_3P_2PtSn$
Hydro(trichlorostannyl)bis(triphenylphosphine)platinum, Pt-00358

$C_{36}H_{32}Ni$
(1,5-Cyclooctadiene)(η^4-1,2,3,4-tetraphenylcyclobutadiene)nickel, Ni-00303

$C_{36}H_{34}BCuP_2$
[Tetrahydroborato(1−)-*H,H'*]bis(triphenylphospine)-copper, Cu-00062

$C_{36}H_{40}NiP_2$
Methyl(2,4,6-trimethylphenyl)-bis(methyldiphenylphosphine)nickel, Ni-00304

$C_{36}H_{44}Ag_4$
Tetrakis(1,3,5-trimethylbenzene)tetrasilver, *in* Ag-00023

$C_{36}H_{46}Cl_2Pd_2$
Di-μ-chlorobis[2-[(2,3-η)-1,2,3,4,5-pentamethyl-2,4-cyclopentadien-1-yl]-2-phenylethyl]dipalladium, Pd-00263

$C_{36}H_{48}Ag_2Li_2N_4$
Tetrakis[μ-[2-[(dimethylamino)methyl]phenyl-*C,C,N*]-bis(silver)dilithium, Ag-00036

$C_{36}H_{48}Au_2Cu_2N_4$
Tetrakis[2-[(dimethylamino)methyl]phenyl]bis(copper)-digold, Au-00089

$C_{36}H_{48}Au_2Li_2N_4$
Tetrakis[μ-[2-[(dimethyamino)methyl]phenyl-*C,C,N*]]-bis(gold)dilithium, Au-00090

$C_{36}H_{52}P_4Pt_2$
Dihydrobis-μ-(diphenylphosphino)bis(triethylphosphine)-diplatinum, Pt-00359

$C_{36}H_{56}Pt_4S_4$
Tetrakis[μ_3-(benzenethiolato)]-dodecamethyltetraplatinum, *in* Pt-00084

$C_{36}H_{60}Li_2N_4Ni$
Cyclododecatrienediphenylnickelate(2−); Di-Li salt, bis(T-MEDA) complex, *in* Ni-00234

$C_{36}H_{66}P_2Pt$
Bis(tricyclohexylphosphine)platinum, Pt-00360

$C_{36}H_{67}ClNiP_2$
Chlorohydrobis(tricyclohexylphosphine)nickel, Ni-00305

$C_{36}H_{67}ClP_2Pd$
Chlorohydrobis(tricyclohexylphosphine)palladium, Pd-00264

$C_{36}H_{68}Ni_2P_4$
Di-μ-*o*-phenylenetetrakis(triethylphosphine)dinickel, Ni-00306

$C_{36}H_{68}P_2Pd$
Dihydrobis(tricyclohexylphosphine)palladium, Pd-00265

$C_{36}H_{68}P_2Pt$
Dihydrobis(tricyclohexylphosphine)platinum, Pt-00361

$C_{36}H_{70}P_2Pt_2$
Di-μ-hydrodihydrobis(tricyclohexylphosphine)diplatinum, Pt-00362

$C_{36}H_{71}BNiP_2$
Hydro[tetrahydroborato(1−)-*H,H'*]-bis(tricyclohexylphosphine)nickel, Ni-00307

$C_{36}H_{71}BP_2Pd$
Hydro[tetrahydroborato(1−)-*H,H'*]-bis(tricyclohexylphosphine)palladium, Pd-00266

$C_{36}H_{72}N_6Ni$
Tetrakis(cyano-*C*)nickelate(2−); Bis(tetrabutylammonium) salt, *in* Ni-00013

$C_{36}H_{84}NiO_{12}P_4$
Tetrakis(triisopropylphosphite)nickel, Ni-00308

$C_{36}H_{87}P_3Pt_3$
Tri-μ-hydrotrihydrotris(tri-*tert*-butylphosphine)-triplatinum, Pt-00363

$C_{36}O_{36}Pt_{18}^{\ominus\ominus}$
Octadeca-μ-carbonyloctadecacarbonyloctadecaplatinate(2−), Pt-00364

$C_{37}H_{30}BClF_4OP_2Pt$
Carbonylchlorobis(triphenylphosphine)platinum(1+); Tetrafluoroborate, *in* Pt-00365

$C_{37}H_{30}ClOP_2Pt^{\oplus}$
Carbonylchlorobis(triphenylphosphine)platinum(1+), Pt-00365

$C_{37}H_{30}Cl_2O_5P_2Pt$
Carbonylchlorobis(triphenylphosphine)platinum(1+); Perchlorate, *in* Pt-00365

$C_{37}H_{30}F_3IP_2Pd$
Iodotrifluoromethylbis(triphenylphosphine)palladium, Pd-00267

$C_{37}H_{30}F_3IP_2Pt$
Iodo(trifluoromethyl)bis(triphenylphosphine)platinum, Pt-00366

$C_{37}H_{30}OP_2PtS$
(Carbon oxysulfide)bis(triphenylphosphine)platinum, Pt-00367

$C_{37}H_{30}P_2PdS_2$
[(*C,S*-η)-Carbon disulfide]bis(triphenylphosphine)-palladium, Pd-00268

$C_{37}H_{30}P_2PtS_2$
(Carbon disulfide-*C,S*)bis(triphenylphosphine)platinum, Pt-00368

$C_{37}H_{30}P_2PtSe_2$
[(*C,Se*-η)-Carbondiselenide]bis(triphenylphosphine)-platinum, Pt-00369

$C_{37}H_{31}BF_4OP_2Pt$
Carbonylhydrobis(triphenylphosphine)platinum(1+); Tetrafluoroborate, *in* Pt-00371

$C_{37}H_{31}ClO_5P_2Pt$
Carbonylhydrobis(triphenylphosphine)platinum(1+); Perchlorate, *in* Pt-00371

$C_{37}H_{31}Cl_3OP_2PtSn$
Carbonylhydrobis(triphenylphosphine)platinum(1+); Trichlorostannate, *in* Pt-00371

$C_{37}H_{31}F_3P_2Pt$
Hydro(trifluoromethyl)bis(triphenylphosphine)platinum, Pt-00370

$C_{37}H_{31}OP_2Pt^{\oplus}$
Carbonylhydrobis(triphenylphosphine)platinum(1+), Pt-00371

$C_{37}H_{33}BrP_2Pt$
Bromo(methyl)bis(triphenylphosphine)platinum, Pt-00372

$C_{37}H_{33}ClP_2Pt$
Chloromethylbis(triphenylphosphine)platinum, Pt-00373

$C_{37}H_{33}IP_2Pd$
Iodomethylbis(triphenylphosphine)palladium, Pd-00269

$C_{37}H_{33}IP_2Pt$
Iodomethylbis(triphenylphosphine)platinum, Pt-00374

$C_{37}H_{33}I_3P_2Pt$
Triiodo(methyl)bis(triphenylphosphine)platinum, Pt-00375

$C_{37}H_{44}O_5P_4Pt_4$
Penta-μ-carbonyltetrakis(dimethylphenylphosphine)-tetraplatinum, Pt-00376

$C_{37}H_{51}BOP_2Pt$
Carbonylhydrobis(triethylphosphine)platinum(1+); Tetraphenylborate, *in* Pt-00145

$C_{37}H_{59}BNiP_4$
Methyltetrakis(trimethylphosphine)nickel(1+); Tetraphenylborate, *in* Ni-00108

$C_{37}H_{66}NiO_2P_2$
[(*C,O*-η)-Carbon dioxide]bis(tricyclohexylphosphine)-nickel, Ni-00309

$C_{37}H_{70}P_2Pt$
Hydromethylbis(tricyclohexylphosphine)platinum, Pt-00377

$C_{38}H_{24}Cl_{10}P_2Pd$
[Ethylenebis[diphenylphosphine]]bis(pentachlorophenyl)-palladium, Pd-00270

$C_{38}H_{26}Cl_5F_5NiP_2$
Bis(methyldiphenylphosphine)(pentachlorophenyl)-(pentafluorophenyl)nickel, Ni-00310

$C_{38}H_{26}F_{10}NiP_2$
Bis(methyldiphenylphosphine)bis(pentafluorophenyl)-nickel, Ni-00311

$C_{38}H_{30}As_2F_4Pt$
(Tetrafluoroethylene)bis(triphenylarsine)platinum, Pt-00378

$C_{38}H_{30}As_2NiO_2$
Dicarbonylbis(triphenylarsine)nickel, Ni-00312

$C_{38}H_{30}AuFeNO_3P_2$
Dicarbonylnitrosyl(triphenylphosphine)-[(triphenylphosphine)aurio]iron, Au-00091

$C_{38}H_{30}Cl_4P_2Pd$
Chloro(trichlorovinyl)bis(triphenylphosphine)palladium, Pd-00271

$C_{38}H_{30}Cl_4P_2Pt$
(Tetrachloroethylene)bis(triphenylphosphine)platinum, Pt-00379

$C_{38}H_{30}F_3NP_2Pt$
[(*N*,1-*η*)-Trifluoroacetonitrile]bis(triphenylphosphine)-platinum, Pt-00380

$C_{38}H_{30}F_4P_2Pt$
(Tetrafluoroethylene)bis(triphenylphosphine)platinum, Pt-00381

$C_{38}H_{30}F_5IP_2Pt$
Iodo(pentafluoroethyl)bis(triphenylphosphine)platinum, Pt-00382

$C_{38}H_{30}NiO_2P_2$
Dicarbonylbis(triphenylphosphine)nickel, Ni-00313

$C_{38}H_{30}NiO_2Sb_2$
Dicarbonylbis(triphenylstibine)nickel, Ni-00314

$C_{38}H_{30}NiO_5P_2$
Dicarbonyl(triphenylphosphine)(triphenylphosphite-*P*)-nickel, Ni-00315

$C_{38}H_{30}NiO_8P_2$
Dicarbonylbis(triphenylphosphite-*P*)nickel, Ni-00316

$C_{38}H_{30}O_2P_2Pt$
Dicarbonylbis(triphenylphosphine)platinum, Pt-00383

$C_{38}H_{31}Cl_3P_2Pd$
Chloro(2,2-dichlorovinyl)bis(triphenylphosphine)-palladium, Pd-00272

$C_{38}H_{32}ClNP_2Pd$
Chloro(cyanomethyl)bis(triphenylphosphine)palladium, Pd-00273

$C_{38}H_{32}ClNP_2Pt$
Chloro(cyanomethyl)bis(triphenylphosphine)platinum, Pt-00384

$C_{38}H_{32}Cl_2P_2Pd$
Chloro(2-chlorovinyl)bis(triphenylphosphine)palladium, Pd-00274

$C_{38}H_{32}F_2NiP_2$
(1,1-Difluoroethylene)bis(triphenylphosphine)nickel, Ni-00317

$C_{38}H_{32}N_2Ni_9O_{18}$
Octadecacarbonylnonanickelate(2−); Bis(benzyltrimethylammonium) salt, *in* Ni-00172

$C_{38}H_{32}P_2Pt$
Acetylenebis(triphenylphosphine)platinum, Pt-00385

$C_{38}H_{33}ClOP_2Pd$
Acetylchlorobis(triphenylphosphine)palladium, Pd-00275

$C_{38}H_{33}NP_2Pt$
Cyanomethylhydrobis(triphenylphosphine)platinum, Pt-00386

$C_{38}H_{34}AgClP_2$
Bis[(triphenylphosphonio)methyl]silver(1+); Chloride, *in* Ag-00037

$C_{38}H_{34}AgP_2^{\oplus}$
Bis[(triphenylphosphonio)methyl]silver(1+), Ag-00037

$C_{38}H_{34}NiP_2$
Ethylenebis(triphenylphosphine)nickel, Ni-00318

$C_{38}H_{34}P_2Pd$
Ethylenebis(triphenylphosphine)palladium, Pd-00276

$C_{38}H_{34}P_2Pt$
[1,2-Ethanediylbis[diphenylphosphine]-*P*,*P*′]-diphenylplatinum, Pt-00387
Ethylenebis(triphenylphosphine)platinum, Pt-00388

$C_{38}H_{35}ClNiP_2$
Chloro(ethyl)bis(triphenylphosphine)nickel, Ni-00319

$C_{38}H_{35}ClP_2PdS$
Chloro[(methylthio)methyl]bis(triphenylphosphine)-palladium, Pd-00277

$C_{38}H_{36}Cl_8P_2PtSn_2$
Dichlorobis(trichlorostannyl)platinate(2−); Bis(triphenylmethylphosphonium) salt, *in* Pt-00474

$C_{38}H_{36}P_2Pd$
Dimethylbis(triphenylphosphine)palladium, Pd-00278

$C_{38}H_{36}P_2Pt$
Dimethylbis(triphenylphosphine)platinum, Pt-00389

$C_{38}H_{41}AgB_8P_2$
Bis(triphenylphosphine)[(7,8,9,-*η*)undecahydro-5,6-dicarbadecaborato(1−)]silver, Ag-00038

$C_{38}H_{55}BP_2Pt$
Ethylene(hydrido)bis(triethylphosphine)platinum(1+); Tetraphenylborate, *in* Pt-00168

$C_{38}H_{66}NiO_2P_2$
Dicarbonylbis(tricyclohexylphosphine)nickel, Ni-00320

$C_{38}H_{70}NiP_2$
Ethylenebis(tricyclohexylphosphine)nickel, Ni-00321

$C_{38}H_{70}P_2Pd$
Ethylenebis(tricyclohexylphosphine)palladium, Pd-00279

$C_{38}H_{84}P_4Pt_2$
Bis[bis(di-*tert*-butylphosphino)propane]diplatinum, Pt-00390

$C_{38}H_{87}P_4Pt_2^{\oplus}$
μ-Hydrodihydrobis[1,3-propanediylbis[bis(1,1-dimethylethyl)phosphine]-*P*,*P*′]diplatinum(1+), Pt-00391

$C_{38}H_{90}N_2Pt$
Hexamethylplatinate(2−); Bis(tetrabutylammonium) salt, *in* Pt-00046

$C_{39}H_{30}F_6NiOP_2$
[Oxy[trifluoro-1-(trifluoromethyl)ethylidene]]-bis(triphenylphosphine)nickel, Ni-00322

$C_{39}H_{30}F_6NiP_2S$
[Thio[trifluoro-1-(trifluoromethyl)ethylidene]]-bis(triphenylphosphine)nickel, Ni-00323

$C_{39}H_{30}F_6OP_2Pd$
(1,1,1,3,3,3-Hexafluoro-2-propanone)-bis(triphenylphosphine)palladium, Pd-00280

$C_{39}H_{30}F_6OP_2Pt$
[Oxy[trifluoro-1-(trifluoromethyl)ethylidene]]-bis(triphenylphosphine)platinum, Pt-00392

$C_{39}H_{30}F_7IP_2Pt$
Iodo(heptafluoropropyl)bis(triphenylphosphine)platinum, Pt-00393

$C_{39}H_{31}F_6NP_2Pt$
[(*N*,2-*η*)-1,1,1,3,3,3-Hexafluoro-2-propanimine]-bis(triphenylphosphine)platinum, Pt-00394

$C_{39}H_{31}F_7P_2Pt$
(1,1,1,3,3,3-Hexafluoro-2-propyl)-fluorobis(triphenylphosphine)platinum, Pt-00395

$C_{39}H_{33}NNiP_2$
[(2,3-*η*)-2-Propenenitrile]bis(triphenylphosphine)-nickel, Ni-00324

$C_{39}H_{34}P_2Pt$
[(1,2-η)-1,2-Propadiene]bis(triphenylphosphine)-platinum, Pt-00396

$C_{39}H_{35}BF_4P_2Pd$
(η^3-2-Propenyl)bis(triphenylphosphine)palladium(1+); Tetrafluoroborate, *in* Pd-00282

$C_{39}H_{35}BF_4P_2Pt$
(η^3-2-Propenyl)bis(triphenylphosphine)platinum(1+); Tetrafluoroborate, *in* Pt-00398

$C_{39}H_{35}ClO_4P_2Pd$
(η^3-2-Propenyl)bis(triphenylphosphine)palladium(1+); Perchlorate, *in* Pd-00282

$C_{39}H_{35}ClO_4P_2Pt$
(η^3-2-Propenyl)bis(triphenylphosphine)platinum(1+); Perchlorate, *in* Pt-00398

$C_{39}H_{35}ClP_2Pt$
Chloro-2-propenylbis(triphenylphosphine)platinum, Pt-00397
(η^3-2-Propenyl)bis(triphenylphosphine)platinum(1+); Chloride, *in* Pt-00398

$C_{39}H_{35}Cl_3P_2PtSn$
(η^3-2-Propenyl)bis(triphenylphosphine)platinum(1+); Trichlorostannate, *in* Pt-00398

$C_{39}H_{35}F_6P_3Pt$
(η^3-2-Propenyl)bis(triphenylphosphine)platinum(1+); Hexafluorophosphate, *in* Pt-00398

$C_{39}H_{35}IP_2Pd_2$
μ-Iodo[μ-(1-η:2,3-η)-2-propenyl]bis(triphenylphosphine)-dipalladium, Pd-00281

$C_{39}H_{35}P_2Pd^{\oplus}$
(η^3-2-Propenyl)bis(triphenylphosphine)palladium(1+), Pd-00282

$C_{39}H_{35}P_2Pt^{\oplus}$
(η^3-2-Propenyl)bis(triphenylphosphine)platinum(1+), Pt-00398

$C_{39}H_{39}ClP_2PbPt$
Chloro(trimethylplumbyl)bis(triphenylphosphine)-platinum, Pt-00399

$C_{39}H_{39}ClP_2PtSn$
(Chlorodimethylstannyl)methylbis(triphenylphosphine)-platinum, Pt-00400

$C_{39}H_{43}AgBP$
Tris(methyldiphenylphosphine)[tetrahydroborato(1−)-*H*]-silver, Ag-00039

$C_{39}H_{43}BCuP$
Tris(methyldiphenylphosphine)[tetrahydroborato(1−)-*H*]-copper, Cu-00064

$C_{39}H_{43}BN_2Ni$
(η^5-2,4-Cyclopentadien-1-yl)bis(2-isocyano-2-methylpropane)nickel(1+); Tetraphenylborate, *in* Ni-00132

$C_{39}H_{55}BP_2Pd$
(η^3-2-Propenyl)bis(triethylphosphine)palladium(1+); Tetraphenylborate, *in* Pd-00112

$C_{39}H_{71}F_6P_3Pt$
(η^3-2-Propenyl)bis(tricyclohexylphosphine)platinum(1+); Hexafluorophosphate, *in* Pt-00401

$C_{39}H_{71}P_2Pt^{\oplus}$
(η^3-2-Propenyl)bis(tricyclohexylphosphine)platinum(1+), Pt-00401

$C_{39}H_{81}O_3P_3Pt_3$
Tricarbonyltris(tri-*tert*-butylphosphine)triplatinum, Pt-00402

$C_{39}H_{90}OP_4Pt_2$
μ-Hydrodihydrobis[1,3-propanediylbis[bis(1,1-dimethylethylphosphine]-*P,P′*]diplatinum(1+); Methoxide, *in* Pt-00391

$C_{40}H_{28}N_2Ni$
(1,10-Phenanthroline)(η^4-1,2,3,4-tetraphenylcyclobutadiene)nickel, Ni-00325

$C_{40}H_{30}Au_2FeO_4P_2$
Tetracarbonylbis[(triphenylphosphine)aurio]iron, Au-00092

$C_{40}H_{30}Au_2O_4OsP_2$
Tetracarbonylbis[(triphenylphosphine)gold]osmium, Au-00093

$C_{40}H_{30}Cl_2N_2P_2Pt$
(Dichlorodicyanoethylene)bis(triphenylphosphine)-platinum, Pt-00403

$C_{40}H_{30}F_6P_2Pd$
[(2,3-η)-1,1,1,4,4,4-Hexafluoro-2-butyne]-bis(triphenylphosphine)palladium, Pd-00283

$C_{40}H_{30}F_6P_2Pt$
[(2,3-η)-1,1,1,4,4,4-Hexafluoro-2-butyne]-bis(triphenylphosphine)platinum, Pt-00404

$C_{40}H_{30}F_8NiP_2$
(Octafluoro-1,4-butanediyl)bis(triphenylphosphine)-nickel, Ni-00326

$C_{40}H_{30}F_8P_2Pt$
[(2,3-η)-1,1,1,2,3,4,4,4-Octafluoro-2-butene]-bis(triphenylphosphine)platinum, Pt-00405

$C_{40}H_{30}N_2P_2Pt$
[(2,3-η)-2-Butynedinitrile]bis(triphenylphosphine)-platinum, Pt-00406

$C_{40}H_{32}O_3P_2Pd$
[(3,4-η)-2,5-Furandione]bis(triphenylphosphine)-palladium, Pd-00284

$C_{40}H_{35}ClN_2O_2P_2Pd$
Chloro(1-diazo-2-ethoxy-2-oxoethyl)-bis(triphenylphosphine)palladium, Pd-00285

$C_{40}H_{36}NiP_2$
[(2,3-η)-2-Butyne]bis(triphenylphosphine)nickel, Ni-00327

$C_{40}H_{36}O_4P_2Pd$
Bis(acetato-*O*)bis(triphenylphosphine)palladium, Pd-00286

$C_{40}H_{36}P_2Pd$
(2-Methylene-1,3-propanediyl)bis(triphenylphosphine)-palladium, Pd-00287

$C_{40}H_{36}P_2Pt$
[(1,2-η)-3-Methylcyclopropene]bis(triphenylphosphine)-platinum, Pt-00407

$C_{40}H_{37}BF_4P_2Pd$
[(1,2,3-η)-2-Methyl-2-propenyl]bis(triphenylphosphine)-palladium(1+); Tetrafluoroborate, *in* Pd-00288

$C_{40}H_{37}ClO_4P_2Pt$
[(1,2,3-η)-2-Methyl-2-propenyl]bis(triphenylphosphine)-platinum(1+); Perchlorate, *in* Pt-00408

$C_{40}H_{37}ClP_2Pd$
[(1,2,3-η)-2-Methyl-2-propenyl]bis(triphenylphosphine)-palladium(1+); Chloride, *in* Pd-00288

$C_{40}H_{37}ClP_2Pt$
[(1,2,3-η)-2-Methyl-2-propenyl]bis(triphenylphosphine)-platinum(1+); Chloride, *in* Pt-00408

$C_{40}H_{37}F_6P_3Pd$
[(1,2,3-η)-2-Methyl-2-propenyl]bis(triphenylphosphine)-palladium(1+); Hexafluorophosphate, *in* Pd-00288

$C_{40}H_{37}F_6P_3Pt$
[(1,2,3-η)-2-Methyl-2-propenyl]bis(triphenylphosphine)-platinum(1+); Hexafluorophosphate, *in* Pt-00408

$C_{40}H_{37}P_2Pd^{\oplus}$
[(1,2,3-η)-2-Methyl-2-propenyl]bis(triphenylphosphine)-palladium(1+), Pd-00288

$C_{40}H_{37}P_2Pt^{\oplus}$
[(1,2,3-η)-2-Methyl-2-propenyl]bis(triphenylphosphine)-platinum(1+), Pt-00408

$C_{40}H_{40}P_2Pt$
Diethylbis(triphenylphosphine)platinum, Pt-00409

$C_{40}H_{42}P_2PbPt$
Methyl(trimethylplumbyl)bis(triphenylphosphine)-platinum, Pt-00410

$C_{40}H_{52}Ag_2B_{16}P_2$
11-Bis[triphenylphosphine-11-argenta-5,6-dicarbundecaborane(11)], *in* Ag-00032

$C_{40}H_{52}BOP_3Pd$
Benzoyltris(trimethylphosphine)palladium(1+); Tetraphenylborate, *in* Pd-00130

$C_{40}H_{56}Cu_4N_4$
Tetrakis[μ-[2-[(dimethylamino)methyl]-5-methylphenyl-*C*:*C*,*N*]]tetracopper, Cu-00065

$C_{40}H_{57}BP_2Pd$
[(1,2,3-η)-2-Butenyl]bis(triethylphosphine)-palladium(1+); Tetraphenylborate, *in* Pd-00131

$C_{40}H_{57}BP_2Pt$
[(1,2,3-η)-2-Butenyl]bis(triethylphosphine)platinum(1+); Tetraphenylborate, *in* Pt-00187

$C_{40}H_{60}Li_2NiO_4$
Cyclododecatrienediphenylnickelate(2−); Di-Li salt, tetrakis(THF) complex, *in* Ni-00234

$C_{40}H_{60}NiO_8P_4$
Tetrakis(diethyl phenylphosphonite-*P*)nickel, Ni-00328

$C_{40}H_{60}NiP_4$
Tetrakis(diethylphenylphosphine)nickel, Ni-00329

$C_{40}H_{66}F_6P_2Pt$
[(2,3-η)-1,1,1,4,4,4-Hexafluoro-2-butyne]-bis(tricyclohexylphosphine)platinum, Pt-00411

$C_{40}H_{72}F_{20}N_2Ni$
Tetrakis(pentafluorophenyl)nickelate(2−); Bis(tetrabutylammonium) salt, *in* Ni-00223

$C_{40}H_{72}N_2Ni_3O_8$
Tetra-μ-carbonyltetracarbonyltrinickelate(2−); Bis(tetrabutylammonium) salt, *in* Ni-00062

$C_{40}H_{73}ClP_2Pd_2$
μ-Chloro[μ-[(1-η:2,3-η)-2-methyl-2-propenyl]]-bis(tricyclohexylphosphine)dipalladium, Pd-00289

$C_{40}H_{74}NiP_2$
[(2,3-η)-2-Butene]bis(tricyclohexylphosphine)nickel, Ni-00330

$C_{41}H_{35}As_2F_6PPd$
($η^5$-2,4-Cyclopentadien-1-yl)bis(triphenylarsine)-palladium(1+); Hexafluorophosphate, *in* Pd-00290

$C_{41}H_{35}As_2Pd^{\oplus}$
($η^5$-2,4-Cyclopentadien-1-yl)bis(triphenylarsine)-palladium(1+), Pd-00290

$C_{41}H_{35}BrP_2Pd_2$
μ-Bromo-μ-(2,4-cyclopentadien-1-yl)-bis(triphenylphosphine)palladium, Pd-00291

$C_{41}H_{35}Cl_3NiP_2Sn$
($η^5$-2,4-Cyclopentadien-1-yl)bis(triphenylphosphine)-nickel(1+); Trichlorostannate, *in* Ni-00331

$C_{41}H_{35}F_6PPdSb_2$
($η^5$-2,4-Cyclopentadien-1-yl)bis(triphenylantimony)-palladium(1+); Hexafluorophosphate, *in* Pd-00293

$C_{41}H_{35}F_6P_3Pd$
($η^5$-2,4-Cyclopentadien-1-yl)bis(triphenylphosphine)-palladium(1+); Hexafluorophosphate, *in* Pd-00292

$C_{41}H_{35}INiP_2$
($η^5$-2,4-Cyclopentadien-1-yl)bis(triphenylphosphine)-nickel(1+); Iodide, *in* Ni-00331

$C_{41}H_{35}NiP_2^{\oplus}$
($η^5$-2,4-Cyclopentadien-1-yl)bis(triphenylphosphine)-nickel(1+), Ni-00331

$C_{41}H_{35}P_2Pd^{\oplus}$
($η^5$-2,4-Cyclopentadien-1-yl)bis(triphenylphosphine)-palladium(1+), Pd-00292

$C_{41}H_{35}PdSb_2^{\oplus}$
($η^5$-2,4-Cyclopentadien-1-yl)bis(triphenylantimony)-palladium(1+), Pd-00293

$C_{41}H_{38}P_2Pt$
[(1,2-η)-1,2-Dimethylcyclopropene]-bis(triphenylphosphine)platinum, Pt-00412

$C_{41}H_{42}BClOP_2Pt$
Carbonylchlorobis(dimethylphenylphosphine)platinum(1+); Tetraphenylborate, *in* Pt-00190

$C_{41}H_{72}F_5N_5Pd$
Tricyano(pentafluorophenyl)palladate(2−); Bis(tetrabutylammonium) salt, *in* Pd-00045

$C_{42}H_{30}As_2BrF_5Pd$
Bromo(pentafluorophenyl)bis(triphenylarsine)palladium, Pd-00294

$C_{42}H_{30}BrF_5P_2Pd$
Bromo(pentafluorophenyl)bis(triphenylphosphine)-palladium, Pd-00295

$C_{42}H_{30}Br_2Ni_2$
Di-μ-bromobis[(1,2,3-η)-1,2,3-triphenyl-2-cyclopropen-1-yl]dinickel, Ni-00332

$C_{42}H_{30}ClF_5NiP_2$
Chloro(pentafluorophenyl)bis(triphenylphosphine)nickel, Ni-00333

$C_{42}H_{30}ClF_5P_2Pd$
Chloro(pentafluorophenyl)bis(triphenylphosphine)-palladium, Pd-00296

$C_{42}H_{30}Cl_4Pd_3$
Tetra-μ-chlorobis(1,2,3-triphenylcyclopropenyl)-tripalladium, Pd-00297

$C_{42}H_{30}Cu_2O_4$
Bis[μ-(benzoato-*O*,*O*′)]bis[1,1′-($η^2$-1,2-ethynediyl)-bis[benzene]]dicopper, *in* Cu-00054

$C_{42}H_{30}N_4P_2Pt$
(Tetracyanoethylene)bis(triphenylphosphine)platinum, Pt-00413

$C_{42}H_{31}F_5OP_2Pd$
Hydroxy(pentafluorophenyl)bis(triphenylphosphine)-palladium, Pd-00298

$C_{42}H_{32}ClN_3O_6P_2Pt$
Chloro(2,4,6-trinitrophenyl)bis(triphenylphosphine)-platinum, Pt-00414

$C_{42}H_{34}O_2P_2Pd$
(*p*-Benzoquinone)bis(triphenylphosphine)palladium, Pd-00299

$C_{42}H_{34}P_2Pd$
[1,2-Ethanediylbis(diphenylphosphine)-*P*,*P*′]-bis(phenylethynyl)palladium, Pd-00300

$C_{42}H_{35}Au_2BF_4P_2$
μ-Phenylbis(triphenylphosphine)digold(1+); Tetrafluoroborate, *in* Au-00094

$C_{42}H_{35}Au_2P_2^{\oplus}$
μ-Phenylbis(triphenylphosphine)digold(1+), Au-00094

$C_{42}H_{35}BrNiP_2$
Bromo(phenyl)bis(triphenylphosphine)nickel, Ni-00334

$C_{42}H_{35}BrP_2Pt$
Bromo(phenyl)bis(triphenylphosphine)platinum, Pt-00415

$C_{42}H_{35}ClNiP_2$
Chlorophenylbis(triphenylphosphine)nickel, Ni-00335

$C_{42}H_{35}ClP_2Pd$
Chlorophenylbis(triphenylphosphine)palladium, Pd-00301

$C_{42}H_{35}ClP_2Pt$
Chloro(phenyl)bis(triphenylphosphine)platinum, Pt-00416

$C_{42}H_{35}IP_2Pd$
Iodophenylbis(triphenylphosphine)palladium, Pd-00302

$C_{42}H_{35}IP_2Pt$
Iodophenylbis(triphenylphosphine)platinum, Pt-00417

$C_{42}H_{36}Ni$
Tris[(1,2-η)-1,2-diphenylethene]nickel, Ni-00336

$C_{42}H_{36}O_4P_2Pd$
[(2,3-η)-Dimethyl-2-butynedioate]-bis(triphenylphosphine)palladium, Pd-00303

$C_{42}H_{37}ClOP_2Pd$
Chloro(3-oxo-1-cyclohexen-1-yl)bis(triphenylphosphine)-palladium, Pd-00304

$C_{42}H_{38}NiO_4P_2$
[(2,3-η)-Dimethyl-2-butenedioate]-bis(triphenylphosphine)nickel, Ni-00337

$C_{42}H_{38}P_2Pt$
[(1,4-η)-Bicyclo[2.2.0]hex-1(4)-ene]-bis(triphenylphosphine)platinum, Pt-00418
[(1,2-η)-Cyclohexyne]bis(triphenylphosphine)platinum, Pt-00419

$C_{42}H_{42}NNiP_3$
[Tris(2-diphenylphosphinoethyl)amine]nickel, Ni-00338

$C_{42}H_{43}ClP_2Pt$
Chlorohydrobis(tribenzylphosphine)platinum, Pt-00420

$C_{42}H_{48}As_2Cl_9NP_2PtSn_3$
Tris(trichlorostannyl)bis(trimethylarsine)platinate(1−) ; Bis(triphenylphosphine)iminium salt, *in* Pt-00044

$C_{42}H_{48}N_{12}Ni_4O_6P_4$
Hexacarbonyltetrakis(3,3′,3″-phosphinidynetripropionitrile)tetranickel, Ni-00339

$C_{42}H_{54}Cl_2O_2Pd_2$
Di-μ-chlorobis[(16,17,20-η)-3-methoxy-19-nor-1,3,5(10),-17(20)-pregnatetraene]dipalladium, Pd-00305

$C_{42}H_{62}AsBrP_2Pt_2$
μ-Bromo-μ-(diphenylarsino)-diphenylbis(tripropylphosphine)diplatinum, Pt-00421

$C_{42}H_{62}P_2Pt_2S_2$
Diphenylbis-μ-(phenylthio)bis(tripropylphosphine)-diplatinum, Pt-00422

$C_{42}H_{65}BClF_4P_5Pd_3$
μ-Chlorobis[μ-(diphenylphosphino)]-tris(triethylphosphine)tripalladium(1+); Tetrafluoroborate, *in* Pd-00306

$C_{42}H_{65}ClP_5Pd_3^{\oplus}$
μ-Chlorobis[μ-(diphenylphosphino)]-tris(triethylphosphine)tripalladium(1+), Pd-00306

$C_{42}H_{66}BP_3Pt$
Hydrotris(triethylphosphine)platinum(1+); Tetraphenylborate, *in* Pt-00220

$C_{42}H_{72}NiP_2$
Hydrido(phenyl)bis(tricyclohexylphosphine)nickel, Ni-00340

$C_{43}H_{30}ClF_5O_5P_2Pd$
Carbonylbis(triphenylphosphine)(pentafluorophenyl)-palladium(1+); Perchlorate, *in* Pd-00307

$C_{43}H_{30}F_5OP_2Pd^{\oplus}$
Carbonylbis(triphenylphosphine)(pentafluorophenyl)-palladium(1+), Pd-00307

$C_{43}H_{35}ClNiOP_2$
Benzoylchlorobis(triphenylphosphine)nickel, Ni-00341

$C_{43}H_{35}ClOP_2Pd$
Benzoylchlorobis(triphenylphosphine)palladium, Pd-00308

$C_{43}H_{37}ClP_2Pd$
Benzylchlorobis(triphenylphosphine)palladium, Pd-00309

$C_{43}H_{40}P_2Pt$
[(1,2-η)-Cycloheptyne]bis(triphenylphosphine)platinum, Pt-00423

$C_{43}H_{63}BOP_2Pt$
Carbonyl(hydrido)bis(triisopropylphosphine)platinum(1+) ; Tetraphenylborate, *in* Pt-00239

$C_{44}H_{30}Ni_8O_8P_6$
Octacarbonylhexakis[μ_4-(phenylphosphinidine)]-octanickel, Ni-00342

$C_{44}H_{35}ClP_2Pd$
Chloro(phenylethynyl)bis(triphenylphosphine)palladium, Pd-00310

$C_{44}H_{35}ClP_2Pt$
[[Benzo[*c*]phenanthrene-2,11-diylbis(methylene)]-bis[diphenylphosphine]-*P*,*P′*]chlorohydroplatinum, Pt-00424

$C_{44}H_{36}NiOP_2$
[α-[(Diphenylphosphinomethylene)]benzenemethanolato-*O*,*P*]phenyl(triphenylphosphine)nickel, Ni-00343

$C_{44}H_{36}P_2Pd$
Hydrido(phenylethynyl)bis(triphenylphosphine)palladium, Pd-00311

$C_{44}H_{36}P_2Pt$
(Phenylacetylene)bis(triphenylphosphine)platinum, Pt-00425

$C_{44}H_{38}NiP_2$
Styrenebis(triphenylphosphine)nickel, Ni-00344

$C_{44}H_{40}P_2Pd_2$
[μ-[(1-η:2,3-η)-2,4-Cyclopentadien-1-yl]][μ-[(1-η:2,3-η)-2-propenyl]]bis(triphenylphosphine)-dipalladium, Pd-00312

$C_{44}H_{42}Cl_9NP_2PtSn_3$
[(1,2,3,4-η)-1,2,3,4-Tetramethyl-1,3-cyclobutadiene]-tris(trichlorostannyl)platinate(1−); Bis(triphenylphosphine)-iminium salt, *in* Pt-00065

$C_{44}H_{42}NiP_2$
[(1,2,5,6-η)-1,5-Cyclooctadiene]bis(triphenylphosphine)-nickel, Ni-00345

$C_{44}H_{42}P_2Pt$
[(1,2-η)-Cyclooctyne]bis(triphenylphosphine)platinum, Pt-00426

$C_{44}H_{46}NiO_6P_2$
(η^2-Ethene)bis[tris(2-methylphenyl)phosphite-*P*]nickel, Ni-00346

$C_{44}H_{46}O_6P_2Pd$
(η^2-Ethene)bis[tris(2-methylphenyl)phosphite-*P*]-palladium, Pd-00313

$C_{44}H_{48}P_2Pt$
Dibutylbis(triphenylphosphine)platinum, Pt-00427

$C_{44}H_{57}BCu_2N_4O_3$
(μ-Carbonyl)(μ-benzoato-*O*,*O′*)bis(*N*,*N*,*N′*,*N′*-tetramethylethylenediamine)dicopper(1+); Tetraphenylborate, *in* Cu-00053

$C_{44}H_{58}F_6P_4Pd$
[Ethylenebis[diphenylphosphine]]-hydro(tricyclohexylphosphine)palladium(1+); Hexafluorophosphate, *in* Pd-00314

$C_{44}H_{58}P_3Pd^{\oplus}$
[Ethylenebis[diphenylphosphine]]-hydro(tricyclohexylphosphine)palladium(1+), Pd-00314

$C_{44}H_{80}P_2Pd_2$
Bis[μ-[(1-η:2,3-η)-2-methyl-2-propenyl]]-bis(tricyclohexylphosphine)dipalladium, Pd-00315

$C_{45}H_{35}F_5P_2Pt$
(Pentafluorophenyl)-2-propenylbis(triphenylphosphine)-platinum, Pt-00428

$C_{45}H_{55}Au_5$
Pentakis(1,3,5-trimethylbenzene)pentagold, *in* Au-00061

$C_{45}H_{55}Cu_5$
Pentakis(1,3,5-trimethylbenzene)pentacopper, *in* Cu-00035

$C_{46}H_{35}BrNiP$
Bromo(η^4-1,2,3,4-tetraphenylcyclobutadiene)-(triphenylphosphine)nickel, Ni-00347

$C_{46}H_{38}Au_2FeP_2$
1,1′-[Bis[triphenylphosphine]aurio]ferrocene, Au-00095

$C_{46}H_{39}Au_2BF_4FeP_2$
[Bis(triphenylphosphine)digold](η^5-2,4-cyclopentadien-1-yl)[μ_3-[(1-η:1-η:1,2,3,4,5-η)-2,4-cyclopentadien-1-ylidene]]iron(1+); Tetrafluoroborate, *in* Au-00096

$C_{46}H_{39}Au_2FeP_2^{\oplus}$
[Bis(triphenylphosphine)digold](η^5-2,4-cyclopentadien-1-yl)[μ_3-[(1-η:1-η:1,2,3,4,5-η)-2,4-cyclopentadien-1-ylidene]]iron(1+), Au-00096

$C_{46}H_{40}N_2O_{30}Pt_{15}$
Pentadeca-μ-carbonylpentadecacarbonylpentadecaplatinate(2−); Bis-(tetraethylammonium) salt, *in* Pt-00347

$C_{46}H_{66}Cl_2O_4Pd_2$
Bis[(16,17-20-η)-(3β)-3-(acetyloxy)-pregna-5,16-dien-20-yl]di-μ-chlorodipalladium, Pd-00316

$C_{46}H_{72}F_{10}N_4Pd$
Dicyanobis(pentafluorophenyl)palladate(2−); Bis(tetrabutylammonium) salt, *in* Pd-00091

$C_{47}H_{35}Cl_5NP_2Pd^{\oplus}$
Pentachlorophenyl(pyridine)bis(triphenylphosphine)-palladium(1+), Pd-00317

$C_{47}H_{35}Cl_6NO_4P_2Pd$
Pentachlorophenyl(pyridine)bis(triphenylphosphine)-palladium(1+); Perchlorate, *in* Pd-00317

$C_{47}H_{38}O_2P_2Pt$
[(3,4-η)-3-Methyl-4-phenyl-3-cyclobutene-1,2-dione]-bis(triphenylphosphine)platinum, Pt-00429

$C_{47}H_{38}P_2Pt$
(Methylene-1,8-naphthalenediyl)bis(triphenylphosphine)-platinum, Pt-00430

$C_{48}H_{30}Cl_2F_{10}P_2Pd_2$
Di-μ-chlorobis(pentafluorophenyl)-bis(triphenylphosphine)dipalladium, Pd-00318

$C_{48}H_{30}Cl_{12}Ni_2P_2$
Di-μ-chlorobis(pentachlorophenyl)-bis(triphenylphosphine)dinickel, Ni-00348

$C_{48}H_{30}F_{10}P_2Pt$
Bis(pentafluorophenyl)bis(triphenylphosphine)platinum, Pt-00431

$C_{48}H_{30}F_{18}NiP_2$
[Hexatris(trifluoromethyl)benzene]-bis(triphenylphosphine)nickel, Ni-00349

$C_{48}H_{40}Li_2NiP_2$
Diphenylbis(triphenylphosphine)nickelate(2−); Di-Li salt, *in* Ni-00351

$C_{48}H_{40}N_2NiP_2$
(Azobenzene)bis(triphenylphosphine)nickel, Ni-00350

$C_{48}H_{40}NiP_2^{\ominus\ominus}$
Diphenylbis(triphenylphosphine)nickelate(2−), Ni-00351

$C_{48}H_{40}P_2Pt$
Diphenylbis(triphenylphosphine)platinum, Pt-00432

$C_{48}H_{47}As_3NNi^{\oplus}$
[Tris(2-diphenylarsinoethyl)amine]phenylnickel(1+), Ni-00352

$C_{48}H_{60}Ge_2P_2Pd$
Bis(triethylphosphine)bis(triphenylgermyl)palladium, Pd-00319

$C_{48}H_{60}Ge_2P_2Pt$
Bis(triethylphosphine)bis(triphenylgermyl)platinum, Pt-00433

$C_{48}H_{60}P_2Pb_2Pt$
Bis(triethylphosphine)bis(triphenyllead)platinum, Pt-00434

$C_{48}H_{60}P_2PtSn_2$
Bis(triethylphosphine)bis(triphenylstannyl)platinum, Pt-00435

$C_{48}H_{68}Na_4Ni_2O_5$
Bis[(η^2-ethene)diphenylnickel]pentakis(tetrahydrofuran)-tetrasodium, *in* Ni-00112

$C_{48}H_{83}BP_4Pt_2$
Di-μ-hydrohydrotetrakis(triethylphosphine)-diplatinum(1+); Tetraphenylborate, *in* Pt-00307

$C_{48}H_{84}P_4Pt_4$
Octahydrotetrakis(phenyldiisopropylphosphine)-tetraplatinum, Pt-00436

$C_{48}H_{108}Cu_4I_4P_4$
▷Tetraiodotetrakis(tributylphosphine)tetracopper, *in* Cu-00043

$C_{48}H_{108}NiP_3$
Tetrakis(tributylphosphine)nickel, Ni-00353

$C_{48}H_{110}P_4Pt_4$
Dihydrotetrakis(tri-*tert*-butylphosphine)tetraplatinum, Pt-00437

$C_{49}H_{77}N_7Ni_4$
Heptakis(isocyanocyclohexane)tetranickel, Ni-00354

$C_{50}H_{40}P_2Pt$
(Diphenylacetylene)bis(triphenylphosphine)platinum, Pt-00438

$C_{50}H_{42}Au_2P_4$
Bis[μ-[methylenebis[diphenylphosphinato]](1−)-*P*:*P*′]-digold, Au-00097

$C_{50}H_{42}NiP_2$
Diphenylethylenebis(triphenylphosphine)nickel, Ni-00355

$C_{50}H_{44}Cl_2P_2Pd_2$
Dibenzyldi-μ-chlorobis(triphenylphosphine)dipalladium, Pd-00320

$C_{50}H_{44}P_2PtSn_2$
Dichlorobis(trichlorostannyl)platinate(2−); Bis(triphenylbenzyl-phosphonium) salt, *in* Pt-00474

$C_{50}H_{46}O_2P_2Pd$
[(5,6-η-1-Ethenyl-1,2,3,3*a*,3*b*,7*a*,8,8*a*-octahydrocyclopent[*a*]indene-4,7-dione]-bis(triphenylphosphine)palladium, Pd-00321

$C_{50}H_{47}ClP_4Pt_2$
μ-Hydrodihydrobis[μ-[methylenebis[diphenylphosphine]-*P*:*P*′]diplatinum(1+); Chloride, *in* Pt-00439

$C_{50}H_{47}F_6P_5Pt_2$
μ-Hydrodihydrobis[μ-[methylenebis[diphenylphosphine]-*P*:*P*′]diplatinum(1+); Hexafluorophosphate, *in* Pt-00439

$C_{50}H_{47}P_4Pt_2^{\oplus}$
μ-Hydrodihydrobis[μ-[methylenebis[diphenylphosphine]-*P*:*P*′]diplatinum(1+), Pt-00439

$C_{50}H_{54}Cu_6N_4$
Tetrakis[μ_3-[2-(dimethylaminophenyl)-*C*:*C*:*N*]]bis[μ-[(4-methylphenyl)ethenyl]]hexacopper, Cu-00066

$C_{51}H_{42}O_3Pd$
Tris[(1,2-η)-1,5-diphenyl-1,4-pentadien-2-one]-palladium, Pd-00322

$C_{51}H_{42}O_3Pd_2$
Tris[μ-[(1,2-η:4,5-η)-1,5-diphenyl-1,4-pentadien-3-one]]-dipalladium, Pd-00323

$C_{51}H_{43}BF_4OP_2Pt$
[(1,2,3-η)-6-Ethoxy-1*H*-phenalen-1-yl]-bis(triphenylphosphine)platinum; Tetrafluoroborate, *in* Pt-00440

$C_{51}H_{43}OP_2Pt^{\oplus}$
[(1,2,3-η)-6-Ethoxy-1*H*-phenalen-1-yl]-bis(triphenylphosphine)platinum, Pt-00440

$C_{51}H_{46}Cl_2P_4Pt_2$
Dichloro-μ-methylenebis[μ-[methylenebis[diphenylphosphine]-*P*:*P*′]]-diplatinum, Pt-00441

$C_{51}H_{49}P_4Pt_2^{\oplus}$
μ-Hydrohydromethylbis[μ-[methylenebis(diphenylphosphine)-*P*:*P*′]]-diplatinum(1+), Pt-00442

$C_{51}H_{72}F_{15}N_3Pd$
(Cyano-*C*)tris(pentafluorophenyl)palladate(2−); Bis(tetrabutylammonium) salt, *in* Pd-00161

$C_{52}H_{40}P_2Pd$
Bis(phenylethynyl)bis(triphenylphosphine)palladium, Pd-00324

$C_{52}H_{40}P_2Pt$
Bis(phenylethynyl)bis(triphenylphosphine)platinum, Pt-00443

$C_{52}H_{44}F_{12}O_2P_6Pt_2$
Dicarbonylbis[μ-[methylenebis[diphenylphosphine]-*P*:*P'*]]-diplatinum(2+); Bis(hexafluorophosphate), *in* Pt-00444

$C_{52}H_{44}O_2P_4Pt_2^{\oplus\oplus}$
Dicarbonylbis[μ-[methylenebis[diphenylphosphine]-*P*:*P'*]]-diplatinum(2+), Pt-00444

$C_{52}H_{44}O_4Pd_3$
Bis(2,4-pentanedionato-*O*,*O'*)bis[μ-[(1,2,3-η:1,3-η)-1,2,3-triphenyl-1-propen-1-yl-3-ylidene]]-tripalladium, Pd-00325

$C_{52}H_{48}NiP_4$
Bis[1,2-bis(diphenylphosphino)ethane]nickel, Ni-00356

$C_{52}H_{49}BNNiP$
(η⁵-2,4-Cyclopentadien-1-yl)(2-isocyano-2-methylpropane)(triphenylphosphine)nickel(1+); Tetraphenylborate, *in* Ni-00262

$C_{52}H_{49}ClNiO_4P_4$
Bis[1,2-ethanediylbis[diphenylphosphine]-*P*,*P'*]-hydronickel(1+); Perchlorate, *in* Ni-00357

$C_{52}H_{49}Cl_3NiP_4Si$
Bis[1,2-ethanediylbis[diphenylphosphine]-*P*,*P'*]-hydronickel(1+); Trichlorosiliconate, *in* Ni-00357

$C_{52}H_{49}F_6NiP_5$
Bis[1,2-ethanediylbis[diphenylphosphine]-*P*,*P'*]-hydronickel(1+); Hexafluorophosphate, *in* Ni-00357

$C_{52}H_{49}NiP_4^{\oplus}$
Bis[1,2-ethanediylbis[diphenylphosphine]-*P*,*P'*]-hydronickel(1+), Ni-00357

$C_{52}H_{50}ClF_6P_5Pt_2$
μ-Chlorodimethylbis[μ-[methylenebis[diphenylphosphine]-*P*:*P'*]]diplatinum(1+); Hexafluorophosphate, *in* Pt-00445

$C_{52}H_{50}ClP_4Pt_2^{\oplus}$
μ-Chlorodimethylbis[μ-[methylenebis[diphenylphosphine]-*P*:*P'*]]diplatinum(1+), Pt-00445

$C_{52}H_{50}Cl_2P_4Pt_2$
μ-Chlorodimethylbis[μ-[methylenebis[diphenylphosphine]-*P*:*P'*]]diplatinum(1+); Chloride, *in* Pt-00445

$C_{52}H_{50}P_4Pt$
Dimethylbis[methylenebis(diphenylphosphine)-*P*]platinum, Pt-00446

$C_{52}H_{51}F_6P_5Pt_2$
Di-μ-hydrodimethylbis[μ-[methylenebis[diphenylphosphine]-*P*:*P'*]]-diplatinum(1+); Hexafluorophosphate, *in* Pt-00447

$C_{52}H_{51}P_4Pt_2^{\oplus}$
Di-μ-hydrodimethylbis[μ-[methylenebis[diphenylphosphine]-*P*:*P'*]]-diplatinum(1+), Pt-00447

$C_{52}H_{52}NiO_4P_4$
Tetrakis(methyldiphenylphosphinite-*P*)nickel, Ni-00358

$C_{52}H_{52}NiP_4$
Tetrakis(methyldiphenylphosphine)nickel, Ni-00359

$C_{52}H_{54}P_2PtSn_2$
Bis(dimethylphenylphosphine)dihydridobis(triphenyltin)-platinum, Pt-00448

$C_{52}H_{62}Cu_5LiO_4$
Hexa-μ-phenylpentacuprate(1−); Li salt, tetra-THF complex, *in* Cu-00060

$C_{52}H_{64}P_2Pt$
Dioctylbis(triphenylphosphine)platinum, Pt-00449

$C_{52}H_{80}P_4Pt_3$
Bis(μ-diphenylacetylene)tetrakis(triethylphosphine)-triplatinum, Pt-00450

$C_{53}H_{53}ClO_4P_4Pt_2$
Trimethylbis[μ-[methylenebis[diphenylphosphine]-*P*:*P'*]]-diplatinum(1+); Perchlorate, *in* Pt-00451

$C_{53}H_{53}F_6P_4Pt_2Sb$
Trimethylbis[μ-[methylenebis[diphenylphosphine]-*P*:*P'*]]-diplatinum(1+); Hexafluoroantimonate, *in* Pt-00451

$C_{53}H_{53}F_6P_5Pt_2$
Trimethylbis[μ-[methylenebis[diphenylphosphine]-*P*:*P'*]]-diplatinum(1+); Hexafluorophosphate, *in* Pt-00451

$C_{53}H_{53}P_4Pt_2^{\oplus}$
Trimethylbis[μ-[methylenebis[diphenylphosphine]-*P*:*P'*]]-diplatinum(1+), Pt-00451

$C_{53}H_{108}O_5P_4Pd_4$
Pentacarbonyltetrakis(tributylphosphine)tetrapalladium, Pd-00326

$C_{54}H_{44}NiP_2$
[Ethylenebis[diphenylphosphine]](η⁴-1,2,3,4-tetraphenylcyclobutadiene)nickel, Ni-00360

$C_{54}H_{45}K_3NiSi_3$
Tris(triphenylsilyl)nickelate(3−); Tri-K salt, *in* Ni-00362

$C_{54}H_{45}NiP_3$
Tris(triphenylphosphine)nickel, Ni-00361

$C_{54}H_{45}NiSi_3^{\ominus\ominus\ominus}$
Tris(triphenylsilyl)nickelate(3−), Ni-00362

$C_{54}H_{45}P_3Pt$
Tris(triphenylphosphine)platinum, Pt-00452

$C_{54}H_{46}BrNiP_2$
Bromohydrotris(triphenylphosphine)nickel, Ni-00363

$C_{54}H_{46}ClO_4P_3Pt$
Hydrotris(triphenylphosphine)platinum(1+); Perchlorate, *in* Pt-00453

$C_{54}H_{46}P_3Pt^{\oplus}$
Hydrotris(triphenylphosphine)platinum(1+), Pt-00453

$C_{54}H_{51}BNNiP$
(η⁵-2,4-Cyclopentadien-1-yl)(isocyanocyclohexane)-(triphenylphosphine)nickel(1+); Tetraphenylborate, *in* Ni-00281

$C_{54}H_{56}P_4Pt_2$
Bis[μ-[methylenebis[diphenylphosphine]-*P*:*P'*]]-tetramethyldiplatinum, *in* Pt-00325

$C_{54}H_{72}P_4Pt_2$
Bis-μ-(diphenylphosphido)-diphenylbis(tripropylphosphine)diplatinum, Pt-00454

$C_{54}H_{82}F_6P_4Pt$
Hydrobis(tricyclohexylphosphine)(triphenylphosphine)-platinum(1+); Hexafluorophosphate, *in* Pt-00455

$C_{54}H_{82}P_3Pt^{\oplus}$
Hydrobis(tricyclohexylphosphine)(triphenylphosphine)-platinum(1+), Pt-00455

$C_{54}H_{86}Cl_2O_2Pd_2$
Di-μ-chlorobis[(4,5,6-η)-3-oxo-5-cholesten-4-yl]-dipalladium, Pd-00327

$C_{54}H_{87}BP_4Pt_2$
μ-Hydrohydrophenyltetrakis(triethylphosphine)-diplatinum(1+); Tetraphenylborate, *in* Pt-00346

$C_{54}H_{94}P_2Pt_2Si_2$
Di-μ-hydrobis(benzyldimethylsilyl)-bis(tricyclohexylphosphine)diplatinum, Pt-00456

$C_{54}H_{102}Ni_2P_4$
Di-μ-hydrobis[1,3-propanediylbis[dicyclohexylphosphine]-*P*,*P'*]dinickel, Ni-00364

$C_{54}H_{108}O_6P_4Pd_4$
Hexa-μ-carbonyltetrakis(tributylphosphine)-tetrapalladium, Pd-00328

$C_{55}H_{45}NiOP_3$
Carbonyltris(triphenylphosphine)nickel, Ni-00365

$C_{55}H_{45}NiO_{10}P_3$
Carbonyltris(triphenylphosphite-*P*)nickel, Ni-00366

$C_{55}H_{45}OP_3Pd$
Carbonyltris(triphenylphosphine)palladium, Pd-00329

$C_{55}H_{45}OP_3Pt$
Carbonyltris(triphenylphosphine)platinum, Pt-00457

$C_{55}H_{45}OP_3Pt_2S$
Carbonyl(μ-sulfido)tris(triphenylphosphine)diplatinum, Pt-00458

$C_{55}H_{48}BF_4P_3Pt$
Methyltris(triphenylphosphine)platinum(1+); Tetrafluoroborate, *in* Pt-00459

$C_{55}H_{48}CuP_3$
Methyltris(triphenylphosphine)copper, Cu-00067

$C_{55}H_{48}FO_3P_3PtS$
Methyltris(triphenylphosphine)platinum(1+); Fluorosulfonate, *in* Pt-00459

$C_{55}H_{48}P_3Pt^{\oplus}$
Methyltris(triphenylphosphine)platinum(1+), Pt-00459

$C_{55}H_{52}O_3P_4Pt_3$
Tri-μ-carbonyltetrakis(methyldiphenylphosphine)-triplatinum, Pt-00460

$C_{56}H_{40}Br_4Ni_2$
Di-μ-bromodibromobis(1,2,3,4-tetraphenyl-1,3-cyclobutadiene)dinickel, *in* Ni-00256

$C_{56}H_{40}Br_4Pd_2$
Dibromodi-μ-bromobis(tetraphenylcyclobutadiene)-dipalladium, Pd-00330

$C_{56}H_{40}Cl_4Pd_2$
Di-μ-chlorodichlorobis(tetraphenylcyclobutadiene)-dipalladium, Pd-00331

$C_{56}H_{40}Cl_4Pt_2$
Di-μ-chlorodichlorobis[1,2,3,4-tetraphenyl-1,3-cyclobutadiene]diplatinum, Pt-00461

$C_{56}H_{40}Cl_6Pd_3$
Tetra-μ-chlorodichlorobis(tetraphenyl-1,3-cyclobutadiene)tripalladium, Pd-00332

$C_{56}H_{40}Ni$
Bis(η^4-1,2,3,4-tetraphenylcyclobutadiene)nickel, Ni-00367

$C_{56}H_{40}Pd$
Bis(tetraphenylcyclobutadiene)palladium, Pd-00333

$C_{56}H_{49}BF_4NNiP_3$
Acetonitrilehydrotris(triphenylphosphine)nickel(1+); Tetrafluoroborate, *in* Ni-00368

$C_{56}H_{49}NNiP_3^{\oplus}$
Acetonitrilehydrotris(triphenylphosphine)nickel(1+), Ni-00368

$C_{56}H_{50}BF_4P_3Pt$
Ethyltris(triphenylphosphine)platinum(1+); Tetrafluoroborate, *in* Pt-00462

$C_{56}H_{50}P_3Pt^{\oplus}$
Ethyltris(triphenylphosphine)platinum(1+), Pt-00462

$C_{56}H_{56}Cu_8O_8$
Octakis[μ_3-(2-methoxyphenyl-*C*:*C*:*O*)]octacopper,10CI, *in* Cu-00026

$C_{56}H_{64}B_2Cu_2N_6O_2$
Dicarbonyl[μ-(1,2-ethanediamine-*N*,*N'*)]bis(1,2-ethanediamine-*N*,*N'*)dicopper(2+); Bis(tetraphenylborate), *in* Cu-00033

$C_{56}H_{72}Br_2F_{20}N_2Pd_2$
Di-μ-bromotetrakis(pentafluorophenyl)dipalladate(2−); Bis(tetrabutylammonium) salt, *in* Pd-00193

$C_{56}H_{72}Cl_2F_{20}N_2Pd_2$
Di-μ-chlorotetrakis(pentafluorophenyl)dipalladate(2−); Bis(tetrabutylammonium) salt, *in* Pd-00194

$C_{56}H_{72}F_{20}N_2Pd$
Tetrakis(pentafluorophenyl)palladate(2−); Bistetrabutylammonium salt, *in* Pd-00195

$C_{56}H_{72}N_2O_{24}Pt_{12}$
Dodeca-μ-carbonyldodecacarbonyldodecaplatinate(2−); Bis(tetrabutylammonium) salt, *in* Pt-00311

$C_{56}H_{100}CuN_{18}O_{24}S_2$
▷Zorbamycin, Cu-00068

$C_{57}H_{45}ClNiO_4P_2$
[(1,2,3-η)-1,2,3-Triphenyl-2-cyclopropen-1-yl]-bis(triphenylphosphine)nickel(1+); Perchlorate, *in* Ni-00369

$C_{57}H_{45}F_6NiP_3$
[(1,2,3-η)-1,2,3-Triphenyl-2-cyclopropen-1-yl]-bis(triphenylphosphine)nickel(1+); Hexafluorophosphate, *in* Ni-00369

$C_{57}H_{45}F_6P_3Pt$
[(2,3-η)-1,2,3-Triphenyl-2-cyclopropen-1-ylium]-bis(triphenylphosphine)platinum(1+); Hexfluorophosphate, *in* Pt-00463

$C_{57}H_{45}NiP_2^{\oplus}$
[(1,2,3-η)-1,2,3-Triphenyl-2-cyclopropen-1-yl]-bis(triphenylphosphine)nickel(1+), Ni-00369

$C_{57}H_{45}O_3P_3Pd_3$
Tri-μ-carbonyltris(triphenylphosphine)tripalladium, Pd-00334

$C_{57}H_{45}P_2Pt^{\oplus}$
[(2,3-η)-1,2,3-Triphenyl-2-cyclopropen-1-ylium]-bis(triphenylphosphine)platinum(1+), Pt-00463

$C_{57}H_{54}Cl_{15}P_3PtSn_5$
Pentakis(trichlorostannyl)platinate(3−); Tris(triphenylmethylphosphonium) salt, *in* Pt-00476

$C_{58}H_{40}NiO_2$
Bis[(2,3,4,5-η)-2,3,4,5-tetraphenyl-2,4-cyclopentadien-1-one]nickel, Ni-00370

$C_{58}H_{47}F_6O_4P_3Pt$
Hydrotris(triphenylphosphine)platinum(1+); Hydridobis(trifluoroacetate), *in* Pt-00453

$C_{58}H_{90}CuN_{18}O_{24}S_2$
Zorbanomycin *B*, Cu-00069

$C_{60}H_{40}Ni_6O_{12}P_2$
Dodecacarbonylhexanickelate(2−); Bis(tetraphenylphosphonium) salt, *in* Ni-00102

$C_{60}H_{45}As_3ClF_5O_4Pd$
(Pentafluorophenyl)tris(triphenylarsine)palladium(1+); Perchlorate, *in* Pd-00335

$C_{60}H_{45}As_3F_5Pd^{\oplus}$
(Pentafluorophenyl)tris(triphenylarsine)palladium(1+), Pd-00335

$C_{60}H_{45}ClF_5NiO_4P_3$
Pentafluorophenyltris(triphenylphosphine)nickel(1+); Perchlorate, *in* Ni-00371

$C_{60}H_{45}F_5NiP_3^{\oplus}$
Pentafluorophenyltris(triphenylphosphine)nickel(1+), Ni-00371

$C_{60}H_{50}Cl_2O_2Pd_2$
Di-μ-chlorobis[(1,2,3-η)-4-ethoxy-1,2,3,4-tetraphenyl-2-cyclobuten-1-yl]dipalladium, Pd-00336

$C_{60}H_{50}P_2PbPt$
Phenylbis(triphenylphosphine)triphenylplumbylplatinum, Pt-00464

$C_{60}H_{60}Br_2Ni_2P_4$
Dibromobis[1,2-ethanediylbis(diphenylphosphine)-*P*,*P'*]-[μ-[(1,2,3-η:6,7,8-η)-2,6-octadiene-1,8-diyl]]-dinickel, Ni-00372

$C_{61}H_{52}BF_4P_3Pt$
Benzyltris(triphenylphosphine)platinum(1+); Tetrafluoroborate, *in* Pt-00465

$C_{61}H_{52}P_3Pt^{\oplus}$
Benzyltris(triphenylphosphine)platinum(1+), Pt-00465

$C_{62}H_{56}P_4Pt_2$
Bis[μ-[methylenebis[diphenylphosphine]-*P:P'*]]-tetrapropyne-1-yldiplatinum, Pt-00466

$C_{62}H_{58}P_2PtSn_2$
Dihydrobis(methyldiphenylphosphine)-bis(triphenylstannyl)platinum, Pt-00467

$C_{62}H_{72}N_2O_{30}Pt_{15}$
Pentadeca-μ-carbonylpentadecacarbonylpentadecaplatinate(2−); Bis(tetrabutylammonium) salt, *in* Pt-00347

$C_{62}H_{107}BP_4Pt_2$
μ-Hydrodihydrobis[1,3-propanediylbis[bis(1,1-dimethylethylphosphine]-*P,P'*]diplatinum(1+); Tetraphenylborate, *in* Pt-00391

$C_{62}H_{108}O_{14}P_4Pd_{10}$
Tetradecacarbonyltetrakis(tributylphosphine)-decapalladium, Pd-00337

$C_{63}H_{63}NiO_9P_3$
Tris[tris(2-methylphenyl)phosphite-*P*]nickel, Ni-00373

$C_{63}H_{63}NiP_3$
Tris[tris(4-methylphenyl)phosphine]nickel, Ni-00374

$C_{64}H_{44}F_{10}N_2P_2Pd$
Dicyanobis(pentafluorophenyl)palladate(2−); Bis(benzyltriphenylphosphonium) salt, *in* Pd-00091

$C_{64}H_{48}Ni_2$
μ-Cyclooctatetraenebis[η^4-1,2,3,4-tetraphenylcyclobutadiene]dinickel, Ni-00375

$C_{64}H_{56}Cl_4Pd_2$
Di-μ-chlorodichlorobis[tetrakis(4-methylphenyl)-cyclobutadiene]dipalladium, Pd-00338

$C_{64}H_{57}BP_2Pd$
[(1,2,3-η)-2-Methyl-2-propenyl]bis(triphenylphosphine)-palladium(1+); Tetraphenylborate, *in* Pd-00288

$C_{64}H_{57}BP_2Pt$
[(1,2,3-η)-2-Methyl-2-propenyl]bis(triphenylphosphine)-platinum(1+); Tetraphenylborate, *in* Pt-00408

$C_{66}H_{40}Ni_9O_{18}P_2$
Octadecacarbonylnonanickelate(2−); Bis(tetraphenylphosphonium) salt, *in* Ni-00172

$C_{72}H_{60}As_4Ni$
Tetrakis(triphenylarsine)nickel, Ni-00376

$C_{72}H_{60}As_4Pd$
Tetrakis(triphenylarsine)palladium, Pd-00339

$C_{72}H_{60}Au_4I_2P_4$
Di-μ-iodotetrakis(triphenylphosphine)tetragold, Au-00098

$C_{72}H_{60}N_2O_2P_4Pd_2$
Dinitrosyltetrakis(triphenylphosphine)dipalladium, *in* Pd-00261

$C_{72}H_{60}NiO_{12}P_4$
Tetrakis(triphenyl phosphite-*P*)nickel, Ni-00377

$C_{72}H_{60}NiP_4$
Tetrakis(triphenylphosphine)nickel, Ni-00378

$C_{72}H_{60}O_2P_4Pt_3S$
[μ-(Diphenylphosphino)]-μ-phenyl-μ-sulfonyltris(triphenylphosphine)triplatinum, Pt-00468

$C_{72}H_{60}O_{12}P_4Pt$
Tetrakis(triphenylphosphite-*P*)platinum, Pt-00469

$C_{72}H_{60}P_2Pb_2Pd$
Bis(triphenylphosphine)bis(triphenylplumbyl)palladium, Pd-00340

$C_{72}H_{60}P_2Pb_2Pt$
Bis(triphenylphosphine)bis(triphenylplumbyl)platinum, Pt-00470

$C_{72}H_{60}P_4Pd$
Tetrakis(triphenylphosphine)palladium, Pd-00341

$C_{72}H_{60}P_4Pt$
Tetrakis(triphenylphosphine)platinum, Pt-00471

$C_{72}H_{60}PdSb_4$
Tetrakis(triphenylstibine)palladium, Pd-00342

$C_{72}H_{67}As_3BNNi$
[Tris(2-diphenylarsinoethyl)amine]phenylnickel(1+); Tetraphenylborate, *in* Ni-00352

$C_{75}H_{60}O_3P_4Pd_3$
Tri-μ-carbonyltetrakis(triphenylphosphine)tripalladium, Pd-00343

$C_{75}H_{60}O_3P_4Pt_3$
Tri-μ-carbonyltetrakis(triphenylphosphine)triplatinum, Pt-00472

$C_{75}H_{66}P_6Pt_2$
Tris[methylenebis(diphenylphosphine)]diplatinum, Pt-00473

$C_{78}H_{66}BP_3Pt$
Hydrotris(triphenylphosphine)platinum(1+); Tetraphenylborate, *in* Pt-00453

$C_{84}H_{40}O_{36}P_2Pt_{18}$
Octadeca-μ-carbonyloctadecacarbonyloctadecaplatinate(2−); Bis(tetraphenylphosphonium) salt, *in* Pt-00364

$C_{84}H_{60}Ni_2$
(π-Pentaphenylcyclopentadienyl)(π-tetraphenylcyclobutadiene)(μ-π-triphenylpropenyl)-dinickel, Ni-00379

$C_{84}H_{60}Pd_2$
μ-Diphenylacetylenebis(η^5-pentaphenylcyclopentadienyl)-dipalladium, Pd-00344

$C_{84}H_{162}O_{12}P_6Pd_{10}$
Octa-μ-carbonyltetra-μ_3-carbonylhexakis(tributylphosphine)decapalladium, Pd-00345

$C_{86}H_{144}N_4O_{22}Pt_{19}$
Deca-μ-carbonyldodecacarbonylnonadecaplatinate(4−); Tetrakis(tetrabutylammonium) salt, *in* Pt-00278

$C_{92}H_{78}Au_4Fe_2O_4P_4S$
[Bis(triphenylphosphine)digold](η^5-2,4-cyclopentadien-1-yl)[μ_3-[(1-η:1-η:1,2,3,4,5-η)-2,4-cyclopentadien-1-ylidene]]iron(1+); Sulfate, *in* Au-00096

$C_{108}H_{96}Cu_6P_6$
Hexa-μ-hydridohexakis(triphenylphosphine)hexacopper, *in* Cu-00050

$C_{118}H_{80}O_{22}P_4Pt_{19}$
Deca-μ-carbonyldodecacarbonylnonadecaplatinate(4−); Tetrakis(tetraphenylphosphonium) salt, *in* Pt-00278

$C_{126}H_{84}Au_{11}F_{21}I_3P_7$
Triiodoheptakis[tris(4-fluorophenyl)phosphine]-undecagold, Au-00099

$C_{144}H_{120}Au_9N_3O_9P_8$
Octakis(triphenylphosphine)nonagold(3+); Nitrate, *in* Au-00100

$C_{144}H_{120}Au_9P_8^{\oplus\oplus\oplus}$
Octakis(triphenylphosphine)nonagold(3+), Au-00100

$Cl_8PtSn_2^{\ominus\ominus}$
Dichlorobis(trichlorostannyl)platinate(2−), Pt-00474

$Cl_{12}HPtSn_4^{\ominus\ominus\ominus}$
Hydrotetrakis(trichlorostannyl)platinate(3−), Pt-00475

$Cl_{12}NiP_4$
Tetrakis(phosphorous trichloride)nickel, Ni-00380

$Cl_{15}PtSn_5^{\ominus\ominus\ominus}$
Pentakis(trichlorostannyl)platinate(3−), Pt-00476
$F_{12}NiP_4$
Tetrakis(phosphorous trifluoride)nickel, Ni-00381
$F_{12}P_4Pd$
Tetrakis(trifluorophosphine)palladium, Pd-00346
$F_{12}P_4Pt$
Tetrakis(trifluorophosphine)platinum, Pt-00477

CAS Registry Number Index

27661-80-9 (Octafluoro-1,4-butanediyl)-bis(triphenylphosphine)nickel, Ni-00326

27664-43-3 Carbonyl(μ-sulfido)tris(triphenylphosphine)diplatinum, Pt-00458

27711-50-8 Chloro[ethylenebis[diphenylphosphine]]methylplatinum, Pt-00323

27711-51-9 Chloro[ethylenebis(diphenylphosphine)]phenylplatinum, Pt-00350

27776-75-6 Bis(dimethylphenylphosphine)-methyl[methyl(methoxy)methylene]platinum(1+); *trans-form*, Hexafluorophosphate, *in* Pt-00253

27776-77-8 Bis(dimethylphenylphosphine)-methyl[methoxy(phenylmethyl)methylene]platinum(1+); *trans-form*, Hexafluorophosphate, *in* Pt-00317

27776-78-9 [Dihydro-2(3*H*)-furanylidene]-bis(dimethylphenylphosphine)methylplatinum(1+); Hexafluorophosphate, *in* Pt-00263

27892-37-3 Chloro(dimethyl sulfide)gold, Au-00012

27900-91-0 Chlorohydrobis(triisopropylphosphine)palladium, Pd-00160

28016-71-9 Chlorohydrobis(tricyclohexylphosphine)palladium, Pd-00264

28042-59-3 Dicarbonylbis(triphenylstibine)nickel, Ni-00314

28069-69-4 Tetrakis(trimethylphosphine)nickel, Ni-00099

28101-79-3 Tetrakis(tributylphosphine)nickel, Ni-00353

28377-73-3 Di-μ-chlorobis(8-quinolinylmethyl-*C*,*N*)dipalladium, Pd-00169

28775-98-6 Bis(dimethylphenylphosphine)bis(phenylethynyl)-platinum; *trans-form*, *in* Pt-00352

28796-12-5 Dicarbonylbis(tricyclohexylphosphine)nickel, Ni-00320

28829-00-7 Tris[tris(2-methylphenyl)phosphite-*P*]nickel, Ni-00373

28850-19-3 Iodomethylbis(triphenylphosphine)platinum; *trans-form*, *in* Pt-00374

28850-20-6 Bromo(methyl)bis(triphenylphosphine)platinum; *trans-form*, *in* Pt-00372

28850-21-7 Chloromethylbis(triphenylphosphine)platinum; *trans-form*, *in* Pt-00373

28855-35-8 Diethylbis(triphenylphosphine)platinum, Pt-00409

28855-38-1 Dibutylbis(triphenylphosphine)platinum, Pt-00427

28966-81-6 Dichlorobis(triphenylphosphine)palladium; *trans-form*, *in* Pd-00260

29012-89-3 [(2,3-η)-2-Butynedinitrile]-bis(triphenylphosphine)platinum, Pt-00406

29158-92-7 Bromomethylbis(triethylphosphine)palladium, Pd-00090

29187-01-7 (2,2′-Bipyridine-*N*,*N*′)chlorophenylnickel, Ni-00141

29259-31-2 Chloro[2-(phenylazo)phenyl]-bis(triethylphosphine)palladium; *trans-form*, *in* Pd-00207

29718-65-8 Iodomethylbis(triethylphosphine)platinum, Pt-00148

29826-91-3 Trichloro(dimethylsulfide)gold, Au-00014

29827-42-7 Dichloro(isocyanobenzene)(triphenylphosphine)palladium, Pd-00215

29827-43-8 Dichloro(isocyanobenzene)(triphenylarsine)palladium, Pd-00214

29827-46-1 Dichlorobis(isocyanocyclohexane)palladium, Pd-00099

29893-78-5 Chlorohydrobis(triphenylphosphine)palladium, Pd-00262

29961-88-4 Chloro(2-methylphenyl)bis(triethylphosphine)platinum; *trans-form*, *in* Pt-00237

30123-12-7 (Pentafluorophenyl)silver, Ag-00011

30142-19-9 Phenyl(triphenylphosphine)gold, Au-00081

30179-97-6 Chloro(methyl)bis(trimethylarsine)platinum; *trans-form*, *in* Pt-00056

30179-98-7 Chlorobis(dimethylphenylphosphine)methylpalladium, Pd-00135

30180-03-1 Acetylchlorobis(dimethylphenylphosphine)platinum; *trans-form*, *in* Pt-00202

30376-85-3 Chlorohydrobis(triisopropylphosphine)nickel; *trans-form*, *in* Ni-00171

30376-90-0 Dichloro(isocyanobenzene)(triethylphosphine)platinum; *cis-form*, *in* Pt-00142

30394-37-7 Dichloro[ethoxy(phenylamino)methylene]-(triethylphosphine)platinum; *cis-form*, *in* Pt-00174

30394-40-2 Dichloro[ethoxy(phenylamino)methylene]-(tripropylphosphine)platinum; *cis-form*, *in* Pt-00211

30645-13-7 1-Propynylcopper, Cu-00010

30676-27-8 Di-μ-chlorotetramethyldigold, *in* Au-00011

30812-03-4 Chlorobis(dimethylphenylphosphine)methylplatinum; *cis-form*, *in* Pt-00192

30916-06-4 Hydro[tetrahydroborato(1−)-*H*,*H*′]-bis(tricyclohexylphosphine)palladium, Pd-00266

31306-07-7 Hydrotetrakis(triethylphosphite-*P*)nickel(1+), Ni-00241

31323-25-8 ▷Fluopsin *C*, Cu-00012

31386-94-4 Bis(4-phenyl-1,3-butadiynyl)-bis(triethylphosphine)nickel, Ni-00290

31386-97-7 Bis(phenylethynyl)bis(triethylphosphine)palladium, Pd-00230

31387-03-8 Bis(phenylethynyl)bis(triphenylphosphine)palladium; *trans-form*, *in* Pd-00324

31387-20-9 Bromo(methyl)bis(triisopropylphosphine)nickel; *trans-form*, *in* Ni-00179

31666-47-4 (η^2-Ethene)bis[tris(2-methylphenyl)phosphite-*P*]-nickel, Ni-00346

31666-77-0 Di-μ-chlorobis[(1,2,3-η)-2-methyl-2-penten-1-yl]dipalladium, Pd-00080

31666-78-1 Di-μ-chlorobis[(2,3,4-η)-3-methyl-3-penten-2-yl]dipalladium, Pd-00081

31724-99-9 [(1,2,5,6-η)-1,5-Cyclooctadiene](2,4-pentadionato-*O*,*O*′)palladium(1+); Tetrafluoroborate, *in* Pd-00087

31725-00-5 [(1,2,5,6-η)-1,5-Cyclooctadiene](2,4-pentanedionato-*O*,*O*′]platinum(1+); Tetrafluoroborate, *in* Pt-00141

31725-11-8 [(1,2,5,6-η)-1,5-Cyclooctadiene](η^5-2,4-cyclopentadien-1-yl)platinum(1+); Tetrafluoroborate, *in* Pt-00139

31741-68-1 (η^5-2,4-Cyclopentadien-1-yl)-phenyl(triethylphosphine)palladium, Pd-00137

31741-69-2 (η^5-2,4-Cyclopentadien-1-yl)-phenyl(triethylphosphine)platinum, Pt-00194

31741-89-6 Bromo(η^5-2,4-cyclopentadien-1-yl)-(triphenylphosphine)palladium, Pd-00192

31742-08-2 Dichloro(4-methylaniline)[(3,4-η)-2,2,5,5-tetramethyl-3-hexyne]platinum; *trans-form*, *in* Pt-00195

31760-65-3 Bromo(η^5-2,4-cyclopentadien-1-yl)-(triethylphosphine)palladium, Pd-00066

31760-66-4 (η^5-2,4-Cyclopentadien-1-yl)-iodo(triethylphosphine)platinum, Pt-00103

31760-68-6 [(1,2,5,6-η)-1,5-Cyclooctadiene][(1,2-η)-hexafluoropropene]nickel, Ni-00078

31781-20-1 [(1,2,3-η)-2-Butenyl]bis(triethylphosphine)platinum(1+), Pt-00187

31781-38-1 Ethylene(hydrido)bis(triethylphosphine)platinum(1+); *trans-form*, Tetraphenylborate, *in* Pt-00168

31781-67-6 (η^5-2,4-Cyclopentadien-1-yl)triphenylphosphinecopper, Cu-00055

31781-68-7 Dichlorobis(ethylene)platinum, Pt-00026

31811-17-3 (η^5-2,4-Cyclopentadien-1-yl)[(1,2,3-η)-2-cyclopenten-1-yl]nickel, Ni-00070

31832-92-5 (η^5-2,4-Cyclopentadien-1-yl)[(1,2,3-η)-1,2,3-triphenyl-2-cyclopropen-1-yl]nickel, Ni-00245

31854-76-9 Hydro-η^3-propenyl(triphenylphosphine)nickel, Ni-00199

31869-34-8 Di-μ-chlorobis[(1,2,3-η)-2-phenyl-2-propenyl]dipalladium, Pd-00143

31871-49-5 Chloro(2,2-dichlorovinyl)-bis(triphenylphosphine)palladium, Pd-00272

31901-96-9 [Ethylenebis[diphenylphosphine]]-hydro(tricyclohexylphosphine)palladium(1+); Hexafluorophosphate, *in* Pd-00314

33635-00-6 Chloro(triethyl phosphite-*P*)gold, Au-00040
33635-47-1 Trimethyl(triphenylphosphine)gold, Au-00076
33637-36-4 [Methoxy[(4-methylphenyl)imino]methyl]-(triphenylphosphine)gold(I), Au-00084
33661-17-5 Bis(dimethylphenylphosphine)[ethoxy(ethylamino)-methylene](isocyanoethane)platinum(2+); Bishexafluorophosphate, *in* Pt-00293
33677-20-2 Dimethylbis(triphenylphosphine)platinum; *trans-form*, *in* Pt-00389
33677-56-4 Bis[(C^3,O^3-η)-1,5-diphenyl-1,4-pentadien-3-one]platinum, Pt-00353
33677-86-0 Dichloro[(1,2,3,4-η)-1,2,3,4,5-pentamethyl-1,3-cyclopentadiene]platinum, Pt-00093
33679-79-7 Carbonyltrichloroplatinate(1−); (2,2′-Bipyridine-*N*,*N*′)carbonylchloroplatinum(1+) salt, *in* Pt-00002
33808-30-9 Bromo(2-methylphenyl)bis(triethylphosphine)nickel, Ni-00177
33914-65-7 (Cyano-*C*)phenylbis(triethylphosphine)platinum; *trans-form*, *in* Pt-00235
33915-25-2 Carbonylhydrobis(triethylphosphine)platinum(1+); *trans-form*, Tetrafluoroborate, *in* Pt-00145
33915-36-5 Carbonylchlorobis(dimethylphenylphosphine)platinum(1+); *trans-form*, Tetrafluoroborate, *in* Pt-00190
33915-37-6 Carbonylhydrobis(triphenylphosphine)platinum(1+); *trans-form*, Tetrafluoroborate, *in* Pt-00371
33915-46-7 Chloro(methoxocarbonyl)bis(triethylphosphine)platinum; *trans-form*, *in* Pt-00163
33937-26-7 Tetrakis(triethylphosphine)platinum, Pt-00306
33937-92-7 Chlorobis(dimethylphenylphosphine)-(trimethylsilylmethyl)platinum; *cis-form*, *in* Pt-00254
33989-32-1 Tricarbonylnitrosyl[(trimethylphosphine)aurio]iron, Au-00033
33989-35-4 Tricarbonylnitrosyl[(triphenylphosphine)aurio]iron, Au-00075
33989-39-8 Dicarbonylnitrosyl(triphenylphosphine)-[(triphenylphosphine)aurio]iron, Au-00091
33989-89-8 Tetrakis(isocyanomethane)platinum(2+); Bis-(tetrafluoroborate), *in* Pt-00068
33989-94-5 Dichloro(isocyanomethane)(triphenylphosphine)platinum; *cis-form*, *in* Pt-00243
34031-29-3 (1-Thioglucopyranosato-*S*)(triethylphosphine)gold; *β*-D-*form*, *in* Au-00066
34031-32-8 ▷[1-Thioglucopyranose-2,3,4,6-tetrakis(methylcarbamato)-*S*]triethylphosphinegold; *β*-D-*form*, *in* Au-00074
34088-91-0 Tricarbonylnitrosyl[(trimethyl phosphite-*P*)aurio]iron, Au-00034
34230-58-5 Diethynylbis(triethylphosphine)platinum; *trans-form*, *in* Pt-00186
34230-61-0 Di(1-propynyl)bis(triethylphosphine)platinum; *trans-form*, *in* Pt-00217
34247-44-4 [1,2-Ethanediylbis[diphenylphosphine]-*P*,*P*′]dimethylgold(1+); Chloride, *in* Au-00086
34275-23-5 Methyl(triethylphosphine)gold, Au-00047
34439-98-0 Tetracarbonyl(trimethylgermyl)-[(triphenylphosphine)aurio]ruthenium; *cis-form*, *in* Au-00082
34664-23-8 Trichloro(ethylene)palladate(1−), Pd-00007
34675-89-3 *π*-Allylchlorobis(triethylphosphine)palladium, *in* Pd-00112
34679-27-1 (Phenylethynyl)gold, Au-00052
34710-35-5 Diiodobis(2-isocyano-2-methylpropane)palladium; *trans-form*, *in* Pd-00059
34710-54-8 (1-Acetyl-2-oxopropyl)(2,4-pentanedionato-*O*,*O*′)-(triphenylphosphine)palladium, Pd-00227
34742-01-3 [Ethylenebis[diphenylphosphine]]-(tetracyanoethylene)palladium, Pd-00245
34742-93-3 Di-*μ*-chlorotetrakis[2-isocyano-2-methylpropane]dipalladium, Pd-00178
34808-06-5 Trichloro[(1,2-η)-1-propene]platinate(1−); Tetrabutylammonium salt, *in* Pt-00017
34829-33-9 Di-*μ*-chlorobis(η^3-6,6-dimethyl-4-methylenebicyclo[3.1.1]hept-3-yl)dipalladium, Pd-00174
34850-19-6 (η^5-2,4-Cyclopentadien-1-yl)-bis(triethylphosphine)palladium(1+); Bromide, *in* Pd-00141
34850-24-3 (η^5-2,4-Cyclopentadien-1-yl)-bis(triethylphosphine)platinum(1+); Chloride, *in* Pt-00196
34850-25-4 (η^5-2,4-Cyclopentadien-1-yl)-bis(triethylphosphine)platinum(1+); Perchlorate, *in* Pt-00196
34852-80-7 Bromo-*π*-cyclopentadienyl(triisopropylphosphine)palladium, Pd-00104
34854-20-1 Chloro(η^5-2,4-cyclopentadien-1-yl)-(triethylphosphine)palladium, Pd-00067
34854-21-2 (η^5-2,4-Cyclopentadien-1-yl)-iodo(triethylphosphine)palladium, Pd-00068
34872-49-6 [(1,2-η)-Cycloheptyne]bis(triphenylphosphine)platinum, Pt-00423
34872-50-9 [(1,2-η)-Cyclohexyne]bis(triphenylphosphine)platinum, Pt-00419
34964-16-4 Carbonyltrichloroplatinate(1−); Tetrabutylammonium salt, *in* Pt-00002
35004-41-2 1-[(Triphenylphosphine)aurio]ferrocene, Au-00085
35428-96-7 Dichloro(η^3-2-propenyl)palladate(1−), Pd-00008
35502-73-9 Di-*μ*-chlorobis[(1,4,5-η)-8-methoxy-4-cycloocten-1-yl]dipalladium, Pd-00153
35655-02-8 Iodomethylbis(triphenylphosphine)palladium; *cis-form*, *in* Pd-00269
35744-03-7 (Tricyclohexylphosphine)[(1,2,2′,5,5′,6-η)-2,3,5-tris(methylene)-1,6-hexanediyl]nickel, Ni-00255
35768-61-7 [(1,2-η)-1,2-Dimethylcyclopropene]-bis(triphenylphosphine)platinum, Pt-00412
35770-09-3 Chloro(η^3-2-propenyl)(triphenylphosphine)platinum, Pt-00262
35770-29-7 (η^5-2,4-Cyclopentadien-1-yl)(η^3-2-propenyl)platinum, Pt-00061
35770-30-0 (η^5-2,4-Cyclopentadien-1-yl)[(1,2,3-η)-2-methyl-2-propenyl]platinum, Pt-00082
35770-41-3 [(1,2,3-η)-2-Methyl-2-propenyl]-bis(triphenylphosphine)platinum(1+); Tetraphenylborate, *in* Pt-00408
35770-44-6 Di-*μ*-chlorobis[(1,2,3,-η)-2-methyl-2-propenyl]diplatinum, Pt-00069
35797-58-1 [(2,3-η)-2-Butyne]bis(dimethylphenylphosphine)methylplatinum(1+); *trans-form*, Hexafluorophosphate, *in* Pt-00264
35798-01-7 *N*,*N*,*N*-Tributyl-1-butanaminium trichlorophenylaurate, *in* Au-00031
35828-66-1 Di-*π*-cyclopentadienyl(*μ*-diphenylacetylene)dinickel, Ni-00228
35828-71-8 [(1,2,5,6-η)-1,5-Cyclooctadiene](η^5-2,4-cyclopentadien-1-yl)palladium(1+); Tetrafluoroborate, *in* Pd-00085
35872-05-0 Carbonyldiiodobis(trimethylphosphine)nickel, Ni-00041
35914-81-9 [*μ*-[η^3:η^3-2,3-Bis(methylene)-1,4-butanediyl]]-bis[(1,2,3-η)-2,4-cyclopentadien-1-yl]dinickel, Ni-00146
35915-74-3 Chloro[methylenebis[diphenylphosphine]-*P*,*P*′]-(η^3-2-propenyl)palladium, *in* Pd-00226
36005-15-9 [(2,3-η)-Bicyclo[2.2.1]hept-2-ene]-chloro[(1,2,3-η)-2-methyl-2-propenyl]nickel, Ni-00080
36180-73-1 [(2,3-η)-2-Butene]bis(tricyclohexylphosphine)nickel, Ni-00330
36180-76-4 Dicarbonylbis(η^5-2,4-cyclopentadien-1-yl)[*μ*-(dibromostannylene)]dinickel, Ni-00083
36222-40-9 (η^5-2,4-Cyclopentadien-1-yl)(2-isocyano-2-methylpropane)copper, Cu-00039
36344-80-6 Tetracarbonylpalladium, Pd-00013
36351-87-8 Chlorobis(pyridine)[(1,2,3-η)-1,2,3-triphenyl-2-cyclopropen-1-yl]nickel, Ni-00286
36351-96-9 [(2,3-η)-Dimethyl-2-butenedioate]-bis(triphenylphosphine)nickel; (*E*)-*form*, *in* Ni-00337
36421-86-0 Tetrakis(phosphorous trichloride)nickel, Ni-00380
36427-01-7 Methyl(2,4-pentanedionato-*O*,*O*′)tricyclohexylphosphinenickel, Ni-00238
36454-23-6 Dicarbonyl(1,10-phenanthroline-N^1,N^{10})nickel, Ni-00109
36484-04-5 (η^3-2-Propenyl)bis(triphenylphosphine)platinum(1+); Tetrafluoroborate, *in* Pt-00398

39929-04-9 Tribromo(dimethyl sulfide)gold, Au-00010
39958-10-6 Bis(benzonitrile)dichloropalladium; *cis-form*, *in* Pd-00094
40575-23-3 (3,3-Dimethyl-1-butynyl)copper, Cu-00021
40587-17-5 Chlorodimethyl(dimethyl sulfide)gold, Au-00022
40696-73-9 Tetra-μ_3-chlorotetrakis(trimethylphosphine)tetrasilver, *in* Ag-00008
40696-74-0 Di-μ-chlorotetrakis(trimethylphosphine)disilver, *in* Ag-00016
40696-88-6 Tris(trimethylphosphine)(trimethylsilanolato)copper, Cu-00044
40696-91-1 Tris(trimethylphosphine)(trimethylsilanolato)silver, Ag-00028
40770-13-6 Pentakis(trichlorostannyl)platinate(3−), Pt-00476
40810-33-1 Hexakiscyanodinickelate(4−); Tetrapotassium salt, *in* Ni-00036
40894-89-1 Bis(dimethylphenylphosphine)iodotrimethylplatinum, Pt-00232
40895-04-3 Dichlorodihydrobis(triethylphosphine)platinum, Pt-00131
40927-17-1 Dichlorobis(isocyanobenzene)palladium; *cis-form*, *in* Pd-00095
40982-03-4 [(1,2-η)-Hexakis(trifluoromethyl)benzene]-bis(triethylphosphine)platinum, Pt-00287
40982-14-7 [(1,2-η)-3-Methylcyclopropene]-bis(triphenylphosphine)platinum, Pt-00407
40988-97-4 Bis[(trimethylsilylmethyl)]cuprate(1−), Cu-00032
41021-81-2 Bis(isocyanobenzene)palladium, Pd-00096
41071-60-7 Dichlorobis(trichlorostannyl)platinate(2−); Bis(triphenylbenzylphosphonium) salt, *in* Pt-00474
41071-62-9 Pentakis(trichlorostannyl)platinate(3−); Tris-(tetramethylammonium) salt, *in* Pt-00476
41101-20-6 Dichloro(isocyanobenzene)(triphenylphosphine)platinum; *cis-form*, *in* Pt-00312
41127-49-5 Hydrotetrakis(trichlorostannyl)platinate(3−); Tris-(tetraethylammonium) salt, *in* Pt-00475
41232-31-9 Bis[μ-(dicyclohexylphosphino)]bis(η^2-ethene)dinickel, Ni-00269
41365-09-7 (η^5-2,4-Cyclopentadien-1-yl)-(isocyanocyclohexane)(triphenylphosphine)-nickel(1+); Trichlorogermanate, *in* Ni-00281
41509-20-0 (η^5-2,4-Cyclopentadien-1-yl)(trichlorogermyl)-(triphenylphosphine)nickel, Ni-00217
41509-54-0 Tetracarbonylbis[(triphenylphosphine)gold]osmium; *cis-form*, *in* Au-00093
41517-22-0 (π-Cyclopentadienyl)-[ethylenebis[diphenylphosphine]]nickel(1+); Tetrachloronickelate, *in* Ni-00287
41517-23-1 (π-Cyclopentadienyl)-[ethylenebis[diphenylphosphine]]nickel(1+); Tetrabromonickelate, *in* Ni-00287
41517-40-2 (π-Cyclopentadienyl)-[ethylenebis[diphenylphosphine]]nickel(1+); Iodide, *in* Ni-00287
41517-41-3 (π-Cyclopentadienyl)-[ethylenebis[diphenylphosphine]]nickel(1+); Hexafluorophosphate, *in* Ni-00287
41559-20-0 1,1′-[Bis[triphenylphosphine]aurio]ferrocene, Au-00095
41572-71-8 Di-μ-chlorobis(η^3-1,2,4,5,6-pentamethyl-3-methylenebicyclo[2.2.0]hex-5-en-1-yl)diplatinum, Pt-00290
41588-04-9 Bromo(pentafluorophenyl)bis(triphenylphosphine)-palladium; *trans-form*, *in* Pd-00295
41600-73-1 [(1,2,3,6,7,8-η)-2,6-Octadiene-1,8-diyl]-(triphenylphosphine)nickel, Ni-00249
41619-36-7 Dibromo[(2,3,5,6-η)-1,2,3,4,5,6-hexamethylbicyclo[2.2.0]hexa-2,5-diene]platinum, Pt-00110
41619-37-8 [(2,3,5,6-η)-1,2,3,4,5,6-Hexamethylbicyclo[2.2.0]hexa-2,5-diene]diiodoplatinum, Pt-00112
41620-22-8 Methyl(trimethylplumbyl)bis(triphenylphosphine)-platinum, Pt-00410
41620-24-0 Bromo(phenyl)bis(triphenylphosphine)platinum; *trans-form*, *in* Pt-00415
41620-25-1 Bromo(methyl)bis(triphenylphosphine)platinum; *cis-(?)-form*, *in* Pt-00372
41630-44-8 Bis(1,3-dimethyl-2-imidazolidinylidene)gold(1+), Au-00063
41649-55-2 Di-μ-chlorobis[(1,2,3-η)-4-hydroxy-1-methyl-1-pentenyl]dipalladium, Pd-00079
41676-86-2 Chloro(1-isocyano-4-methylbenzene)silver, Ag-00019
41685-57-8 Tetrakis(methyldiphenylphosphinite-*P*)nickel, Ni-00358
41685-59-0 Ethylenebis(tricyclohexylphosphine)nickel, Ni-00321
41685-72-7 (Cyano-*C*)phenylbis(triethylphosphine)nickel, Ni-00176
41702-08-3 Di-μ-bromobis(η^3-1,2,4,5,6-pentamethyl-3-methylenebicyclo[2.2.0]hex-5-en-2-yl)diplatinum, Pt-00288
41705-71-9 Bis(triphenylphosphine)bis(triphenylplumbyl)palladium, Pd-00340
41705-72-0 Bis(triphenylphosphine)bis(triphenylplumbyl)platinum, Pt-00470
41762-42-9 Dichlorobis(isocyanobenzene)palladium, Pd-00095
41766-21-6 (Trinitromethyl)silver, Ag-00001
41798-98-5 Bromo(phenyl)bis(triphenylphosphine)nickel, Ni-00334
41820-43-3 Dichlorobis(ethylene)palladium, Pd-00010
41867-97-4 Chloro[selenobis(methane)]gold, Au-00013
41910-22-9 Acetylchlorobis(triphenylphosphine)palladium, Pd-00275
41948-83-8 Tetra-μ-carbonyltetracarbonyltrinickelate(2−); Bis-(tetrabutylammonium) salt, *in* Ni-00062
41970-28-9 Ethyl(2,4-pentanedionato-*O*,*O*′)triphenylphosphinenickel, Ni-00244
42012-03-3 [(2,3-η)-1,2,3-Triphenyl-2-cyclopropen-1-ylium]-bis(triphenylphosphine)platinum(1+); Hexafluorophosphate, *in* Pt-00463
42029-75-4 [(2,3-η)-1,1,1,4,4,4-Hexafluoro-2-butyne]-bis(triethylphosphine)platinum, Pt-00184
42088-00-6 [(2,3,5,6-η)-Bicyclo[2.2.1]hepta-2,5-diene](η^5-2,4-cyclopentadien-1-yl)nickel(1+); Tetrafluoroborate, *in* Ni-00087
42088-01-7 [(1,2,5,6-η)-1,5-Cyclooctadiene](η^5-2,4-cyclopentadien-1-yl)nickel(1+); Tetrafluoroborate, *in* Ni-00104
42152-44-3 Trifluoromethanesulfonic acid copper(1+) salt, Cu-00001
42161-77-3 [μ-[η^3:η^3-2,3-Bismethylene-1,4-butanediyl]]-bis(η^5-2,4-cyclopentadien-1-yl)dipalladium, Pd-00121
42167-76-0 Dibenzylbis(triethylphosphine)platinum; *cis-form*, *in* Pt-00319
42187-62-2 [(1,2,5,6-η)-1,5-Cyclooctadiene](η^5-1-methyl-2,4-cyclopentadien-1-yl)nickel(1+); Tetrafluoroborate, *in* Ni-00119
42402-13-1 Bis(dimethylphenylphosphine)diiododimethylplatinum; *af*-diphosphine-*bc*-diiodo-*de*-dimethyl-*form*, *in* Pt-00206
42443-78-7 Bis[(7,8,9,10,11-η)-undecahydro-7,9-dicarbaundecaborato(2−)]nickelate(1−); Rb salt, *in* Ni-00012
42481-62-9 Chloro(cyanomethyl)bis(triphenylphosphine)platinum; *trans-form*, *in* Pt-00384
42481-73-2 Acetylchlorobis(trimethylphosphine)nickel, Ni-00059
42495-71-6 Chlorodimethylgold, Au-00011
42495-72-7 Bromodimethylgold, Au-00008
42495-73-8 Iododimethylgold, Au-00015
42531-32-8 Di-μ-hydroxydimethylbis(trimethylphosphine)dinickel, Ni-00061
42535-16-0 [(*N*,1-η)-Trifluoroacetonitrile]-bis(triphenylphosphine)platinum, Pt-00380
42562-12-9 Di-μ-chlorodimethylbis(trimethylphosphine)dinickel, Ni-00060
42562-13-0 Methyl(2,4-pentanedionato-*O*,*O*′)-(trimethylphosphine)nickel, Ni-00066
42582-38-7 Bis(dimethylphenylphosphine)iodo(methyl)palladium; *trans-form*, *in* Pd-00136
42582-39-8 Iodomethylbis(trimethylphosphine)palladium, Pd-00029

54845-68-0 (1,2-Ethanediamine-*N,N′*)bis(pentafluorophenyl)palladium, Pd-00093
54845-71-5 Tetrakis[μ-[2-[(dimethyamino)methyl]phenyl-*C,C,N*]]bis(gold)dilithium, Au-00090
54865-84-8 Di-μ-chlorobis[2-(phenylazo)phenyl]dipalladium, Pd-00196
54891-36-0 (2,2′-Bipyridine-*N,N′*)diphenylplatinum, Pt-00269
54936-74-2 Di-μ-chlorodichlorobis(1-isocyano-4-methylbenzene)dipalladium, Pd-00119
55009-50-2 Pentakis(trimethylphosphite)nickel(2+); Diperchlorate, *in* Ni-00138
55015-50-4 Chloro[(1,2-η)-1,3,5,7-cyclooctatetraene]gold, Au-00053
55031-59-9 Bis(acetonitrile)silver(1+), Ag-00010
55046-35-0 Carbonyl(η^5-2,4-cyclopentadien-1-yl)iodonickel, Ni-00023
55046-52-1 [(1,2,5,6-η)-1,5-Cyclooctadiene][1,2-ethanediylbis[diphenylphosphine]-*P,P′*]palladium(2+); Bis(hexafluorophosphate), *in* Pd-00255
55123-60-9 Iodophenylbis(triphenylphosphine)palladium; *trans-form*, *in* Pd-00302
55145-55-6 Chloro(isocyanocyclohexane)silver, Ag-00017
55147-09-6 Bis[1,2-ethanediylbis[diphenylphosphine]-*P,P′*]hydronickel(1+); Perchlorate, *in* Ni-00357
55257-10-8 Bis(cyanomethyl)[1,2-ethanediylbis[diphenylphosphine]-*P,P′*]palladium, Pd-00239
55293-69-1 Tetrakis(diethylphenylphosphine)nickel, Ni-00329
55298-20-9 Chloro(cyanomethyl)bis(triphenylphosphine)palladium, Pd-00273
55333-49-8 Dicarbonyl(triphenylphosphine)(triphenylphosphite-*P*)nickel, Ni-00315
55425-72-4 (2,2′-Bipyridine-*N,N′*)[(1,2,5,6-η)-1,5-cyclooctadiene]nickel, Ni-00162
55451-36-0 Chloro[(1,2,5,6-η)-1,5-cyclooctadiene]-[(phenylsulfonyl)methyl]palladium, Pd-00110
55466-93-8 Tetrakis[2-[(dimethylamino)methyl]phenyl]-bis(copper)digold, Au-00089
55622-77-0 [(3,4-η)-3-Methyl-4-phenyl-3-cyclobutene-1,2-dione]bis(triphenylphosphine)platinum, Pt-00429
55630-32-5 [3-(Trimethylsilyl)-2-propynyl]copper, Cu-00023
55642-26-7 (η^5-2,4-Cyclopentadien-1-yl)-bis(triphenylphosphine)nickel(1+); Trichlorostannate, *in* Ni-00331
55664-26-1 Tris-μ-(2-isocyano-2-methylpropane)tris(2-isocyano-2-methylpropane)triplatinum, Pt-00345
55664-33-0 Bis(tricyclohexylphosphine)platinum, Pt-00360
55684-63-4 Di-μ-chlorobis(η^3-2-ethylidene-6,6-dimethylbicyclo[3.1.1]hept-3-yl)dipalladium, Pd-00189
55744-44-0 Dichlorobis[μ-[(dimethylphosphinidenio)-bis(methylene)]]digold, Au-00057
55744-46-2 Tetrachlorobis[μ-[(dimethylphosphinidenio)-bis[methylene]]]digold, Au-00058
55744-48-4 Trimethyl(trimethylphosphonium η-methylide)gold, Au-00048
55758-63-9 [[Benzo[*c*]phenanthrene-2,11-diylbis(methylene)]-bis[diphenylphosphine]-*P,P′*]chlorohydroplatinum, Pt-00424
55787-57-0 (Trimethylphosphine)[(trimethylsilyl)methyl]gold, Au-00049
55804-42-7 Methyl(trimethylphosphonium η-methylide)gold, Au-00029
55906-24-6 Bis[μ-(acetato-*O:O′*)]disilver, *in* Ag-00006
55927-69-0 Bis[μ-(dimethylphosphinidenio)bis[methylene]iodomethyldigold, Au-00062
55927-91-8 (η^3-2-Propenyl)bis(tricyclohexylphosphine)platinum(1+); Hexafluorophosphate, *in* Pt-00401
55940-14-2 Di-μ-chlorobis(η^3-5-*tert*-butyl-2-methylenecyclohexyl)dipalladium, Pd-00190
55997-54-1 (η^5-2,4-Cyclopentadien-1-yl)-iodo(trimethylphosphine)nickel, Ni-00053
56009-87-1 Tris(ethylene)platinum, Pt-00041
56050-88-5 [η^3-6-(Diphenylmethylene)-2,4-cyclohexadien-1-yl](2,4-pentanedionato-*O,O′*)palladium, Pd-00199
56050-89-6 Acetylacetonato(η^3-triphenylmethyl)platinum, Pt-00282
56116-47-3 Hexakis(isocyanomethane)dipalladium(2+), Pd-00078
56116-48-4 Hexakis(isocyanomethane)dipalladium(2+); Bis(hexafluorophosphate), *in* Pd-00078
56191-55-0 Tribromo(ethylene)platinate(1−), Pt-00009
56200-09-0 [(1,2,5,6-η)-1,5-Cyclooctadiene](2,4-cyclopentadien-1-yl)methylplatinum, Pt-00158
56213-22-0 Trichloro(triethylphosphine)gold, Au-00042
56213-25-3 Tribromo(triethylphosphine)gold, Au-00039
56231-80-2 Carbonylhydrobis(triphenylphosphine)platinum(1+); *trans-form*, Trichlorostannate, *in* Pt-00371
56272-19-6 Chloro(pentafluorophenyl)-bis(triphenylphosphine)palladium; *trans-form*, *in* Pd-00296
56298-20-5 Chlorobis(methyldiphenylphosphine)-(pentafluorophenyl)palladium, Pd-00246
56550-78-8 Hydrido(phenylethynyl)bis(triphenylphosphine)palladium, Pd-00311
56553-44-7 Iodo(phenyl)bis(triethylphosphine)platinum; *cis-form*, *in* Pt-00215
56664-78-9 (2,4-Pentanedionato-*O,O′*)-phenyl(triphenylphosphine)nickel, Ni-00273
56667-47-1 Iodo(triethylphosphine)copper, Cu-00025
56801-51-5 Bis(benzene)di-μ-chlorobis(μ-chloropentachlorodialuminum)dipalladium, Pd-00071
56845-26-2 Dichloro[[2-(η^2-ethenyl)phenyl]diphenylarsine-*As*]platinum, Pt-00242
56870-45-2 Bis[μ-[(dimethylarsinidenio)bis[methylene]]]dicopper, Cu-00031
56931-35-2 Bis[μ-(dimethylarsinidenio)bis[methylene]]disilver, Ag-00021
56938-71-7 Dodecacarbonylpentanickelate(2−), Ni-00101
56960-34-0 Cyano(phenyl)bis(triethylphosphine)palladium, Pd-00167
56960-35-1 Bromo(2-propenyl)bis(triethylphosphine)palladium, Pd-00111
56964-06-8 3-Methyl-3-buten-1-ynylcopper, Cu-00016
56995-59-6 Bis(triethylphosphine)bis(triphenylstannyl)platinum; *trans-form*, *in* Pt-00435
56995-62-1 Bis(dimethylphenylphosphine)-dihydridobis(triphenyltin)platinum, Pt-00448
57029-73-9 Bromo(phenyl)bis(triethylphosphine)palladium, Pd-00158
57048-81-4 Dihydrobis(methyldiphenylphosphine)-bis(triphenylstannyl)platinum, Pt-00467
57108-14-2 Dodecacarbonylpentanickelate(2−); Bis(triphenylphosphine)imminium salt, *in* Ni-00101
57111-08-7 Bis[(triphenylphosphonio)methyl]silver(1+), Ag-00037
57127-90-9 [(5,6-η-1-Ethenyl-1,2,3,3*a*,3*b*,7*a*,8,8*a*-octahydrocyclopent[*a*]indene-4,7-dione]-bis(triphenylphosphine)palladium, Pd-00321
57145-95-6 Bis(dimethylphenylphosphine)bis(3-methoxy-1-propenyl)platinum; *trans-form*, *in* Pt-00292
57158-82-4 Bis(ethylene)(trimethylphosphine)platinum, Pt-00055
57158-83-5 Bis(ethylene)(tricyclohexylphosphine)platinum, Pt-00277
57158-85-7 Tris(ethylene)palladium, Pd-00024
57173-43-0 Chloro[1,2-bis(trifluoromethyl)vinyl]-bis(triethylphosphine)platinum; (*E*)-*cis-form*, *in* Pt-00185
57194-51-1 Di-μ-chlorobis[(1,2,3-η)-4-ethoxy-1,2,3,4-tetraphenyl-2-cyclobuten-1-yl]dipalladium, Pd-00336
57197-50-9 Bis[(1,2,5,6-η)-1,5-cyclooctadiene][μ-[(1,1,1,3,3,3-hexafluoro-2-propanolato(2−)-C^2,*O*]diplatinum, Pt-00227
57204-17-8 Dichloro(1,2-ethanediamine-*N,N′*)-bis(pentafluorophenyl)palladium, Pd-00092
57209-02-6 Dichloro(2,2′-bipyridine)bis(pentafluorophenyl)palladium, Pd-00182
57286-37-0 Bis[2-phenylazo(phenyl)-*C,N*]palladium, Pd-00197
57300-11-5 Chloro[(methylthio)methyl-*C,S*]-(triphenylphosphine)palladium, Pd-00170

63371-86-8 Tris(methyldiphenylphosphine)-[tetrahydroborato(1−)-*H*]copper, Cu-00064

63455-39-0 [Ethylenebis[diphenylphosphine]]dimethylpalladium, Pd-00228

63455-40-3 Diethyl[ethylenebis[diphenylphosphine]]palladium, Pd-00240

63511-32-0 (π-Cyclopentadienyl)(2-methyl-2-propenyl)-(triisopropylphosphine)palladium, Pd-00156

63528-03-0 [(Diethylphosphinidenio)bis(methylene)]-[[methylenebis(diphenylphosphinato)](1−)-*P*,*P*′]palladium, Pd-00243

63600-82-8 [μ-[(1-η:2,3-η)-2,4-Cyclopentadien-1-yl]][μ-[(1-η:2,3-η)-2-propenyl]]-bis(triphenylphosphine)dipalladium, Pd-00312

63643-19-6 (Pentachlorophenyl)(pentafluorophenyl)-bis(triethylphosphine)palladium, Pd-00201

63688-68-6 [(2,3-η)-2-Propenenitrile]-bis(triphenylphosphine)nickel, Ni-00324

63700-76-5 Chloro(pentachlorophenyl)bis(triethylphosphine)-palladium, Pd-00154

63700-80-1 Bromo(pentafluorophenyl)bis(triethylphosphine)palladium; *trans-form*, *in* Pd-00152

63701-76-8 Chloro(phenyl)bis(triethylphosphine)palladium, Pd-00159

63816-42-2 [(*C*,*O*-η)-Carbon dioxide]bis(triethylphosphine)-nickel, Ni-00107

63910-98-5 μ-Hydrodihydrobis[μ-[methylenebis[diphenylphosphine]-*P*:*P*′]diplatinum(1+); Chloride, *in* Pt-00439

63911-00-2 μ-Hydrodihydrobis[μ-[methylenebis[diphenylphosphine]-*P*:*P*′]diplatinum(1+); Hexafluorophosphate, *in* Pt-00439

63936-77-6 [(1,2,5,6-η)-1,5-Cyclooctadiene]dimethylpalladium, Pd-00062

63936-85-6 Chloro[(1,2,5,6-η)-1,5-cyclooctadiene]methylpalladium, Pd-00048

63946-61-2 Nitrosyl[(1,2,3,4,5-η)-1,2,3,4,5-pentaphenyl-2,4-cyclopentadien-1-yl]palladium, Pd-00257

63993-21-5 Tri-μ-carbonyltricarbonyltriplatinate(2−), Pt-00048

64040-88-6 Carbonyl(η^5-2,4-cyclopentadien-1-yl)-(triphenylphosphine)palladium(1+); Perchlorate, *in* Pd-00198

64040-90-0 ▷(π-Cyclopentadienyl)-ethylene(triphenylphosphine)palladium(1+); Perchlorate, *in* Pd-00217

64040-94-4 ▷Carbonyl(η^5-2,4-cyclopentadien-1-yl)-(triphenylphosphine)platinum(1+); Perchlorate, *in* Pt-00281

64040-96-6 ▷Cyclopentadienyl(ethylene)(triphenylphosphine)platinum(1+); Perchlorate, *in* Pt-00314

64065-88-9 [η^5-2,4-Cyclopentadien-1-yl]-(dimethylphenylphosphine)(η^2-ethene)nickel(1+); Perchlorate, *in* Ni-00131

64396-20-9 Diethynylbis(triethylphosphine)platinum; *cis-form*, *in* Pt-00186

64397-36-0 Chloro[1,2-bis(trifluoromethyl)vinyl]-bis(triethylphosphine)platinum, Pt-00185

64424-50-6 (2,2′-Bipyridine-*N*,*N*′)-trichloro(pentafluorophenyl)palladium, Pd-00117

64522-77-6 Biscyclopropylbis(dimethylphenylphosphine)platinum; *cis-form*, *in* Pt-00276

64522-78-7 Chloro(cyclopropyl)bis(dimethylphenylphosphine)-platinum; *trans-form*, *in* Pt-00228

64756-57-6 Bis[η^5-2,4-cyclopentadien-1-yl][μ-[(1,2,3-η:6,7,8-η)-2,6-octadien-1,8-diyl]]dipalladium, Pd-00145

64848-96-0 Pentafluorophenyltris(triphenylphosphine)nickel(1+); Perchlorate, *in* Ni-00371

64913-26-4 [2-[1-(Dimethylamino)ethyl]ferrocenyl-*C*,*N*](2,4-pentanedionato-*O*,*O*′)palladium, Pd-00162

64933-37-5 Hydro(trifluoromethyl)bis(triphenylphosphine)platinum; *trans-form*, *in* Pt-00370

65098-10-4 Chloroethyl[ethylenebis[diphenylphosphine]]platinum, Pt-00330

65106-71-0 Bis[(1,2,3-η)-2-cycloocten-1-yl]nickel, Ni-00152

65153-42-6 Tri(aqua)trimethylplatinum(1+); Fluoride, *in* Pt-00022

65153-45-9 Tri(aqua)trimethylplatinum(1+); Hexafluoroplatinate(2−), *in* Pt-00022

65153-46-0 Tri(aqua)trimethylplatinum(1+); Hexafluorosilicate(2−), *in* Pt-00022

65286-18-2 [2-[(Dimethylamino)methyl]ferrocenyl-*C*,*N*]silver, Ag-00030

65337-71-5 Dioctylbis(triphenylphosphine)platinum, Pt-00449

65391-83-5 Dibenzylbis(triethylphosphine)platinum, Pt-00319

65400-05-7 [(2,3-η)-1,1,1,4,4,4-Hexafluoro-2-butyne]-bis(tricyclohexylphosphine)platinum, Pt-00411

65466-58-2 Carbonyldichloro(triethylphosphine)platinum; *cis-form*, *in* Pt-00054

65832-81-7 [*N*-(2-Aminoethyl)-1,2-ethanediamine-*N*,*N*′,*N*″]-carbonylcopper)(1+), Cu-00018

65877-85-2 Phenylbis(triphenylphosphine)triphenylplumbylplatinum; *cis-form*, *in* Pt-00464

65916-06-5 μ-Chlorobis[μ-(diphenylphosphino)]-tris(triethylphosphine)tripalladium(1+); Tetrafluoroborate, *in* Pd-00306

66197-14-6 [(1,2,3,4,5,6-η)-Methylbenzene]-bis(pentafluorophenyl)nickel, Ni-00173

66197-25-9 Tribromocarbonylplatinate(1−), Pt-00001

66213-26-1 Carbonyltriiodoplatinate(1−), Pt-00005

66213-27-2 Carbonyltriiodoplatinate(1−); Tetrabutylammonium salt, *in* Pt-00005

66213-28-3 Tribromocarbonylpalladate(1−), Pd-00001

66213-29-4 Tribromocarbonylpalladate(1−); Tetrabutylammonium salt, *in* Pd-00001

66219-24-7 Carbonyldichloro(trimethylphosphine)platinum; *cis-form*, *in* Pt-00028

66302-88-3 Tetrakis(pentafluorophenyl)palladate(2−); Bistetrabutylammonium salt, *in* Pd-00195

66302-98-5 Tetrakis(pentafluorophenyl)nickelate(2−); Bis(tetrabutylammonium) salt, *in* Ni-00223

66320-83-0 [(1,2,5,6-η)-1,5-cyclooctadiene][(2,3-η)-1,1,1,4,4,4-hexafluoro-2-butyne]platinum, Pt-00106

66467-51-4 Bis[bis(di-*tert*-butylphosphino)propane]diplatinum, Pt-00390

66674-76-8 [α-[(Diphenylphosphinomethylene)]-benzenemethanolato-*O*,*P*]-phenyl(triphenylphosphine)nickel, Ni-00343

66752-80-5 Azobenzene(1,5-cyclooctadiene)nickel, Ni-00184

66916-62-9 Bis(μ-diphenylacetylene)-tetrakis(triethylphosphine)triplatinum, Pt-00450

66986-71-8 [1,2-Ethanediylbis(diphenylphosphine)-*P*,*P*′]diethynylpalladium, Pd-00238

66986-72-9 [1,2-Ethanediylbis(diphenylphosphine)-*P*,*P*′]-bis(phenylethynyl)palladium, Pd-00300

67087-65-4 Bromo(phenyl)bis(triphenylphosphine)platinum; *cis-form*, *in* Pt-00415

67145-29-3 Dihydro-μ-phosphinotetrakis(triethylphosphine)diplatinum(1+); *cis-trans-form*, Chloride, *in* Pt-00308

67254-04-0 Iodophenylbis(triphenylphosphine)platinum, Pt-00417

67336-53-2 Chlorohydrobis(ethyldiphenylphosphine)platinum; *trans-form*, *in* Pt-00332

67352-53-8 Chloro[dimethylamino(3-hydroxypropyl)methylene]-bis(dimethylphenylphosphine)platinum(1+); *trans-form*, Hexafluorophosphate, *in* Pt-00275

67409-71-6 (η^5-2,4-Cyclopentadien-1-yl)-bis(triphenylphosphine)nickel(1+); Iodide, *in* Ni-00331

67423-87-4 [1,2-Ethanediylbis[diphenylphosphine]-*P*,*P*′](η^3-2-methylenecyclohexyl)palladium(1+); Tetrafluoroborate, *in* Pd-00251

67450-36-6 Bis(η^3-1-acetyl-4-ethylidenepiperidinyl)di-μ-chlorodipalladium, Pd-00151

67483-95-8 [(1,2,3-η)-6-Ethoxy-1*H*-phenalen-1-yl]-bis(triphenylphosphine)platinum, Pt-00440

67551-89-7 Hydrobis(tricyclohexylphosphine)-(triphenylphosphine)platinum(1+); *trans-form*, Hexafluorophosphate, *in* Pt-00455